Pediatric Dermatology

A Quick Reference Guide

3rd Edition

Section on Dermatology
American Academy of Pediatrics

Editors
Anthony J. Mancini, MD, FAAP, FAAD
Daniel P. Krowchuk, MD, FAAP

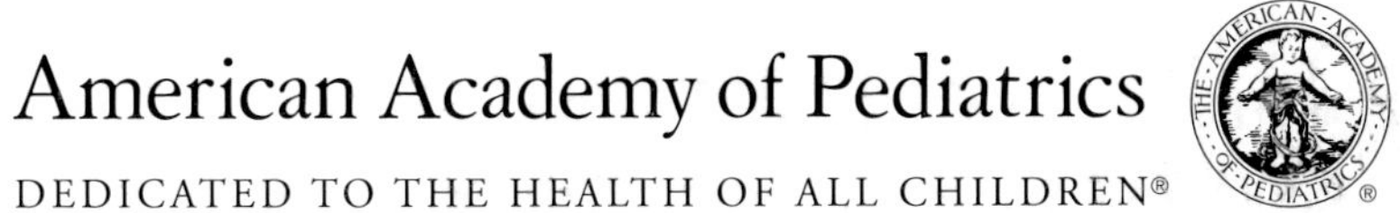

American Academy of Pediatrics Publishing Staff
Mark Grimes, *Director, Department of Publishing*
Peter Lynch, *Manager, Digital Strategy and Product Development*
Theresa Wiener, *Manager, Publishing and Production Services*
Jason Crase, *Manager, Editorial Services*
Linda Diamond, *Manager, Art Direction and Production*
Mary Lou White, *Director, Department of Marketing and Sales*
Linda Smessaert, MSIMC, *Marketing Manager, Professional Publications*

Published by the American Academy of Pediatrics
141 Northwest Point Blvd, Elk Grove Village, IL 60007-1019
Telephone: 847/434-4000
Facsimile: 847/434-8000
www.aap.org

The recommendations in this publication do not indicate an exclusive course of treatment or serve as a standard of medical care. Variations, taking into account individual circumstances, may be appropriate.

Listing of resources does not imply an endorsement by the American Academy of Pediatrics (AAP). The AAP is not responsible for the content of external resources. Information was current at the time of publication.

Products and Web sites are mentioned for informational purposes only and do not imply an endorsement by the American Academy of Pediatrics. Web site addresses are as current as possible but may change at any time.

This publication has been developed by the American Academy of Pediatrics. The contributors are expert authorities in the field of pediatrics. No commercial involvement of any kind has been solicited or accepted in the development of the content of this publication.

Every effort is made to keep *Pediatric Dermatology: A Quick Reference Guide* consistent with the most recent advice and information available from the American Academy of Pediatrics. Special discounts are available for bulk purchases of this publication. E-mail our Special Sales Department at aapsales@aap.org for more information.

First edition published 2006; second, 2012.

Printed in the United States of America
3-332/Rep0517 2 3 4 5 6 7 8 9 10
MA0794
ISBN: 978-1-61002-020-6
eBook: 978-1-61002-021-3
Cover design by Linda Diamond
Publication design by Linda Diamond
Library of Congress Control Number: 2015956185

Reviewers/Contributors

Editors

Anthony J. Mancini, MD, FAAP, FAAD
Professor of Pediatrics and Dermatology
Northwestern University Feinberg School of Medicine
Head, Division of Pediatric Dermatology
Ann & Robert H. Lurie Children's Hospital of Chicago
Chicago, IL

Daniel P. Krowchuk, MD, FAAP
Professor of Pediatrics and Dermatology
Chief, General Pediatrics and Adolescent Medicine
Wake Forest School of Medicine
Winston-Salem, NC

Associate Editors

Anna L. Bruckner, MD, FAAP, FAAD
Associate Professor of Dermatology and Pediatrics
University of Colorado School of Medicine
Children's Hospital Colorado
Anschutz Medical Campus
Aurora, CO

Fred Ghali, MD, FAAP, FAAD
Clinical Associate Professor
Department of Dermatology
UT Southwestern Medical Center
Baylor University Medical Center
Dallas, TX
Pediatric Dermatology of North Texas
Grapevine, TX

Amy Jo Nopper, MD, FAAP, FAAD
Professor of Pediatrics/Dermatology
University of Missouri–Kansas City School of Medicine
Division Director, Dermatology
Children's Mercy Hospitals & Clinics
Kansas City, MO

Michael L. Smith, MD, FAAP, FAAD
Associate Professor of Medicine and Pediatrics
Division of Dermatology
Vanderbilt University Medical Center
Nashville, TN

Patricia A. Treadwell, MD, FAAP, FAAD
Professor of Pediatrics
Indiana University School of Medicine
Riley Hospital for Children
Indianapolis, IN

The editors wish to thank J. Thomas Badgett, MD, PhD, FAAP, for his contributions to the first 2 editions of this text.

American Academy of Pediatrics Board of Directors Reviewer

Pamela K. Shaw, MD, FAAP

Reviewers

Committee on Continuing Medical Education
Committee on Practice and Ambulatory Medicine
Council on Children With Disabilities
Council on School Health
Section on Allergy and Immunology
Section on Breastfeeding
Section on Child Abuse and Neglect
Section on Developmental and Behavioral Pediatrics
Section on Endocrinology
Section on Hematology/Oncology
Section on Infectious Diseases
Section on Neonatal-Perinatal Medicine
Section on Nephrology
Section on Ophthalmology
Section on Plastic Surgery
Section on Rheumatology

American Academy of Pediatrics

Lynn Colegrove, MBA
Manager, Section on Dermatology

To our families—Nicki, Mallory, Christopher, Mackenzie, and Alexander; Heidi and Will—whose understanding and support made this project possible.

Contents

Skin Infections *(continued)*

Localized Bacterial Infections

Systemic Bacterial, Rickettsial, or Spirochetal Infections With Skin Manifestations

Fungal and Yeast Infections

Infestations

Papulosquamous Diseases

Vascular Lesions

Disorders of Pigmentation

Hypopigmentation

Hyperpigmentation

Lumps and Bumps

Bullous Diseases

Genodermatoses

Hair Disorders

Skin Disorders in Neonates/Infants

Acute Drug/Toxic Reactions

Cutaneous Manifestations of Rheumatologic Diseases

Nutritional Dermatoses

Other Disorders

Foreword

Concerns relating to the skin are common reasons for parents to seek medical care for their children. Data from several sources indicate that up to 20% of child visits to pediatricians or family physicians involve a dermatologic problem as the primary reason for the visit, a secondary concern, or an incidental finding on physical examination. The volume of skin-related concerns and the supply-demand crunch for dermatologic referrals mandate that primary care physicians who care for children are prepared to recognize, diagnose, and treat common cutaneous disorders.

This guide was originally designed to be a practical, easy-to-use tool for the busy practitioner, and we hope that this third edition continues to meet these goals. It is not an exhaustive reference; instead, it provides a concise summary of many common dermatologic disorders, with a standardized format that includes a brief background, physical findings, diagnostic modalities, and treatment approaches. Each chapter includes a useful Look-alikes table to assist in differential diagnosis and, when applicable, a Resources for Families section that provides links to patient information or support groups. Chapters to help enhance skills in recognizing and describing skin disorders, performing and interpreting diagnostic tests, and managing skin disease also are included. The accompanying color photographs have been selected to illustrate some cardinal features of each disorder. In this edition, we have added new chapters on acrodermatitis enteropathica; aplasia cutis congenita; dermoid cysts; epidermal nevi; erythema nodosum; Henoch-Schönlein purpura; juvenile plantar dermatosis; kwashiorkor; Langerhans cell histiocytosis; pigmentary mosaicism, hyperpigmented; pigmentary mosaicism, hypopigmented; pityriasis lichenoides; and polymorphous light eruption. We have also updated the text throughout, supplied new links to useful patient resources, and replaced or added numerous clinical images.

We hope this guide continues to fulfill an important need for the pediatric provider who wants a quick dermatology reference.

A.J.M.
D.P.K.

Editors' Note

The information contained in this text has been gleaned from reviews of multiple scientific papers and textbooks. The materials have been synthesized into what we hope is a coherent, easy-to-read style. Individual references have not been included in an effort to keep the size of this work practical for a quick reference guide. Some textbook references are listed here, and we invite the reader to refer to updated medical publications for further information or contemporary scientific updates.

Anthony J. Mancini, MD
Daniel P. Krowchuk, MD

Textbook References

Bolognia JL, Jorizzo JL, Schaffer JV, eds. *Dermatology.* 3rd ed. London, United Kingdom: Elsevier; 2012

Cohen BA. *Pediatric Dermatology.* 3rd ed. Edinburgh, United Kingdom: Elsevier Mosby; 2005

Eichenfield LF, Frieden IJ. *Neonatal and Infant Dermatology.* 3rd ed. Philadelphia, PA: Elsevier Saunders; 2014

Paller AS, Mancini AJ. *Hurwitz Clinical Pediatric Dermatology.* 5th ed. London, United Kingdom: Elsevier; 2016

Schachner LA, Hansen RC. *Pediatric Dermatology.* 4th ed. Edinburgh, United Kingdom: Mosby; 2011

Weston WL, Lane AT, Morelli JG. *Color Textbook of Pediatric Dermatology.* 4th ed. St Louis, MO: Mosby; 2007

Figure Credits

All figures not included in the following list are courtesy of the American Academy of Pediatrics. Special thanks to Anthony J. Mancini, MD; Daniel P. Krowchuk, MD; J. Thomas Badgett, MD, PhD; Anna L. Bruckner, MD; Amy Jo Nopper, MD; Steven D. Resnick, MD; Michael L. Smith, MD; and Patricia A. Treadwell, MD.

AAP
Figure 110.3. Reprinted with permission from Leonard D, Koca R, Acun C, et al. Visual diagnosis: three infants who have perioral and acral skin lesions. *Pediatr Rev.* 2007;28(8):312–318.

Centers for Disease Control and Prevention
Figure 20.1

Rebecca Collins, MD
Figure 75.2

Elsevier
Figures 2.7, 35A.2, 37.2, 37.3, 45.4, 55.8, 57.1, 57.2, 91.9, 114.4, 114.6. Reprinted with permission from Elsevier. From Paller AS, Mancini AJ. *Hurwitz Clinical Pediatric Dermatology: A Textbook of Skin Disorders of Childhood and Adolescence.* 3rd ed. Philadelphia, PA: Elsevier Saunders; 2006.

Figure 114.5. Reprinted with permission from Elsevier. From Mancini AJ. Childhood exanthems: a primer and update for the dermatologist. *Adv Dermatol.* 2000;16:3–38.

Alan B. Fleischer Jr, MD
Figure 78.1

Laurence Givner, MD
Figure 91.11

Chad Haldeman-Englert, MD
Figures 111.1, 111.2, 111.3

Kimberly Horii, MD
Figures 85.3, 88.1

Brandon Newell, MD
Figures 85.5, 87.1, 109.2, 116.1

Howard Pride, MD
Figures 13.1, 13.2, 15.1, 15.2, 17.2, 22.2, 56.1

Mary Rimsza, MD
Figures 20.2, 98.1

Paul J. Sagerman, MD
Figures 93.2, 98.3

Walter W. Tunnesen Jr, MD
Figure 1.10

Anthony J. Vivian, FRCS, FRCOphth
Figure 83.5

Albert Yan, MD
Figures 7.8, 91.5

Approach to the Patient With a Rash

Introduction

- Recognizing and describing skin lesions accurately is essential to the diagnosis and differential diagnosis of skin disorders.
- The first step is to identify the primary lesion, defined as the earliest lesion and the one most characteristic of the disease.
- Next note the distribution, arrangement, and color of primary lesions, along with any secondary change (eg, crusting or scaling).

Types of Primary Lesions

- Flat lesions
  - Macule: a small (<1 cm), circumscribed area of color change without elevation or depression of the skin (Figure 1.1)
  - Patch: a larger (≥1 cm) area of color change without skin elevation or depression (Figure 1.2)
- Elevated lesions
  - Solid lesions
    - Papules (<1 cm in diameter) (Figure 1.3)
    - Nodules: lesion measuring 0.5 to 2.0 cm in diameter, most of which resides below the skin surface (Figure 1.4)
    - Tumor: deeper than a nodule and measuring larger than 2 cm in diameter
    - Wheals: pink, rounded, or flat-topped elevations due to edema in the skin (Figure 1.5)
    - Plaques: plateau-shaped structures often formed by the coalescence of papules; larger than 1 cm in diameter (Figure 1.6)

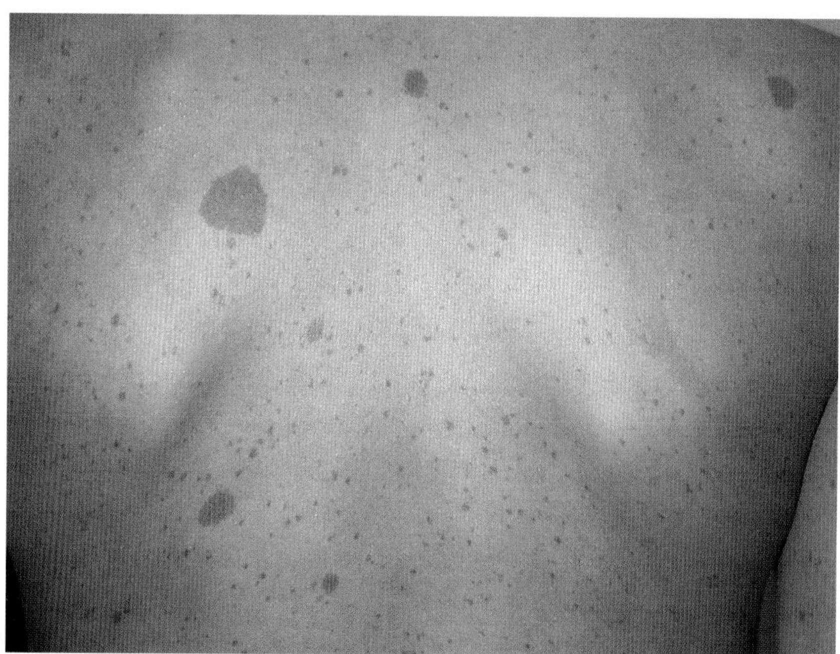

Figure 1.1. Café au lait macules in a patient who has neurofibromatosis type 1.

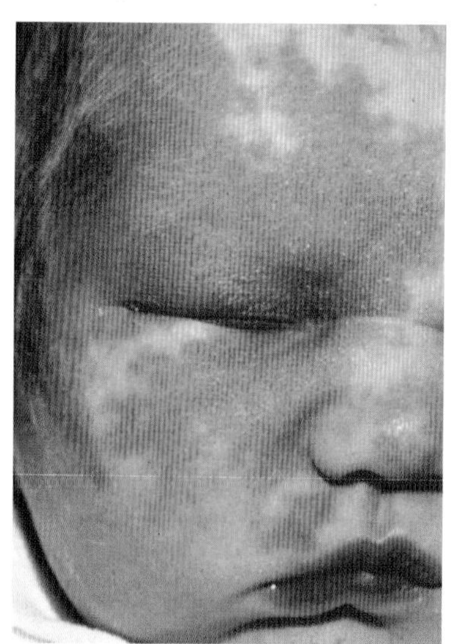

Figure 1.2. A port-wine stain—a vascular patch.

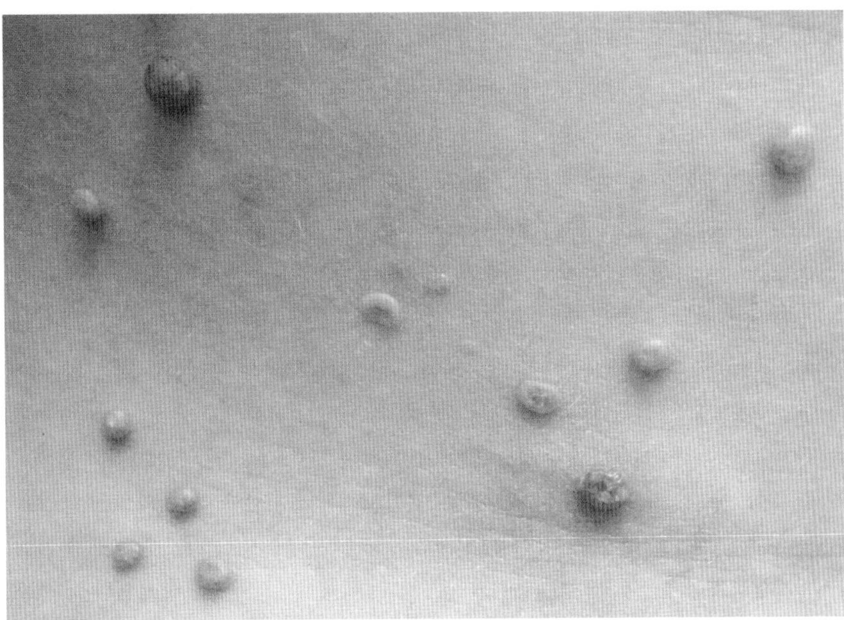

Figure 1.3. Molluscum contagiosum. There are erythematous and skin-colored papules.

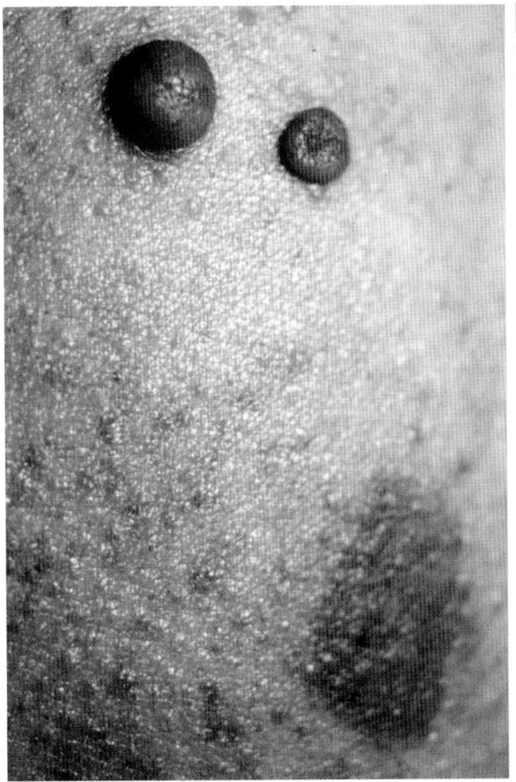

Figure 1.4. Nodules representing neurofibromas in a patient who has neurofibromatosis type 1.

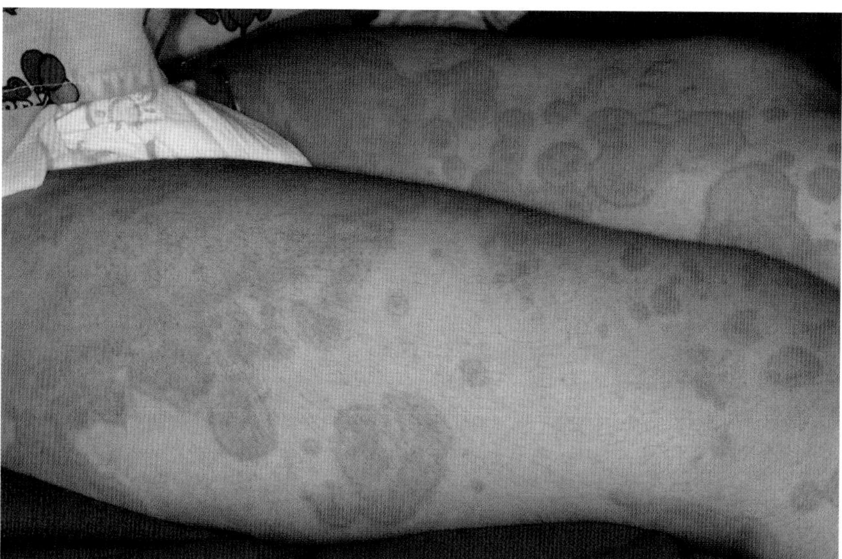

Figure 1.5. Pink wheals in a patient who has urticaria.

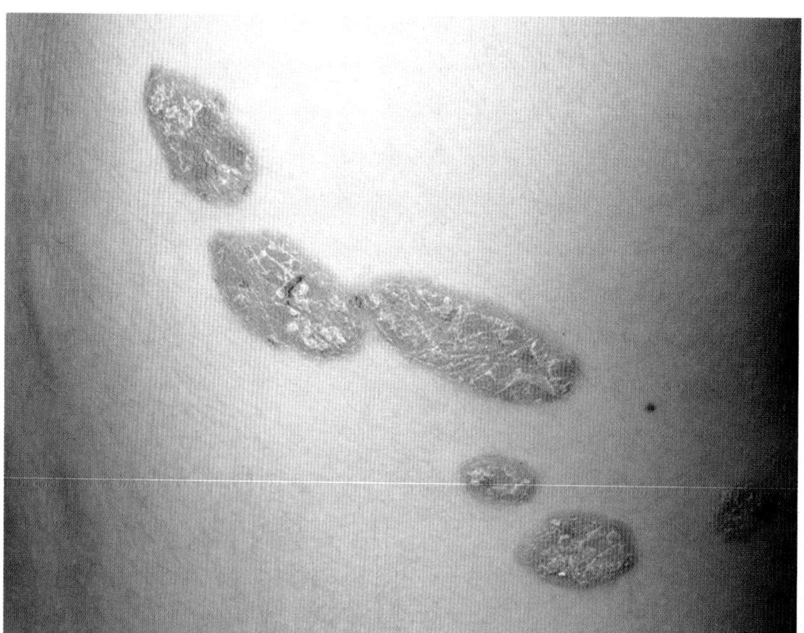

Figure 1.6. Scaling plaques, plateau-like lesions, are observed in psoriasis.

- Fluid-filled lesions
  - Vesicles: smaller than 1 cm in diameter and filled with serous or clear fluid (Figure 1.7)
  - Bullae: 1 cm or larger in diameter and typically filled with serous or clear fluid (Figure 1.8)
  - Pustules: smaller than 1 cm in diameter and filled with purulent material (Figure 1.9)
  - Abscess: 1 cm or larger and filled with purulent material
  - Cysts: 0.5 cm or larger in diameter; represent sacs containing fluid or semisolid material (Unlike in bullae, the material within a cyst is not visible from the surface.)
- Depressed lesions
  - Erosions: superficial loss of epidermis with a moist base (Figure 1.10)
  - Ulcers: deeper lesions extending into the dermis or below (Figure 1.11)

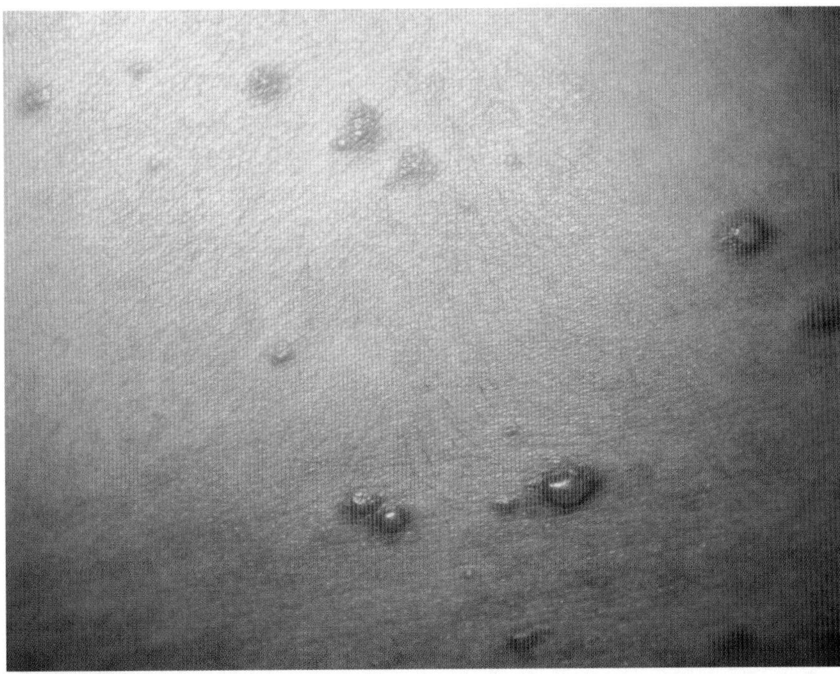

Figure 1.7. Vesicles, as seen here in varicella, are filled with clear or serous fluid.

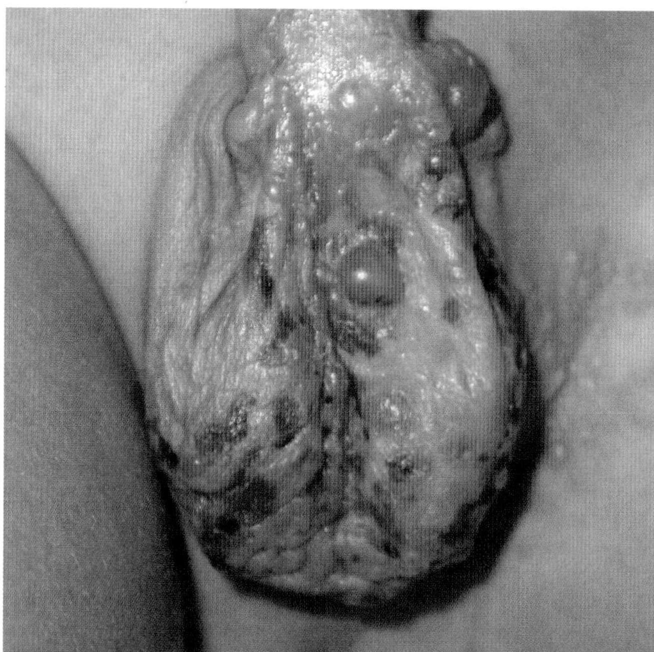

Figure 1.8. Bullae, filled with clear fluid, are observed in chronic bullous disease of childhood.

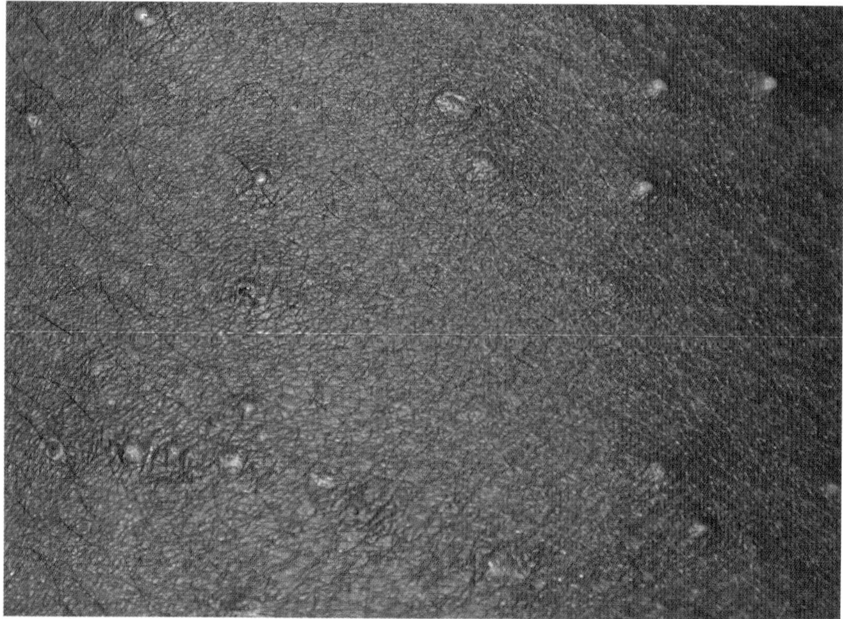

Figure 1.9. Pustules are filled with purulent material. This patient has folliculitis.

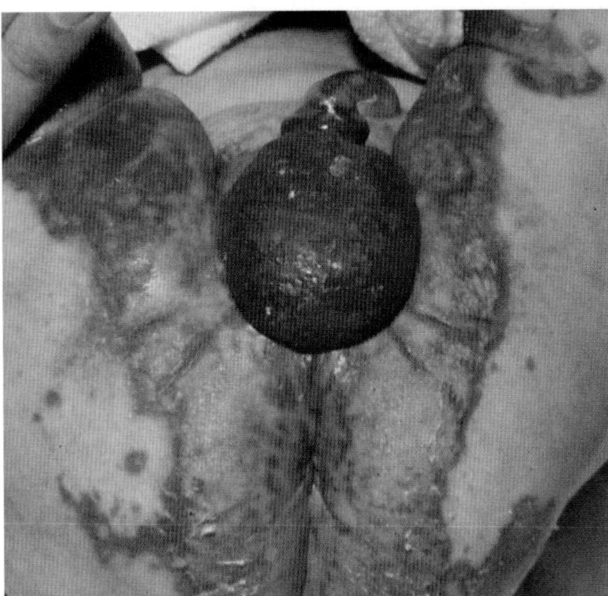

Figure 1.10. Erosions, as seen in this infant who has acrodermatitis enteropathica, represent a superficial loss of epidermis.

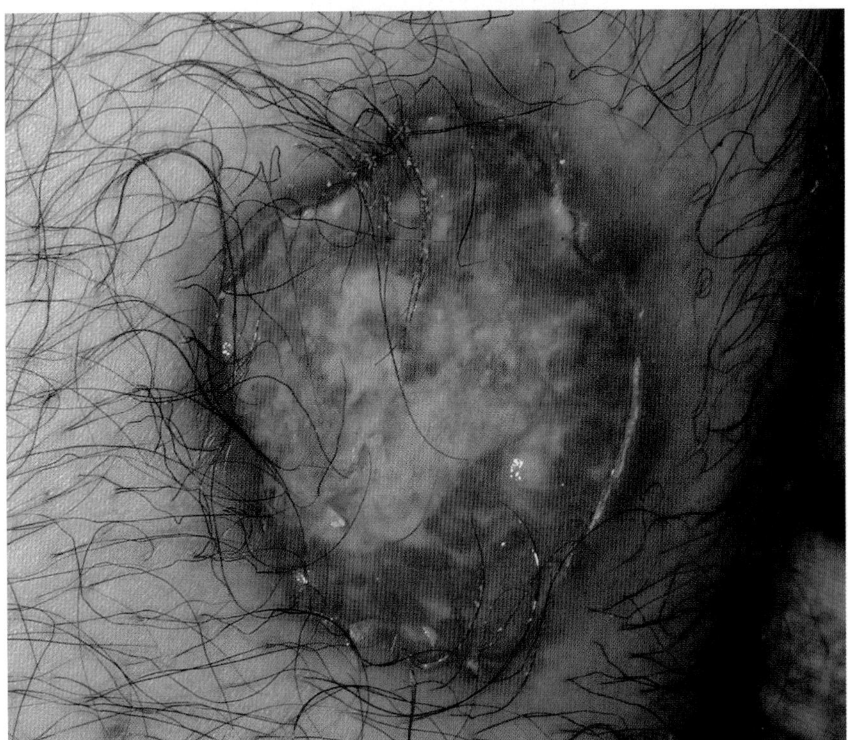

Figure 1.11. An ulcer occurs when there has been loss of epidermal and dermal tissues. In the patient shown here, the ulcer is the result of pyoderma gangrenosum.

Distribution of Lesions

Certain disorders are characterized by unique patterns of lesion distribution. For example,

- Atopic dermatitis in children and adolescents typically involves the antecubital or popliteal fossae.
- Seborrheic dermatitis in adolescents commonly involves not only the scalp but also the eyebrows and nasolabial folds.
- Lesions of psoriasis are often seen in areas that are traumatized, such as the extensor surfaces of the elbows and knees.
- Acne is limited to the face, back, shoulders, and chest, sites of the highest concentrations of pilosebaceous follicles.

Arrangement of Lesions

The arrangement of lesions also may provide a clue to diagnosis. Some examples include

- Linear: contact dermatitis due to plants (eg, poison ivy) (Figure 1.12), lichen striatus, and incontinentia pigmenti; may also occur in epidermal nevi, psoriasis, and warts
- Grouped: herpes simplex virus infection (Figure 1.13), warts, molluscum contagiosum
- Dermatomal: herpes zoster (Figure 1.14)
- Annular (ie, ring-shaped): tinea corporis (Figure 1.15), granuloma annulare, erythema migrans, lupus erythematosus

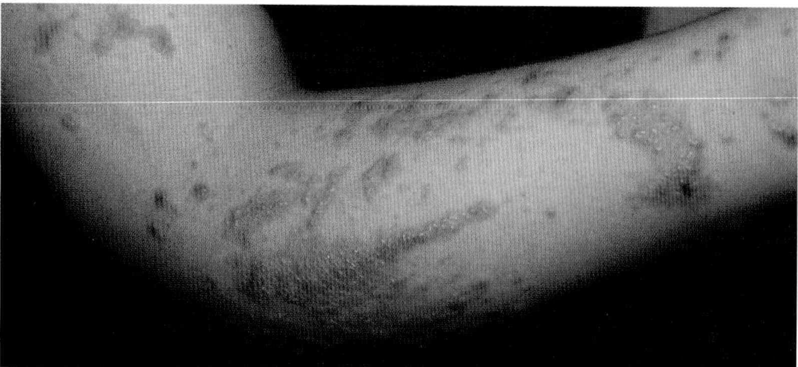

Figure 1.12. A linear arrangement of papules or vesicles often occurs in contact dermatitis due to poison ivy.

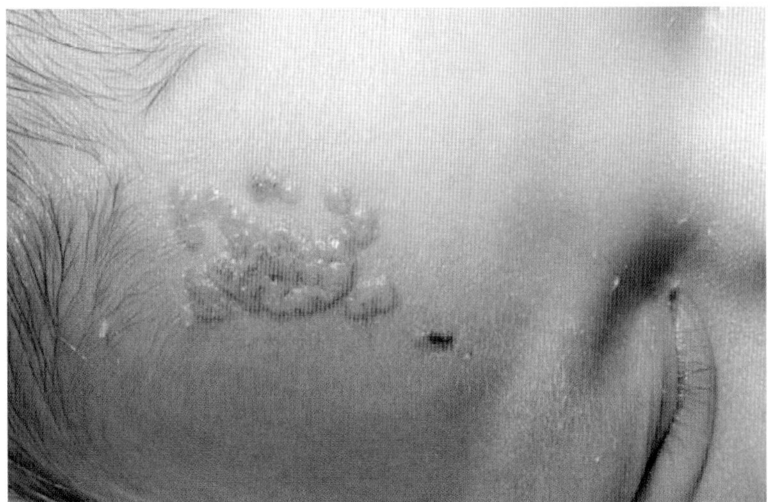

Figure 1.13. Grouped vesicles are characteristic of herpes simplex virus infection on the skin.

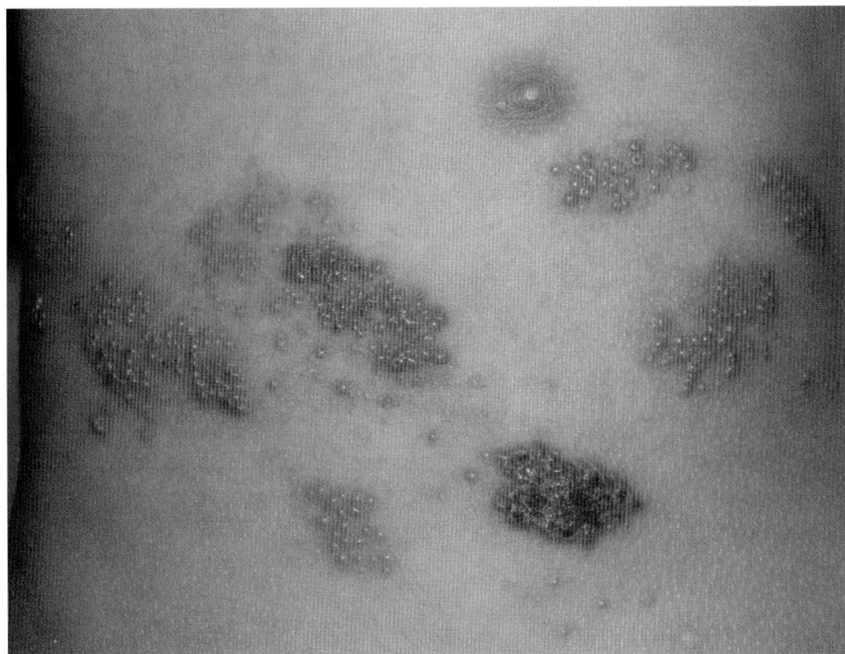

Figure 1.14. The lesions of herpes zoster appear in a dermatomal distribution.

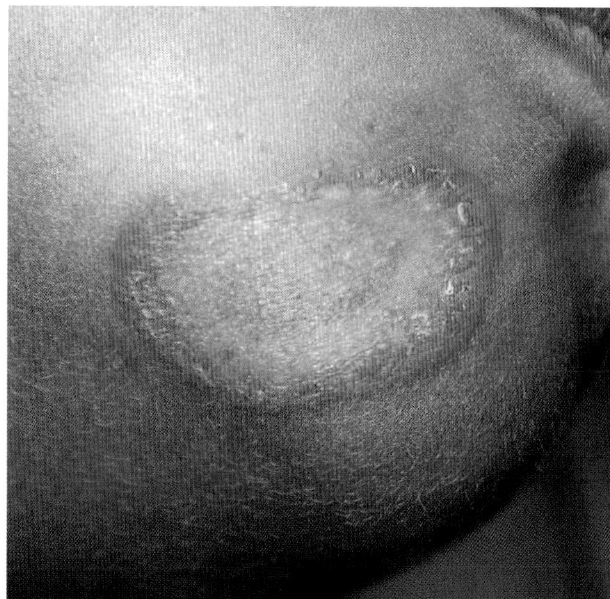

Figure 1.15. An annular plaque (ie, ring-shaped lesion) is typical of tinea corporis.

Color

- Erythematous: pink or red. When erythematous lesions are observed, it is important to note if they blanch. If the red cells are within vessels, as occurs in urticaria, compression of the skin forces the cells into deeper vessels and blanching occurs. However, if the cells are outside vessels, as occurs in forms of vasculitis, blanching will not occur. Non-blanching lesions are termed petechiae, purpura, or ecchymoses. Also note that in individuals with more deeply pigmented skin erythema may be more difficult to appreciate.
- Hyperpigmented: tan, brown, or black.
- Hypopigmented: amount of pigment decreased but not entirely absent (as seen with postinflammatory pigmentary alteration).
- Depigmented: all pigment absent (as occurs in vitiligo).

Secondary Changes

Alterations in the skin that may accompany primary lesions include

- Crusting: dried fluid; commonly seen following rupture of vesicles or bullae (as occurs with the "honey-colored" crust of impetigo).
- Scaling: represents epidermal fragments that are characteristic of several disorders, including fungal infections (eg, tinea corporis) and psoriasis.
- Atrophy: an area of surface depression due to absence of the epidermis, dermis, or subcutaneous fat; atrophic skin often is thin and wrinkled.
- Lichenification: thickening of the skin from chronic rubbing or scratching (as occurs in atopic dermatitis); as a result, normal skin markings and creases appear more prominent (Figure 1.16).

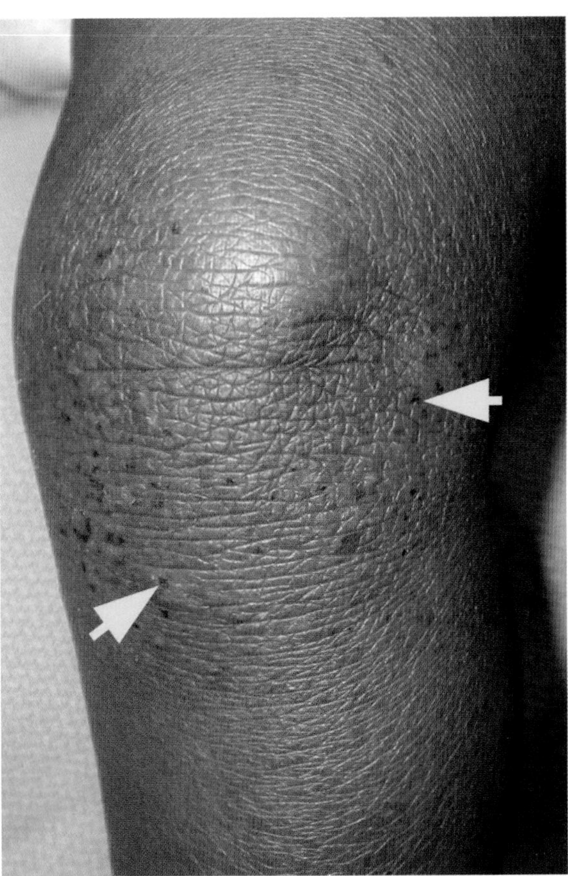

Figure 1.16. Lichenification. The normal skin markings are very prominent due to chronic scratching. Also note the tiny erosions (arrows), some of which have formed crust.

Diagnostic Techniques

Introduction

Several procedures can assist the clinician in diagnosing skin problems. Discussed here are the potassium hydroxide (KOH) preparation, fungal culture, mineral oil preparation for scabies, and Wood light examination.

Potassium Hydroxide (KOH) Preparation

Used to identify fungal elements (eg, spores, hyphae, pseudohyphae) in skin, hair, or nail samples. The procedure is as follows:

- Using the edge of a glass microscope slide or #15 scalpel blade, scrape the skin and collect fragments or hair remnants on a second glass microscope slide. Preparing the area first with alcohol may be useful in helping debris stick to blade or slide.
- If sampling a nail, use a scalpel blade to scrape the underside of the nail (or its surface if superficial infection is suspected) and collect the debris obtained.
- Cover the specimen on the glass slide with a cover slip.
- Apply 1 to 2 drops of 10% to 20% KOH to the edge of the cover slip. Capillary action will draw the liquid under the entire cover slip.
- Gently heat the slide with an alcohol lamp or match, taking care to avoid boiling (which causes the KOH to crystallize and makes interpretation of the preparation difficult).
- Gently compress the cover slip to further separate skin fragments.
- Scan the preparation initially under low power (using the 10x objective lens).

- Examine any suspicious areas under higher power (using a 40x objective lens) for
  - Branching hyphae or spores: characteristic of dermatophyte infections of the skin or nails (eg, tinea corporis, tinea pedis, tinea cruris, onychomycosis) (Figure 2.1).
  - Spores within hair fragments (ie, an endothrix infection): characteristic of the most common form of tinea capitis in the United States caused by *Trichophyton tonsurans* (Figure 2.2). If tinea capitis is caused by *Microsporum canis* (approximately 5% of all cases), hyphae or spores will be seen on the outside of hair shafts (ie, an ectothrix infection).
  - Pseudohyphae and spores: seen in infections with *Candida* species (Figure 2.3).
  - Spores and short hyphae (ie, "spaghetti and meatballs"): seen in tinea versicolor (Figure 2.4).

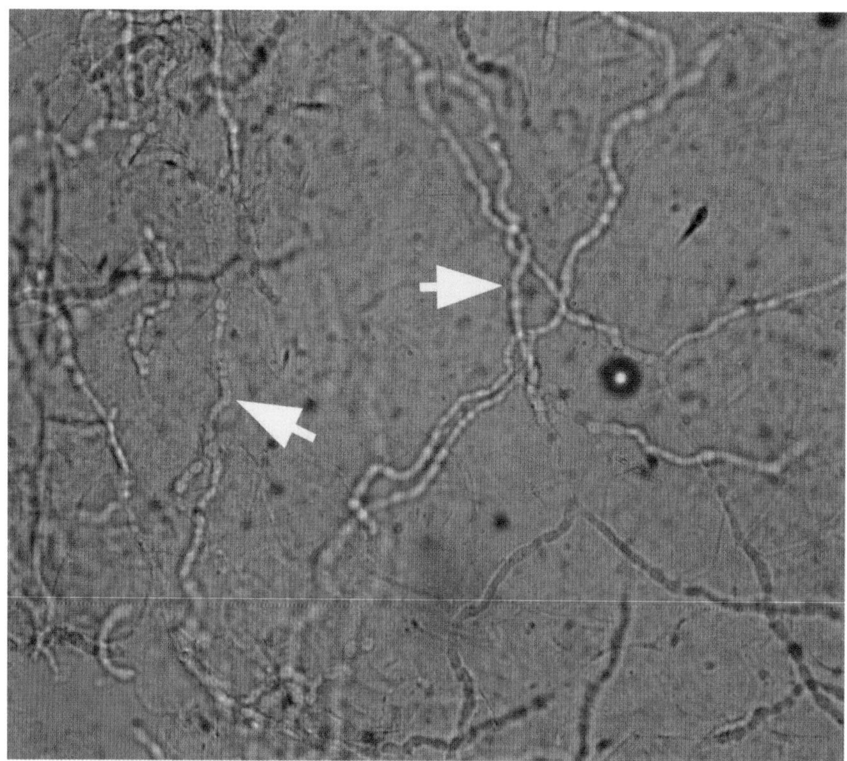

Figure 2.1. Potassium hydroxide preparation showing branching hyphae (arrows).

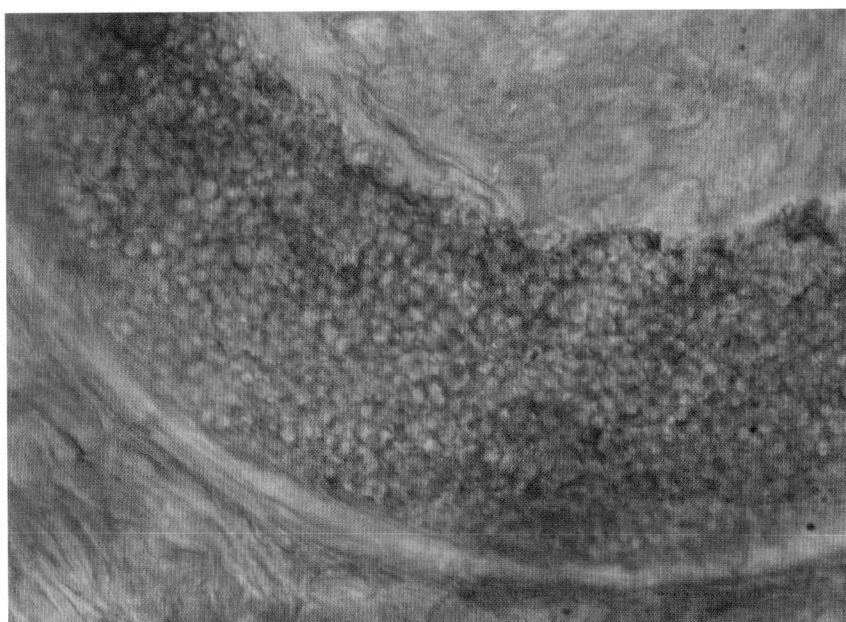

Figure 2.2. Potassium hydroxide preparation in tinea capitis caused by *Trichophyton tonsurans*. The hair fragment is filled with small spheres (ie, arthrospores).

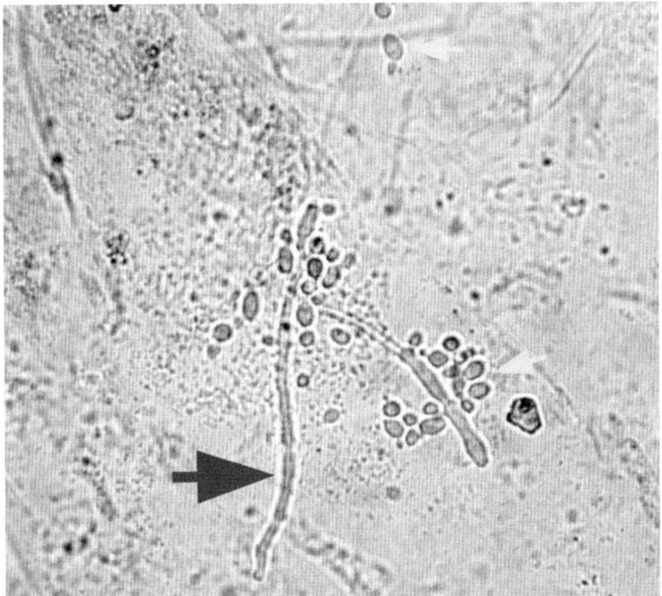

Figure 2.3. Pseudohyphae (red arrow) and spores (yellow arrows) are characteristic of infection caused by *Candida* species.

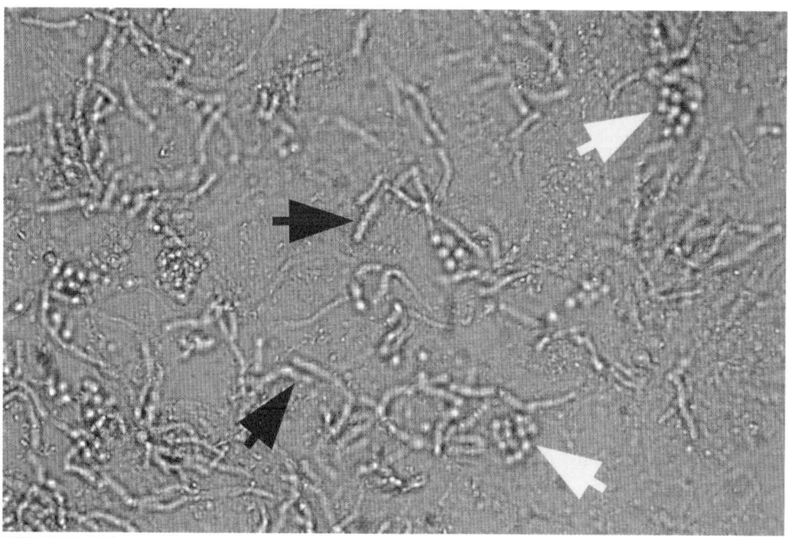

Figure 2.4. In tinea versicolor, the potassium hydroxide preparation reveals short hyphae (red arrows) and spores (yellow arrows) ("spaghetti and meatballs").

Fungal Culture

- Sampling techniques
  - If sampling the skin: Using the edge of a glass microscope slide or #15 scalpel, scrape the lesion and collect scale on a glass microscope slide.
  - If sampling a nail: Use a scalpel blade to scrape the underside of the nail (or its surface if superficial infection is suspected), and collect the debris on a glass microscope slide or folded sheet of paper; alternatively, use a nail clipper to obtain nail clippings.
  - If sampling the scalp
    - Use the edge of a glass microscope slide or #15 scalpel to scrape the affected area, collecting scale and hair remnants (ie, black dot hairs) onto a glass microscope slide.
    - Alternatively, moisten a cotton-tipped applicator with tap water, rub the affected area of the scalp, and inoculate the fungal culture medium with the swab. (If fungal culture medium is not available, a Culturette swab system may be used to collect and transport the specimen to the laboratory.)

- Transfer the material collected to the fungal medium (typically dermatophyte test medium [DTM] or Mycosel agar) and process appropriately.
  - Leave the cap slightly loose to permit air entry.
  - If fungal culture medium is not available, transfer the specimen in a sterile glass tube or other container to the laboratory.
- In the presence of a pathogenic fungus, DTM will change from yellow to red in 1 to 2 weeks (Figure 2.5).

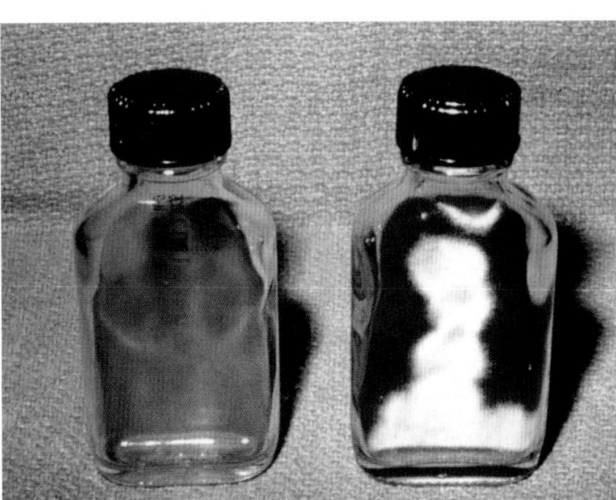

Figure 2.5. Uninoculated dermatophyte test medium is yellow (left). In the presence of a pathogenic fungus the medium becomes red (right).

Mineral Oil Preparation for Scabies

- Place a small drop of mineral oil on a suspicious burrow, papule, or vesicle that has not been traumatized by the patient.
- Using a #15 scalpel blade oriented parallel to the skin surface, scrape the lesion. Because scabies mites live in the epidermis, it is not necessary to scrape deeply; however, some bleeding is common with the procedure.
- Transfer the material to a drop of mineral oil on a glass microscope slide.
- Repeat the process for several other suspicious lesions.
- Cover the sample on the glass slide with a cover slip.
- Examine at low power for the presence of mites, eggs, or fecal material (Figures 2.6 and 2.7).

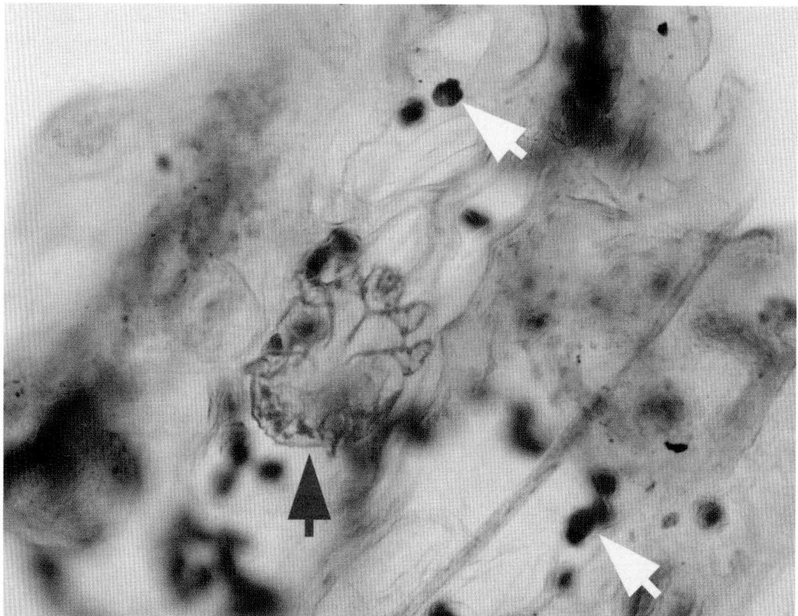

Figure 2.6. Newly hatched mite (red arrow) and fecal material (yellow arrows) on a mineral oil preparation.

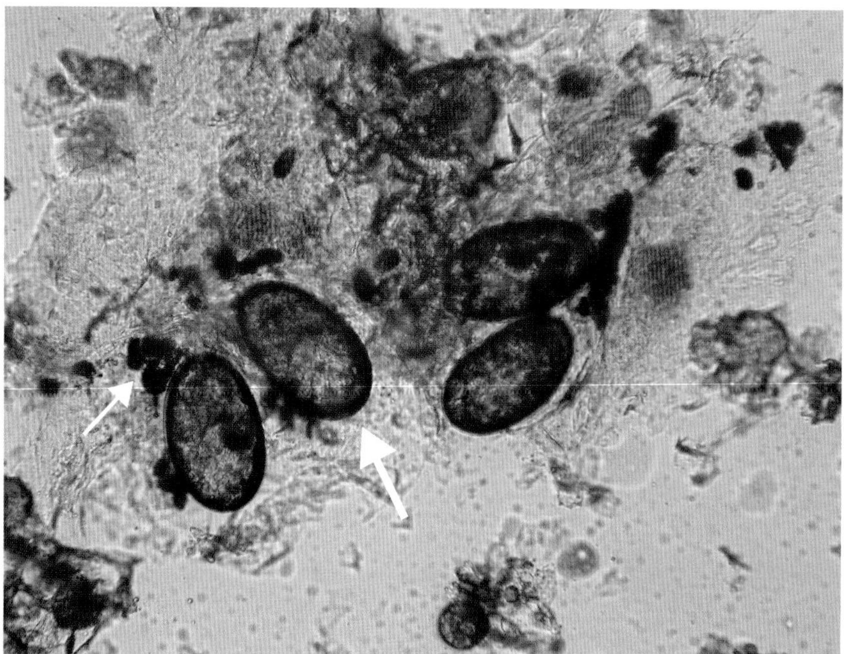

Figure 2.7. A mineral oil preparation in a patient who has scabies reveals eggs (large arrow) and mite fecal material (ie, scybala) (small arrow).

Wood Light Examination

Examination of the skin using Wood light in a darkened room may assist in the diagnosis of several conditions.

- Erythrasma (a superficial *Corynebacterium* infection): Affected areas fluoresce a coral-red color.
- Tinea capitis: Wood light examination is only useful in the recognition of a minority of cases (perhaps 5%) of tinea capitis caused by *Microsporum* species. Green fluorescence does not occur when infections are caused by *T tonsurans*.
- Tinea versicolor (caused by yeasts of the genus *Malassezia* [formerly *Pityrosporum*]): Affected areas may fluoresce a yellow-gold color.
- Diseases characterized by hypopigmentation or depigmentation: In lightly pigmented individuals, examining the skin with Wood light may assist in identifying lesions of vitiligo or ash-leaf macules of tuberous sclerosis.

CHAPTER 3

Therapeutics

I. Selection and Use of Topical Corticosteroids

Introduction

- Topical corticosteroids exert their effect through many mechanisms, including anti-inflammatory, immunosuppressive, antiproliferative, and vasoconstrictive effects.
- Preparations may be grouped according to relative potency (Table 3.1). Differences in potency between groups are not linear. For example, hydrocortisone (group 7) has a relative potency of less than 1; triamcinolone (eg, Kenalog, group 4), 75; and clobetasol propionate (eg, Temovate, group 1), 1,869.

Table 3.1. Selected Topical Corticosteroids by Potency

Group	Generic Name (Brand Name, Vehicle, Concentration)
Group 1 (most potent)	Clobetasol propionate (Temovate, cream or ointment, 0.05%; Olux, foam, 0.05%) Betamethasone dipropionate (Diprolene, ointment, 0.05%) Halobetasol propionate (Ultravate, cream or ointment, 0.05%) Diflorasone diacetate (Psorcon, ointment, 0.05%) Fluocinonide (Vanos, cream, 0.1%)
Group 2	Mometasone furoate (Elocon, ointment, 0.1%) Amcinonide (Cyclocort, ointment, 0.1%) Fluocinonide (Lidex, cream, ointment, gel, or solution, 0.05%) Betamethasone dipropionate (Diprosone, cream, ointment, 0.05%) Betamethasone valerate (Luxiq, foam, 0.12%)
Group 3	Triamcinolone acetonide (Aristocort, ointment, 0.1%) Amcinonide (Cyclocort, cream or lotion, 0.1%) Fluticasone propionate (Cutivate, ointment, 0.005%) Diflorasone diacetate (Psorcon, cream, 0.05%)
Group 4	Mometasone furoate (Elocon, cream, lotion, 0.1%) Triamcinolone acetonide (Kenalog, cream, 0.1%) Fluocinolone acetonide (Synalar, ointment, 0.025%) Hydrocortisone valerate (Westcort, ointment, 0.2%)

Table 3.1. Selected Topical Corticosteroids by Potency *(continued)*

Group	Generic Name (Brand Name, Vehicle, Concentration)
Group 5	Fluticasone propionate (Cutivate, cream, 0.05%) Fluocinolone acetonide (Synalar, cream, 0.025%) Betamethasone valerate (Valisone, cream, 0.1%) Hydrocortisone valerate (Westcort, cream, 0.2%) Prednicarbate (Dermatop, cream, 0.1%)
Group 6	Fluocinolone acetonide (Synalar, solution, 0.01%; Derma-Smoothe/FS, oil, 0.01%) Desonide (Tridesilon, cream, 0.05%; DesOwen, cream or ointment, 0.05%; Desonate, gel, 0.05%; Verdeso, foam, 0.05%) Alclometasone dipropionate (Aclovate, cream or ointment, 0.05%)
Group 7 (least potent)	Hydrocortisone (Hytone, cream or ointment, 1%, 2.5%)

Adapted with permission from Eichenfield LF, Friedlander SF. Coping with chronic dermatitis. *Contemp Pediatr.* 1998;15:53–80.

Selecting and Prescribing a Topical Corticosteroid

Consider the following factors when selecting a topical corticosteroid (see also Table 3.2):

- How old is the patient?
  In general, a less potent preparation is required in infants than in older children or adolescents. For example, for the management of flares of atopic dermatitis, a low-potency preparation (eg, hydrocortisone ointment 1% or 2.5%) usually is sufficient in an infant, while in an adolescent, a mid-potency (eg, triamcinolone 0.1%) or high-potency (eg, mometasone 0.1%) product is needed.
- What area will be treated?
  - Absorption of steroids varies with the thickness of the skin in various regions of the body.
  - Absorption is greatest in areas where the skin is thin (eg, face, perineum) and lowest where the skin is thick (eg, palms, soles). Thus, only a low-potency preparation should be used on the face, while a mid-potency (or high-potency) product will be needed to manage dermatitis on the feet.
- What vehicle should be selected?
  - Creams: tolerated by most patients but can be drying and, occasionally, their ingredients may cause contact or irritant dermatitis

- Ointments: the most effective vehicle, especially for thickened or lichenified skin; increase the absorption and potency ranking of the steroid; generally are preservative-free and less likely to cause contact or irritant dermatitis; have a greasy feel that may not be tolerated by some patients
- Lotions: cosmetically pleasing because they do not leave a greasy feel; tend to sting on open or damaged skin
- Gels: usually for hair-bearing areas; may cause stinging or burning

▶ How much should you dispense?
For treatment of a self-limited condition involving a small area, prescribing a small tube (eg, 15 g) will be sufficient; however, if the process is more extensive or chronic, larger amounts will be needed. Some rules that will help

- One gram of product will cover a 10-cm by 10-cm area (perhaps 30% more coverage if an ointment is used rather than a cream). Note that 0.5 g is the amount of cream dispensed from a standard tube that extends from the tip of the adult finger to the flexural crease overlying the distal volar interphalangeal joint.
- In an older child (6–10 years of age), it takes
  - 1 g to cover the face and neck
  - 1.25 g to cover the hand and arm
  - 1.75 g to cover the chest and abdomen
  - 2.25 g to cover the foot and leg
- Thus, when managing a chronic condition like atopic dermatitis that involves a significant portion of the body, prescribing amounts of 0.5 or 1 lb (227 or 454 g), rather than small tubes, may be necessary.

▶ Cost
As with other medications, the cost of topical corticosteroids varies widely and often is influenced by the patient's insurance formulary. Although proprietary corticosteroids typically are more expensive than generics, generics are not always inexpensive. Consider the cost of these generic moderate-potency steroids: 60 g of hydrocortisone valerate costs as much as $150.12; 80 g of triamcinolone acetonide costs $4. There are insufficient data, however, to enable direct comparison of efficacy and bioavailability of branded versus generic preparations.

Table 3.2. Guidelines for Selecting Corticosteroid Potency

Potency	Guideline
Low	• Infant (any body site) or young child • Face, perineum, axillae in patient of any age
Moderate	• Child (exclusive of face) with moderate to severe disease • Adolescent (exclusive of face or anatomically occluded areas [eg, axillae, genitalia])
High	• Used primarily by dermatologists • Most often used in the management of severe or lichenified dermatoses or those involving the feet or hands

Adverse Effects

When used appropriately topical corticosteroids are very safe; however, using too potent a preparation, particularly in an inappropriate location or for too long, may result in adverse effects.

- Local adverse effects: atrophy, striae, pigmentary changes, easy bruising, hypertrichosis, and acne-like eruptions. To prevent these effects, use only low-potency preparations on the face, axillae, and groin (including the diaper area); limit the duration of use of all corticosteroids; and use high-potency preparations very discriminately.
- Systemic adverse effects: hypothalamic-pituitary-adrenal axis suppression, Cushing syndrome, growth retardation, glaucoma, and cataracts. Systemic adverse effects are most likely to occur when very potent agents are used (even for short periods) or when moderately potent preparations are used over large areas of the body for long periods, especially in young infants, where the ratio of skin to body surface area is larger.

Frequency of Application

- Typically twice daily as needed

II. Selection and Use of Moisturizers

Introduction

- Moisturizers (also known as emollients or lubricants) are designed to hydrate the skin by creating a barrier and preventing evaporation.
- In patients who have atopic dermatitis, moisturizers can reduce the need for corticosteroids.

Selecting a Moisturizer

Traditional moisturizers are available as ointments, creams, or lotions. Barrier repair agents also are available.

- Ointments
  - Water-in-oil emulsions are most occlusive and are the best moisturizers.
  - Have a greasy feel that some patients find unpleasant.
  - Because they generally are preservative-free, they are less likely to cause contact or irritant dermatitis.
  - Some examples include Aquaphor ointment and petrolatum (eg, Vaseline petroleum jelly).
- Creams
  - Oil-in-water emulsions that often are more cosmetically pleasing than ointments.
  - Some examples include Aveeno cream, CeraVe cream, Cetaphil cream, Eucerin cream, and Vanicream.
- Lotions
  - Oil-in-water emulsions containing more water than creams.
  - Cosmetically pleasing but least effective as moisturizers.
  - Some examples include CeraVe lotion, Cetaphil lotion, Curel lotion, DML lotion, Eucerin lotion, Keri lotion, Lubriderm lotion, and Moisturel lotion.
- Barrier repair agents
  - A variety of over-the-counter (eg, CeraVe, Cetaphil RestoraDerm) and prescription (eg, Atopiclair, EpiCeram, Hylatopic, and others) barrier repair agents exist that may help reduce the severity of atopic dermatitis and play an adjunctive therapeutic role. These agents include products with ceramides, filaggrin degradation products, natural moisturizing factor, avenanthramides, glycyrrhetinic acid, shea nut derivatives, and palmitamide monoethanolamine.

- While the exact role of these agents is not yet clarified, they may play a role in active disease (usually in conjunction with anti-inflammatory agents like corticosteroids and calcineurin inhibitors) and as maintenance agents.
- Prescription barrier repair agents typically are expensive.

Adverse Effects

Preservatives, antimicrobial agents, or fragrances contained in moisturizers, or products that are lanolin-based, may cause allergic or irritant contact dermatitis.

Frequency of Application

- Apply 2 to 3 times daily if needed (application should immediately follow a bath or shower while the skin is still damp).
- Lotions and creams may need to be applied more often than ointments.
- If the patient is being treated with a topical corticosteroid or calcineurin inhibitor, apply these agents first, followed by the moisturizer.

III. Cryotherapy

Introduction

Cryotherapy employs liquid nitrogen (or another cryogen) to destroy skin lesions through tissue necrosis. In pediatrics it is commonly used to treat warts.

Selecting a Cryogen

- Liquid nitrogen is the most effective cryogen, with an achieved temperature of approximately -195°C.
- If cryotherapy will be performed infrequently, products that employ other cryogens (eg, dimethyl ether and propane [eg, Histofreezer]) may prove more economical because they have a long shelf life, although their effectiveness and freeze effect (temperature around -57°C) are significantly lower than liquid nitrogen.
- Cryotherapy devices can also be purchased by patients without a prescription. They employ dimethyl ether and propane.

Procedure

- Liquid nitrogen usually is applied with a spray device or a cotton swab that is dipped into the liquid nitrogen and then applied to the skin.
  - Standard cotton-tipped applicators do not work well because the tight wrap of the cotton does not allow liquid nitrogen to be absorbed.
  - To make an applicator, wrap additional cotton onto the tip of an applicator, shaping it to a point.
- Liquid nitrogen should be applied to the lesion until a white ring (the ice ball) extends 1 to 3 mm beyond the margin of the wart. The freeze should be maintained for 10 to 30 seconds. Some experts advise a second treatment following initial thawing.
- Patients should be advised that within 1 to 2 days a blister may form. Once the blister ruptures, the area should be cleansed twice daily and a topical antibiotic and a bandage applied.
- Any remaining wart should be treated with a keratolytic that contains salicylic acid. Repeat cryotherapy may be performed in 2 to 3 weeks if necessary.

IV. Sun Protection

Elements of Sun Protection

- Minimize prolonged outdoor activities between 10:00 am and 4:00 pm when possible.
- Wear protective clothing, such as a wide-brimmed hat, long-sleeved shirt, and long pants. Many manufacturers produce sun-protective clothing with an ultraviolet (UV) protection factor (approximately equivalent to the sun protection factor [SPF]) of 30 or more.
- Use a sunscreen regularly.
  - Choose a product with an SPF of 30 or more that has UV-A and UV-B protection. Sun protection factor is a better measure of protection from UV-B than UV-A. UV-A protection is designated by the number of stars on the packaging, ranging from 1 star (low protection) to 4 stars (very high protection).
  - Consider a product that is not alcohol-based (will not cause stinging) and that is labeled nonacnegenic or noncomedogenic (to prevent worsening acne in adolescents).
  - Apply liberally (using too little may reduce the SPF), ideally 30 minutes before beginning outdoor activities, even on cloudy days.
  - Apply every 2 hours, as well as after swimming or activities resulting in significant sweating.
  - Although there are limited data on the safety of sunscreen use in infants younger than 6 months, there is no evidence that applying small amounts is associated with adverse long-term effects. Therefore, in situations in which other sun protection strategies may be inadequate or unfeasible, it is reasonable to apply sunscreen to exposed areas of the skin in young infants.
- To prevent cataracts and ocular melanoma, wear sunglasses labeled "block 99% or 100% of UV-A and UV-B rays," "UV absorption up to 400 nm," or "meets ANSI UV requirements."

Dermatitis

CHAPTER 4

Atopic Dermatitis

Introduction/Etiology/Epidemiology

- Most common chronic pediatric skin disorder, affecting as many as 15% of children.
- Cause unknown but appears to be the result of a complex inflammatory process.
- Strong genetic predisposition; many patients have personal or family history of atopy.
- Generally begins during infancy or childhood; 90% of those ultimately affected present before 5 years of age.
- Children who have atopic dermatitis are susceptible to certain bacterial and viral infections.
  - Increased adherence of *Staphylococcus aureus* to the skin and reduced production of antimicrobial peptides may explain the high rates of colonization with and infection due to this bacterium.
  - Altered T-cell function may explain the predisposition of children to develop molluscum contagiosum, eczema herpeticum, and eczema vaccinatum.

Signs and Symptoms

- Characterized by pruritus with resultant scratching that leads to excoriations and lichenification.
- The appearance of lesions varies with the patient's age and racial background.
  - Infants and toddlers: involvement of the face, trunk, and extensor extremities (Figures 4.1 and 4.2).
  - Childhood: Lesions are concentrated in flexural areas, such as the antecubital and popliteal fossae, wrists, and ankles (Figures 4.3 and 4.4). Some children exhibit round, crusted lesions (ie, nummular [coin-shaped] eczema, Figure 4.5); in older children, the feet may be involved (Figure 4.6).

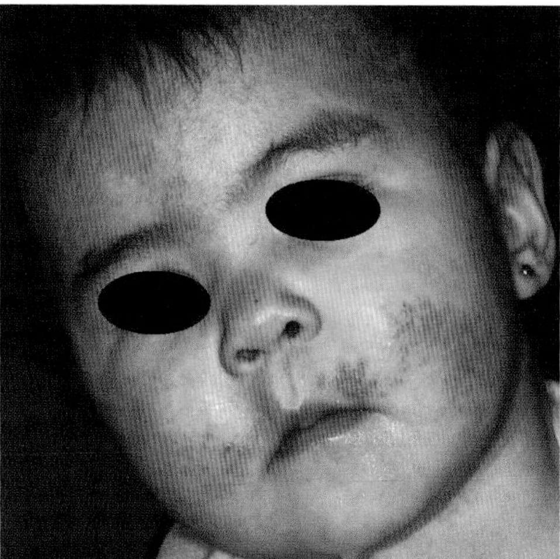

Figure 4.1. Erythematous patches on the face of an infant who has atopic dermatitis.

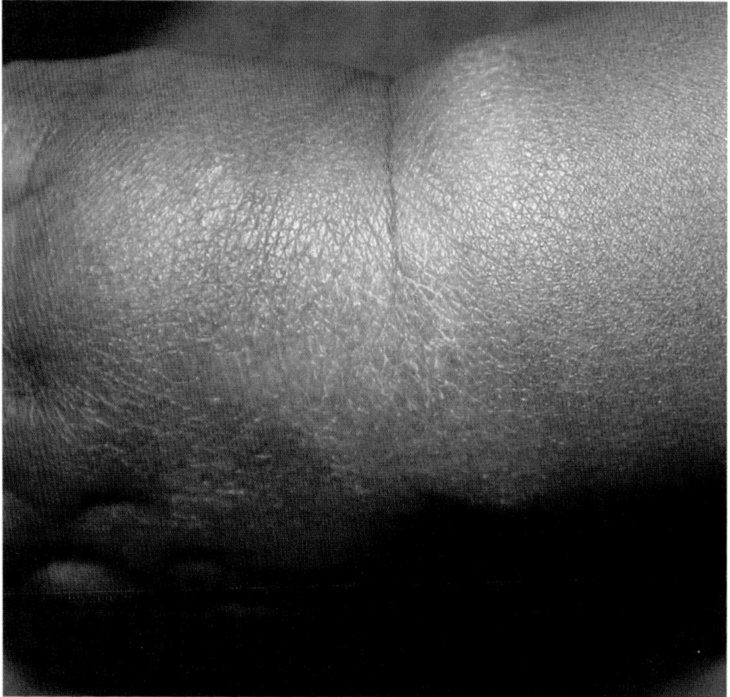

Figure 4.2. Hypopigmented patch on the dorsum of the wrist in an infant who has atopic dermatitis.

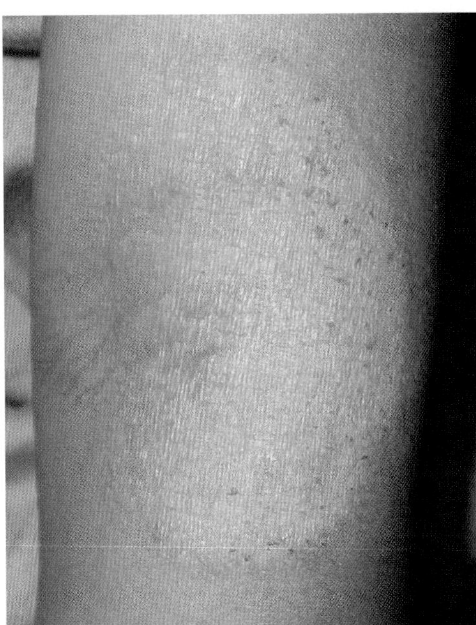

Figure 4.3. Erythematous lichenified patch in the antecubital fossa in childhood atopic dermatitis.

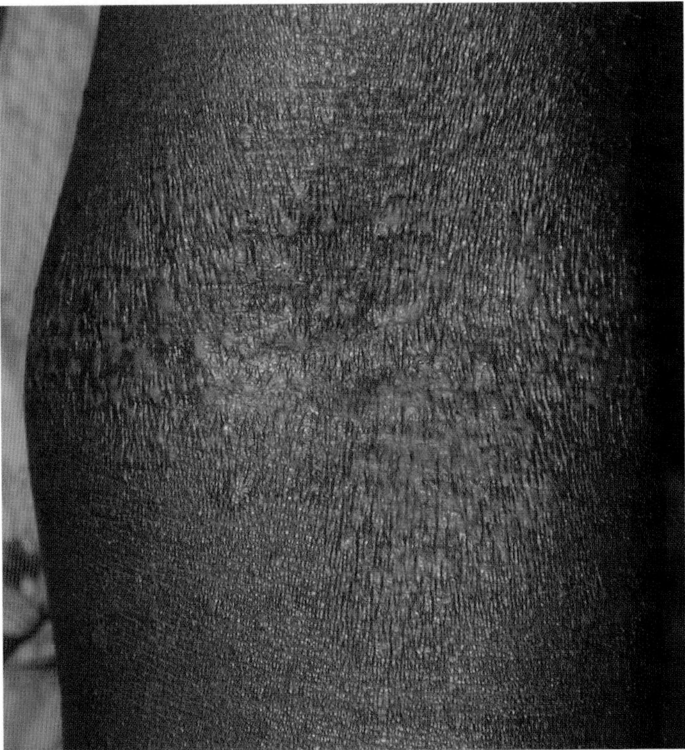

Figure 4.4. Chronic atopic dermatitis in the antecubital fossa.

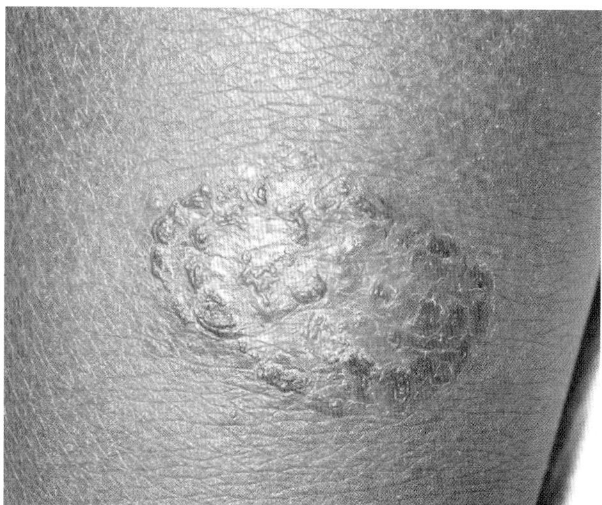

Figure 4.5. Oval crusted lesion of nummular eczema.

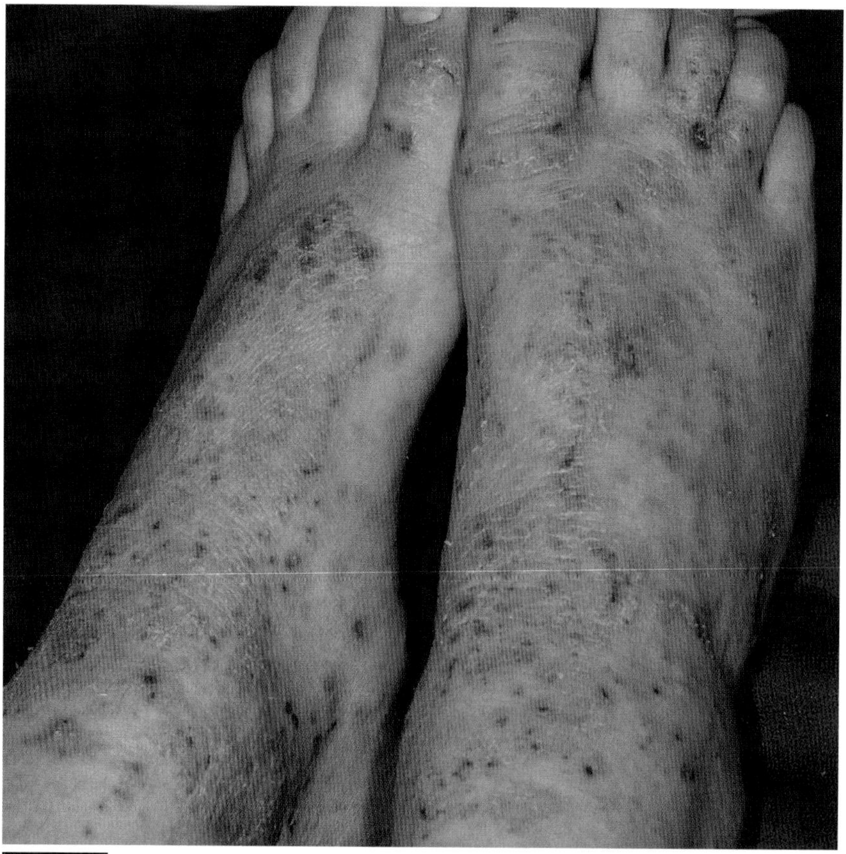

Figure 4.6. Involvement of the feet in atopic dermatitis: erythema, lichenification, scaling, and numerous erosions.

- Adolescents continue to exhibit a flexural distribution but often develop lesions on the hands, face, and neck (Figure 4.7).
- In lightly pigmented individuals, lesions are erythematous, somewhat scaly or crusted papules, patches, or thin plaques. In people of color, erythema is less obvious, the eruption often is more papular, and postinflammatory hypopigmentation or hyperpigmentation often is present (see Figure 4.2).

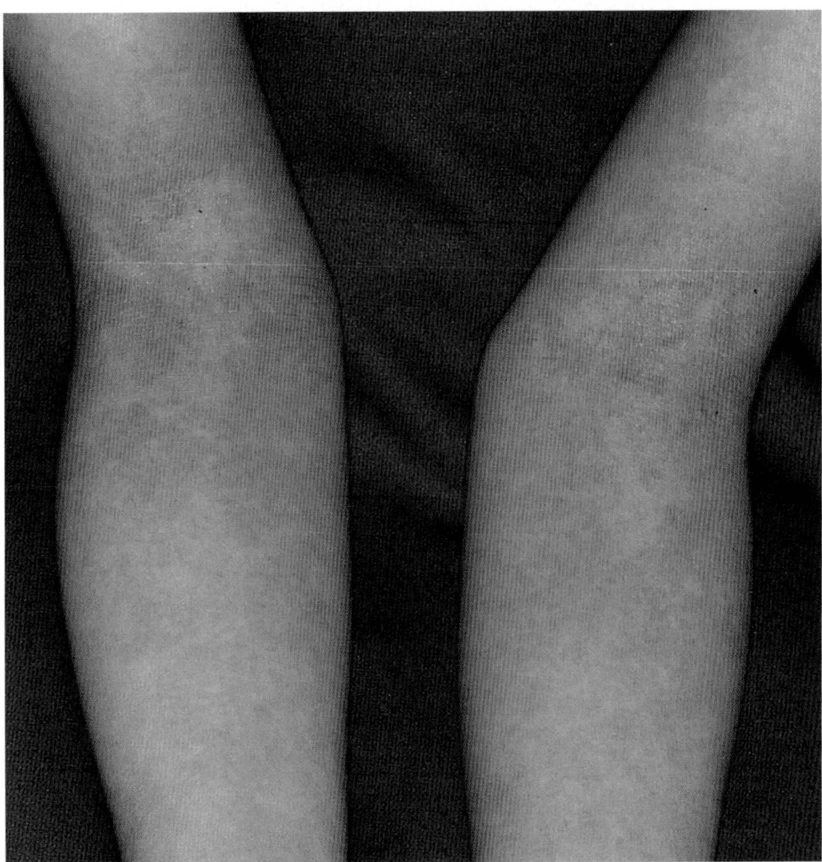

Figure 4.7. Erythematous patches in the antecubital fossae of an adolescent who has atopic dermatitis.

- Other cutaneous abnormalities that serve as clues to diagnosis include
  - Dennie-Morgan folds (atopic pleats): prominent skinfolds located beneath the lower eyelids
  - Dry skin (xerosis)
  - Hyperlinearity of the palms and soles
  - Lichenification: thickened skin with prominent creases (see Figure 4.3)
  - Keratosis pilaris: papules centered about follicles that have a central core of keratin debris and, at times, surrounding erythema (Figure 4.8); lesions usually located on the upper outer arms, face, and thighs
  - Pityriasis alba: small, poorly defined areas of hypopigmentation located on the face or elsewhere (Figure 4.9)
  - Ichthyosis vulgaris: polygonal scales, most commonly involving the lower extremities (Figure 4.10)

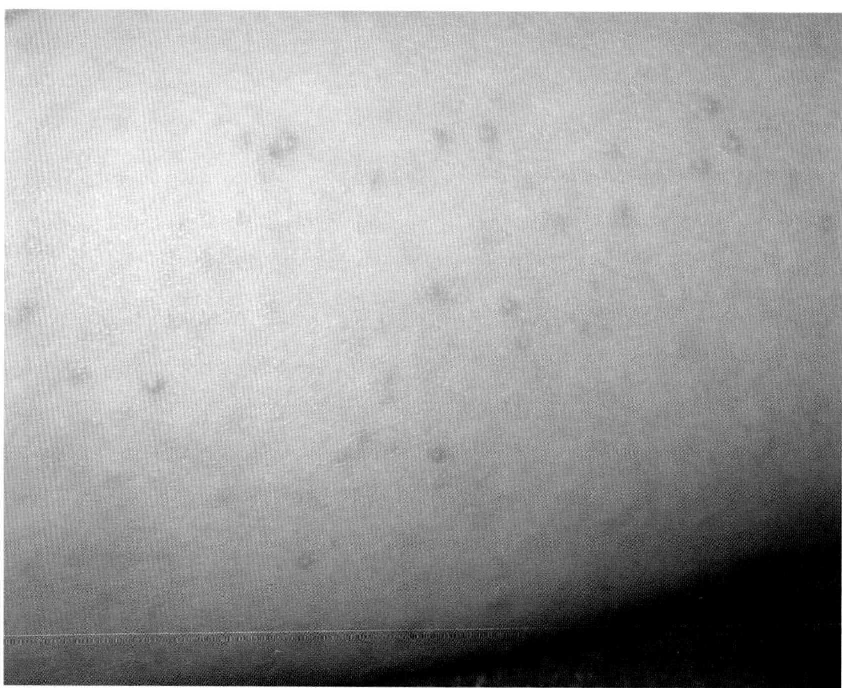

Figure 4.8. Keratosis pilaris: follicular papules that have a central core of keratin debris.

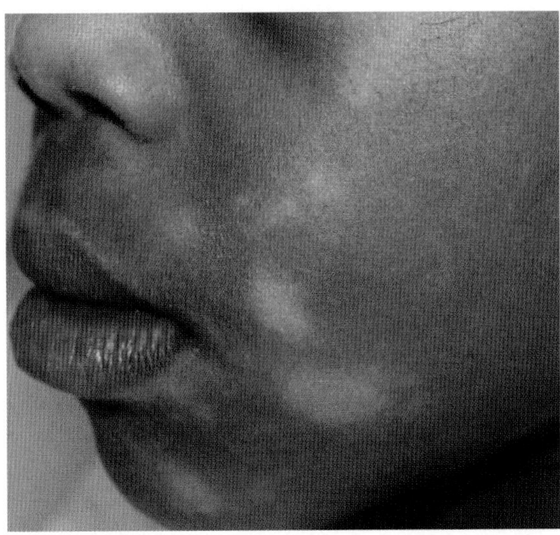

Figure 4.9. Ill-defined hypopigmented macules are characteristic of pityriasis alba.

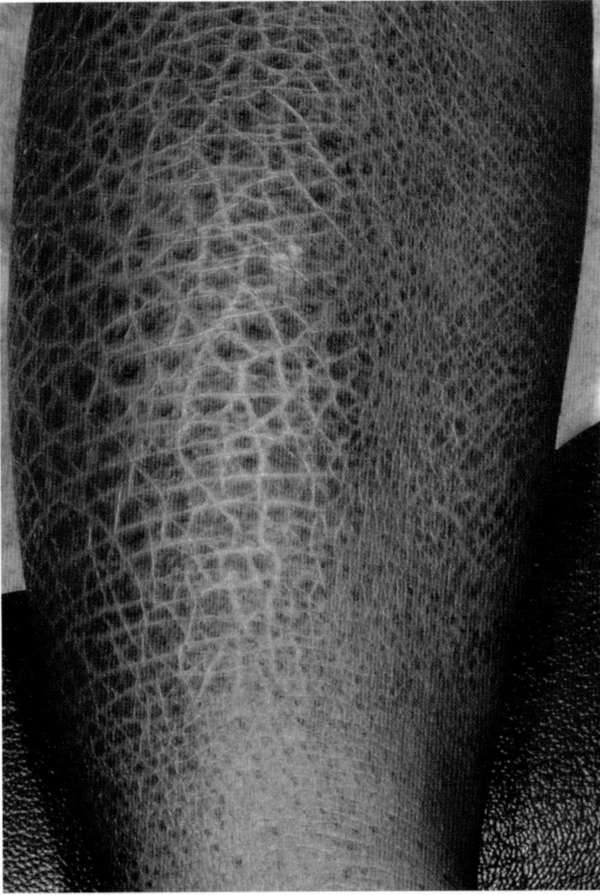

Figure 4.10. Polygonal scales with a pasted-on appearance located on the lower extremities are characteristic of ichthyosis vulgaris, a condition commonly associated with atopic dermatitis.

Look-alikes

Disorder	Differentiating Features
Contact dermatitis	• Location corresponds to exposure to contact allergen (eg, ear lobules in those with sensitivity to nickel used in earrings). • Configuration may be unusual (eg, linear in plant dermatitis).
Psoriasis	• Erythematous papules and plaques with thick, silvery scale. • Scaling of scalp common, pitting of nails may be observed. • Pruritus much less common/less severe than in atopic dermatitis. • Extensor (rather than flexural) surfaces of knees and elbows common sites of involvement.
Scabies	• Papules often larger than those in atopic dermatitis. • Linear burrows present. • Beyond infancy, lesions concentrated in interdigital spaces, wrist flexures, on penis and scrotum, or on areolae. • Other family members may be affected.
Seborrheic dermatitis	• Erythematous, greasy, scaling patches involving the eyebrows, nasolabial folds, and intertriginous areas (eg, retroauricular areas, axillae, and, in infants, the diaper area) • Scaling of scalp common • Most often seen in infants <1 year or after adrenarche; less common in prepubertal children • Pruritus often minimal
Tinea corporis	• Often annular, with central clearing • Pruritus often absent

How to Make the Diagnosis

- The diagnosis is made clinically based on the presence of 3 or more of the following signs or symptoms: typical morphology and distribution of lesions, pruritus, chronic relapsing course, and a family or personal history of atopic disorders.
- The presence of associated features (discussed previously) provides support for the diagnosis.

Treatment

Daily Measures

Hydrate Skin and Prevent Pruritus

- Daily bathing is desirable, if less than 10 minutes and warm (not hot) water is used.
- Apply an emollient as needed to control dry skin; most effective timing is when applied immediately after bathing (while skin is still moist). Application often is recommended at least once daily, but this will vary with the individual and environmental factors (eg, during warm weather months in humid conditions an emollient may not be needed).
  - Lotions (eg, Aveeno, CeraVe, Cetaphil, Curel, Eucerin, Lubriderm, Moisturel, or others) work well for most individuals, although preservatives (found in some) occasionally cause stinging or skin reactions.
  - Creams (eg, Aveeno, CeraVe, Cetaphil, Eucerin, Vanicream, Moisturel, or others) moisturize better than lotions and do not leave as greasy a feel, which may be a benefit in older patients.
  - Ointments (eg, Aquaphor, Vaseline, or others) are very good moisturizers but because of their greasy feel may not be well tolerated by some.
- During colder months when humidity is low one may consider using a vaporizer in the patient's room at night (taking care to cleanse the device regularly and avoid moisture contact with walls [which could promote mold growth]).
- Use a fragrance-free, non-soap cleanser. Examples include synthetic detergent (ie, syndet) cleansers in bar (eg, Cetaphil Bar, Dove Bar) or liquid (eg, Dove Liquid) forms or lipid-free cleansers (eg, Aquanil, CeraVe, Cetaphil).
- Use an additive-free (fragrance and dye-free) detergent for laundering clothes (eg, All Free Clear, Ivory Snow, Tide Free and Gentle). If a fabric softener is used, it too should be additive free.
- Wear cotton clothing next to the skin when possible.

When the Disease Flares

Reduce Inflammation

Apply a topical corticosteroid twice daily as needed. Ointments are preferred over creams because they tend to be more effective and better tolerated (although some patients prefer creams because they are less greasy). The selection and use of these agents is discussed in detail in Chapter 3. Systemic corticosteroids rarely are necessary for the management of atopic dermatitis.

- Infants (or treatment of the face in a patient of any age): Use a low-potency preparation (eg, hydrocortisone 1% or 2.5%).
- Young children (exclusive of the face): Use a low-potency preparation (eg, hydrocortisone 1% or 2.5%) or, if necessary, a mid-potency preparation (eg, triamcinolone 0.025% or 0.1%, fluocinolone 0.025%).
- Older children and adolescents (exclusive of the face): Use a mid-potency preparation (eg, triamcinolone 0.1%); a high-potency agent (eg, mometasone 0.1%, fluocinonide 0.05%) may be needed for resistant, non-facial areas during a flare.
- Once symptoms have improved, the corticosteroid may be withdrawn and a moisturizer continued regularly. However, applying a corticosteroid once or twice weekly at locations prone to exacerbations has been shown to reduce relapses and increase the time to the next flare.

Control Pruritus

Administer a bedtime dose of a first-generation antihistamine (eg, hydroxyzine 0.5–1 mg/kg, diphenhydramine 1.25 mg/kg) to provide sedation, improve sleep, and reduce scratching; daytime doses may occasionally be needed but should be lower (to avoid sedation). Alternatively, some practitioners use a nonsedating agent (eg, cetirizine) for daytime coverage in school-aged children, although evidence of its benefit is controversial.

Control Infection

If there is evidence of secondary bacterial infection (eg, crusting, pustules, oozing [Figure 4.11]), consider administering an oral antistaphylococcal antibiotic (eg, cephalexin or other agent based on local antibiotic resistance patterns) for 7 to 10 days. If no improvement is noted within 48 hours, consider skin swab for bacterial culture to assess for resistant organisms (eg, methicillin-resistant *S aureus*) and treat appropriately. At this time, most *S aureus* isolates from patients with atopic dermatitis in the United States remain methicillin-sensitive.

If infection is limited to very focal areas, a prescription topical antimicrobial agent (eg, mupirocin, retapamulin) may be useful.

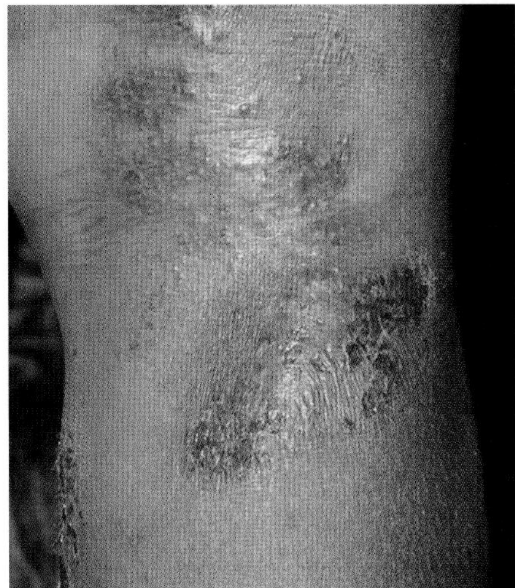

Figure 4.11. Erosions, weeping, and crusting are observed when lesions of atopic dermatitis become secondarily infected.

Other Measures

- Non-corticosteroid topical calcineurin inhibitors (eg, tacrolimus [Protopic], pimecrolimus [Elidel])
  - Reduce inflammation and avoid potential local or systemic corticosteroid adverse effects.
  - Are used as second-line agents in patients older than 2 years for whom topical corticosteroids fail or when avoidance of more potent topical corticosteroid is desired (eg, treatment of the face). The US Food and Drug Administration advises using these agents only for active areas of dermatitis and discourages chronic long-term application.
    - Are generally used in conjunction with topical corticosteroids (eg, a topical corticosteroid is applied morning and afternoon and the topical calcineurin inhibitor at bedtime).
    - Once symptoms have improved, application of a topical calcineurin inhibitor 2 to 3 times weekly at locations prone to exacerbations has been shown to reduce relapses.
- Control *S aureus* colonization: may be useful for those with severe or recalcitrant disease. Consider one of the following options: (1) twice weekly 5- to 10-minute baths to which household bleach (6%) is added (½ cup in a full tub of water [40 gallons]), (2) use of a sodium hypochlorite body wash (like CLn BodyWash) in the bath or shower, or (3) intranasal mupirocin (twice a day for 5 days). Although some favor the use of an antibacterial soap containing triclosan (eg, Cetaphil Antibacterial Bar, Liquid Dial Antibacterial), evidence of their efficacy in atopic dermatitis is lacking and concerns about safety have been raised.

- Wet-wrap therapy: This method may be useful during severe flares of atopic dermatitis. A topical corticosteroid is applied to affected areas and covered with a moistened cotton suit, wet gauze strips, or a specially designed, commercially available garment, which is then covered with a dry outer layer (eg, dry pajamas). The wrap may be worn for several hours or up to 24 hours; on removal, emollient is applied. Once the disease flare improves, wet-wrap therapy is discontinued.
- Barrier repair agents
  - A variety of over-the-counter (eg, CeraVe, Cetaphil RestoraDerm) and prescription (eg, Atopiclair, EpiCeram, Hylatopic) barrier repair agents exist that may help reduce the severity of atopic dermatitis and play an adjunctive therapeutic role. These agents include products with ceramides, filaggrin degradation products, natural moisturizing factor, avenanthramides, glycyrrhetinic acid, shea nut derivatives, and palmitamide monoethanolamine.
  - While the exact role of these agents is not yet clarified, they may play a role in active disease (usually in conjunction with anti-inflammatory agents like corticosteroids and calcineurin inhibitors) and as maintenance agents.
  - The prescription barrier repair agents typically are expensive.
- Dietary manipulation
  - Breastfeeding for the first 4 months of life reduces the incidence and severity of atopic dermatitis in high-risk children (ie, those with a first-degree relative who has atopic dermatitis). However, this risk reduction is modest (at most 33%). Maternal antigen avoidance during pregnancy or lactation is not recommended.
  - Food allergy should be considered in those children with moderate to severe disease that is recalcitrant to standard therapies or when there is a history of pruritus or rash occurring within 30 minutes of ingesting a food. However, most patients with atopic dermatitis do not have food as a trigger of their atopic dermatitis. Guidelines for the diagnosis and management of food allergy in the United States have been published (*J Allergy Clin Immunol.* 2010;126[6 Suppl]:S1–S58).
  - Egg, peanut, and milk account for 72% of food allergies, but soy, fish, and wheat also may be responsible. Children suspected of having food allergy contributing to atopic dermatitis are best referred to an allergist.
- House dust mite avoidance: Avoidance through frequent vacuuming and encasing pillows and mattresses with allergen-proof products may result in a modest reduction in the severity of atopic dermatitis. Such recommendations are reserved for patients with severe or recalcitrant disease.

Treating Associated Conditions

- Keratosis pilaris and ichthyosis vulgaris
  - Advise patients and families there is no cure and the course may be variable.
  - Use of an emollient or emollient with a keratolytic agent (eg, AmLactin, Lac-Hydrin, Carmol), applied twice daily as needed, may soften papules and make them less noticeable.
  - Good dry skin care is vital.
- Pityriasis alba
  - Apply an appropriate topical corticosteroid twice daily (eg, for the face, hydrocortisone 1%) for 2 to 3 weeks to treat any existing inflammation (topical calcineurin inhibitors may also be useful in this regard).
  - Sun protection should be recommended to reduce the contrast between normal skin (which will become darker with sun exposure) and affected skin (in which there is temporary melanocyte dysfunction).
  - The patient and family should be counseled that several months might be required for normal pigmentation to return.

Prognosis

- The prognosis for children with atopic dermatitis is good; 80% to 90% of infants experience a spontaneous resolution or improvement in symptoms by adolescence. However, until this time the course is chronic and relapsing, an issue that should be discussed with patients and parents.

When to Worry or Refer

- Consider referral to a dermatologist for patients who have severe or extensive disease, do not respond to standard treatment, or have chronic or recurrent bacterial or viral (eg, molluscum contagiosum, herpes simplex virus) infections.

Resources for Families

- American Academy of Pediatrics: HealthyChildren.org.
  www.HealthyChildren.org/eczema
- American Academy of Dermatology: Atopic dermatitis.
  https://www.aad.org/public/diseases/eczema/atopic-dermatitis
- American Academy of Dermatology: Dyshidrotic eczema.
  https://www.aad.org/public/diseases/eczema/dyshidrotic-eczema
- MedlinePlus: Information for patients and families (in English and Spanish) sponsored by the National Library of Medicine and National Institutes of Health.
  https://www.nlm.nih.gov/medlineplus/eczema.html
- National Eczema Association (NEA): NEA is a national patient-oriented organization. The site contains information for patients and families (primarily in English but some in Spanish), education for practitioners, and links to other resources.
  www.nationaleczema.org
- Society for Pediatric Dermatology: Patient handout on atopic dermatitis.
  http://pedsderm.net/for-patients-families/patient-handouts
- WebMD: Information for families is contained in Health A-Z topics.
  www.webmd.com/skin-problems-and-treatments/eczema/default.htm

Contact Dermatitis (Irritant and Allergic)

I. Irritant Contact Dermatitis

Introduction/Etiology/Epidemiology

- Inflammatory reaction of the skin caused by physical contact with an irritating substance.
- Occurs in any individual exposed to sufficient amount of offending agent.
- Modified by local physical factors (eg, diapering) and individual susceptibility (eg, diminished skin barrier function, as in atopic dermatitis).
- Common forms of irritant contact dermatitis
  - Irritant diaper dermatitis: most common pediatric presentation of irritant contact dermatitis (occurs in up to 20% of all infants); caused by friction, moisture, maceration, and occlusion
  - Dry skin dermatitis (ie, asteatotic eczema): caused by low relative humidity and aggravated by soaps, excessive bathing, and alcohol-containing lotions
  - Lip-licking dermatitis and thumb-sucking dermatitis: caused by wetting the skin frequently with saliva
- Irritant contact dermatitis is more common in children with underlying atopic dermatitis, presumably related to their diminished skin barrier function.

Signs and Symptoms

Irritant Diaper Dermatitis

- Affects convex surfaces of buttocks, upper inner thighs (Figure 5.1)
- Characteristically spares creases/folds
- Sharply marginated erythema that becomes more deeply red with a "glazed" appearance
- May have "tide mark" dermatitis at edge of diaper

Asteatotic Eczema

- Dry, rough skin with white, sometimes rectangular, scaling and variable erythema (Figure 5.2)
- Often associated with keratosis pilaris

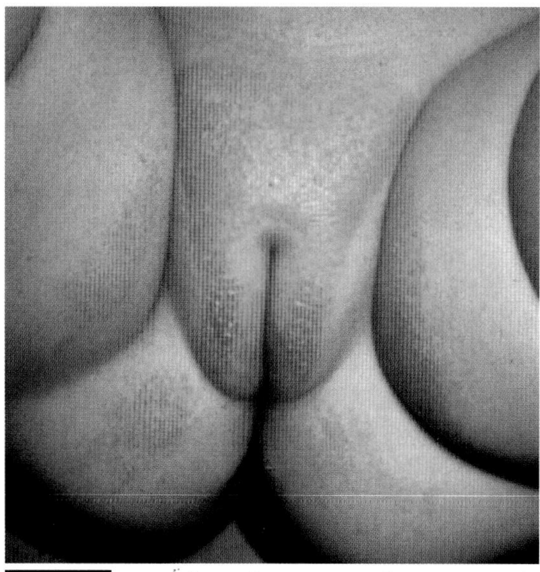

Figure 5.1. Irritant diaper dermatitis. Erythematous patches sparing the skinfolds.

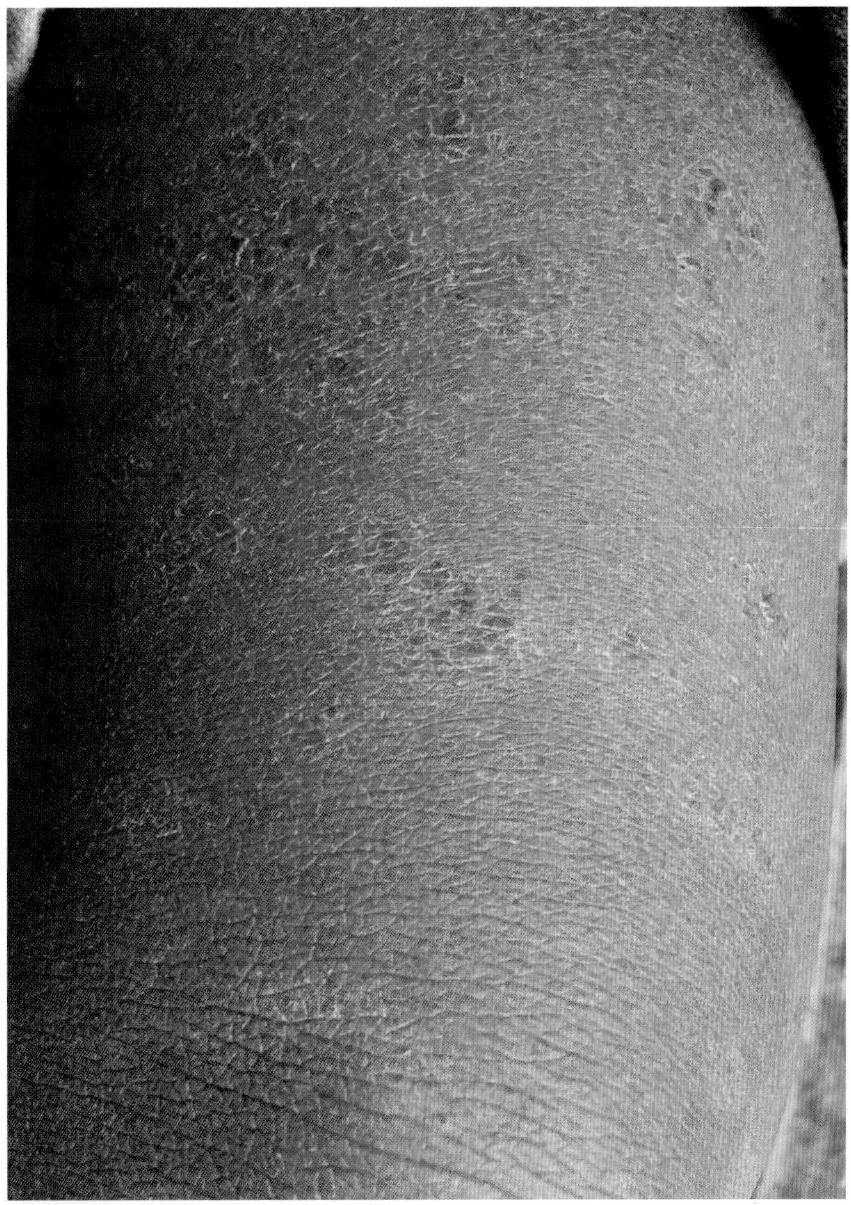

Figure 5.2. Asteatotic eczema is characterized by dry, rough skin with white rectangular scaling.

Look-alikes *(See also Chapter 91, Diaper Dermatitis.)*

Disorder	Differentiating Features
Irritant Diaper Dermatitis	
Candidiasis	• Erythematous patches that involve convexities and inguinal creases • Satellite papules and pustules • Scaling at margins of involved areas
Seborrheic dermatitis	• Salmon-pink patches with greasy scale that involve the convexities and inguinal creases. • Involvement of scalp, face, retroauricular creases, or chest may be present.
Bullous impetigo	• Flaccid blisters filled with clear or purulent fluid. • Blisters rupture rapidly, leaving round or oval crusted erosions with a rim of scale.
Folliculitis	• Pustules with surrounding erythema centered around hair follicles
Intertrigo	• Erythema and superficial erosions in inguinal creases
Jacquet erosive dermatitis	• Well-defined shallow ulcers or ulcerated diaper dermatitis nodules
Perianal bacterial dermatitis	• Well-defined, moist erythema surrounding anus. • Pain and constipation may be present.
Langerhans cell histiocytosis	• Involves skin creases. • Erosions, petechiae, and hemorrhagic papules often present on scalp. • Seborrheic dermatitis-like eruption may be present. • Lymphadenopathy often present.
Nutritional or metabolic disorders (eg, zinc deficiency, cystic fibrosis, biotin-dependent multiple carboxylase deficiency)	• Sharply marginated plaques with shiny, peeling scale • Eruption often located in a periorificial (eg, perioral, perianal) and acral distribution • Secondary bacterial, candidal infection common • Unresponsive to typical therapies • May have associated diarrhea, alopecia, or failure to thrive
Asteatotic Eczema	
Nummular eczema	• Well-defined crusted patches or erosions • History of atopic dermatitis often present
Allergic contact dermatitis	• Rash located at site of antigen exposure. • Characteristic (eg, linear) or geographic patterns may be present. • History of exposure to antigen.
Atopic dermatitis	• History of atopic dermatitis usually present • Eruption located in typical areas (eg, antecubital fossae in a child)

How to Make the Diagnosis

- Irritant diaper dermatitis: The diagnosis usually is made clinically based on the typical appearance and distribution of the eruption.
- Asteatotic dermatitis: The diagnosis is made clinically based on the appearance of lesions; the observation of keratosis pilaris; a history of using harsh, drying soaps; and its occurrence during times of low environmental humidity.

Treatment of Irritant Contact Dermatitis

General Principles for All Types of Irritant Contact Dermatitis

- Decrease or eliminate contact with the irritant, when feasible.
- Restore skin barrier function with emollients.
- Decrease inflammation with anti-inflammatory measures (typically topical corticosteroids).
- Treat secondary infection, if present.

Irritant Diaper Dermatitis

- Remove/diminish contactants (urine and feces) from skin surface.
- Decrease skin maceration by keeping skin surface free of aqueous material (keep skin surface dry).
- Specific measures
  - Change diapers frequently.
  - Use super-absorbing disposable diapers.
  - Gently cleanse with tap water or fragrance-free diaper wipes; avoid soaps.
  - Use emollient ointments or barrier creams to protect skin surface (eg, zinc oxide ointment or paste, petrolatum).
  - Selectively use 1% to 2.5% hydrocortisone ointment or cream for active inflammation (apply a thick layer prior to application of emollient or barrier ointments).
  - Selectively use anticandidal creams (eg, nystatin, an imidazole antifungal agent) if there is evidence of candidiasis (apply a thin layer prior to application of emollient or barrier ointments).
  - Do not use combination topical therapies that contain potent topical steroids (eg, betamethasone/clotrimazole).

Asteatotic Dermatitis

- Restore skin barrier function and diminish transepidermal water loss.
- Apply emollients/moisturizers at least 1 to 2 times daily.
- Eliminate use of soaps as much as possible; when improved, reintroduce soaps that are superfatted or contain emollient ingredients.
- Selectively use low- or mid-potency topical corticosteroids for more severe cases.

Prognosis

- The prognosis for irritant dermatitis is excellent providing appropriate treatment is instituted.
- Recurrences are common.

When to Worry or Refer

- Uncertainty about the diagnosis
- Failure to respond to therapy

II. Allergic Contact Dermatitis

Introduction/Etiology/Epidemiology

- Allergic contact dermatitis is an inflammatory immune reaction in the skin.
- Results from cell-mediated immunity and the pathogenesis involves a sensitization phase and an elicitation phase.
- A wide variety of natural and synthetic substances can produce allergic contact dermatitis.
- Up to 10% of childhood dermatitis may represent allergic contact dermatitis.
- Some sources of contact allergens in children include
  - Plants, especially poison ivy, poison oak, and poison sumac (Urushiol is the antigen in these plants.)
  - Jewelry, belt buckles, clothing snaps, toys or devices with metal (nickel)
  - Shoes (potassium dichromate)
  - Toilet seats (lacquered or painted wood, plastic, cleaning products; can represent irritant or allergic contact dermatitis)
  - Topical medications, creams, lotions (quaternium-15, formaldehyde, lanolin, topical antimicrobials)
    - Premoistened hygienic wipes containing preservatives methylisothiazolinone or methylchloroisothiazolinone

Signs and Symptoms

- Usually an acute, intensely pruritic, exudative dermatitis.
- Vesiculation and blister formation may be prominent in allergic contact dermatitis to very potent sensitizers like poison ivy (Figure 5.3). Less potent antigens (eg, nickel) produce features of a subacute or chronic dermatitis with lichenification and scaling (Figure 5.4).

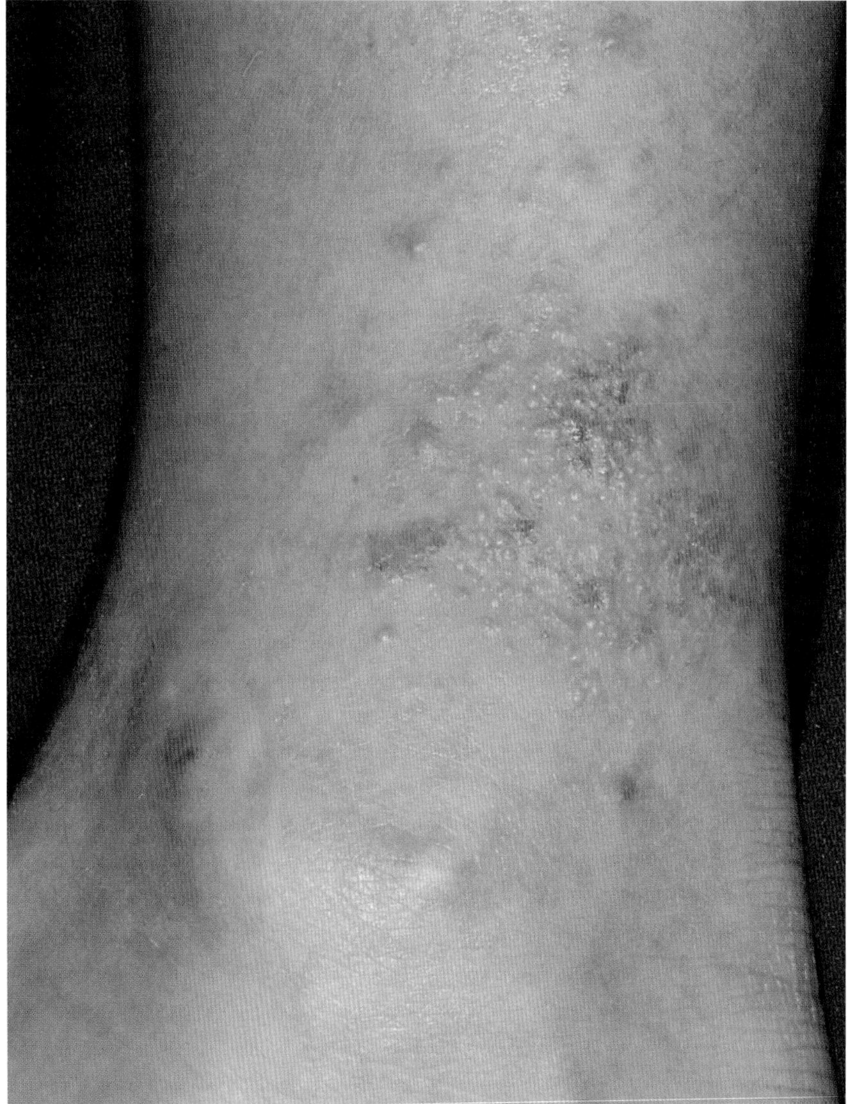

Figure 5.3. Multiple small vesicles overlying an erythematous plaque in a boy exposed to poison ivy.

- Dermatitis typically is limited to the area(s) of skin in contact with the allergen.
  - Involvement at the site of contact with a wristwatch, clothing snap, belt buckle (see Figure 5.4), earring (Figure 5.5), or necklace suggests nickel allergy.
  - Involvement of the dorsa of the feet occurs in shoe dermatitis (often due to potassium dichromate in leather).
  - Symmetric involvement of the posterior thighs and buttocks in a circular pattern occurs in toilet seat dermatitis (Figure 5.6), which can arise due to allergic sensitization (essential oils in wood, varnish, paint), irritants (harsh cleaning products), or a combination of the two.
  - Linearly arranged dermatitis or vesicles are characteristic of plant dermatitis, with distribution corresponding to the plant brushing in a streaky fashion against the skin (Figure 5.7).
  - Distribution can sometimes be misleading or confusing. Eyelid dermatitis may be caused by allergic contact sensitivity to components of nail polish. The fingers are spared, but the sensitive skin of the eyelids is affected.
  - An associated hypersensitivity or id reaction may occur in association with the primary allergic contact dermatitis and presents with symmetrically placed pruritic papules on the extensor arms (Figure 5.8), legs, and cheeks.

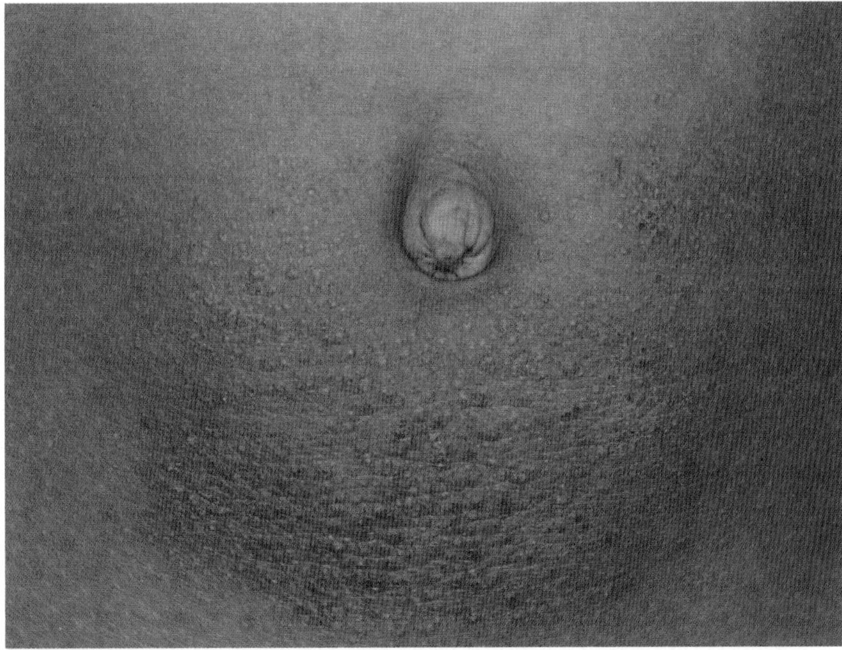

Figure 5.4. Contact dermatitis caused by nickel in a clothing snap or belt buckle affects the lower abdomen.

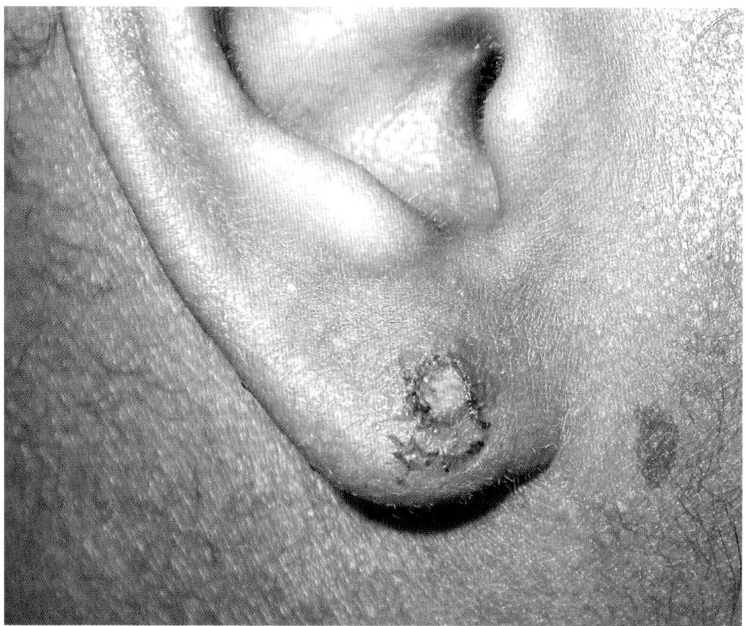

Figure 5.5. Nickel contact dermatitis at the site of an earring.

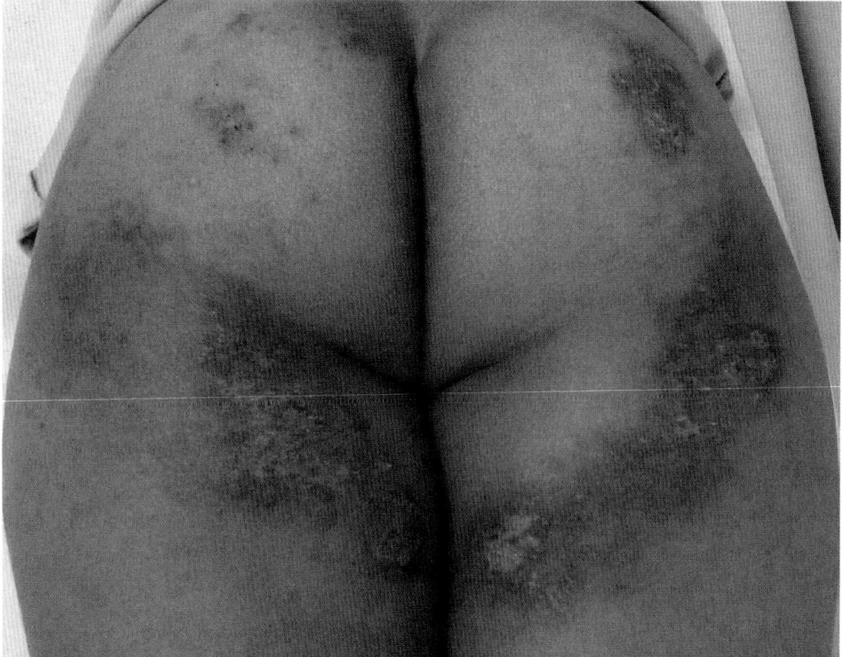

Figure 5.6. In toilet seat dermatitis, symmetric, eczematous lesions are seen on the posterior thighs and buttocks.

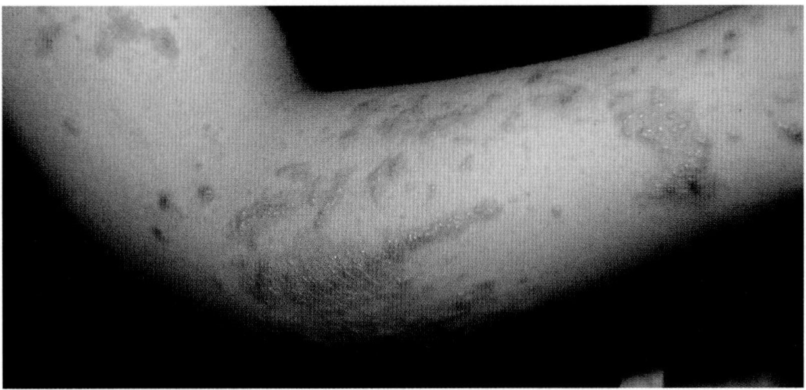

Figure 5.7. Vesicles and erythematous papules in a linear arrangement are often seen in allergic contact dermatitis caused by plants.

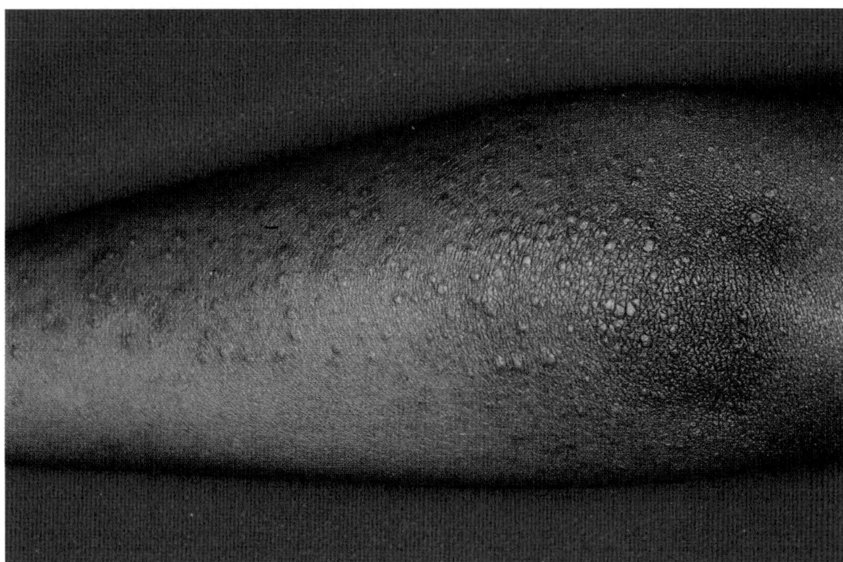

Figure 5.8. Id reaction. These itchy papules occurred on the extensor arms and legs in a young girl with allergic contact dermatitis to nickel.

- Once the allergic contact dermatitis reaction occurs, the response to a strong allergen lasts 2 to 3 weeks, even without further exposure.
- Continued appearance of new areas of dermatitis in episodes of poison ivy represent more slowly evolving reactions in areas that received a lower dose or exposure to allergen. The blister fluid of poison ivy lesions does not contain allergen and cannot spread the eruption.

Look-alikes

Disorder	Differentiating Features
Atopic dermatitis	• Typical distribution based on age of patient (eg, antecubital fossae in a child or adolescent) • History of atopic dermatitis often present
Irritant contact dermatitis	• Area of involvement often not as well defined as in allergic contact dermatitis
Seborrheic dermatitis	• Located in typical areas (eg, nasolabial folds, eyebrows, scalp). • Scale is greasy. • Sites of involvement may not be consistent with allergen exposure.
Herpes zoster	• May be confused with contact dermatitis due to plants. • Pain usually more prominent than pruritus. • Lesions typically distributed along a dermatome. • Viral culture or direct fluorescent antibody testing may be valuable in differentiating the 2 conditions.

How to Make the Diagnosis

- Acute onset, extreme pruritus, and localized distribution of the dermatitis are often sufficient to make a clinical diagnosis.
- Chronic dermatitis caused by contact allergens can be more challenging to diagnose, but distribution of the eruption is key.
- Chronic, lichenified subumbilical dermatitis is virtually always related to nickel allergy from buckles or pant snaps.
- Patch testing is the gold standard for establishing the diagnosis. It is not needed for straightforward plant dermatitis or nickel allergy but may be essential to evaluate for other forms of allergic contact dermatitis when the offending agent is less clear.

Treatment

- Topical corticosteroids are the mainstay of treatment for allergic contact dermatitis.
  - Moderate- or high-potency agents are often necessary to produce a therapeutic response and may be needed 2 times daily for 1 to 2 weeks.
  - Wet dressings are a helpful adjunct for more severe cases.

- Facial, genital, and extensive allergic contact dermatitis from potent allergens, such as poison ivy, require systemic corticosteroids. Prednisone at a dose of 1 mg/kg (up to 60 mg) as a single daily dose is prescribed and tapered over 2 to 3 weeks. (This prolonged treatment course is necessary to avoid rebound exacerbation.)
- Id reactions may be treated with low- to mid-potency topical corticosteroids and generally resolve concomitantly with successful treatment of the primary contact dermatitis.
- Identification and avoidance of the offending allergen is the goal of long-term management and, in some cases, requires patch testing to help identify the allergen involved.

Prognosis

- The prognosis is good, providing the responsible antigen is identified and avoided.

When to Worry or Refer

- Refer patients to a dermatologist when the diagnosis is uncertain.
- Refer patients who have recurrent or treatment-resistant contact dermatitis or those for whom an antigen has not been identified (patch testing may be indicated).

Resources for Families

- American Academy of Dermatology: Contact dermatitis. **https://www.aad.org/public/diseases/eczema/contact-dermatitis**

Juvenile Plantar Dermatosis

Introduction/Etiology/Epidemiology

- Juvenile plantar dermatosis (also known as "sweaty sock syndrome") is a dermatitis thought to be the result of friction (applied by footwear) and excessive sweating. Cycles of foot moisture (due to excessive sweating and occlusion of the feet by socks and shoes) and evaporative drying (when footwear is removed) likely contribute.
- Usually affects young children and resolves by adolescence. The course is chronic and relapsing.

Signs and Symptoms

- Scaling and erythema of the plantar forefeet and toes (especially the great toes) with sparing of the interdigital spaces (Figure 6.1).
- Fissures may occur (Figure 6.2) that at times may be deep and painful.

Look-alikes

Disorder	Differentiating Features
Tinea pedis	• Most commonly involves the interdigital spaces with scaling and fissuring. • Relapsing course uncommon. • Relatively uncommon before adolescence. • Concomitant onychomycosis may be present. • Potassium hydroxide examination of scrapings positive for fungal elements.
Contact dermatitis	• Usually affects the dorsum of the foot (although plantar foot may be involved as well)
Psoriasis	• Usually presents as erythematous plaques with thicker scale. • Lesions of psoriasis may be present elsewhere.
Pityriasis rubra pilaris	• Usually involves the soles diffusely (not just the distal feet) and the palms with thickening of the skin, scaling, and a yellow-orange color • Lesions usually present elsewhere (especially elbows, knees)

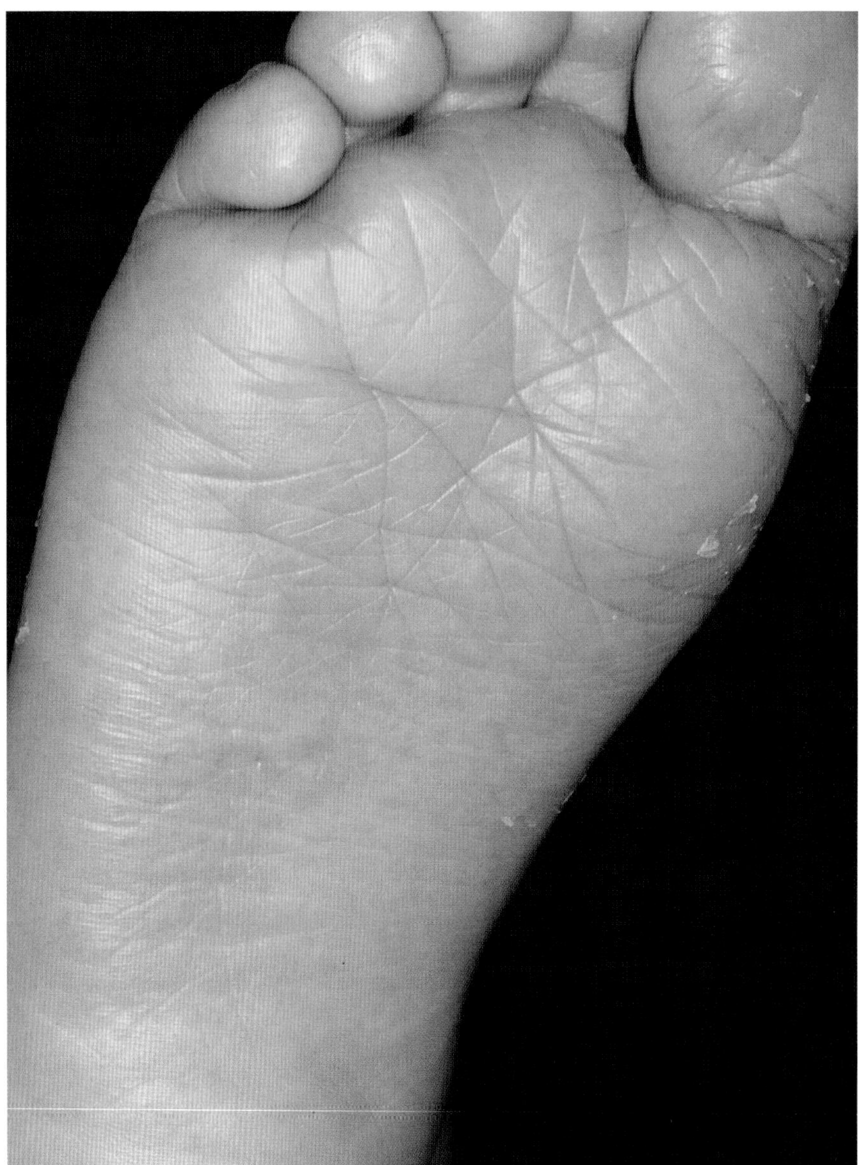

Figure 6.1. Lichenification, erythema, and scaling of the forefoot in juvenile plantar dermatosis.

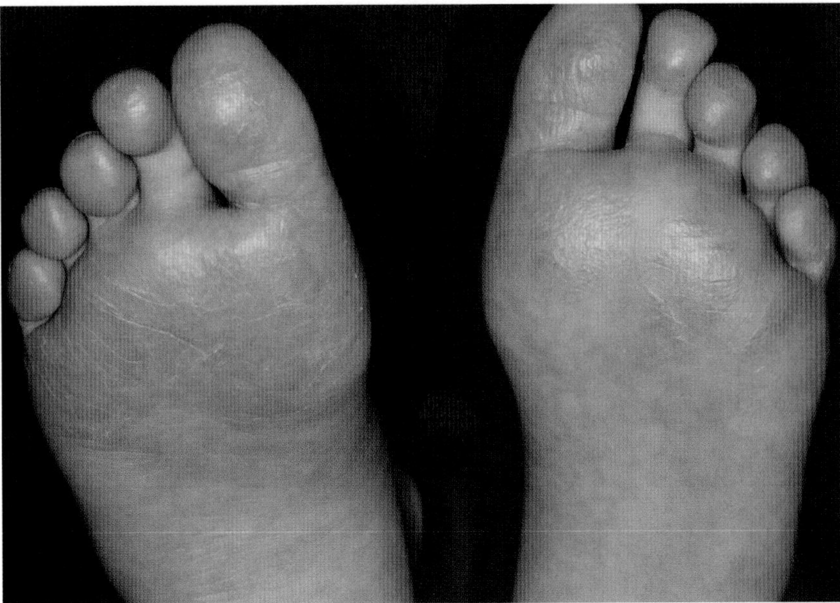

Figure 6.2. Erythema and scaling of the forefeet in juvenile plantar dermatosis. There is superficial fissuring of the right lateral foot.

Treatment

- The goal of treatment is to reduce foot moisture and cycles of excessive moisture and drying.
    - Wear absorbent socks, preferably cotton.
    - Avoid occlusive shoes or boots.
    - Sprinkle absorbent powder in shoes.
    - Remove socks and shoes after arriving home and apply a moisturizing cream or ointment.
- A medium-potency (eg, triamcinolone) or high-potency (eg, fluocinonide) topical corticosteroid may be applied to control inflammation or pruritus.
- If painful fissures appear, a cyanoacrylate adhesive (eg, Super Glue, Krazy Glue) may be applied to seal the fissure (thereby reducing pain).
- If crusting or pustules appear, suggesting secondary staphylococcal infection, treat with an oral antibiotic based on local antibiotic resistance patterns.
- Topical antiperspirants or oral anticholinergic agents are occasionally utilized; the former may be limited by increased irritation.

Prognosis

- The prognosis is excellent because the disorder typically resolves by adolescence.

When to Worry or Refer

- Consider referral for patients who do not respond to standard treatment measures.

Acne

Acne Vulgaris

Introduction/Etiology/Epidemiology

- Most common skin disease that is treated by physicians
- Affects approximately 45 million individuals in the United States, including at least 85% of all teenagers and young adults
- Most often self-limited and tends to remit during early adulthood but can be a continuing problem for a significant subset of young and middle-aged adults
- Has the potential for significant negative effect on quality of life
- Successful treatment is generally associated with improved psychologic well-being

Pathophysiology

- Result of a complex interaction between hormonal changes and their effects on the pilosebaceous apparatus (specialized structures consisting of a hair follicle and sebaceous glands concentrated on the face, chest, and back).
- Onset at puberty as a result of increased androgen production.
- End-organ androgen hyperresponsiveness of the follicle probably also plays a role.

Multifactorial Pathogenesis

- Disordered function of the pilosebaceous unit with abnormal follicular keratinization (tendency toward increased follicular plugging).
- Increased sebum production, under the influence of adrenal and gonadal androgens.
- Increased density of *Propionibacterium acnes,* a normal resident of the skin. Although the exact role of *P acnes* is unclear, it likely contributes to the pathogenesis of acne via bacterial overgrowth, activation of the innate immune response via toll-like receptors, and release of several degrading enzymes.

Factors That May Exacerbate Acne

- Trauma: scrubbing the skin too vigorously or picking of lesions
- Comedogenic cosmetics or other skin care products
- Tight-fitting sports equipment
- Medications: corticosteroids (topical, inhaled, and oral) and anabolic steroids, antiepileptic drugs, lithium, and certain contraceptives
- Hormonal dysregulation as occurs with polycystic ovarian syndrome and Cushing syndrome (may be associated with more severe acne)

Signs and Symptoms

Early on, acne lesions often appear on the forehead and middle third of the face (T-zone) and are obstructive (ie, comedones); inflammatory lesions tend to develop later and may occur on all areas of the face, neck, chest, and back.

- Comedonal lesions: often the first sign of acne, appearing before other signs of puberty.
  - Open comedones (blackheads): dilated follicles (Figure 7.1).
  - Closed comedones (whiteheads): white or skin-colored papules without surrounding erythema (Figure 7.2).
  - Recent data suggest these lesions may be accompanied by inflammation, although it is not clinically apparent.
- Inflammatory lesions typically appear later in the course of acne vulgaris and vary from 1- to 2-mm micro-papules to nodules larger than 5 mm (Figure 7.3).
- Large (5–15 mm) inflammatory nodules and cysts occur in the most severe cases, and such nodulocystic presentations are most likely to lead to permanent scarring.
  - Mild, moderate, and severe inflammatory acne can be associated with disfiguring postinflammatory discoloration, which can be red, violaceous, or gray-brown hyperpigmentation.
  - Pigmentary changes may persist for many months to years (Figure 7.4).

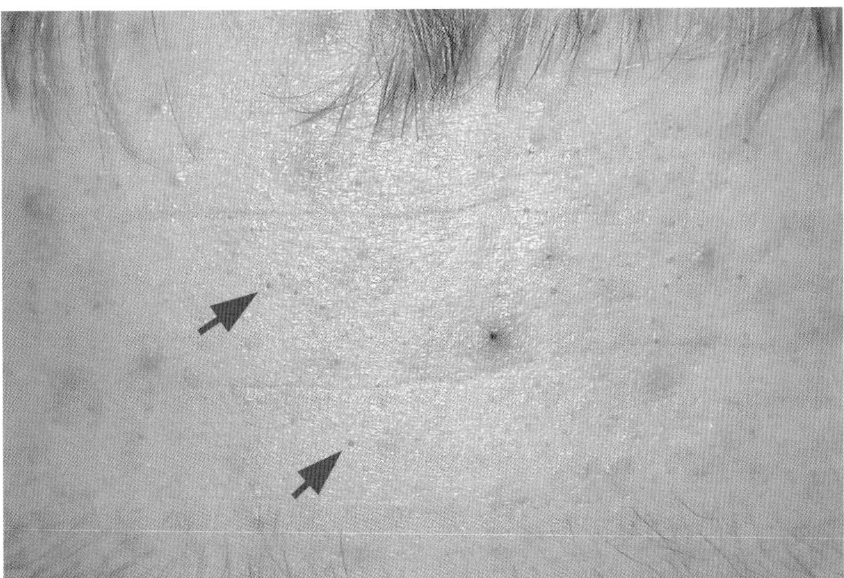

Figure 7.1. Open comedones (ie, blackheads) on the forehead (arrows).

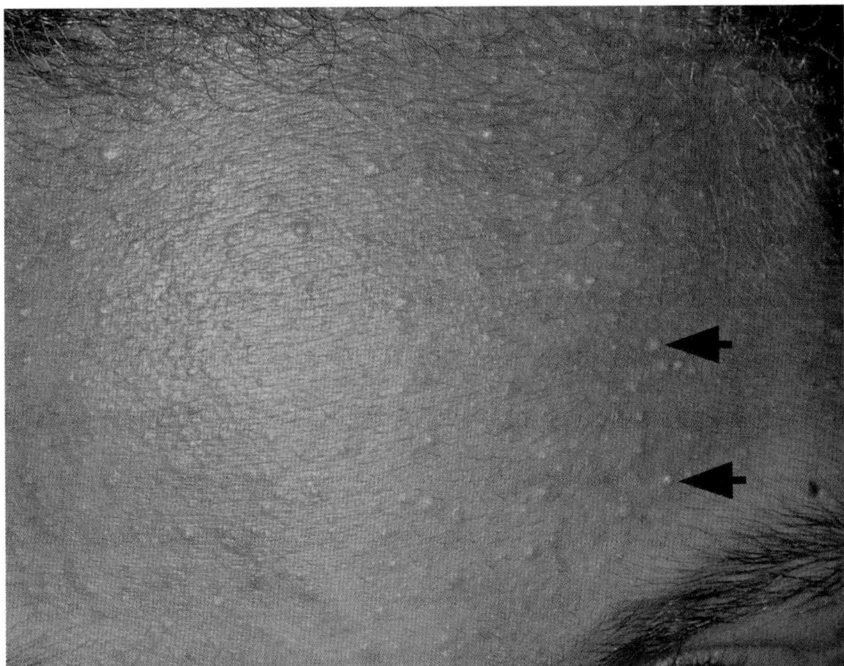

Figure 7.2. Closed comedones are small white or flesh-colored papules without surrounding erythema (arrows). This patient has mild acne.

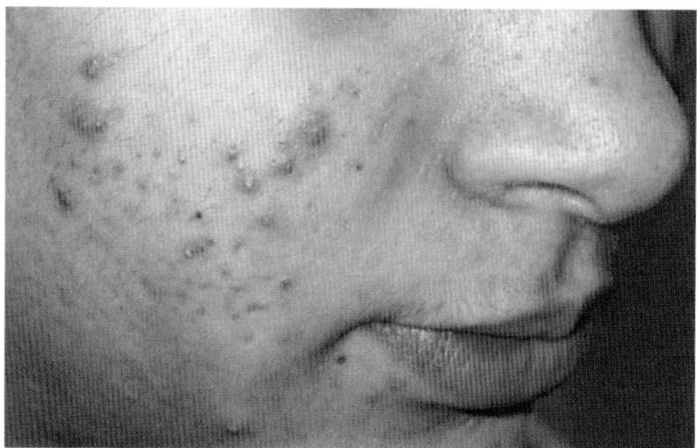

Figure 7.3. Inflammatory lesions are erythematous papules, pustules, or nodules. This patient has moderate acne. Note some mild early scarring.

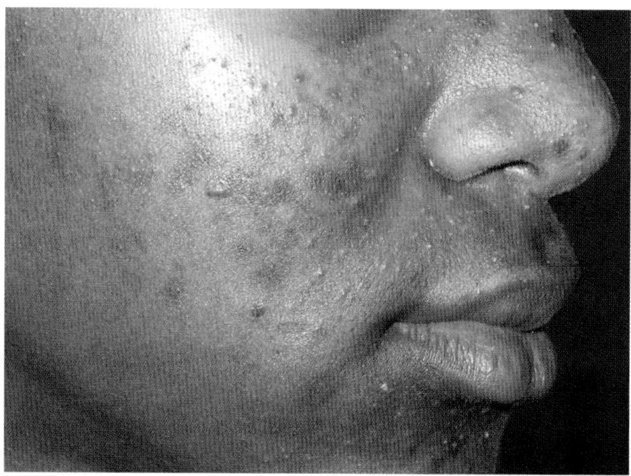

Figure 7.4. Patient with moderate acne. As inflammatory lesions resolve, areas of hyperpigmentation persist.

Look-alikes

In each of the conditions listed herein, comedones are absent.

Disorder	Differentiating Features
Acne rosacea	• Flushing and telangiectasias
Angiofibromas (ie, adenoma sebaceum)	• Appears during childhood (earlier than acne) • Favors nose and medial cheeks • Associated with tuberous sclerosis or multiple endocrine neoplasia type 1
Flat warts	• Flesh-colored to tan papules or small, thin plaques
Gram-negative folliculitis	• Sudden worsening of acne in patient receiving long-term antibiotic treatment for acne vulgaris
Keratosis pilaris	• Presents during infancy or early childhood. • Presence of a central keratin plug differentiates keratosis pilaris from acne. • Favors lateral cheeks (rather than T-zone) and may also be present on the extensor upper arms, dorsal thighs.
Miliaria rubra	• Erythematous, small papules often in occluded areas (eg, skinfolds) • Resolves rapidly
Molluscum contagiosum	• Translucent papules, often with central umbilication
Periorificial dermatitis	• Concentrated around mouth, nares, or, less commonly, eyes • Often (but not always) history of preceding use of topical corticosteroids
Pityrosporum folliculitis	• Typically spares the face. • Potassium hydroxide preparation performed on pustule roof will demonstrate budding yeast.
Steroid acne	• Lesions have monomorphous appearance (ie, only papules without comedones). • Temporal relationship between onset or worsening of acne and corticosteroid therapy.

How to Make the Diagnosis

- The clinical diagnosis of acne vulgaris is usually straightforward.

Treatment

(Options for acne treatment based on lesion type and disease severity are summarized in Figures 7.5 through 7.7.)

- Adolescents are anxious for improvement in their acne, but 4 to 6 weeks or longer may be required to observe a benefit from treatment.
- Acne treatment is facilitated by optimizing skin care and appropriate pharmacologic intervention tailored to the lesion type and severity of disease.
  - Drying of the skin by therapeutic cleansers (eg, those containing salicylic acid) may be aggravated by prescription acne medications containing a retinoid (tretinoin, adapalene, tazarotene), benzoyl peroxide, and some antibiotic formulations. If these prescription products will be used, a mild cleanser should be recommended.
  - For those who develop dryness when using acne medications, judicious application of a noncomedogenic moisturizer may be useful.

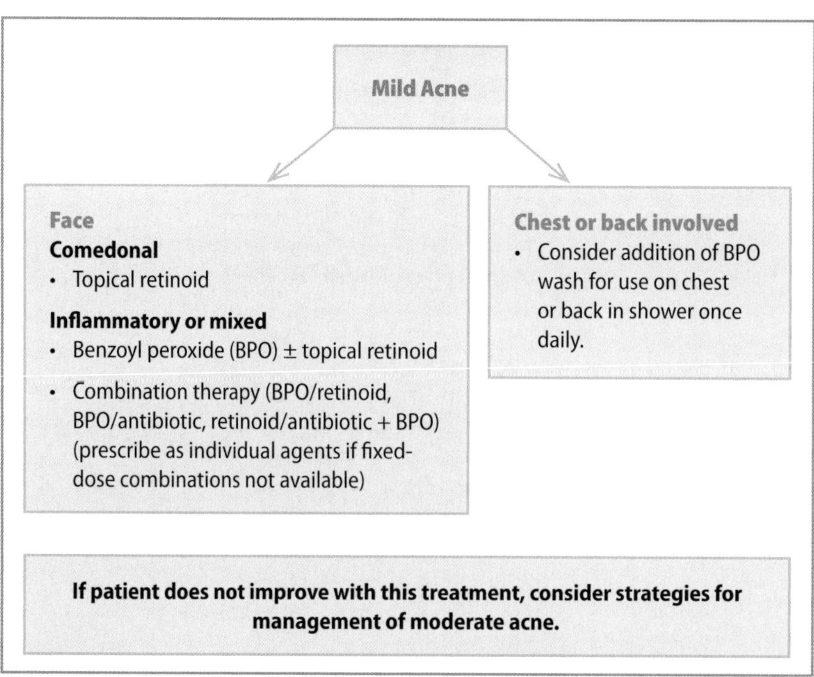

Figure 7.5. Treatment options for mild acne based on lesion type.

Moderate Acne

Only face involved

- Combination therapy (benzoyl peroxide [BPO]/retinoid, BPO/antibiotic + retinoid, retinoid/antibiotic + BPO) (prescribe as individual agents if fixed-dose combinations not available).
- Consider oral antibiotic (doxycycline or minocycline 50–100 mg twice a day) along with topical regimen if inflammatory lesions are numerous.

Face and chest or back involved

- Oral antibiotic plus topical regimen (See box at left.)
- BPO wash for use on chest or back in shower

If patient does not improve with this treatment

- **Add oral antibiotic (if not already done) or try alternative antibiotic or dosing regimen.**
- **Consider hormonal therapy (eg, combined oral contraceptive) for females.**
- **Refer to dermatologist.**

Figure 7.6. Treatment options for moderate acne.

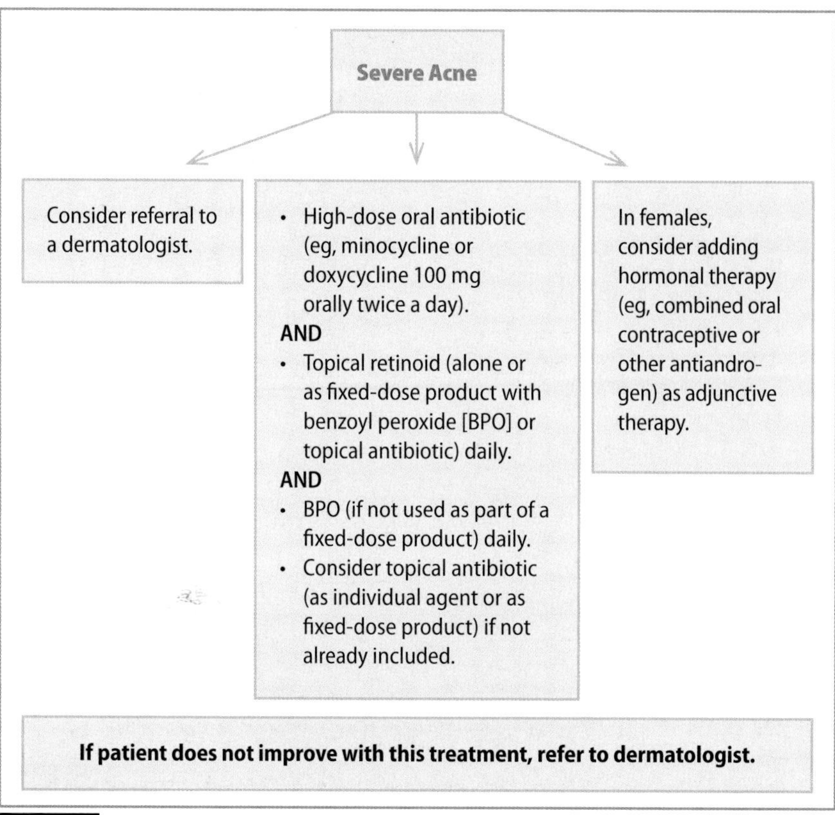

Figure 7.7. Treatment options for severe acne.

- Therapy falls into 4 categories.
  - Topical agents: retinoids, benzoyl peroxide, antibiotics, and fixed-dose combination products (Table 7.1), which combine 2 of these agents
  - Oral antibiotics: minocycline, doxycycline, tetracycline, erythromycin (latter 2 used less often in the current era); occasionally others
  - Hormonal therapy: oral contraceptives, antiandrogens such as spironolactone
  - Isotretinoin

Table 7.1. Topical Retinoids and Fixed-Dose Combination Products for Acne

Product Type/Active Ingredients	Recommended Dosing
Retinoids[a]	
Adapalene 0.1% cream, gel, lotion/0.3% gel	Daily at bedtime
Tretinoin 0.025% cream, gel/0.01% gel/0.04%, 0.1% micro-gel/ 0.05% cream, gel/0.1% cream	Daily at bedtime
Tazarotene 0.05% cream, gel/0.1% cream, gel	Daily at bedtime
Antibiotic/BPO	
Clindamycin 1.2%/BPO 2.5% gel	Daily
Clindamycin 1.2%/BPO 3.75% gel	Daily
Clindamycin 1%/BPO 5% gel	Daily to twice daily
Erythromycin 3%/BPO 5% gel	Twice daily
Retinoid-containing	
Clindamycin 1.2%/Tretinoin 0.025% gel	Daily at bedtime
Adapalene 0.1%/BPO 2.5% gel	Daily

Abbreviation: BPO, benzoyl peroxide.
[a]If prescribing a retinoid, consider beginning with adapalene or tretinoin cream 0.025% to reduce the potential for drying or irritation.

- Treatment strategies are based on lesion type and severity of disease.
  - Mild acne (Face: approximately one-fourth of the face is involved; lesions are comedones or a mixture of comedones and few to several papules or pustules; no nodules or scarring.) (see Figure 7.2)
    - Topical retinoids or fixed-dose combination products containing a retinoid are ideal for comedonal and mild inflammatory acne, but correct use is essential to minimize problems of irritation. Benzoyl peroxide or fixed-dose combination products containing benzoyl peroxide are an alternative option.
    - Retinoid pearls
      - Apply to a dry face.
      - Apply no more than a pea-sized amount for the entire face.
        1. If the entire face is to be covered, advise the patient to divide the pea-sized aliquot and dab equal amounts on each side of the forehead, each cheek, nose, and chin and then to rub it into the skin.
        2. Apply to all areas, rather than spot therapy (remember that topical retinoids [and benzoyl peroxide] play a preventive as well as therapeutic role in acne).
      - Use a noncomedogenic moisturizer, if needed, to counteract extreme dryness associated with topical retinoid therapy.

- Moderate acne (Face: approximately one-half of the face is involved; there are several to many papules or pustules and a few to several nodules; a few scars may be present.) (see Figures 7.3 and 7.4)
  - The initial combination of a retinoid, benzoyl peroxide, and an antibiotic is recommended for the synergy of addressing different aspects of disease pathogenesis. Retinoids are comedolytic and prevent comedogenesis, antibiotics decrease *P acnes* and reduce inflammation, and benzoyl peroxide—a nonantibiotic antimicrobial—lowers the likelihood of developing antibiotic-resistant *P acnes*. The ultimate choice of products depends on disease severity, likelihood of patient adherence (fixed-dose combination products may increase adherence), and medication cost/access (branded fixed-dose combination products are more expensive).
  - Examples of effective topical therapy for moderate acne include
    - Fixed-dose topical combination product containing a retinoid and an antibiotic, along with benzoyl peroxide (in the form of a wash or leave-on product)
    - Fixed-dose topical combination product containing benzoyl peroxide and an antibiotic, along with a topical retinoid
    - Topical retinoid, antibiotic, and benzoyl peroxide prescribed as individual agents
  - Oral antibiotics should be added if significant numbers of inflammatory lesions are present or the chest and back are significantly involved. Again, concomitant use of benzoyl peroxide is recommended because it appears to decrease the risk of developing antibiotic resistance. Systemic antibiotics are not recommended as monotherapy for acne. The duration of oral antibiotic use should be as short as feasible, with consideration for discontinuation at 3- to 6-month intervals.
  - Female patients who have significant inflammatory acne, particularly those who have premenstrual or menstrual flares, may benefit from hormonal intervention, such as a combined oral contraceptive or spironolactone.
- Severe acne (Face: approximately three-fourths or more of the face is involved; there are many papules, pustules, cysts, and nodules; scarring often is present.) (Figure 7.8)
  - Nodulocystic acne or the presence of scarring warrants prompt consideration for isotretinoin therapy (with referral to a dermatologist).
  - High-dose oral antibiotics in combination with topical therapy (eg, benzoyl peroxide and topical retinoid) is an option while considering isotretinoin.

- In female patients, hormonal or antiandrogen therapies can also be considered; however, if they fail and the patient continues to have nodulocystic or scarring lesions, isotretinoin should be strongly considered.

- Topical retinoids or the combination of topical retinoids and benzoyl peroxide is recommended as maintenance therapy to minimize the likelihood of relapse.

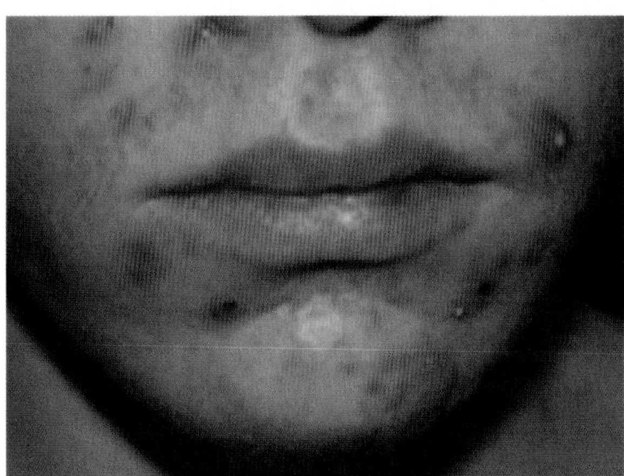

Figure 7.8. In severe acne, nodules and scarring are present.

Prognosis

- Acne vulgaris is often, but not always, self-limited and resolves by the late teenage or early adult years.
- Treatment is warranted during periods of disease activity to alleviate disfigurement, enhance well-being, and prevent permanent scarring.
- Management can be challenging because patient expectations are high, efficacy of treatment is variable, and potential medication side effects need to be weighed against benefits, with appropriate matching of therapeutic aggressiveness and severity of disease.
- Patients require periodic clinical assessments to evaluate response to therapy and provide ongoing support and encouragement.

When to Worry or Refer

- Failure to respond to topical or oral therapies after 2 to 3 months of appropriate use.
- Severe acne with presence of nodules, cysts, or scarring.
- Early-onset acne at younger than 7 years (or other signs of androgen excess) warrants hormonal evaluation.

Resources for Families

- American Academy of Pediatrics: HealthyChildren.org.
  www.HealthyChildren.org/acne
- American Academy of Dermatology: Acne.
  https://www.aad.org/public/diseases/acne-and-rosacea/acne
- MedlinePlus: Information for patients and families (in English and Spanish) sponsored by the National Library of Medicine and National Institutes of Health.
  https://www.nlm.nih.gov/medlineplus/acne.html
- Society for Pediatric Dermatology: Patient handout on acne.
  http://pedsderm.net/for-patients-families/patient-handouts
- Society for Pediatric Dermatology: Patient handout on isotretinoin.
  http://pedsderm.net/for-patients-families/patient-handouts
- WebMD: Information for families is contained in Health A-Z topics.
  www.webmd.com/skin-problems-and-treatments/acne/default.htm

CHAPTER
8

Neonatal and Infantile Acne

Introduction/Etiology/Epidemiology

Neonatal Acne

- Neonatal acne may present at birth but more commonly appears during the first few weeks of life.
- There are likely several etiologies for acneiform eruptions in neonates, including maternal and fetal androgens and, in patients with markedly pustular lesions, a hypersensitivity response to resident yeast (eg, *Malassezia* species).
- The term *neonatal cephalic pustulosis* has been proposed to describe the more pustular presentation (Figure 8.1).

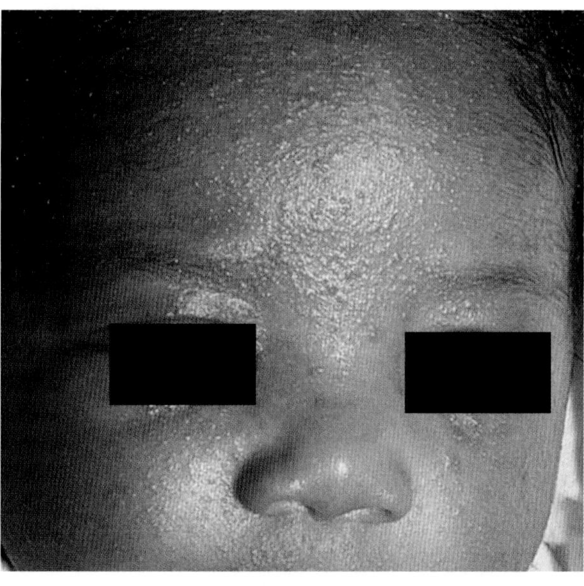

Figure 8.1. Erythematous papules and pustules distributed widely on the face and scalp in neonatal cephalic pustulosis, often considered a variant of neonatal acne.

Infantile Acne

- Later onset than neonatal acne, usually after 4 to 6 weeks of age
- Considered to be androgen-driven with associated sebaceous gland hyperactivity
- Spontaneously resolves between 6 and 12 months in most patients
- Occasionally more persistent or more severe with the potential for scarring

Signs and Symptoms

Neonatal Acne

- Inflammatory, erythematous papules and pustules (Figure 8.2)
- Primarily on the cheeks but also scattered on the entire face, extending into the scalp (see Figure 8.1)
- Comedones typically absent; truncal involvement rare

Infantile Acne

- Full range of typical acneiform lesions may be seen: papules, pustules, open and closed comedones, and occasionally nodules (Figure 8.3).
- Occurs primarily on the face.
- Scarring may be present.

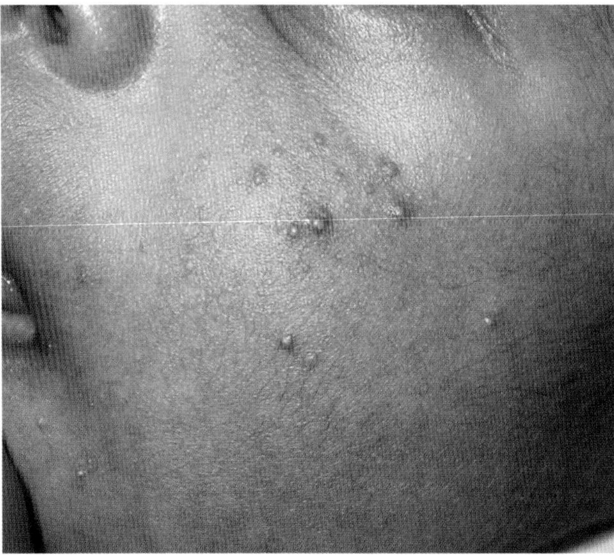

Figure 8.2. Papules and pustules on the cheek of an infant who has neonatal acne; comedones are absent.

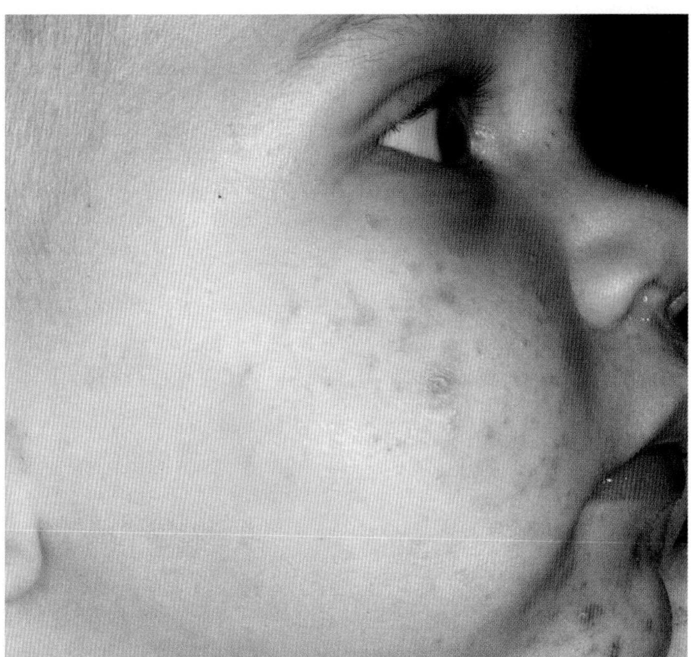

Figure 8.3. Erythematous papules and pustules on the cheek in infantile acne.

Look-alikes

Disorder	Differentiating Features
Neonatal Acne	
Miliaria rubra or pustulosa	• Erythematous papules (miliaria rubra) or pustules (miliaria pustulosa); may be difficult to differentiate from neonatal acne • Often in areas of occlusion (eg, skinfolds) or those covered by clothing
Milia	• White papules without surrounding erythema
Sebaceous hyperplasia	• Yellow (not erythematous) papules, typically on the nose
Seborrheic dermatitis	• Erythematous, scaling patches (typically lacks discrete papules)
Infantile Acne	
Lesions that may mimic infantile acne include all of those listed for neonatal acne. The presence of typical acne lesions, especially comedones, helps confirm the diagnosis.	
Keratosis pilaris	• Inflammatory type may mimic acne lesions. • Papules have central keratotic plug. • Typically limited to lateral cheeks. • Other atopic history may be present.

Treatment

Neonatal Acne

- Neonatal acne spontaneously resolves without treatment; watchful waiting with reassurance is appropriate.
- If treatment is requested, 2.5% benzoyl peroxide, 2% erythromycin solution or gel, or 1% clindamycin lotion can be applied sparingly on a nightly to every other night basis until resolution is noted. Alternatively, 2% ketoconazole cream may be used if neonatal cephalic pustulosis is suspected.

Infantile Acne

- More severe or persistent infantile acne may lead to scarring, and treatment is often indicated.
- Topical 2.5% benzoyl peroxide, topical 2% erythromycin solution or gel, or topical 1% clindamycin lotion may be useful for inflammatory papules and pustules. (These may be applied once or twice daily as tolerated.)
- Topical retinoids (eg, tretinoin 0.025% cream, adapalene 0.1% cream) may be helpful for comedones as well as inflammatory lesions, but side effects of erythema and irritation can be problematic in some patients. Begin topical retinoid with application every second or third night, progressing to nightly application, if tolerated, over 2 to 3 weeks.
- More severe variants of infantile acne may require oral erythromycin.
- In rare cases of severe nodulocystic disease in infants, isotretinoin has been used safely and successfully; such patients merit referral to a pediatric dermatologist.

Prognosis

- Neonatal acne is a self-limited disorder with no long-term sequelae.
- Infantile acne is typically self-limited, but more persistent or severe disease may result in long-term scarring.
- The relationship of severe infantile acne to later risk of acne vulgaris is unclear, but some investigators believe it is a risk factor for more significant adolescent and adult acne.

When to Worry or Refer

- Unusually severe neonatal or infantile acne.
- Severe or unresponsive disease may require endocrine testing to assess for excess androgens.

Resources for Families

- American Academy of Pediatrics: HealthyChildren.org. **www.HealthyChildren.org/infantrashes**

Periorificial Dermatitis

Introduction/Etiology/Epidemiology

- Periorificial dermatitis is an acneiform disorder of facial skin commonly seen in older teenagers and young adult women but also in younger children (Figure 9.1).
- The "adult" or "classic" presentation is best characterized as an acne variant in a spectrum between acne vulgaris and acne rosacea, displaying a combination of acneiform papules/pustules along with varying degrees of erythema.
- A granulomatous juvenile variant of "classic" periorificial dermatitis exists. It is sometimes referred to as granulomatous periorificial dermatitis.
- The cause is unknown, but it has been associated with chronic application of topical corticosteroids, as well as bubble gum, oils, greases, and toothpastes.
- Boys and girls are equally affected; it is more common in African American children.

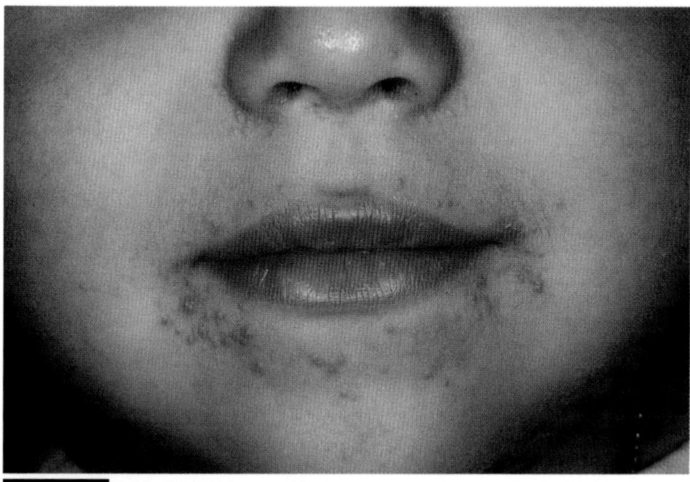

Figure 9.1. Periorificial dermatitis.

Signs and Symptoms

- Flesh-colored to red, monomorphous papules and papulopustules on a red background, distributed around the mouth, with a narrow zone of sparing around the vermillion border (see Figure 9.1).
- Scaling is commonly present.
- Other periorificial areas are commonly affected, including the perinasal and periorbital regions.
- The granulomatous variant presents in a similar fashion but with prominence of translucent, pink papules (Figure 9.2) and often a history of prior corticosteroid application.

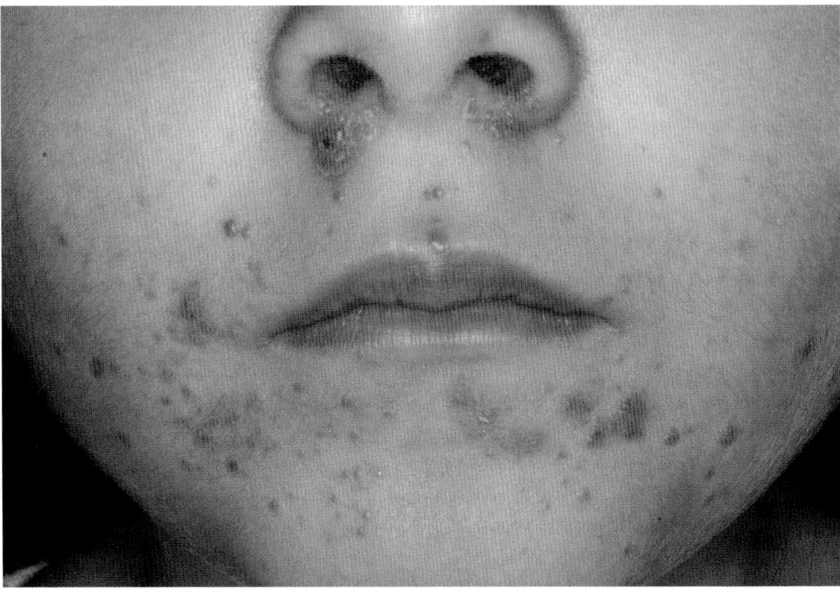

Figure 9.2. Granulomatous periorificial dermatitis. Translucent pink papules and pustules in the perioral and perinasal locations in a young girl who was initially treated with topical corticosteroids.

Look-alikes

Disorder	Differentiating Features
Atopic dermatitis	• Less papular • Other areas of body usually affected
Acne vulgaris	• Distribution of early lesions more commonly in the T-zone (forehead, nose, and chin). • Comedones present. • Onset rarely occurs between 1 and 7 years of age.
Allergic contact dermatitis	• Less papular. • History of exposure to antigen may be present. • Pruritus usually present.
Irritant contact dermatitis (eg, caused by lip licking or pacifier)	• Less papular. • History of lip licking or pacifier use present. • Involved areas often have sharp geometric borders.
Flat warts	• Small, flesh-colored to tan, flat-topped papules and plaques. • Erythema absent. • May be present elsewhere. • Koebnerization (distribution of lesions in a linear fashion following skin trauma or scratching) may be evident.
Sarcoidosis	• When limited to face, may be difficult to distinguish from periorificial dermatitis • Papules often red-brown in color • Often in other locations (eg, neck, upper trunk, extremities)
Benign cephalic histiocytosis	• Usually occurs in children 3 years or younger. • Papules may be erythematous, but often yellow-brown, and may simulate flat warts.

How to Make the Diagnosis

- The diagnosis is made clinically based on lesion morphology and characteristic distribution.
- Skin biopsy may be useful in questionable cases but is rarely necessary.

Treatment

- Mild cases: topical antibiotics, most commonly metronidazole or erythromycin, applied once to twice daily; topical sulfacetamide with or without sulfur may also be useful.
- Severe cases: oral antibiotic therapy (eg, with erythromycin; in patients >8 years, doxycycline or minocycline).
- Topical corticosteroids lead to initial improvement, but rapid flaring is seen on their discontinuation. If the patient has been treated with these agents, gradually taper the potency of the agent over 2 to 4 weeks or consider use of a topical calcineurin inhibitor such as pimecrolimus cream while concurrently initiating appropriate therapy as outlined previously.

Prognosis

- The condition improves slowly (often requires 4–12 weeks) but steadily with appropriate therapy.
- Treatments should be used until clearing has occurred, with gradual tapering to prevent rebound.
- Postinflammatory hyperpigmentation or hypopigmentation may be seen and generally resolves over several months.

When to Worry or Refer

- Consider referral if the diagnosis is in question or the patient has not responded to appropriate therapy.

Resources for Families

- WebMD: Information for families is contained in Health A-Z topics. **www.webmd.com/skin-problems-and-treatments/perioral-dermatitis**

Skin Infections

Localized Viral Infections

Herpes Simplex

Introduction/Etiology/Epidemiology

- Herpes simplex virus (HSV) 1 and HSV-2 are 2 members of the *Herpesviridae* family of viruses that also includes varicella-zoster virus (VZV), Epstein-Barr virus, cytomegalovirus, and human herpesviruses 6, 7, and 8.
- Primary HSV infection is generally a childhood disease involving the mouth (herpetic gingivostomatitis), lips, or eyes.
  - Serologic evidence of HSV-1 infection increases steadily with age, and 18% to 35% of children are estimated to have infection by 5 years of age.
  - In many cases, acquisition of infection is asymptomatic.
  - If acquisition of infection is accompanied by clinical disease, it is characterized as primary clinical disease. Such syndromes (eg, primary HSV gingivostomatitis) are typically moderate to severe illnesses accompanied by fever, lymphadenopathy, constitutional symptoms, and more severe or prolonged cutaneous or mucocutaneous disease.
- HSV infections are characterized by the phenomenon of latency. Following initial infection, individuals are prone to subsequent recurrences of localized cutaneous disease at the site of initial infection resulting from reactivation of latent virus in regional sensory or autonomic nerve ganglia. Recurrent HSV is generally a more limited clinical syndrome than primary HSV.
- Asymptomatic acquisition of primary HSV infection may subsequently lead to clinically recognized disease, often with features of recurrent HSV (ie, milder disease).
- HSV infections are typically transmitted by direct contact with skin lesions or infectious mucous membrane secretions.

- HSV-2 infection is most commonly acquired by sexual contact; however, HSV-1 prevalence in genital infections has been increasing.
    - Genital HSV-2 infection in prepubertal children should raise suspicion of child abuse.
    - HSV-2 is the most common cause of neonatal HSV infection, which occurs in as many as 1 per 3,000 deliveries in the United States.
- Neonatal HSV (Figure 10.1) most commonly occurs as a result of transmission during passage through the birth canal, less often via ascending infection, and is usually associated with premature rupture of membranes. It rarely follows postnatal transmission from a caregiver.
    - Infants born to mothers who have a primary genital infection are at the highest risk (25%–60%) of becoming infected.
    - Risk of transmission to newborns by mothers shedding HSV as the result of a reactivated infection is significantly lower (2%).
    - Approximately two-thirds of neonates with disseminated or central nervous system disease have skin lesions, but these lesions may not be present at onset of symptoms.

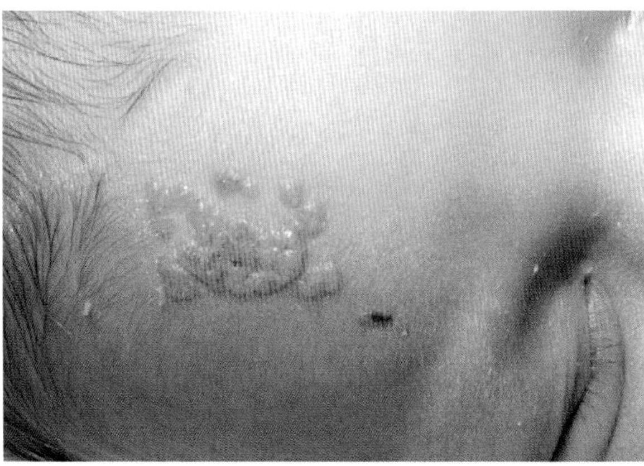

Figure 10.1. Clustered vesicles on an erythematous base in an infant with neonatal herpes simplex virus infection.

Signs and Symptoms

- Grouped 1- to 2-mm vesicles on an erythematous base are the classic lesions of HSV skin infection (see Figure 10.1).
- Skin vesicles evolve to form pustules, erosions, and crusts.
- Mucosal vesicles in areas of friction (eg, mouth, vulvovaginal, anorectal) are rapidly unroofed and form small ulcers.
- Coalescent vesicles or erosions may appear as larger bullae or superficial ulcerations.
- Lesions may occur on any cutaneous or mucocutaneous site but are most common on the face.
- Distinctive regional distributions of HSV infection are recognized as the following clinical syndromes:
    - Primary HSV gingivostomatitis: Affected children develop fever and ulcers on the buccal mucosae, tongue, gingivae, and perioral skin (Figure 10.2).
    - Herpes labialis ("cold sore"): Lesions occur on the lips, most often at the vermilion border; most common type of recurrent herpes infections overall (Figure 10.3).
    - Herpetic whitlow: primary or recurrent HSV infection of a finger (Figure 10.4).
    - Genital HSV infection.
    - Ocular HSV infection.
    - Eczema herpeticum: widespread HSV infection in an individual with preexisting generalized skin disease, most often atopic dermatitis (Figure 10.5).
    - Traumatic HSV infection (eg, herpes gladiatorum, herpetic whitlow).
    - Zosteriform herpes simplex: manifest as "recurrent shingles."
- Skin lesions are sometimes pruritic but typically painful. Primary infection syndromes may have severe pain.
- Regional lymphadenopathy is common, particularly with primary HSV infection.
- Recurrent HSV infection is often preceded by a characteristic brief prodrome of itching or dysesthesia at the site of impending recurrence.

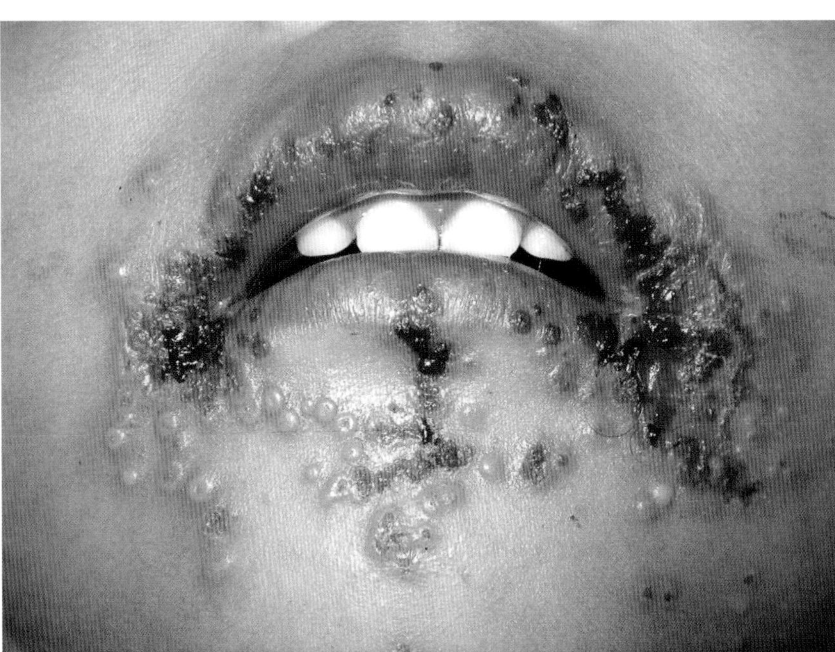

Figure 10.2. Vesicles and ulcers affecting the perioral skin are observed in herpes gingivostomatitis.

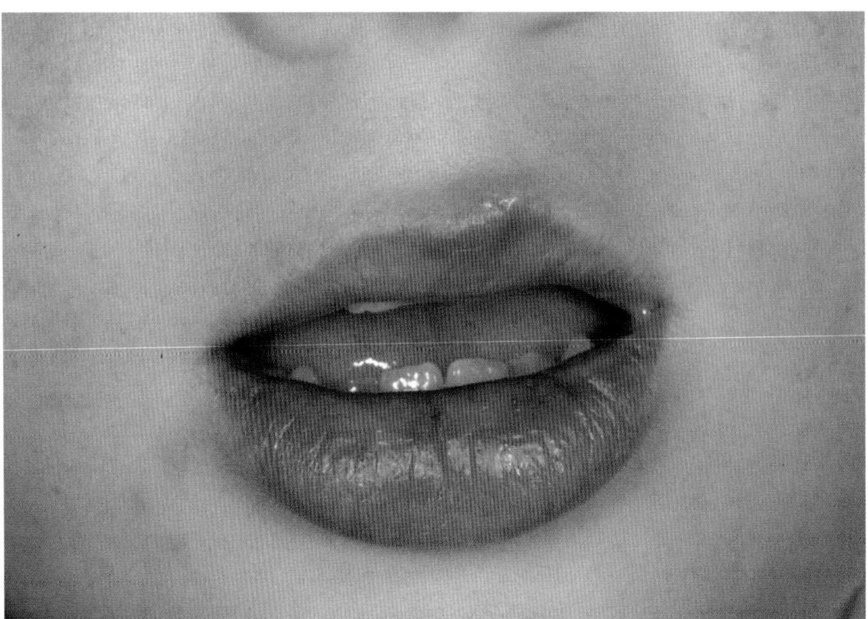

Figure 10.3. Herpes labialis ("cold sore"). Vesicles occur on the lips, most often at the vermilion border.

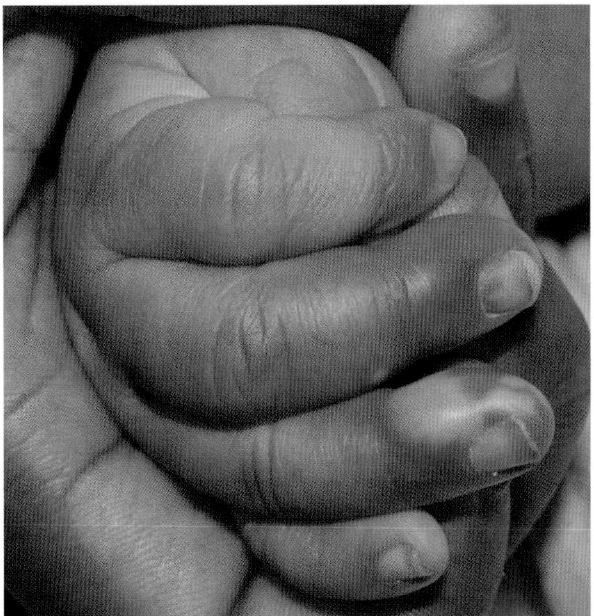

Figure 10.4. Vesicles located on the finger are characteristic of herpetic whitlow.

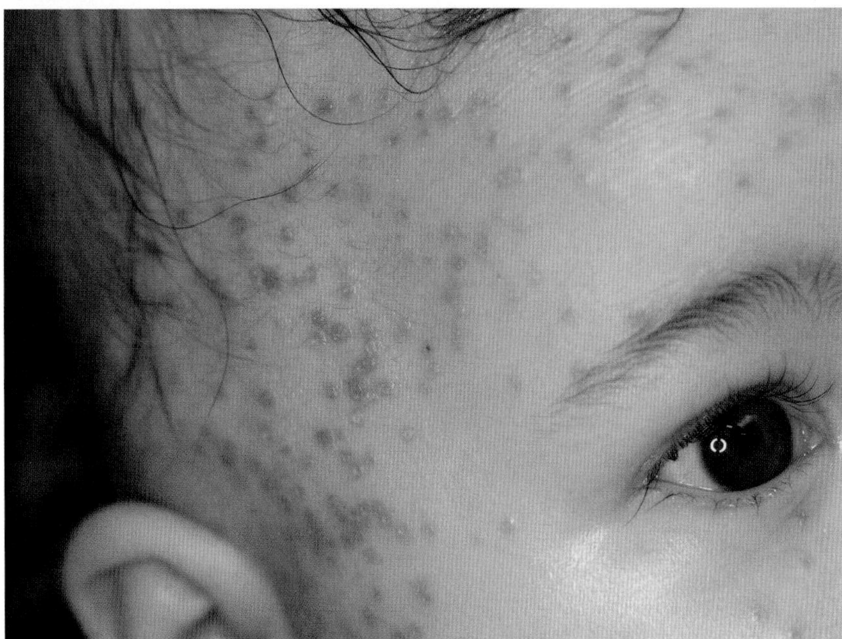

Figure 10.5. Eczema herpeticum is characterized by vesicles and monomorphous erosions with a "punched out" appearance, typically in areas of active dermatitis.

Look-alikes

Disorder	Differentiating Features
Herpes zoster	• Usually presents as multiple lesions in a dermatomal distribution (can be difficult to distinguish clinically from HSV infection if the dermatomal distribution is absent [ie, if there is only one group of vesicles])
Allergic contact dermatitis	• May appear in a linear distribution (if due to plants) • Pruritus a common feature
Hand-foot-and-mouth disease	• Individual (not grouped) vesicles. • Palm and sole involvement a prominent feature. • Vesicles often oval shaped. • With severe disease, larger bullae may be present. • In "eczema Coxsackium," lesions may predominate in areas prone to atopic dermatitis (ie, may simulate eczema herpeticum).
Herpangina	• Vesicles and erosions primarily involve the palate, uvula, and tonsillar pillars. • No involvement of surrounding perioral skin or lips.
Aphthous stomatitis (canker sores)	• Single or multiple (usually ≤3) discrete, shallow ulcers, 3–6 mm in size, affecting the oral mucosa. • Lesions have gray-white membrane and sharp, slightly raised, red borders.
Bullous impetigo	• Flaccid bullae or round, superficial erosions with a rim of surrounding scale • No deep-seated vesicles as seen in HSV infection
Blistering dactylitis	• May be difficult to distinguish clinically from herpetic whitlow • Solitary bulla, whereas the lesions of HSV infection often are smaller vesicles
Thermal burn	• May mimic herpetic whitlow, but history of injury usually is present.
Bullous mastocytoma	• Peau d'orange appearance of surface • History of localized blistering, which becomes less likely after infancy • Positive Darier sign (urtication following firm stroking of lesion)

How to Make the Diagnosis

- The diagnosis usually is made clinically based on the classic clinical morphology and distribution of lesions, especially when supported by history of recurrence.
- Laboratory investigations can be useful when the diagnosis is uncertain.
  - Viral culture is a reliable method for confirming the diagnosis and is considered the gold standard, although, in many settings, it has been replaced by polymerase chain reaction testing.
  - Polymerase chain reaction, when available, is a highly sensitive and specific diagnostic test.
  - Direct immunofluorescence examination of lesional swabs offers rapid diagnosis and can distinguish HSV and VZV infection with high sensitivity, but such testing may not be available in many office settings.
  - Serologic studies are less useful clinically.
  - Tzanck smear of a fresh vesicle can provide rapid information, but utility of the test is limited by experience/expertise of the clinician and hampered by suboptimal sensitivity and specificity (Figure 10.6). A positive Tzanck smear result cannot distinguish between HSV and VZV infection.

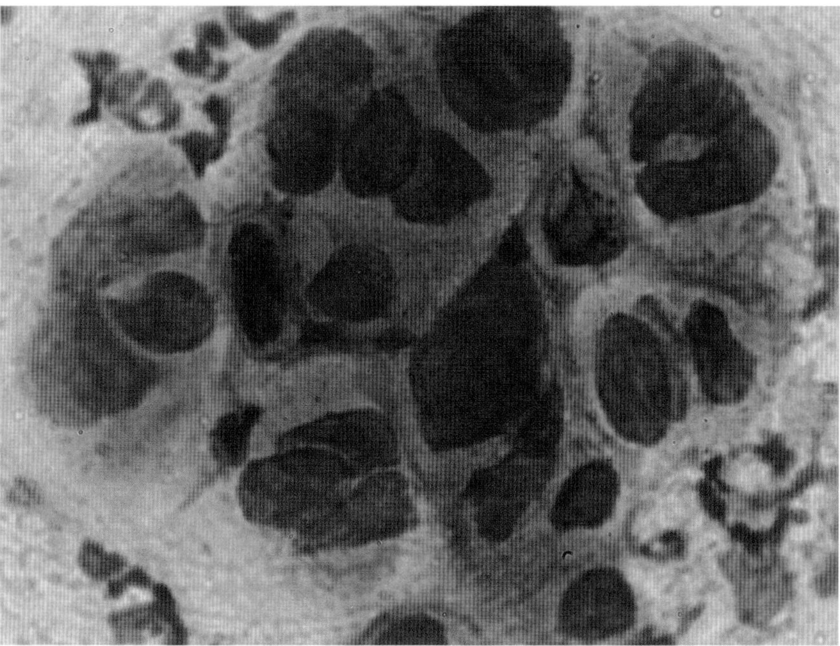

Figure 10.6. Tzanck smear in herpes simplex virus infection; multinucleated giant cells are present.

Treatment

- Supportive therapy suffices in most cases, using simple cleansing and comfort measures, astringent gels, soothing moisturizers, or topical antibiotic ointments (to prevent secondary bacterial infection).
- Oral analgesics (eg, viscous lidocaine solution, benzocaine lozenges, compounded mouthwashes) may be useful for associated pain.
- Oral antiviral therapy is indicated for severe disease, frequently recurrent disease, and individuals who are immunosuppressed. Oral acyclovir, valacyclovir, or famciclovir may be used. Treatment is more effective when started earlier (eg, in the first 48 hours) in the outbreak.
- Severe primary infections, infections in immunocompromised hosts, recurrences associated with erythema multiforme, and eczema herpeticum should be treated systemically (oral or intravenous, depending on severity and host risk factors); some of these patients may merit inpatient hospitalization.
- Neonatal HSV infection requires parenteral acyclovir therapy.
- The decision to treat less severe or recurrent outbreaks is based on the frequency and severity of the lesions and level of distress to the patient or family.
- Current treatment guidelines are summarized in the current edition of *Red Book: Report of the Committee on Infectious Diseases* (**www.aapredbook.org**).

Prognosis

- In most immunocompetent individuals, HSV infections beyond the neonatal period are mild and self-limited and have an excellent prognosis.
- Circumstances in which disease may be more severe and require more aggressive therapy are discussed in the next section.

When to Worry or Refer

- Infants 6 weeks or younger who have evidence of HSV infection should be evaluated immediately and treated with intravenous acyclovir. Consultation with a pediatric infectious disease specialist is desirable.
- Widespread lesions over eczematous skin (ie, eczema herpeticum) or infection in an immunocompromised child can be severe, often requiring hospitalization and treatment with intravenous acyclovir.

- Widespread oral lesions (ie, herpes gingivostomatitis) with resulting mouth pain and dehydration require hydration, antiviral therapy, and analgesia.
- Patients who develop erythema multiforme or Stevens-Johnson syndrome following HSV infection should be referred to a dermatologist and often require suppressive antiviral therapy in an effort to prevent recurrences.
- Involvement in or around the eye should be immediately evaluated by an ophthalmologist.
- Evidence of central nervous system involvement (eg, seizures, behavioral changes, lethargy).
- Sexual abuse should be suspected in children with anogenital herpes infection if there is no clear history of autoinoculation as the source of infection.

Resources for Families

- American Academy of Pediatrics: HealthyChildren.org.
www.HealthyChildren.org/coldsores
- American Academy of Dermatology: Herpes simplex.
https://www.aad.org/public/diseases/contagious-skin-diseases/herpes-simplex
- American Sexual Health Association: Nonprofit organization that provides information for patients in English and Spanish on sexually transmitted infections, including HSV infection. Web site provides links to support groups for those who have genital HSV infection.
www.ashasexualhealth.org/stdsstis/herpes
- MedlinePlus: Information for patients and families (in English and Spanish) sponsored by the National Library of Medicine and National Institutes of Health.
https://www.nlm.nih.gov/medlineplus/herpessimplex.html
- WebMD: Information for families is contained in the Health A-Z topics.
www.webmd.com/skin-problems-and-treatments/tc/cold-sores-topic-overview

Herpes Zoster

Introduction/Etiology/Epidemiology

- Herpes zoster (shingles) represents reactivation of latent varicella-zoster virus (VZV) infection in the sensory nerve root ganglia, which persists after preceding varicella infection (chickenpox).
- May occur at any age, but incidence increases with age.
- Incidence in children is low; higher risk of herpes zoster exists in young children whose mothers had varicella during pregnancy or who themselves had primary varicella early in life (ie, within the first year of life).
- Higher incidence in children with HIV infection, acute lymphocytic leukemia, or congenital (or other acquired) immunodeficiency disorders.
- May occur in children who have received past varicella vaccination but at lower rates than following wild-type primary VZV infection.
- Individuals who have active herpes zoster lesions may transmit VZV by direct contact to those without immunity. If infected, the nonimmune individual would develop varicella, not herpes zoster.

Signs and Symptoms

- Pain, itching, or paresthesia in a localized distribution may precede the skin eruption, but this is more common in adults than in children.
- Malaise, headache, and fever may precede or accompany the eruption, but mild itching is often the only associated symptom.
- The eruption is characteristically unilateral, following the distribution of 1 to 3 dermatomes (Figure 11.1).
- Thoracic dermatomes are most commonly involved in children, followed by the ophthalmic branch of the trigeminal nerve.

- Nasal tip involvement implies involvement in the nasociliary branch of the ophthalmic branch of the trigeminal nerve; this is a predictor of possible ocular disease (eg, keratitis, conjunctivitis, scleritis).
- Individual lesions may appear as grouped erythematous papules or circumscribed erythematous patches that evolve to discrete grouped vesicles on an erythematous base.
- Vesicles may become cloudy pustules before rupturing and forming crusts (analogous to the evolution observed in varicella and herpes simplex virus [HSV] infections).
- The entire process lasts from 1 to 3 weeks.
- Severe symptoms, extensive disease (beyond the primary dermatomes), and scarring may occur in immunosuppressed patients. Such individuals also are at risk for viral dissemination and visceral complications.
- Postherpetic neuralgia is uncommon in children and is usually limited to those who have had severe disease in the setting of immunosuppression.

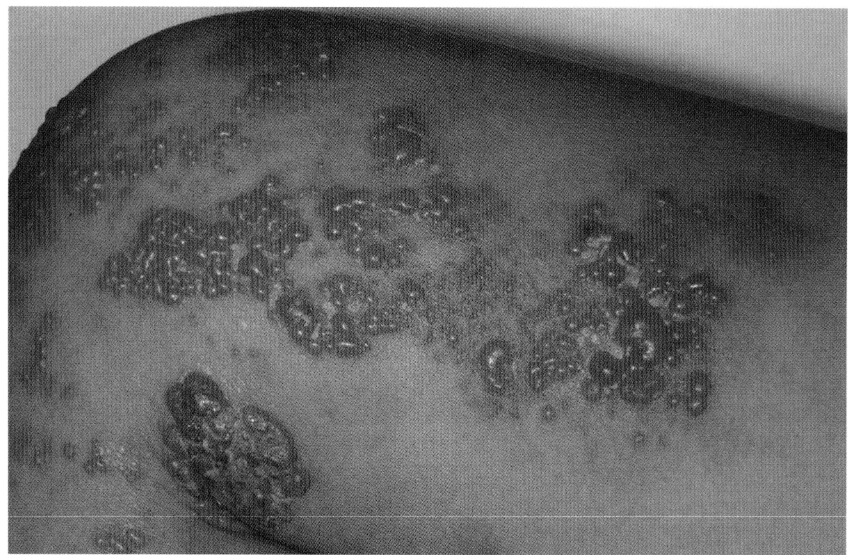

Figure 11.1. Herpes zoster is characterized by grouped vesicles in a dermatomal distribution.

Look-alikes

Disorder	Differentiating Features
Herpes simplex virus (HSV) infection	• Usually localized without dermatomal distribution. • Dermatomal HSV infection tends to be recurrent (but may otherwise be very difficult to distinguish clinically).
Allergic contact dermatitis	• Not usually dermatomal in distribution • Itch more prominent than pain

How to Make the Diagnosis

- Clinical appearance of lesions, dermatomal distribution, and history usually provide sufficient information for accurate diagnosis.
- Laboratory investigations can be useful when the diagnosis is uncertain.
  - Polymerase chain reaction, when available, is a specific, sensitive, and useful diagnostic tool.
  - Direct immunofluorescence of lesional swabs offers rapid diagnosis and can distinguish HSV and VZV infection with high sensitivity, but such testing may not be available in many office settings.
  - Viral culture from skin lesions can be performed but is limited by difficulty in isolating VZV in cell culture.
  - Serologic tests are of limited usefulness.
  - Tzanck smear of a fresh vesicle can provide rapid information, but utility of the test is limited by experience/expertise of the clinician and hampered by suboptimal sensitivity and specificity. A positive Tzanck smear result cannot distinguish between HSV and VZV infection.
- A history of "recurrent zoster" usually indicates the patient has HSV infection, not zoster.
- Attempts to elicit history of exposure to contact allergens, especially poison ivy, should be made to exclude the possibility of allergic contact dermatitis in patients in whom pruritus is the prominent symptom.

Treatment

- Specific therapy is unnecessary in children with mild symptoms and limited involvement.
- Topical antipruritics (menthol/camphor lotions) and oral antihistamines are useful for symptomatic relief of itching.
- Antiviral therapy with acyclovir (oral or intravenous) or other oral antiviral agents (eg, famciclovir, valacyclovir) should be considered in high-risk patients who have disease in proximity to the eye or are immunosuppressed or in any patient with more severe disease or significant symptoms.
- Aluminum acetate solution compresses may be soothing and help to speed drying and healing of blisters.

When to Worry or Refer

- Complicated infection in an immunocompromised patient may require hospitalization.
- Referral is indicated if the diagnosis is uncertain.
- An ophthalmologist should be consulted for zoster in the distribution of the ophthalmic branch (V1) of the trigeminal nerve or if nasal tip involvement is present.

Resources for Families

- American Academy of Dermatology: Shingles.
https://www.aad.org/public/diseases/contagious-skin-diseases/shingles
- Centers for Disease Control and Prevention: About shingles (herpes zoster).
www.cdc.gov/shingles/about/index.html
- MedlinePlus: Information for patients and families (in English and Spanish) sponsored by the National Library of Medicine and National Institutes of Health.
https://www.nlm.nih.gov/medlineplus/shingles.html
- WebMD: Information for families is contained in Health A-Z topics.
www.webmd.com/skin-problems-and-treatments/shingles/default.htm

CHAPTER 12

Molluscum Contagiosum

Introduction/Etiology/Epidemiology

- Discrete papular eruption
- Common in infants and children
- Caused by a poxvirus
- Usually not associated with sexual abuse or immunodeficiency in infants and children
- May occur as a sexually transmitted infection in sexually active adolescents and young adults

Signs and Symptoms

- Usually asymptomatic.
- Lesions are 1- to 6-mm, discrete, skin-colored, erythematous, or translucent (may mimic vesicles) papules; some lesions are umbilicated (ie, have a central dell or depression) (Figure 12.1).
- Widespread or sometimes "giant" (8–15 mm) lesions may occur in immunosuppressed individuals.
- Extensive lesions often are observed in children with atopic dermatitis.
- Can occur on any cutaneous location but commonly seen on face, eyelids, neck, chest, axillae, folds of extremities, and genital region.
- Eyelid lesions may be associated with chronic conjunctivitis or keratitis.
- May be associated with a mild to moderate dermatitis occurring in the vicinity of the papules, known as "molluscum dermatitis" (Figure 12.2).

- Linear arrangement of lesions may be present due to autoinoculation (Koebner phenomenon).
- Genital location most common when occurring as a sexually transmitted infection in sexually active adolescents or young adults but may also be seen in younger children.

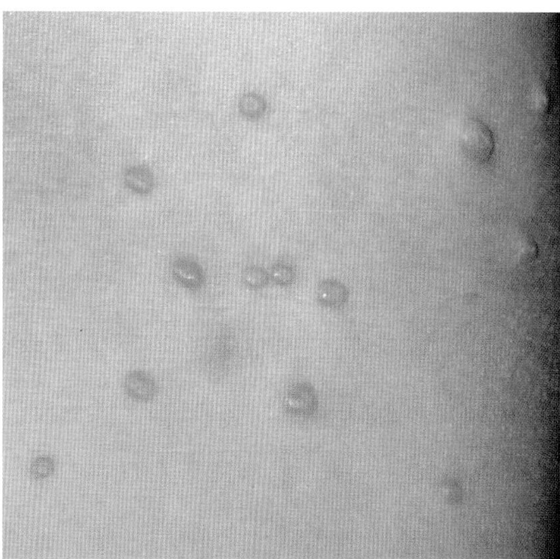

Figure 12.1. Somewhat erythematous, translucent papules are typical of molluscum contagiosum. Note umbilication (ie, central depression) of larger lesions.

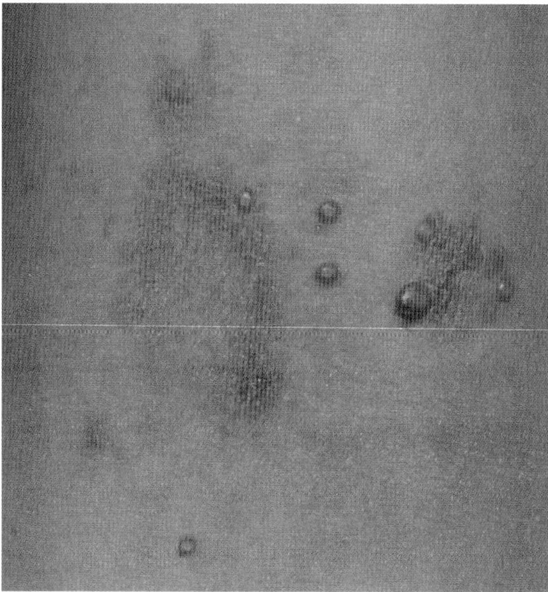

Figure 12.2. Molluscum dermatitis. Erythematous patches with scale surround lesions of molluscum contagiosum.

Look-alikes

Disorder	Differentiating Features
Milia	• Small white papules that lack central umbilication • Often limited to facial distribution
Closed comedones	• Small white papules that lack central umbilication • Occur in older children or adolescents (Molluscum contagiosum typically affects younger children.) • Most often limited to facial distribution
Flat warts	• Flat-topped papules or small thin plaques • Umbilication absent
Cryptococcosis	• Molluscum-like lesions possible in immunocompromised patients • Umbilication of papules usually not present • May have ulcers in addition to papules

How to Make the Diagnosis

- The diagnosis is made clinically based on the appearance of lesions.
- A skin scraping of a characteristic papule can be used for a "crush" preparation and stained with Giemsa or methylene blue, revealing numerous characteristic molluscum (Henderson-Patterson) bodies on direct microscopy; rarely necessary.
- Skin biopsy occasionally is used for large or atypical lesions.

Treatment

- Lesions often resolve spontaneously over several months or years. In one recent study, the mean time to resolution was 13 months.
- Watchful waiting is an acceptable management plan, although treatment is often requested by parents.
- Application of cantharidin (blister beetle extract) is a painless and effective procedure; however, it must be performed by an experienced clinician, it is an off-label therapy, and the agent is becoming more difficult to access in the United States.
- Curettage of individual lesions is effective, but limitations include pain, fear (in young children), and risks of spread and scarring.
- Lesions in close proximity to the eyelid margin, causing chronic conjunctivitis, may require surgical excision.

- Cryotherapy with liquid nitrogen also is effective but may be traumatic for young children in whom it is poorly tolerated.
- Imiquimod cream is another off-label option. Although applied 3 times weekly for genital condylomata, treatment of molluscum generally requires daily application and may require many weeks of application; irritant contact dermatitis is a common limiting side effect of this therapy.
- Topical retinoids (eg, tretinoin) have been used, mainly for facial lesions; mechanism of action is probably induction of irritant dermatitis, which may actually be a limiting side effect.
- Immunotherapy using intralesional injection of skin test antigens (most often *Candida*) may be effective, but published data are limited and the associated pain, anxiety, and need for repeated injections make this option less feasible for young children.

When to Worry or Refer

- When treatment is requested but is not available in your practice
- When diagnosis is uncertain
- When extensive disease is present
- When molluscum is associated with poorly controlled atopic dermatitis

Resources for Families

- American Academy of Pediatrics: HealthyChildren.org. **www.HealthyChildren.org/molluscumcontagiosum**
- American Academy of Dermatology: Molluscum contagiosum. **https://www.aad.org/public/diseases/contagious-skin-diseases/molluscum-contagiosum**
- Society for Pediatric Dermatology: Patient handout on molluscum. **http://pedsderm.net/for-patients-families/patient-handouts**
- WebMD: Information for families is contained in the Health A-Z topics. **www.webmd.com/skin-problems-and-treatments/molluscum-contagiosum**

CHAPTER 13

Warts

Introduction/Etiology/Epidemiology

- Epithelial growths are induced by different subtypes of human papillomavirus (HPV).
- Clinical wart subtypes correlate with different HPV subtypes.
- Very common in children.
- Most spontaneously resolve in 1 to 2 years.
- Often recalcitrant to multiple therapies.
- Transmission may occur person to person, from fomites, or from autoinoculation.
- Usually asymptomatic, but large or multiple plantar lesions may be associated with pain, limitation in activities.
- Can be disfiguring.
- In patients who have immunodeficiency (including HIV infection), lesions may be numerous and widespread.

Signs and Symptoms

- Common warts: discrete, skin-colored papules with characteristic rough (ie, verrucous) surface (Figure 13.1). Lesions exhibit tiny dark specks that represent thrombosed capillaries.
- Plantar warts: rough or smooth papules and plaques localized to the plantar feet, most often over weight-bearing surfaces. Lesions exhibit tiny dark specks that represent thrombosed capillaries.
- Flat warts: smooth, pink or skin-colored, flat-topped papules, 1 to 3 mm, typically seen on the face or legs, but may occur in other locations (Figure 13.2).
- Anogenital warts (ie, condylomata acuminata): discrete papules or confluent plaques; pink to red or skin-colored; localized to genitalia or adjacent skin of inguinal, thigh, suprapubic, or perianal areas (Figure 13.3).

- Periungual warts: often occur in association with common warts; present as papules, confluent plaques, or nodules adjacent to nails, occasionally with destructive involvement of the proximal or lateral nail fold areas. Lesions exhibit tiny dark specks that represent thrombosed capillaries.

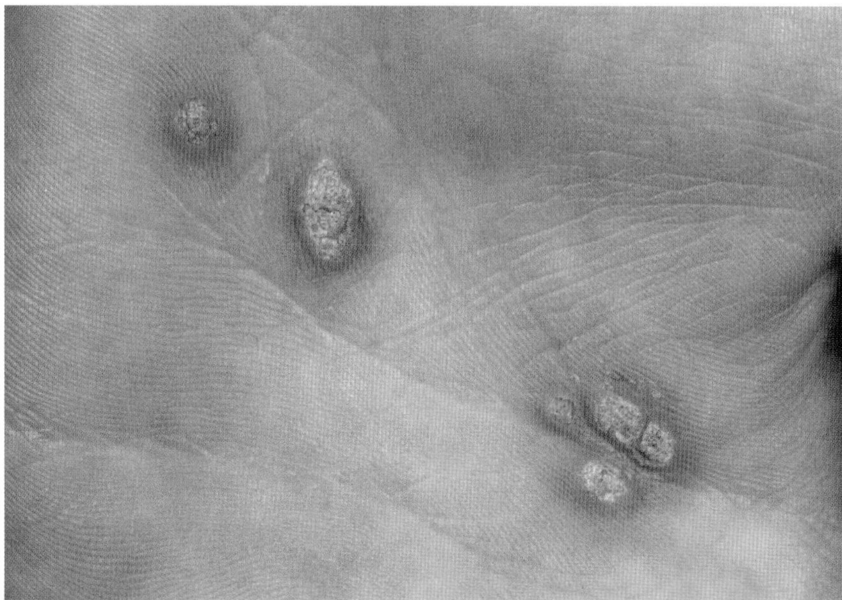

Figure 13.1. Common warts appear as rough (ie, verrucous) papules.

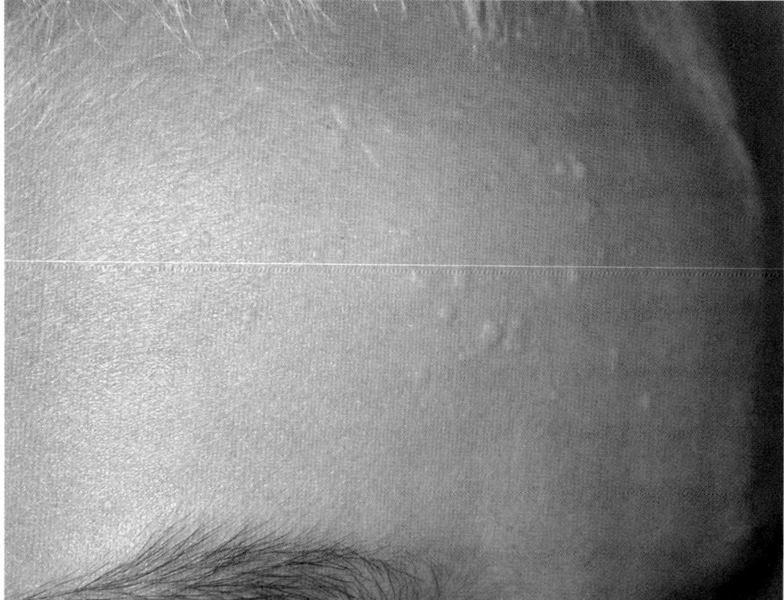

Figure 13.2. Flat warts are small, flat-topped papules.

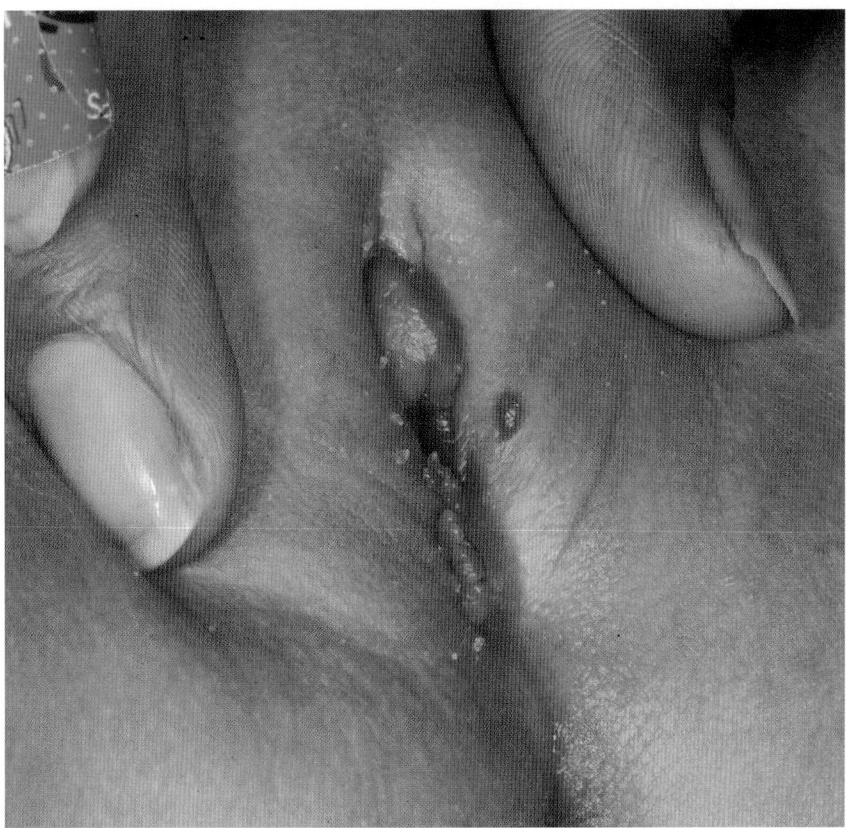

Figure 13.3. Condylomata acuminata appear as skin-colored papules and plaques.

Look-alikes

Disorder	Differentiating Features
Plantar Wart	
Callus	• Located over pressure points • Lacks black specks (ie, thrombosed capillaries) • Dermatoglyphics often preserved
Condylomata Acuminata	
Condylomata lata	• Appear as moist white plaques • Associated with secondary syphilis
Molluscum contagiosum	• White or translucent papules that may have central umbilication
Flat Warts	
Lichen planus	• Violaceous and may have Wickham striae (a lacy, white pattern) on surface. • White papules or lacy, white plaques may be present on the buccal mucosa.
Lichen nitidus	• White or skin-colored, tiny, flat-topped papules • Atopic history common
Molluscum contagiosum	• White or translucent papules that may have central umbilication
Benign cephalic histiocytosis	• May be difficult to differentiate from flat warts • Limited to face; rarely involves other skin surfaces
Common Warts	
Epidermal nevi	• Present since birth or shortly thereafter. • Linear or whorled distribution may be evident.
Granuloma annulare	• Papules or plaques that usually form rings • Rough (ie, verrucous) surface absent
Knuckle pads	• Plaques or papules overlying interphalangeal joints • Rough (ie, verrucous) surface absent

Treatment

- Warts are self-limited, usually asymptomatic, and do not necessarily require treatment. None of the current treatments are uniformly effective, and patients and parents should understand the potential limitations of therapy.
- The risk-benefit ratio of therapy must be considered, and care should be exercised to avoid overly painful or traumatic treatments in young children.
- First-line therapy is usually a topical salicylic acid plaster or liquid, with or without duct tape occlusion (Table 13.1).

Table 13.1. Optimizing Use of Over-the-Counter Salicylic Acid Therapy for Warts
Apply 17% salicylic acid liquid to wart(s). • May use a plaster impregnated with salicylic acid if desired. • May use a higher concentration of salicylic acid for management of warts on the plantar surface of the foot.
Air-dry for 2 to 3 minutes (develops into a white film).
Occlude surface of wart with duct tape or similar adhesive tape.
Remove tape in the morning.
If further debridement is necessary, file tissue down with an emery board.
Repeat nightly until wart is resolved.
Notes • This treatment is most effective for plantar warts. • Do not apply to facial, fold, or genital area warts. • If area becomes macerated or inflamed, withhold treatment for 1 to 3 nights, then resume. • May take up to 8 weeks to see wart resolution.

- A compounded cream of 5-fluorouracil and salicylic acid applied under tape occlusion nightly may be effective.
- Cryotherapy with spray or cotton swab application of liquid nitrogen or other cryogen is effective if used repeatedly (with treatments separated by 2–4 weeks) but should be reserved for motivated, older children who can tolerate painful procedures. In the interval between cryotherapy treatments, any remaining wart should be treated with salicylic acid as described previously.
- Topical imiquimod may be useful when applied daily to warts; however, its efficacy is often limited by the hyperkeratosis found in common warts, and irritant dermatitis may be seen with its use. Imiquimod is not US Food and Drug Administration (FDA) approved for treatment of common warts.
- Cimetidine (30–40 mg/kg per day orally divided twice a day or 3 times a day) for 6 to 8 weeks or more may be effective in some children; not FDA approved for this indication.
- Other treatment options include intralesional injection of skin test antigens (eg, *Candida, Trichophyton*), intralesional chemotherapy injections (eg, bleomycin), and topical immunotherapy with squaric acid; these are not FDA-approved therapies and published data are limited.
- Treatments such as pulsed-dye laser and surgical excision are occasionally considered but do not necessarily offer greater efficacy. Surgery entails a high risk of permanent scarring.

When to Worry or Refer

- Patients with symptomatic warts that have not responded to standard therapies should be referred for discussion of other treatment options.
- Immunosuppressed patients with multiple lesions merit more aggressive therapy given the potential association between warts and an increased risk of cutaneous malignancy.
- Anogenital warts in children may be a marker for sexual abuse, although autoinoculation, vertical transmission (a consideration primarily in children <3 years), and benign (nonsexual) modes of transmission are also possible. If the history or physical examination raises concern, referral and thorough investigation are vital.

Resources for Families

- American Academy of Pediatrics: HealthyChildren.org.
  www.HealthyChildren.org/warts
- American Academy of Dermatology: Warts.
  https://www.aad.org/public/diseases/contagious-skin-diseases/warts
- MedlinePlus: Information for patients and families (in English and Spanish) sponsored by the National Library of Medicine and National Institutes of Health.
  https://www.nlm.nih.gov/medlineplus/warts.html
- Society for Pediatric Dermatology: Patient handout on warts.
  http://pedsderm.net/for-patients-families/patient-handouts
- WebMD: Information for families is contained in the Health A-Z topics.
  www.webmd.com/skin-problems-and-treatments/guide/warts

Skin Infections

Systemic Viral Infections

CHAPTER 14

Erythema Infectiosum/ Human Parvovirus B19 Infection (Fifth Disease)

Introduction/Etiology/Epidemiology

- Caused by human parvovirus B19.
- Usually affects children between 4 and 10 years of age.
- Most common in the winter and spring with endemic peaks every 6 to 9 years.
- Transmission is via respiratory droplets or via blood and blood products.
- Incubation period is 4 to 14 days.
- Clearance of viremia precedes appearance of the erythema infectiosum rash by several days; thus, patients who have the skin eruption are not considered contagious.

Signs and Symptoms

- Up to 50% of infections may be subclinical.
- Classic finding is a "slapped-cheek" appearance of bright red patches or plaques on the cheeks (Figure 14.1).
- Facial rash may be preceded 1 to 2 weeks by a mild prodrome of low-grade fever, chills, malaise, myalgias, and pharyngitis, which occurs during the viremic phase.
- One to 4 days after the facial rash appears, the exanthem spreads to involve the trunk and extremities (especially the extensor surfaces).
- Over the next 1 to 4 weeks, erythematous patches, papules, and plaques tend to coalesce and then partially clear, leaving a characteristic lacy, reticular pattern of erythema, especially on the flexor surfaces of the arms (Figure 14.2).

- Pruritus is sometimes prominent.
- After the exanthem fades, it is commonly "reactivated" for several weeks to months by physical factors, including sunlight, physical activity, or hot baths.
- Arthralgia and arthritis may be the most common manifestation of parvovirus B19 infection in adolescents and adults, especially females, but occur rarely in younger children. The joint symptoms are typically brief in duration, affect large joints, and may be pauciarticular or polyarticular. Rarely, the arthralgia may persist for months or years.
- Human parvovirus B19 exhibits tropism for erythroid progenitor cells, and individuals with predisposing hematologic conditions resulting in a shortened red blood cell half-life (eg, sickle cell disease, spherocytosis, thalassemias) are at risk for aplastic crises. These crises occur before and in the early periods of the rash phase.
- Susceptible pregnant women who become infected during the first half of pregnancy with human parvovirus B19 may transmit the infection to their developing fetus, with risk of fetal anemia, nonimmune fetal hydrops, and fetal death in 2% to 6% of cases.

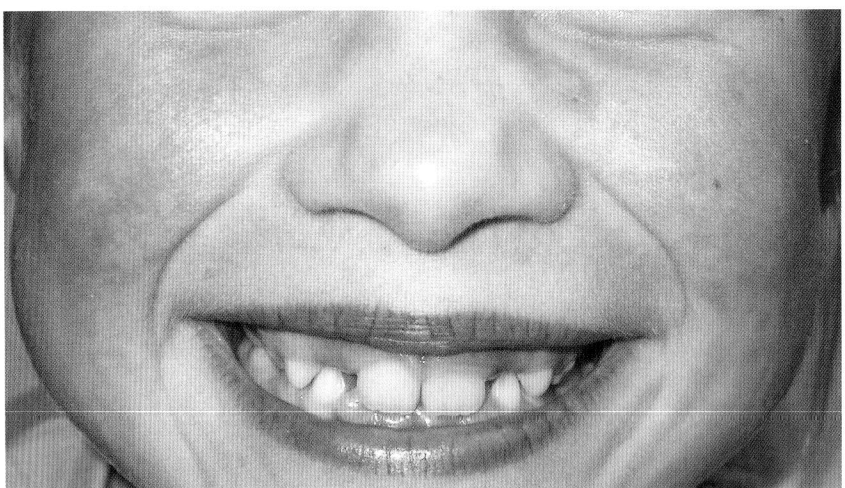

Figure 14.1. Patients who have erythema infectiosum exhibit erythematous cheeks (ie, a "slapped-cheek" appearance).

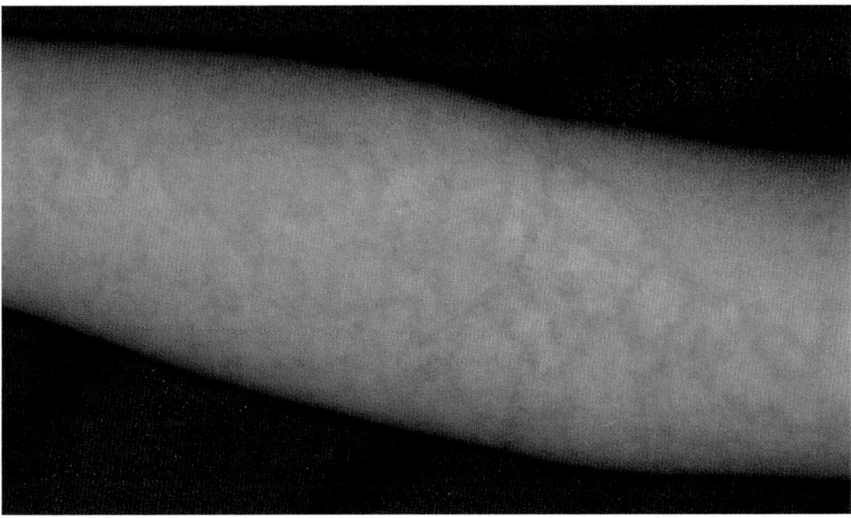

Figure 14.2. Erythema infectiosum produces a lacy, reticulated erythema on the extremities.

Look-alikes

Disorder	Differentiating Features
Exanthematous drug eruption	• History of drug exposure elicited • "Slapped-cheek" appearance absent
Nonspecific viral exanthem	• Fever or other symptoms may be present. • "Slapped-cheek" appearance absent.
Livedo reticularis	• Typically a long-standing finding, not acutely acquired • "Slapped-cheek" appearance absent
Exanthem of juvenile idiopathic arthritis	• Clinical features of juvenile idiopathic arthritis present • "Slapped-cheek" appearance absent • Exanthem most apparent during febrile periods
Scarlet fever	• Circumoral pallor may give "slapped-cheek" appearance. • Generalized, sandpaper-like eruption. • Pharyngitis and lymphadenopathy usually present.
Urticaria	• Acute onset of pruritic and edematous papules, plaques, wheals. • Distribution usually generalized. • Dermatographism may be present. • Lesions last less than 24 hours and "migrate" to other areas.

How to Make the Diagnosis

- The diagnosis is most often made clinically based on characteristic findings.
- Serologic detection of IgM directed against human parvovirus B19 can confirm the diagnosis when obtained within 30 days of the onset of the illness.

Treatment

- No specific treatment is indicated.
- Children with characteristic rash can return to school or child care, as they are no longer considered contagious.
- Nonsteroidal anti-inflammatory drugs may be used for arthritis.
- Hospitalization and red blood cell transfusion may be required in children with transient aplastic crises.

Prognosis

- Erythema infectiosum typically resolves without sequelae.
- Immunodeficient patients with parvovirus B19 infection may develop chronic bone marrow suppression, and intravenous Ig therapy has been used in this setting.
- Exposed pregnant women should be advised to contact their obstetric provider to discuss potential risks and be offered serologic testing. If acute infection is confirmed, serial fetal ultrasound should be considered to monitor for fetal hydrops, congestive heart failure, and intrauterine growth restriction.

When to Worry or Refer

- Referral may be indicated if atypical features are present or the diagnosis is in question.
- Pregnant women exposed to or infected with human parvovirus B19 should consult their obstetric provider (as discussed previously).

Resources for Families

- American Academy of Pediatrics: HealthyChildren.org.
www.HealthyChildren.org/FifthDisease
- Centers for Disease Control and Prevention: Alphabetical listing of diseases and conditions provides information for families in English or Spanish.
www.cdc.gov/parvovirusB19/index.html
- MedlinePlus: Information for patients and families (in English and Spanish) sponsored by the National Library of Medicine and National Institutes of Health.
https://www.nlm.nih.gov/medlineplus/fifthdisease.html

Gianotti-Crosti Syndrome

Introduction/Etiology/Epidemiology

- Also known as papular acrodermatitis of childhood and papulovesicular acrolocated syndrome
- Distinctive exanthem of childhood affecting extensor extremities, face, and buttocks
- Initially described in association with hepatitis B infection
- Subsequently demonstrated to also occur in response to a variety of viral infections
  - Epstein-Barr virus is probably the most common cause worldwide and in the United States.
  - Enteroviruses, hepatitis A, cytomegalovirus, adenovirus, rotavirus, parvovirus, human herpesvirus 6, rubella, and respiratory syncytial virus have all been implicated.

Signs and Symptoms

- Abrupt onset of symmetrically distributed, erythematous, or skin-colored papules.
- May be lichenoid (ie, flat-topped) or firm, dome-shaped edematous papules.
- Localized to face (Figure 15.1), extensor surfaces of the extremities (Figure 15.2), and buttocks (sparing the trunk); occasionally, lesions will be most prominent on the distal extremities and buttocks.
- Lesions range in size from 1 to 10 mm, but their size usually is consistent within an individual patient.
- Confluence of papules may lead to appearance of edematous plaques, especially on the elbows or knees.
- Pruritus is variable.

- Occasional mild constitutional symptoms and low-grade fever; lymphadenopathy common.
- Hepatomegaly and abnormal liver function studies may be present in hepatitis B–associated cases.

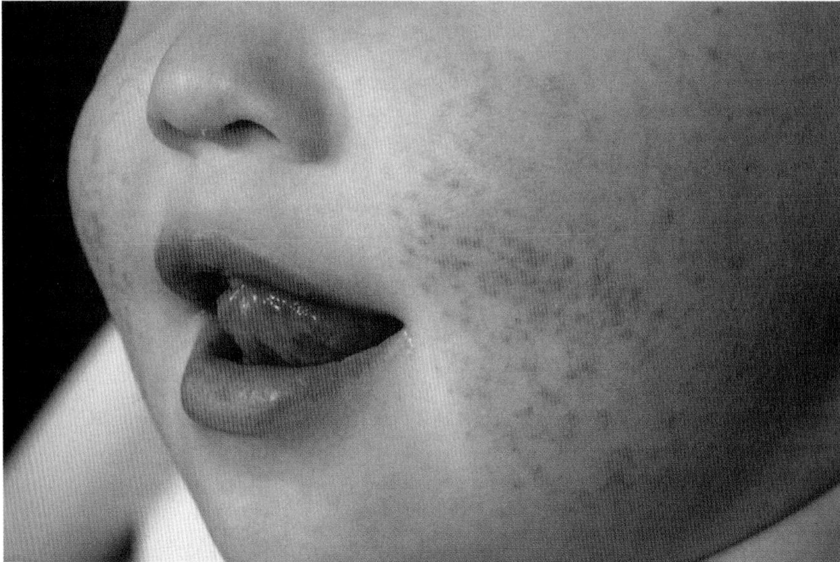

Figure 15.1. Erythematous papules on the face of a child with Gianotti-Crosti syndrome.

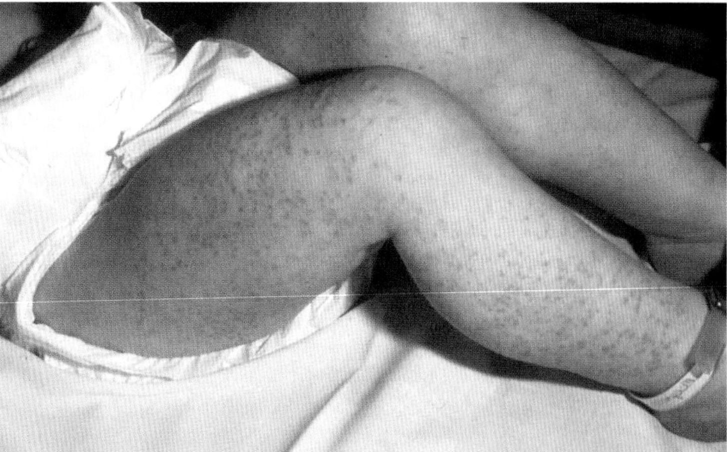

Figure 15.2. The papules of Gianotti-Crosti syndrome often are located on the extensor surfaces of the lower extremities.

Look-alikes

Disorder	Differentiating Features
Insect bites	• Not distributed symmetrically • May exhibit a central punctum
Papular atopic dermatitis	• More likely to present in a chronic, recurrent pattern • Atopic history present
Lichen planus	• Purple polygonal papules that may have fine, white, reticulated scale on surface • Most often distributed on volar wrists, lower legs, and ankles • White, reticulated patches often present on buccal mucosa
Lichenoid drug eruption	• History of medication use • Generalized, with truncal involvement as well
Molluscum contagiosum	• Not distributed symmetrically. • Individual lesions are pearly and translucent and often contain a central punctum or depression. • Acute onset unusual; typically a gradual increase in the number of lesions over weeks to months. • Some reports in the literature suggest occasional coexistence of molluscum and Gianotti-Crosti syndrome, the latter possibly representing an id-type reaction.

How to Make the Diagnosis

- The diagnosis is made clinically based on the unique appearance and distribution of lesions.
- Skin biopsy may occasionally be useful in diagnosis but rarely is necessary.
- Routine serologic evaluations for hepatitis B infection are not indicated; testing should be considered only if there are risk factors or concerning history or examination findings.

Treatment

- Rarely necessary, aside from reassurance and education about the natural history.
- Oral antihistamines for pruritus.
- Topical steroids do not change the natural history of the skin eruption; may be helpful for treating pruritus.

Prognosis

- Self-limited, with eventual complete resolution (sometimes with postinflammatory hypopigmentation).
- Lesions may persist for up to 2 months, in contrast to most other viral exanthems.

Resources for Families

- NORD National Organization for Rare Disorders: Information for patients and families.
  https://rarediseases.org/rare-diseases/gianotti-crosti-syndrome

CHAPTER 16

Hand-Foot-and-Mouth Disease (HFMD) and Other Enteroviral Exanthems

Introduction/Etiology/Epidemiology

Hand-Foot-and-Mouth Disease

- The most distinctive enteroviral exanthem.
- Typical HFMD most often caused by coxsackievirus A16 but may be caused by coxsackieviruses A5, A7, A9, A10, B1, B2, B3, and B5 and enterovirus 71; recently described atypical HFMD caused primarily by coxsackievirus A6.
- Most commonly occurs in the late summer or early fall.
- Incubation period is 4 to 6 days.
- Highly contagious; may occur in epidemics.

Herpangina

- A characteristic enanthem that has clinical overlap with the enanthem of HFMD (without other features of the exanthem).
- Most often caused by coxsackieviruses from groups A and B.

Eruptive Pseudoangiomatosis

- An uncommon exanthem characterized by the sudden appearance of several small, angioma-like lesions in the setting of a viral prodrome or illness.
- Most often seen in infants and children, although reported in adults (often immunocompromised) as well.
- Associated with echovirus subtypes 25 and 32, although other viral etiologies are possible.

Signs and Symptoms

Hand-Foot-and-Mouth Disease

- Brief prodrome of fever, malaise may occur.
- Cough, diarrhea noted infrequently.
- An enanthem precedes the characteristic exanthem.
- Hand-foot-and-mouth disease enanthem
  - Vesicles that erode to form ulcers on a red base; size ranges between 4 and 8 mm (Figure 16.1).
  - Most common on buccal mucosa and tongue.
  - May also involve palate, uvula, and tonsillar pillars.
  - Lesions are often quite painful, sometimes severe enough to lead to anorexia, dehydration.

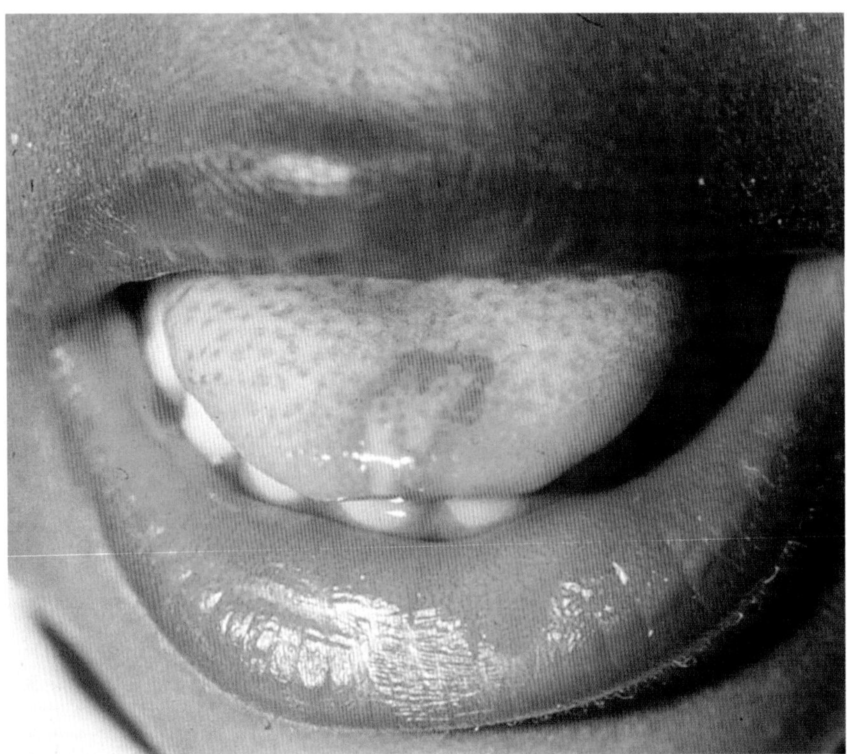

Figure 16.1. Ulcers may occur on the tongue or buccal mucosa in hand-foot-and-mouth disease.

- Hand-foot-and-mouth disease exanthem
  - Deep-seated vesicopustules with gray-white color, 3 to 7 mm in size; often the vesicles are oval (Figures 16.2 and 16.3).
  - Vesicles often have surrounding erythema.
  - Typically, lesions are limited to the palms and soles but also may involve lateral surfaces of hands and feet; involvement of buttocks, elbows, knees, and perineum may also be seen in younger children.
  - In patients with atypical HFMD, vesicles are often larger and more numerous, may enlarge into bullae, become hemorrhagic, or present as erosions (Figure 16.4).
- Distribution of lesions in atypical HFMD may be generalized but often with accentuation around the mouth (Figure 16.5), in the anogenital regions, and on the dorsal extremities.
  - Lesions of atypical HFMD may have a predilection for areas of eczematous dermatitis (hence the term "eczema Coxsackium") and prior skin injury, such as sunburn.
- Cervical and submandibular adenopathy occasionally observed.
- Temporary Beau lines (transverse grooves in the nail plate) or nail shedding (onychomadesis; Figure 16.6) may occur a few weeks to a few months following HFMD, presumably due to nail matrix arrest; these secondary changes are common following atypical HFMD.

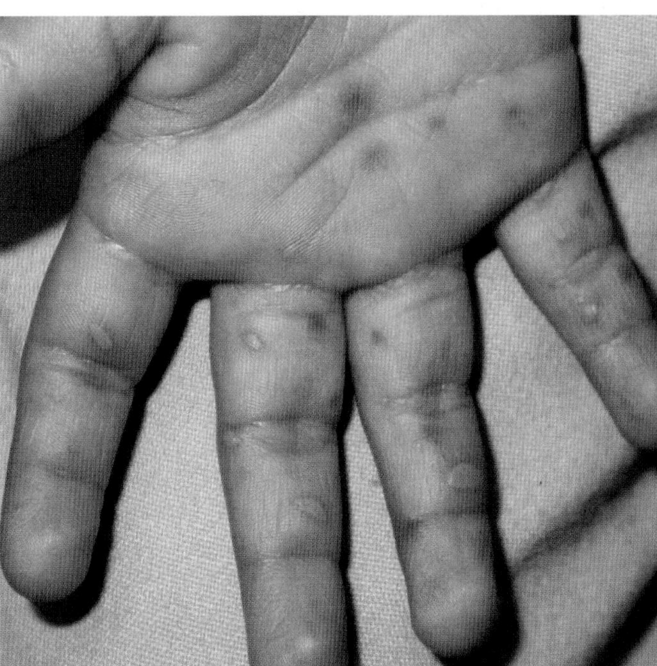

Figure 16.2. Oval vesicles with surrounding erythema on the hand of a child who has hand-foot-and-mouth disease.

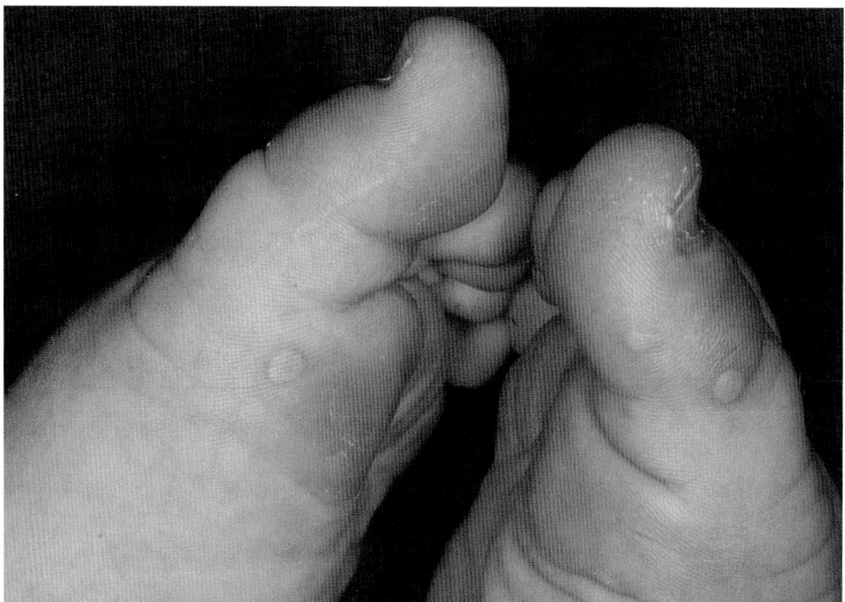

Figure 16.3. Hand-foot-and-mouth disease. Oval vesicles with mild surrounding erythema.

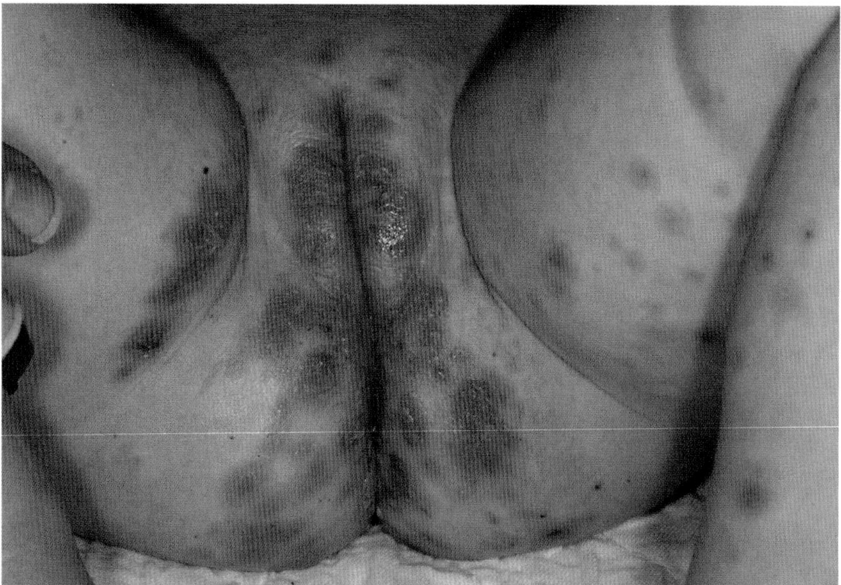

Figure 16.4. Ruptured bullae and large erosions in a young girl with atypical hand-foot-and-mouth disease.

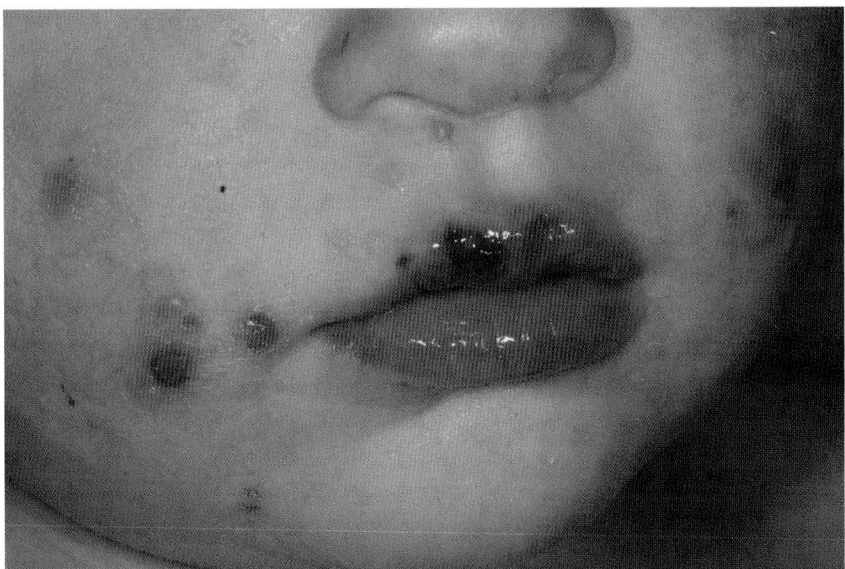

Figure 16.5. Perioral vesicles and erosions in a toddler with atypical hand-foot-and-mouth disease.

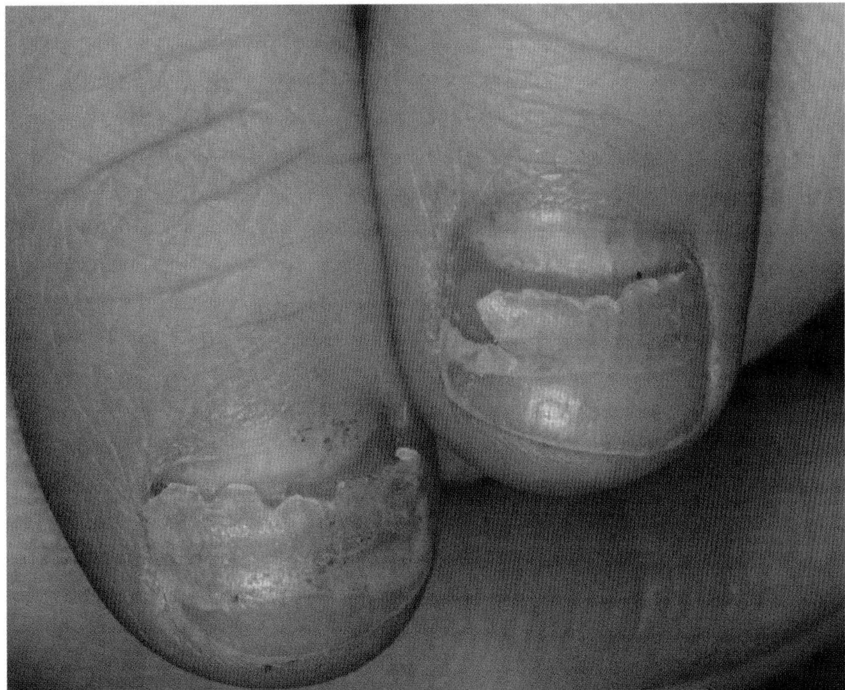

Figure 16.6. Onychomadesis (nail shedding) following hand-foot-and-mouth disease in an otherwise healthy 4-year-old girl.

Herpangina

- Enanthem with painful tiny vesicles and punched-out erosions.
- Distributed on soft palate, uvula, tonsillar pillars, and posterior pharynx.
- Erosions typically have a rim of erythema and a yellow-gray coating.
- Fever is common; 25% may have abdominal pain, vomiting.
- Erosions persist for approximately 7 days.

Eruptive Pseudoangiomatosis

- Acute onset of multiple, small (2–4 mm), bright red ("hemangioma-like") papules with a surrounding pale halo.
- Lesions blanch with pressure.
- Preceding or concurrent fever, headache, upper respiratory symptoms may be present.
- Lesions resolve spontaneously over 1 to 2 weeks without treatment.

How to Make the Diagnosis

- Diagnosis of HFMD, herpangina, and eruptive pseudoangiomatosis is usually made clinically.
- Although rarely necessary, a specific diagnosis of enteroviral infections may be made by viral culture, serologic testing, or polymerase chain reaction–based testing of lesional swabs, oropharyngeal swabs, blood, stool, or urine.
- Viral culture or direct fluorescent examination for herpes simplex virus is relatively rapid and may be clinically helpful to distinguish these infections from atypical HFMD or the oral erosions of herpangina.
- Skin biopsy may be necessary to distinguish eruptive pseudoangiomatosis from other vascular lesions if the process is not resolving spontaneously, as expected.

Treatment

- Generally, simple supportive measures (oral fluids, analgesics, and antipyretics) are adequate for HFMD and herpangina.
- Severe pain may require more aggressive pain management; hospitalization for intravenous hydration and narcotic analgesics occasionally is required.
- Eruptive pseudoangiomatosis usually requires no therapy.

Look-alikes

Disorder	Differentiating Features
Typical Hand-Foot-and-Mouth Disease	
The typical appearance and distribution of lesions usually prevents confusion with other disorders.	
Atypical Hand-Foot-and-Mouth Disease	
Eczema herpeticum	• Uniform, punched-out erosions in areas of atopic dermatitis predominate. • Viral testing positive for herpes simplex virus.
Varicella	• Less common in era of universal vaccination. • Crops of lesions in varying stages (papules, vesicles, crusts) are seen.
Bullous impetigo	• Flaccid blisters and superficial erosions with peripheral collarette of blister roof. • Honey-colored crusts may be present. • Predominance of lesions around the nose, hands, diaper area. • Bacterial culture positive for *Staphylococcus aureus*.
Allergic contact dermatitis	• Localized erythema, papules, and vesicles in a pattern consistent with an "outside job" • Itch (often severe) very common
Autoimmune blistering disorders	• Uncommon • Progressive and unremitting without immunosuppressive therapy
Herpangina	
Herpes gingivostomatitis	• Patients typically ill with fever. • Ulcers involve gingivae and perioral skin.
Aphthous ulcer (canker sores)	• Usually a chronic or recurring problem. • Fever and other symptoms of herpangina typically lacking. • In severe disease (recurrent aphthous ulcer major), ulcers >1 cm may occur.
Eruptive Pseudoangiomatosis	
Infantile hemangioma	• Appear in the first weeks to month after birth and persist for years before spontaneously resolving • Typically solitary, although a diffuse pattern of numerous small lesions can occur
Pyogenic granuloma	• Friable red vascular papule that bleeds easily with minor trauma • Typically solitary
Bacillary angiomatosis	• Occurs in immunocompromised individuals, most often in the setting of HIV infection

Prognosis

- The prognosis for HFMD, herpangina, and eruptive pseudoangiomatosis is excellent; all typically resolve without sequelae.
- Normal nail regrowth is the norm following post-enteroviral onychomadesis.

When to Worry or Refer

- If the diagnosis is in question or lesions are persistent or recurrent.
- Consider hospitalization if fluid intake is inadequate or dehydration is suspected.
- Because enteroviruses are a major cause of meningitis in summer and fall, neck stiffness, lethargy, or severe irritability should prompt a thorough evaluation.

Resources for Families

Hand-Foot-and-Mouth Disease

- American Academy of Pediatrics: HealthyChildren.org. **www.HealthyChildren.org/HandFootMouth**
- Centers for Disease Control and Prevention: Alphabetic listing of diseases and conditions provides information for families in English and Spanish. **www.cdc.gov/hand-foot-mouth/index.html**

Measles

Introduction/Etiology/Epidemiology

- Acute febrile illness caused by measles virus, an RNA virus of the genus *Morbillivirus* in the *Paramyxoviridae* family.
- Humans are the only natural host.
- Transmitted by direct contact with infectious droplets or, less commonly, by airborne spread.
- Immunization program in the United States, started in 1963, has resulted in more than 99% decrease in reported incidence. Two vaccine doses are needed to ensure protection.
- Noteworthy increase in measles cases occurred in the United States from 1989 to 1991 as a result of low immunization rates in preschool-aged children, especially in urban areas.
- Indigenous cases became markedly less common until recently, when increasing numbers of cases began to again be observed; in 2011, 222 cases were reported to the Centers for Disease Control and Prevention, and in 2014, 644 cases were reported.
- A large multistate outbreak occurred in early 2015, linked to an amusement park in California; among the earliest patients, 45% were unvaccinated, 5% had received only one dose, and 43% had unknown or undocumented vaccination status.
- Vaccine failure occurs in up to 5% of children who receive a single dose of vaccine at 12 months or older.
- Patients are contagious from 1 to 2 days before onset of symptoms (3–5 days before the rash) to 4 days after appearance of the rash.
- Incubation period is 10 to 14 days from exposure to onset of symptoms.
- Classically occurs in the winter and spring; sporadic cases can occur year-round.

Signs and Symptoms

- Prodrome of high fever, cough, coryza, and conjunctivitis precedes the exanthem by 2 to 4 days.
- Characteristic enanthem: Koplik spots
  - Appear during the prodrome and fade 2 to 3 days after onset of exanthem
  - White or blue-gray punctate papules superimposed on an erythematous base, located on buccal mucosa, often adjacent to molars (Figure 17.1)
- Exanthem begins behind the ears and at the scalp margin, rapidly spreading downward to involve most of the body (cephalocaudad spread).
- Discrete erythematous papules and macules appear and gradually become confluent (Figure 17.2).
- Pruritus is uncommon.
- Eruption lasts 4 to 7 days before fading, often with fine desquamation.
- Generalized adenopathy and splenomegaly may occur with the exanthem.
- Modified measles may occur in infants with residual maternal antibody.
  - Less severe illness
  - Shortened prodrome
  - Exanthem less confluent
- *Atypical measles* previously occurred in those who received killed measles vaccine and then were exposed to wild-type measles virus. It presents as a syndrome with high fever, abdominal pain, nodular pulmonary lesions, severe headache, and an acral (distal extremities, hands, feet) eruption with vesicular, vesiculopustular, or purpuric lesions.

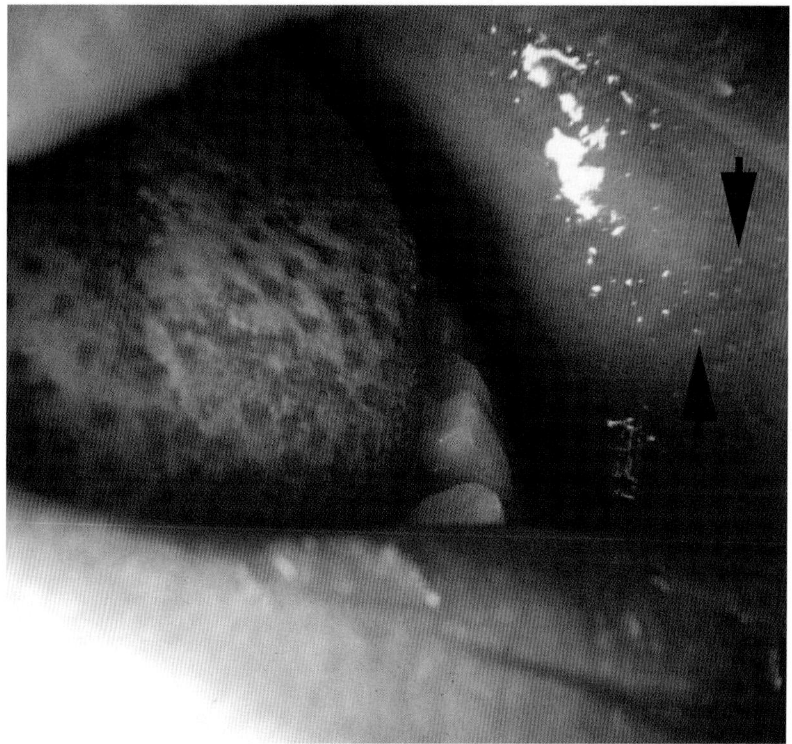

Figure 17.1. Koplik spots (arrows): punctate white-gray papules on an erythematous base that appear on the buccal mucosa.

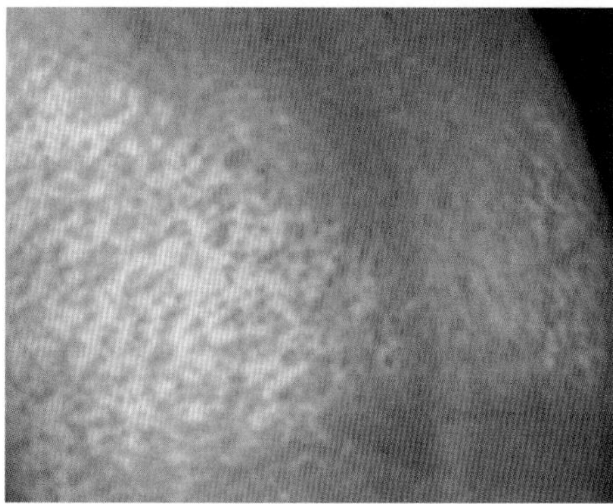

Figure 17.2. Measles produces an erythematous macular and papular eruption.

Look-alikes

A number of viral exanthems may mimic the rash of measles; however, the typical symptoms of measles are lacking.

Disorder	Differentiating Features
Exanthematous drug eruption	• History of drug exposure
Rubella	• Patients generally well with slight fever, arthralgias, or arthritis. • Patients have posterior cervical, suboccipital, or postauricular lymphadenopathy. • Rash typically lighter in color.
Roseola	• Patients often appear well and lack typical symptoms of measles (cough, conjunctivitis, coryza). • Characteristic history of high fever followed by abrupt defervescence (which coincides with onset of exanthem).
Erythema infectiosum	• Patients appear well. • "Slapped-cheek" appearance and presence of a lacy, reticulated, erythematous eruption.
Infectious mononucleosis	• Patients exhibit sore throat and malaise; exudative pharyngitis. • Conjunctivitis absent. • Exanthem classically exacerbated by receipt of penicillin-class antibiotics.
Kawasaki disease	• Lymphadenopathy, fissuring of lips, and induration of hands and feet prominent. • Cough and coryza uncommon symptoms. • Exanthem (especially desquamation) often accentuated in perineum. • BCG vaccination site may develop edema, erythema, crusting.
Rocky Mountain spotted fever	• May mimic atypical measles. • Headache a prominent symptom; history of a tick bite may be elicited. • Rash spreads centripetally.
Meningococcemia	• May mimic atypical measles • Patients seriously ill • Purpura widespread (not limited to acral areas)
Papular-purpuric gloves-and-socks syndrome	• May mimic atypical measles • Characteristically petechial or purpuric erythema of palms and soles with sharp demarcation at wrists and ankles

How to Make the Diagnosis

- The diagnosis is made clinically based on typical symptoms and physical findings (eg, Koplik spots).
- The diagnosis may be confirmed by any one of the following symptoms:
  - Measles IgM antibody
  - Fourfold or greater increase in measles IgG antibody titers in paired acute and convalescent specimens
  - Isolation of measles virus from urine, blood, or nasopharyngeal secretions
  - Polymerase chain reaction–based assays available

Treatment

- No specific antiviral therapy is available.
- Vitamin A supplementation is a consideration in areas with dietary deficiency—low levels of vitamin A have been associated with a higher complication rate. (Consult the current edition of *Red Book: Report of the Committee on Infectious Diseases* [www.aapredbook.org] for supplementation recommendations.)

Prognosis

- Usually good with supportive care.
- Complications include bacterial otitis media, pneumonia, laryngotracheobronchitis, thrombocytopenia, hepatitis, and diarrhea.
- Rare complications include encephalitis (including subacute sclerosing panencephalitis, which may occur years after infection), myocarditis, pericarditis, acute glomerulonephritis, and Stevens-Johnson syndrome.
- Young infants, malnourished children, and immunodeficient children are at highest risk for complications.

When to Worry or Refer

- Consultation with a pediatric infectious disease specialist is recommended if the diagnosis is in question.

Resources for Families

- American Academy of Pediatrics: HealthyChildren.org.
  www.HealthyChildren.org/Measles
- Centers for Disease Control and Prevention: Alphabetic listing of diseases and conditions provides information for families in English and Spanish.
  www.cdc.gov/measles/index.html
- MedlinePlus: Information for patients and families (in English and Spanish) sponsored by the National Library of Medicine and National Institutes of Health.
  https://www.nlm.nih.gov/medlineplus/measles.html

CHAPTER 18

Papular-Purpuric Gloves-and-Socks Syndrome (PPGSS)

Introduction/Etiology/Epidemiology

- Caused by any of multiple viral agents, although parvovirus B19 is the most common cause.
- Other reported etiologic associations include human herpesvirus 6, human herpesvirus 7, measles virus, and cytomegalovirus.
- Most often affects young adults but has occurred in children.
- Most common during the spring and summer.
- There appear to be epidemiologically relevant differences between the immune response to parvovirus B19 in PPGSS compared to patients with erythema infectiosum.
  - Clearance of viremia correlates with appearance of the rash in erythema infectiosum, such that patients with the skin eruption are not considered contagious.
  - The eruption of PPGSS seems to coincide with viremia and, therefore, patients with clinical findings should be considered potentially infectious.

Signs and Symptoms

- Rapidly progressive erythema and edema of the palms and soles (Figure 18.1), with progression to a petechial or purpuric appearance with sharp demarcation at the wrists and ankles.
- Lesions may also occur on the elbows, knees, buttocks, and dorsal surfaces of the hands and feet.
- Associated symptoms include low-grade fever, malaise, myalgias, anorexia, and joint pain.
- Patients often report pruritus, burning discomfort, or pain at sites of involvement.

- Associated enanthem presents as vesicles and small erosions on the palate, posterior pharynx, tongue, and mucosal surfaces of the lips.
- Lymphadenopathy occurs in 16% of patients.

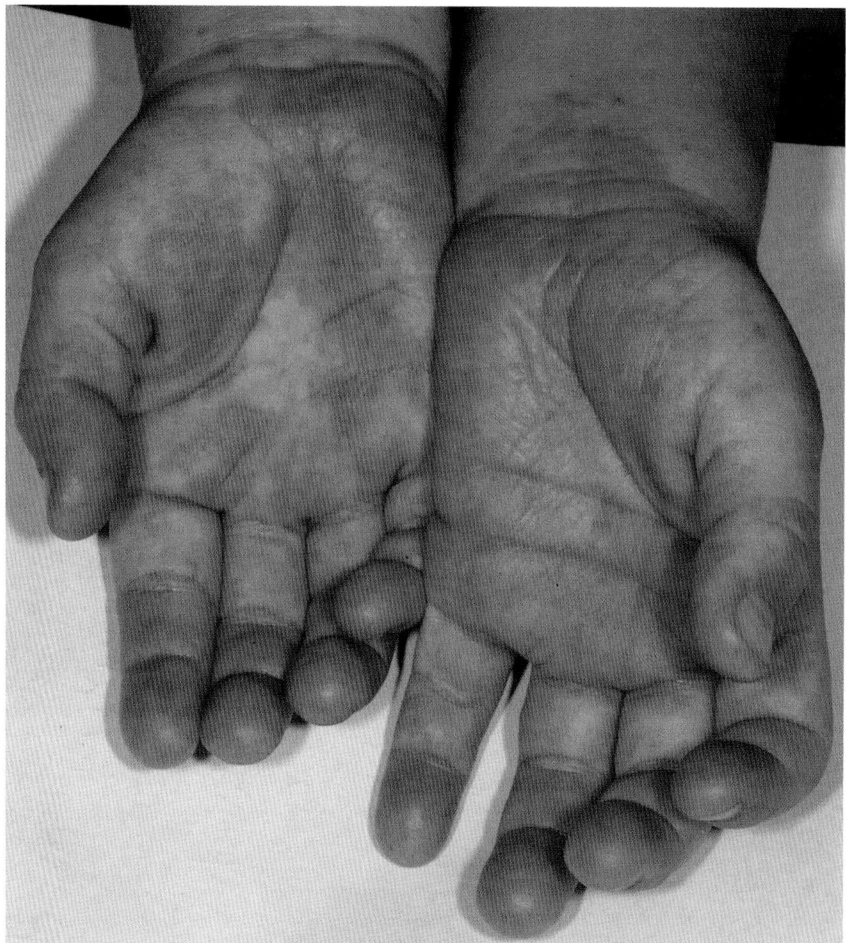

Figure 18.1. Erythema and edema of the palms early in the course of papular-purpuric gloves-and-socks syndrome.

Look-alikes

Disorder	Differentiating Features
Cutaneous vasculitis	• Purpuric papules or nodules (ie, palpable purpura) • Widespread, not typically limited to the hands and feet (although there may be preferential involvement of the lower extremities)
Rocky Mountain spotted fever	• Patients acutely ill with fever and severe headache. • Lesions spread centripetally to involve the arms, legs, and trunk (ie, do not remain limited to the hands and feet). • History of a tick bite may be elicited.
Meningococcemia	• Patients acutely ill with fever and malaise • Purpura usually not limited to the hands and feet • Areas of purpura may develop blistering and/or become necrotic
Hand-foot-and-mouth disease	• Round or oval deep-seated vesicles with surrounding erythema • Petechiae and purpura absent

How to Make the Diagnosis

- The diagnosis is made clinically based on the characteristic appearance and distribution of the eruption.
- Measurement of serum anti-parvovirus B19 IgM may be useful in B19-associated cases in which the diagnosis is in question.

Treatment

- Supportive care with symptomatic treatment for pruritus.
- No specific therapy is available.

Prognosis

- Spontaneous resolution usually occurs over 1 to 2 weeks.
- Exposed pregnant women should be advised to contact their obstetric provider to discuss potential risks and be offered serologic testing. If acute infection is confirmed, serial fetal ultrasound should be considered to monitor for fetal hydrops, congestive heart failure, and intrauterine growth restriction.

When to Worry or Refer

- Consultation with a pediatric dermatologist or infectious disease specialist is indicated when the diagnosis is uncertain.
- Pregnant women exposed to or who have acquired human parvovirus B19 infection should consult their obstetric provider (as discussed previously).

Roseola Infantum (Exanthem Subitum)

Introduction/Etiology/Epidemiology

- Caused by human herpesvirus (HHV) 6 in most cases; occasionally HHV-7.
- Usually affects children between 6 months and 3 years of age (peak age: 6–7 months).
- Occurs throughout the year but may be more common in the spring and fall.
- Transmission is airborne via respiratory droplets.
- Incubation period is 9 to 10 days.

Signs and Symptoms

- The hallmark finding is high fever (38.3°C–41.1°C [101°F–106°F]) without a rash that lasts for 3 to 5 days in an otherwise well-appearing or sometimes irritable infant.
- The exanthem of roseola typically occurs within 1 to 2 days following defervescence.
- Rose-pink macules and papules on the neck and trunk are characteristic; the rash also may involve the proximal extremities and face (Figure 19.1).
- A faint halo of blanching may be seen surrounding each individual lesion.
- An enanthem with red papules on the soft palate and uvula occurs in two-thirds of cases (Nagayama spots).
- Associated findings may include pharyngitis, tonsillitis, and lymphadenopathy (occipital, postauricular, or posterior cervical).
- Neurologic complications of HHV-6 or HHV-7 infection can occur, including febrile seizures and, rarely, encephalitis.

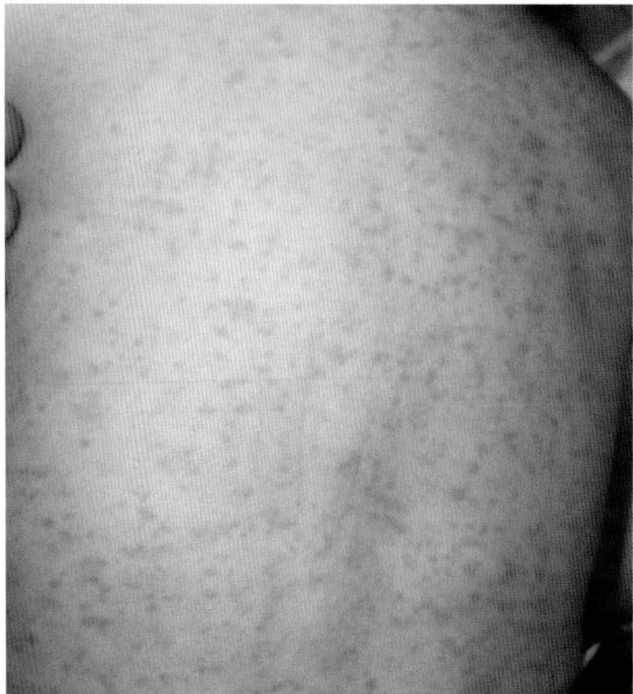

Figure 19.1. Roseola infantum. Erythematous macules and papules in an infant who developed the eruption following several days of high fever.

Look-alikes

A variety of viral agents, including enteroviruses, adenoviruses, parvovirus B19, rubella, rotavirus, and parainfluenza virus, may cause a clinical picture similar in appearance to roseola. The appearance of the rash as the fever resolves is characteristic of roseola.

How to Make the Diagnosis

- Characteristic clinical findings in the appropriate age group, with an exanthem following high fever, are highly suggestive of the diagnosis.
- Laboratory confirmation is usually unnecessary; in atypical or questionable cases where it is indicated, specific serologic and polymerase chain reaction testing are available.

Treatment

- Most cases require only supportive care.
- Immunocompromised patients may warrant consideration for antiviral therapy; ganciclovir, foscarnet, and cidofovir have been used. Referral to a pediatric infectious disease specialist is indicated in this setting.

Prognosis

- Roseola infantum typically resolves without sequelae.

When to Worry or Refer

- Consult a pediatric infectious disease specialist if a patient is immunocompromised.

Resources for Families

- American Academy of Pediatrics: HealthyChildren.org. **www.HealthyChildren.org/roseola**
- WebMD: Information for families is contained in the Health A-Z topics. **www.webmd.com/skin-problems-and-treatments/tc/roseola-topic-overview**

Rubella

Introduction/Etiology/Epidemiology

Classic Rubella

- Mild illness in most children
- Up to half of all cases asymptomatic
- Caused by rubella virus, an RNA virus
- Rare following the institution of universal vaccination; 2 doses administered in combination with measles and mumps

Congenital Rubella

- Embryopathy results from first (or occasionally second) trimester infection.
- Universal vaccination has greatly reduced the incidence.

Signs and Symptoms

Classic Rubella

- Mild lymphadenopathy may precede exanthem by several days; suboccipital and posterior auricular nodes are characteristically involved.
- Faint pink, macular eruption starts on the face and spreads to the trunk and proximal extremities (Figure 20.1).
- Within 48 hours, the face clears and the exanthem spreads in a cephalocaudad fashion to the distal extremities.
- Petechiae and purpura occur rarely.
- Patient usually appears well, but associated pharyngitis and arthritis may be present; the latter may last for several months.
- Fever is usually absent in young children.

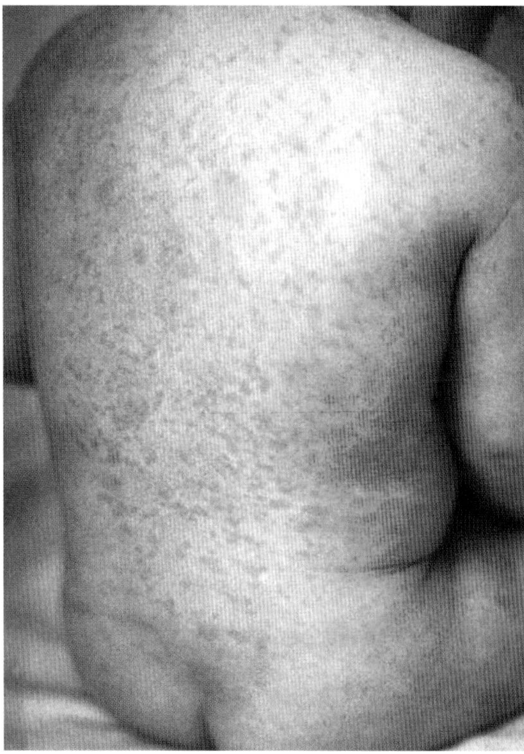

Figure 20.1. An erythematous macular eruption occurs in rubella.

Congenital Rubella

- Neonate may present with disseminated blue-purple nodules ("blueberry muffin" rash) (Figure 20.2) and thrombocytopenia.
- Neonatal hepatitis with jaundice can occur.
- Embryopathy: deafness, congenital heart defects, cataracts, glaucoma, growth and psychomotor retardation.

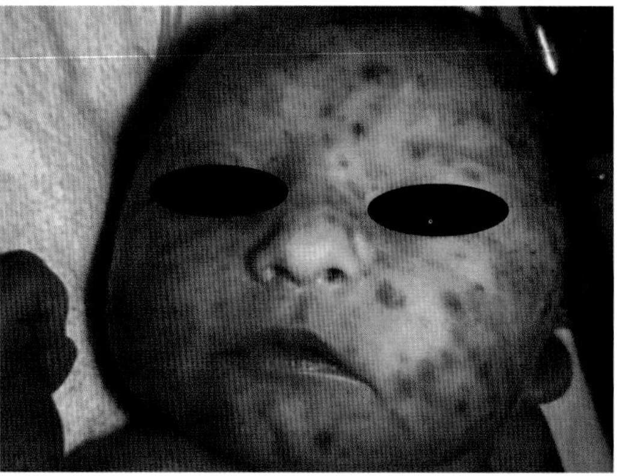

Figure 20.2. Blue-purple nodular eruption ("blueberry muffin" rash) in an infant with congenital rubella infection.

Look-alikes

Disorder	Differentiating Features
Classic Rubella	
Measles (rubeola)	• Patients ill with fever, cough, coryza, and conjunctivitis • Exanthem more intensely red
Enteroviral	• May have characteristic clinical syndrome (eg, hand-foot-and-mouth disease). • Eruption may have a petechial component. • Posterior cervical and suboccipital lymphadenopathy uncommon.
Infectious mononucleosis	• Patients ill with fever, pharyngitis, malaise
Exanthematous drug eruption	• History of drug exposure. • Posterior cervical and suboccipital lymphadenopathy are typically absent.
Congenital Rubella	
Cytomegalovirus infection	• Cataracts (present in congenital rubella) absent
Toxoplasmosis	• Infants often asymptomatic
Congenital syphilis	• Infants have rhinorrhea (often bloody), condylomata lata (flat-topped papules and plaques located at mucocutaneous junctions, including the perineum and angles of the mouth), and scaly, copper-colored papules and plaques. • Exanthem may be vesiculobullous.
Herpes simplex virus infection	• Typical skin lesions often present (eg, clustered vesicles on an erythematous base)
Congenital thrombocytopenia (eg, Wiskott-Aldrich syndrome, neonatal thrombocytopenia)	• Petechiae may be present, but hepatosplenomegaly, cataracts, intrauterine growth retardation, and other features of congenital rubella syndrome are absent.

How to Make the Diagnosis

- The rash of rubella is nonspecific; a clinical diagnosis of rubella cannot be made.
- Diagnostic tests available include
  - Viral culture from nasal mucosa swabs.
  - Viral culture from urine, pharyngeal swabs in congenital rubella.
  - Serologic testing for rubella IgM antibodies or a 4-fold or greater rise in IgG antibodies in paired acute and convalescent specimens may be helpful.
  - Polymerase chain reaction–based assays available.

Treatment

- No specific therapy possible.
- Supportive care includes use of nonsteroidal anti-inflammatory agents for arthritis.
- Affected children should avoid contact with pregnant women and should be excluded from school until 7 days following onset of the rash.
- Multidisciplinary care for congenital rubella (including ophthalmology, cardiology, and developmental pediatrics).

Prognosis

- Rubella is typically a self-limited illness.
- Arthritis may last for several months.
- The prognosis for congenital rubella syndrome is guarded and depends on the extent of involvement.

When to Worry or Refer

- Referral may be warranted if the diagnosis is in question.
- Consult a pediatric infectious disease specialist if a pregnant woman who is susceptible or of unknown serologic status is exposed to rubella.

Resources for Families

- American Academy of Pediatrics: HealthyChildren.org.
  www.HealthyChildren.org/rubella
- Centers for Disease Control and Prevention: Alphabetic listing of diseases and conditions provides information for families in English and Spanish.
  www.cdc.gov/rubella/index.html
- MedlinePlus: Information for patients and families (in English and Spanish) sponsored by the National Library of Medicine and National Institutes of Health.
  https://www.nlm.nih.gov/medlineplus/rubella.html

Unilateral Laterothoracic Exanthem (ULE)

Introduction/Etiology/Epidemiology

- An uncommon exanthem that was rediscovered in 1992–1993 and correlated with earlier published reports.
- Also known as asymmetric periflexural exanthem of childhood.
- Etiology unknown but seems most likely to be a viral exanthem.
- Mean age of reported patients is 2 years.

Signs and Symptoms

- Onset of the eruption often preceded by low-grade fever and mild gastrointestinal or upper respiratory symptoms.
- Most patients develop initial red, patchy exanthem localized on one side of the chest near the axilla.
- In some, the rash may begin in the inguinal region or on an extremity.
- Lesional morphology is variable, including morbilliform, scarlatiniform, urticarial, vesicular, reticulated, and purpuric patterns (Figure 21.1).
- Pruritus is common, but secondary bacterial superinfection is rare.
- Exanthem often generalizes to bilateral involvement but usually maintains a unilateral predominance on initial side of involvement.
- Spontaneous resolution begins during the third week with complete resolution over 5 to 8 weeks.

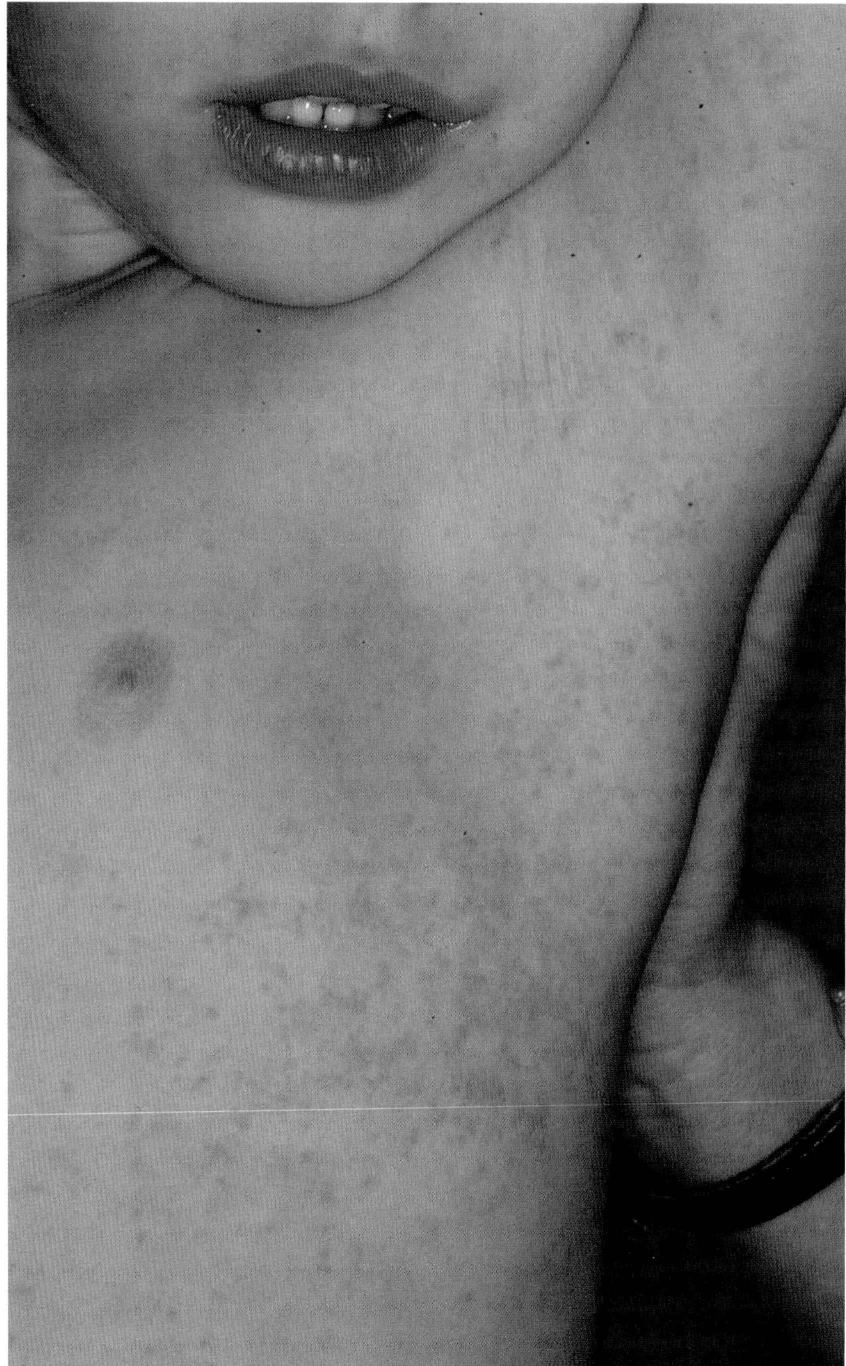

Figure 21.1. Erythematous, fine, papular eruption involving the axilla and lateral chest in unilateral laterothoracic exanthem.

Look-alikes

Disorder	Differentiating Features
Contact dermatitis	• May be difficult to distinguish from early ULE. • History of exposure to an allergen may be obtained. • Does not generalize as typically seen in ULE.
Papular eczema	• Eruption typically is symmetrically distributed (not unilateral) and often involves the extremities. • History of atopic dermatitis may be elicited.
Tinea corporis	• Annular papules and plaques that have an elevated, scaly border and central clearing • Usually more localized than ULE
Pityriasis rosea	• Eruption symmetrically distributed on the trunk (not unilateral). • Typical lesions are oval, thin plaques with long axes oriented parallel to lines of skin stress. • Trailing scale (free edge points inward) is present.
Gianotti-Crosti syndrome	• Concentrated on the cheeks, upper extremities, knees, and buttocks with relative sparing of the trunk

How to Make the Diagnosis

- The diagnosis is made clinically based on the unilateral clinical presentation (or history of unilateral onset), with eventual generalization and prolonged course.

Treatment

- Topical corticosteroids or oral antihistamines may be useful for pruritus but will not alter the natural history of the eruption.

Prognosis

- Spontaneous resolution (in 3–8 weeks) without sequelae is typical.

When to Worry or Refer

- Consider referral when the diagnosis is in question.

CHAPTER 22

Varicella

Introduction/Etiology/Epidemiology

- Acute febrile illness caused by varicella-zoster virus (VZV), a double-stranded DNA virus of the *Herpesviridae* family.
- Humans are the only natural host of VZV.
- Highly contagious disease of childhood, transmitted by person-to-person contact; airborne spread has been documented.
- Immunization with a live, attenuated virus vaccine has been available in the United States since 1995 and is highly effective. Incidence has dropped dramatically since that time.
- Incubation typically is 14 to 16 days (range, 10–21 days) from exposure to onset of symptoms.
- Usually occurs during the winter and spring; sporadic cases may occur year-round.

Signs and Symptoms

- Vesicular exanthem that usually begins on the scalp or trunk.
- Lesions may appear in crops and may first appear as red macules, which quickly develop a surface vesicle (Figures 22.1 and 22.2).
- Individual lesions appear as a clear vesicle on an erythematous base ("dewdrop on a rose petal").
- The lesions usually crust within hours to days and then begin to gradually heal.
- The exanthem spreads centrifugally, so fresh vesicles may be seen on the extremities, with older crusted lesions on the trunk. Lesions in varying stages of development are characteristic of varicella (see Figure 22.2).
- Increased numbers of lesions may be seen in areas of skin injury or irritation (eg, atopic dermatitis sites, areas of sunburn).

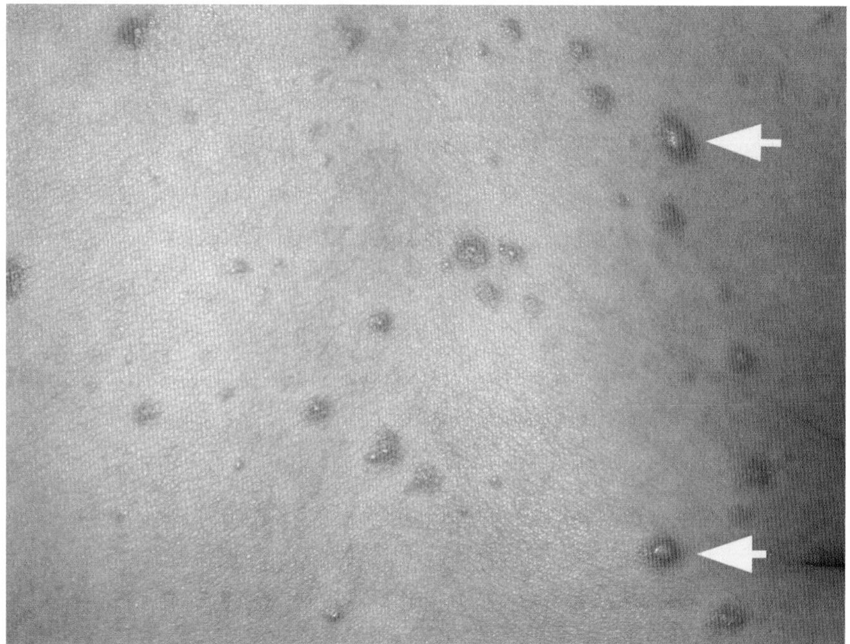

Figure 22.1. Varicella: typical vesicles ("dewdrop on a rose petal") are present (arrows).

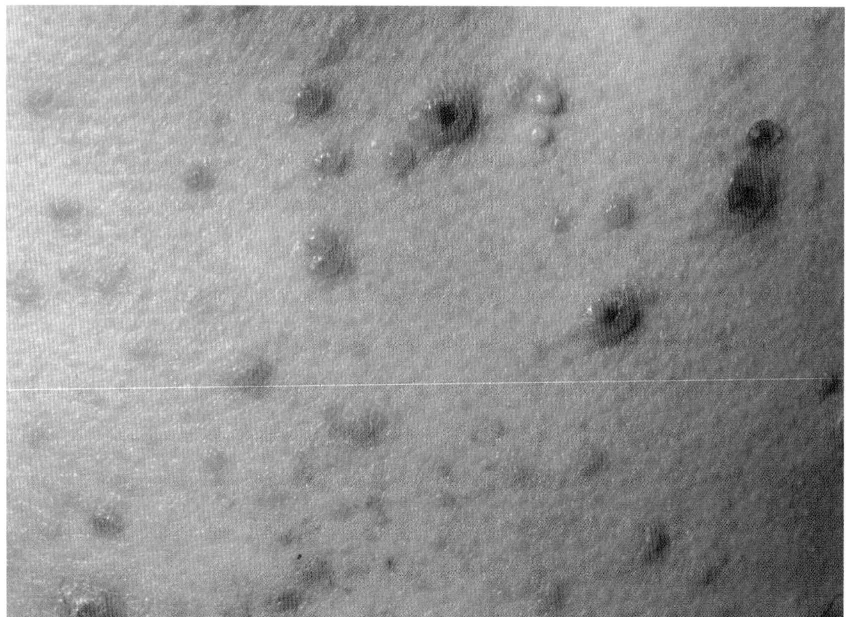

Figure 22.2. In varicella, lesions are in different stages of development. This patient demonstrates papules, vesicles, and crusts.

- Low-grade fever and malaise are typical; more severe disease may occur in adolescents, adults, and immunocompromised individuals.
- Pruritus is common and sometimes severe.
- Complications include staphylococcal and streptococcal superinfection of skin lesions, pneumonia, encephalitis, and purpura fulminans. Streptococcal superinfection usually presents with a reappearance of fever in the patient who is several days into the illness. Reye syndrome may occur in children taking salicylates.
- Chickenpox occurring in a person who has previously received the varicella vaccine generally is a milder illness than in an unvaccinated child, with fewer lesions (<50), lower fever, and shorter disease duration.

Look-alikes

Disorder	Differentiating Features
Hand-foot-and-mouth disease (HFMD)	• Eruption concentrated on the hands, feet, and buttocks (is not generalized). • Oval vesicles with a rim of erythema (classic appearance of "dewdrop on a rose petal") is lacking.
Other enteroviral exanthems	• Erythematous macules and papules that may mimic early varicella; petechiae may be present. • More recently, a severe form of HFMD has been observed and may present with widespread vesicles or bullae; lesions tend to predominate on distal extremities, anogenital region, and face; in some instances, involvement may be concentrated at sites of preceding atopic dermatitis (so-called "eczema Coxsackium").
Herpes simplex virus infection	• Clustered (not single) vesicles on an erythematous base • Eruption typically localized, not generalized
Bullous insect bite reaction	• Eruption not generalized • Lower extremities most often involved • Constitutional symptoms absent
Rickettsialpox	• Black eschar at site of primary mite bite • Absence of "dewdrop on a rose petal" vesicles
Disseminated herpes zoster	• Occurs in immunocompromised patients. • Reactivation of VZV may cause dissemination beyond dermatomal borders, with visceral involvement.
Smallpox (variola)	• Rash begins on face and rapidly spreads to the distal extremities; later involves the trunk (centripetal distribution, unlike centrifugal distribution seen in varicella). • Vesicles and pustules are deep-seated and firm (not fragile as in varicella). • All lesions are simultaneously in the same stage of development.

How to Make the Diagnosis

- Characteristic clinical features of lesional morphology, distribution, and progression usually suggest the diagnosis of varicella.
- Laboratory testing is rarely necessary in uncomplicated disease. If testing is required, the following tests may be available:
  - Vesicular fluid sent for polymerase chain reaction (PCR). This is the preferred method due to superior sensitivity and specificity.
  - Scrapings of the base of intact vesicles with direct fluorescent antibody examination provide rapid diagnosis, but sensitivity is inferior to PCR.
  - Viral culture from skin lesions can be performed, but sensitivity is limited compared with PCR and results may take several days.

Treatment

- In immunocompetent children supportive care is directed at measures to reduce itching and prevent secondary bacterial skin infection.
- Antipruritic lotions with menthol, camphor, colloidal oatmeal, or calamine are helpful, as are antihistamines administered orally.
- Once- to twice-daily baths and trimming of fingernails will minimize trauma from scratching (and risk of secondary bacterial superinfection).
- Oral acyclovir can reduce the duration and severity of varicella in normal children, if initiated in the first 24 hours of rash. It is not recommended for routine use in otherwise healthy children but is indicated for those at risk of serious disease, including those older than 12 years; with chronic cutaneous or pulmonary disease; receiving long-term salicylate therapy; and receiving short, intermittent, or aerosolized steroid therapy. Readers should consult the current edition of *Red Book: Report of the Committee on Infectious Diseases* (www.aapredbook.org) for guidelines.
- Secondary bacterial infections, most often caused by *Staphylococcus aureus* or *Streptococcus pyogenes,* should be treated with a systemic antibiotic, based on local susceptibility patterns.

Prognosis

- Healthy children typically recover uneventfully and scarring is rare.
- Children with uncomplicated chickenpox who have been excluded from school or child care may return when all lesions have crusted. Immunized persons who have not developed crusting may return when no new lesions have appeared in the last 24 hours.
- Permanent cutaneous scars are common, especially in areas of secondary infection.

When to Worry or Refer

- Varicella lesions may become secondarily infected with *S aureus* or *S pyogenes;* these should be managed appropriately. Such infections may progress rapidly and require prompt treatment and close follow-up. Hospitalization is sometimes necessary.
- Immunocompromised individuals, infants, adolescents, adults, pregnant women, and individuals with chronic pulmonary or cutaneous conditions are at risk for severe disease. If exposed to varicella, they should be managed in consultation with a pediatric infectious disease specialist. Postexposure prophylaxis is available and effective if initiated promptly.

Resources for Families

- American Academy of Pediatrics: HealthyChildren.org.
  www.HealthyChildren.org/varicella
- Centers for Disease Control and Prevention: Alphabetic listing of diseases and conditions provides information for families in English and Spanish.
  www.cdc.gov/chickenpox/index.html
- MedlinePlus: Information for patients and families (in English and Spanish) sponsored by the National Library of Medicine and National Institutes of Health.
  https://www.nlm.nih.gov/medlineplus/chickenpox.html

Skin Infections

Localized Bacterial Infections

CHAPTER 23

Acute Paronychia

Introduction/Etiology/Epidemiology

- Paronychia (inflammation of the periungual folds) occurs when the cuticle becomes disrupted by maceration or injury and pathogens enter the space.
- Paronychia occurs more frequently in individuals who often have their hands in water or in children with a habit of finger sucking. In addition, trauma to the periungual folds is another risk factor for its development.
- *Staphylococcus aureus* is the agent primarily responsible for acute paronychia. (*Candida* species most often result in chronic paronychia; see Fungal and Yeast Infections [chapters 35–41].)

Signs and Symptoms

- Periungual folds show erythema, swelling, and tenderness (Figure 23.1).
- Purulent drainage is commonly present.
- Patients with chronic infections may be noted to have dermatitis of the surrounding areas (eg, fingers, hands).

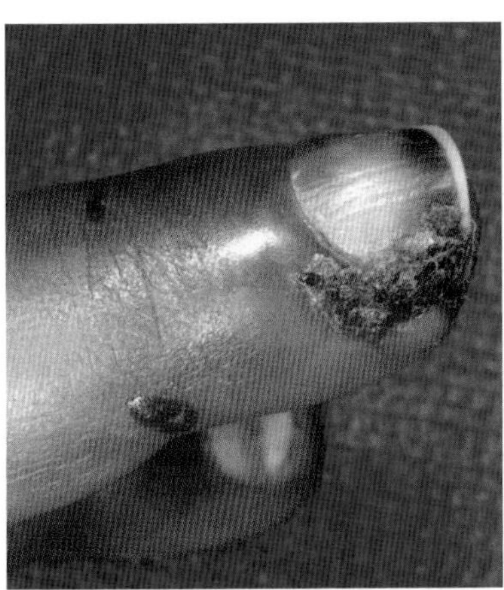

Figure 23.1. Acute paronychia with inflammation, pustule formation, and crusting of the periungual fold.

Look-alikes

Disorder	Differentiating Features
Chronic paronychia	• Problem long-standing (not acute) • Usually asymptomatic • Swelling and erythema of proximal and lateral nail folds with loss of cuticle; purulent drainage absent • May have associated nail dystrophy (ridging, pitting)
Herpes simplex virus infection (ie, herpetic whitlow)	• Usually presents as discrete, deep-seated, often clustered vesicles with surrounding erythema. • Usually very painful. • Regional lymphadenopathy may be present. • Recurrent lesions can be associated with prodromal symptoms. • Viral culture will reveal herpes simplex virus.
Psoriasis	• Pitting is most typical nail change in psoriasis. • Lateral onycholysis may result in disruption of the periungual folds; paronychia may eventually result.
Blistering dactylitis	• Usually presents as a tender, deep-seated blister on the volar surface of the distal finger pad. • Bacterial culture reveals group A ß-hemolytic streptococci (or occasionally *S aureus*).
Trauma	• History of trauma • Absence of purulent discharge • Cuticle usually normal

How to Make the Diagnosis

- The condition is often diagnosed based on the clinical features.
- Gram stain of the drainage can identify the organisms.
- Bacterial culture usually reveals *S aureus*.

Treatment

- An oral antistaphylococcal antibiotic (eg, cephalexin) usually is effective. Failure of response may indicate presence of methicillin-resistant *S aureus*, and changing therapy to clindamycin, doxycycline (in children >8 years), trimethoprim-sulfamethoxazole, or another appropriate agent (based on bacterial culture and sensitivity testing) should be considered.
- Topical antibiotic ointment (eg, mupirocin, retapamulin) may be used in mild cases, but the condition usually requires systemic therapy.
- Warm soaks may hasten resolution.

- Drainage and culture of purulent pockets occasionally is necessary.
- Preventive strategies include
  - Institute drying measures, including minimizing exposure to water and wearing gloves for "wet" work.
  - Avoid trauma, when feasible.

Prognosis

- Acute paronychia usually resolves completely without long-term sequelae.
- Mechanical factors or exposures may result in recurrence.
- Permanent nail ridging or dystrophy may result with severe infections.

When to Worry or Refer

- Consider referral to a dermatologist or infectious disease specialist for patients who have severe or extensive involvement or who do not respond to standard treatment.

Resources for Families

- MedlinePlus: Information for patients and families (in English and Spanish) sponsored by the National Library of Medicine and National Institutes of Health.
  www.nlm.nih.gov/medlineplus/ency/article/001444.htm

CHAPTER 24

Blistering Dactylitis

Introduction/Etiology/Epidemiology

- Blistering dactylitis is a skin infection caused most often by group A ß-hemolytic streptococcus or, less often, by *Staphylococcus aureus* or group B ß-hemolytic streptococcus.
- The peak incidence is in school-aged children.

Signs and Symptoms

- Tender superficial bullae occur on the distal volar (palmar surface of) finger pads (Figure 24.1) or, less often, the plantar surface of the toes; erythema usually surrounds the bullae.
- May involve one or more digits.
- Larger bullae may extend around to involve the nail folds.
- There is generally an absence of systemic symptoms.

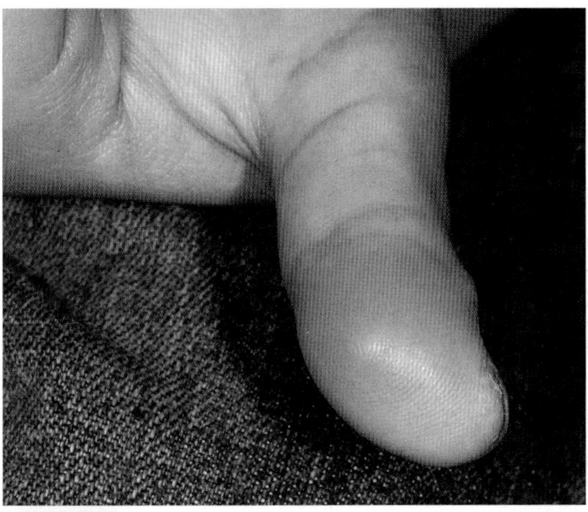

Figure 24.1. Blistering dactylitis. Note tense bulla of the thumb.

Look-alikes

Disorder	Differentiating Features
Herpes simplex virus infection (ie, herpetic whitlow)	• Deep-seated, clustered vesicles with surrounding erythema. • May have a history of recurrent lesions in the same site(s). • Viral culture or polymerase chain reaction testing demonstrates herpes simplex virus. • Regional lymphadenopathy may be present.
Acute paronychia	• Erythema and swelling of lateral or proximal nail folds. • Discrete vesicles or bullae typically absent. • Bacterial culture most often demonstrates *S aureus.*
Hand-foot-and-mouth disease	• Lesions tend to occur on the sides of the fingers/toes as well as palms and soles. • Blisters have an elliptical shape and are more deep-seated. • Multiple, smaller blisters present. • Oral erosions characteristically present.
Burn	• History may be confirmatory. • Clinical signs or historical information concerning for abuse or neglect may be present.
Epidermolysis bullosa (EB)	• Trauma-induced bullae occur recurrently. • Weber-Cockayne variant may be localized to the hands and feet; however, multifocal involvement usually seen (with multiple lesions) and not limited to distal digits. • Other forms of EB have additional lesions located on other areas of the body or mucosae.

How to Make the Diagnosis

- The diagnosis is usually made based on the clinical findings.
- Gram stain or bacterial culture of the bulla is often confirmatory.

Treatment

- Drainage of the bulla(e) can decrease pain if it is present; perform bacterial culture on fluid obtained to confirm the causative organism.
- Although oral penicillin or erythromycin given for 10 days is usually effective, an antistaphylococcal antibiotic (eg, cephalexin) often is selected because some cases may be caused by *S aureus.*
- Failure of response may indicate presence of methicillin-resistant *S aureus* and suggests consideration for a change of therapy to clindamycin, doxycycline (in children >8 years), trimethoprim-sulfamethoxazole, or another appropriate agent (as based on bacterial culture and sensitivity testing).

Prognosis

- The prognosis for children with blistering dactylitis is excellent.
- Lesions heal completely without permanent sequelae.

When to Worry or Refer

- Consider referral to a dermatologist or infectious disease specialist for patients who have severe or extensive involvement, in whom there is a question about the diagnosis, or who do not respond to standard treatment.

CHAPTER 25

Ecthyma

Introduction/Etiology/Epidemiology

- Ecthyma is a deep pyoderma (a deep cutaneous infection) that is most prevalent in tropical climates.
- The most common causative organisms are group A ß-hemolytic streptococcus (GABHS) and *Staphylococcus aureus.*
- Although the lesions may initially seem to be impetigo, the organisms progress to invade the dermis.
- Ecthyma can develop at sites of previous skin disorders, such as insect bites or scabies.

Signs and Symptoms

- The extremities are most often involved.
- Ecthyma lesions may be vesicopustules or crusted erosions; usually there is surrounding erythema. Often lesions will progress to become necrotic in appearance, with deep punched-out ulcers (Figure 25.1).

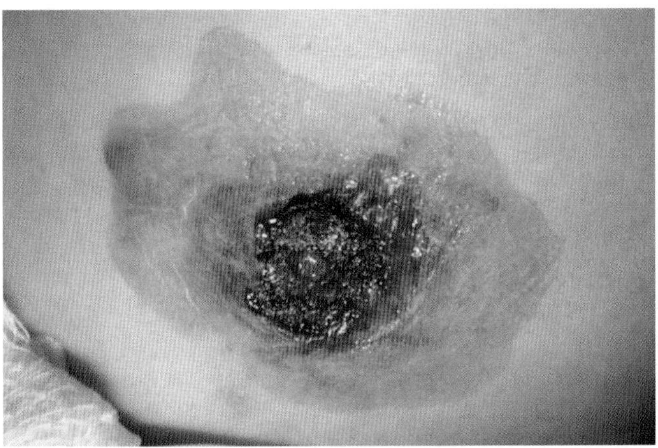

Figure 25.1. Ecthyma lesion with central necrotic crust.

Look-alikes

Disorder	Differentiating Features
Impetigo	**Nonbullous** • Superficial erosions with honey-colored crust **Bullous** • Fragile bullae that rupture rapidly leaving round superficial erosions. • Periphery of lesions may exhibit scale, the remnant of the bulla roof.
Brown recluse spider bite	• Timing of appearance of lesion corresponds to exposure to spider. • Usually becomes painful after a few hours. • Usually a single location rather than a multifocal process. • Initial lesion noted to have central hemorrhagic area with surrounding edema and erythema; may produce the "red, white, and blue sign" (ie, rings of color surrounding the lesion). • Rapidly progresses, resulting in large necrotic plaque, commonly with eschar formation.
Ecthyma gangrenosum	• Localized septic vasculitis usually associated with *Pseudomonas aeruginosa* bacteremia. • Lesions initially present as hemorrhagic papules. • Subsequently progress into deep ulcer with necrosis and, occasionally, eschar formation. • Often accompanied by high fever, myalgias. • Most affected children are immunosuppressed.
Cutaneous anthrax	• Spores enter through a cut or an abrasion. • Initial lesion is a painless, pruritic papule that subsequently develops a central clear bulla. • When bulla ruptures, necrosis and an ulcer develop, surrounded by massive edema and multiple smaller lesions.
Vasculitis	• Many vasculitic processes can present with hemorrhagic papules with necrosis, including leukocytoclastic vasculitis, Henoch-Schönlein purpura, and polyarteritis nodosa. • Associated symptoms (fever) and signs (painful regional lymphadenopathy) assist in diagnosis and help to differentiate these disorders from ecthyma.
Cigarette burns	• History or findings on clinical examination often arouse suspicion for child abuse. • Lesions in various stages of healing commonly noted.

How to Make the Diagnosis

- The clinical findings usually lead to the correct diagnosis.
- Bacterial culture often reveals GABHS.
- Skin biopsy (usually unnecessary) shows an intense polymorphonuclear infiltrate and organisms on tissue Gram stain.

Treatment

- Systemic antibiotic therapy is the treatment of choice.
- The chosen antibiotic should have activity against GABHS and *S aureus* (because the latter is an occasional cause or may be present as a secondary infectious agent). Failure to respond to therapy indicates the need to review culture and sensitivity results for presence of methicillin-resistant *S aureus* or to reconsider the diagnosis.

Prognosis

- Because of the penetration into the dermis, ecthyma lesions often heal with permanent scarring.
- Rapid healing usually occurs with appropriate antibiotic therapy.

When to Worry or Refer

- Consider referral to a dermatologist for patients who have severe or extensive disease or do not respond to standard treatment.

Resources for Families

- MedlinePlus: Information for patients and families (in English and Spanish) sponsored by the National Library of Medicine and National Institutes of Health.
  www.nlm.nih.gov/medlineplus/ency/article/000864.htm

CHAPTER 26

Folliculitis/Furunculosis/Carbunculosis

Introduction/Etiology/Epidemiology

- Definitions
  - Folliculitis: superficial inflammation centered around a follicle
  - Furuncle: bacterial folliculitis of a single follicle that involves a deeper portion of the follicle
  - Carbuncle: bacterial folliculitis that involves the deeper portions of several contiguous follicles
- Types of folliculitis include
  - Bacterial folliculitis (the most common type) is most often caused by *Staphylococcus aureus.* While many of these isolates are still methicillin-sensitive *S aureus* (MSSA), some may be methicillin-resistant *S aureus* (MRSA).
  - Hot tub folliculitis is usually caused by gram-negative bacteria (most often *Pseudomonas aeruginosa*).
  - Gram-negative bacteria can also cause folliculitis in acne patients receiving long-term antibiotic therapy.
  - *Pityrosporum* (a yeast) may be a cause of folliculitis localized to the back, upper chest, shoulders, and upper arms.
  - *Demodex* (a skin mite) folliculitis presents as erythematous follicular papulopustules on the face, usually in immunocompromised hosts (eg, children receiving chemotherapy for leukemia).
- Predisposing conditions for furuncles and carbuncles include obesity, diabetes, and immunodeficiency, as well as warm, humid climates.

Signs and Symptoms

- Folliculitis is characterized by discrete follicular-centered pustules with surrounding erythema (Figures 26.1 and 26.2).
  - The most common locations are the buttocks and thighs, especially in young children.
  - Occasionally, folliculitis can be seen in areas that are subject to occlusion and irritation from clothing.
  - Lesions are most often painless; however, they can be mildly tender and are often pruritic.
  - Hot tub folliculitis often presents with localization of lesions to areas covered by the bathing garment.
- Furuncles/carbuncles present as erythematous papulonodules or nodules, often with a central punctum (Figure 26.3).
  - The central area tends to be the point where fluctuance will develop.
  - Pain is common, and fever may be present.
  - Pain diminishes following drainage of the lesion.

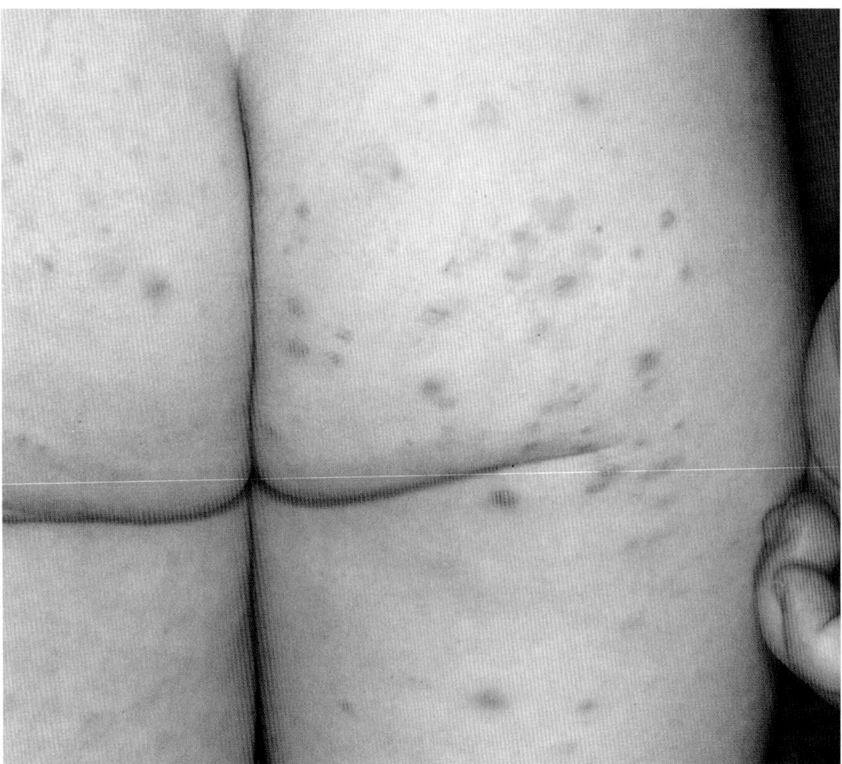

Figure 26.1. Folliculitis with erythematous papules and papulopustules of the buttocks.

- Skin and soft tissue infections due to community-acquired MRSA often present as furuncles and carbuncles.
  - Lesions typically are erythematous, fluctuant, and painful.
  - They may reveal purulent drainage.
  - Other family or household members may have (or previously have had) similar lesions.

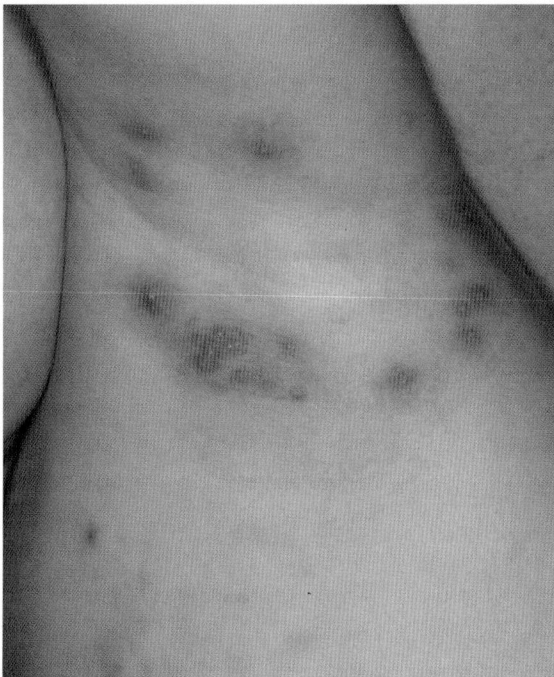

Figure 26.2. The lesions of folliculitis are erythematous papules and pustules centered around follicles.

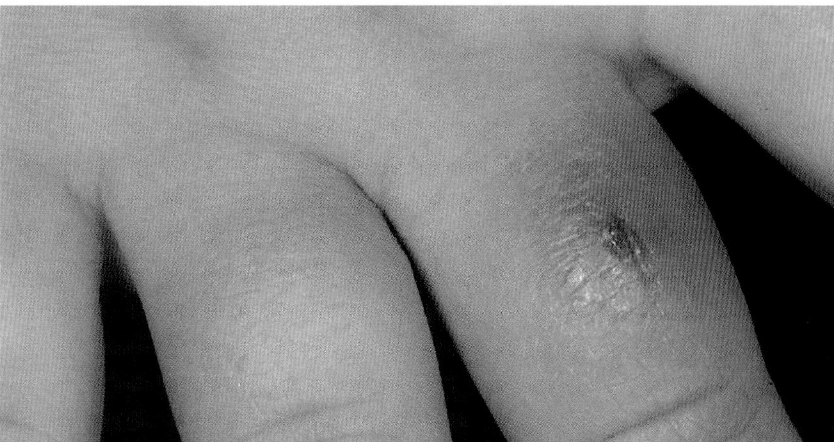

Figure 26.3. Furuncle. This nodular lesion may drain from the central portion.

Look-alikes

Disorder	Differentiating Features
Folliculitis from opportunistic organisms (especially in immunocompromised patients)	• Persistent despite appropriate therapy. • Patients with leukopenia may show less erythema than expected.
Viral exanthem	• Erythematous papules and macules. • Pustules usually lacking. • Lesions not centered around hair follicles. • Other symptoms (eg, upper respiratory, gastrointestinal) may be present.
Insect bites	• Usually have a central punctum present on close inspection • Most often occur on exposed areas • Extreme pruritus common • May see linear groupings ("breakfast, lunch, and dinner" sign) • Pustules rare • Lesions not centered around hair follicles
Acne nodule	• May look very similar to a carbuncle, but typical acne lesions (eg, open and closed comedones) usually also present • Lesions usually limited to face, chest, shoulders, and back
Hidradenitis suppurativa	• Recurrent papules, cysts, sinus tracts, and nodules that heal with scarring • Typically located in axillary and inguinal regions; occasionally involve posterior auricular area

How to Make the Diagnosis

- The diagnosis is usually made clinically.
- Skin swab for bacterial culture will usually reveal the causative agent.
- When furuncles or carbuncles are drained, a swab of the contents should be sent for bacterial culture and sensitivities.

Treatment

- Preventive measures include
  - Avoid tight-fitting clothing.
  - Lose weight (if applicable).
  - Use antibacterial cleansers that contain chlorhexidine (avoid ears) or triclosan (>18 months).
  - For nasal carriers of *S aureus*, intranasal mupirocin (for patient and family contacts) for 1 week may diminish recurrences.
  - Patients who are prone to frequent recurrences may benefit from bleach baths: ¼ to ½ cup of sodium hypochlorite solution (eg, Clorox liquid bleach) added to a full bathtub of water and used as a soak for 10 minutes once or twice weekly. Use of a sodium hypochlorite cleanser is another option.
- Treatment for folliculitis
  - Antibacterial skin cleansers, including chlorhexidine (avoid ears), sodium hypochlorite, or triclosan (>18 months).
  - Topical antibiotic for mild cases (eg, clindamycin, mupirocin, retapamulin).
  - Oral antistaphylococcal antibiotic (eg, cephalexin, dicloxacillin) for 7 to 10 days for severe cases. If MRSA is suspected or isolated, use of clindamycin, doxycycline (in children >8 years), trimethoprim-sulfamethoxazole, or another appropriate agent (as determined by antibiotic sensitivity testing) is indicated.
  - Culture of purulent material whenever possible.
- Treatment for furunculosis and carbunculosis
  - Warm, moist compresses to promote or facilitate drainage.
  - Incision and drainage may be necessary for larger or more fluctuant lesions or if the process is due to MRSA. Incision and drainage is recommended as initial therapy for MRSA-associated furuncles and carbuncles, with or without antibiotics.
  - Skin swab of pustular fluid should be sent for bacterial culture.
  - Oral antistaphylococcal antibiotic (eg, cephalexin, dicloxacillin) for 7 to 10 days for MSSA; if MRSA is suspected or isolated, use of clindamycin, doxycycline (in children >8 years), trimethoprim-sulfamethoxazole, or another appropriate agent (as determined by antibiotic sensitivity testing) is indicated.
  - Intermittent short courses of rifampin are recommended by some for patients with frequent or moderate to severe recurrences.

Prognosis

- In children with normal immunity the prognosis is excellent.
- Recurrence is common, especially in the continued presence of common risk factors.
- Immunocompromised individuals may have infections with unusual organisms that are more difficult to diagnose and treat.

When to Worry or Refer

- Consider referral to a dermatologist for patients who have severe or extensive disease or do not respond to standard treatments. If the patient develops a severe infection with MRSA that requires hospitalization, an infectious disease specialist should be consulted.

Resources for Families

- Centers for Disease Control and Prevention: Patient information on hot tub folliculitis.
  www.cdc.gov/healthywater/swimming/rwi/illnesses/hot-tub-rash.html
- MedlinePlus: Information for patients and families (in English and Spanish) sponsored by the National Library of Medicine and National Institutes of Health.
  www.nlm.nih.gov/medlineplus/ency/article/000823.htm
- Centers for Disease Control and Prevention: MRSA in health care settings. Has patient information materials.
  www.cdc.gov/mrsa

Impetigo

Introduction/Etiology/Epidemiology

- Impetigo is a superficial bacterial infection of the skin.
- In North America, the etiologic agent is primarily *Staphylococcus aureus.* In some cases, group A ß-hemolytic streptococcus may be cultured; however, it is most often present as a secondary agent. *Streptococcus* is the primary cause in only a small percentage of cases.
- Increased incidence in the summer is due to disruptions in the skin barrier from cuts, scrapes, and insect bites.

Signs and Symptoms

- Nonbullous (ie, crusted or common) impetigo: Initial lesion is a superficial vesicle that ruptures easily; exudate dries to form a honey-colored crust (Figure 27.1).
- Bullous impetigo: A superficial fragile bulla containing serous fluid or pus forms and then ruptures to form a round, very erythematous erosion, often with a surrounding collarette of scale (remnant of the blister roof) (Figure 27.2).
- Lesions tend to be located in exposed areas, especially the face and extremities.
- Diaper area involvement is common in infants.
- Lesions often spread due to autoinoculation.

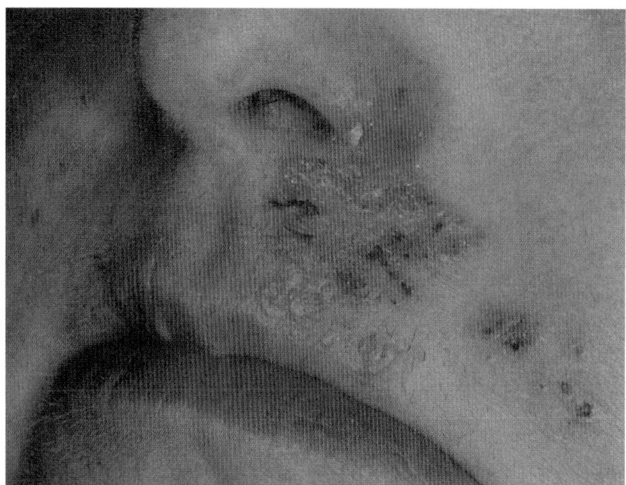

Figure 27.1. Nonbullous impetigo. Note honey-colored crusting.

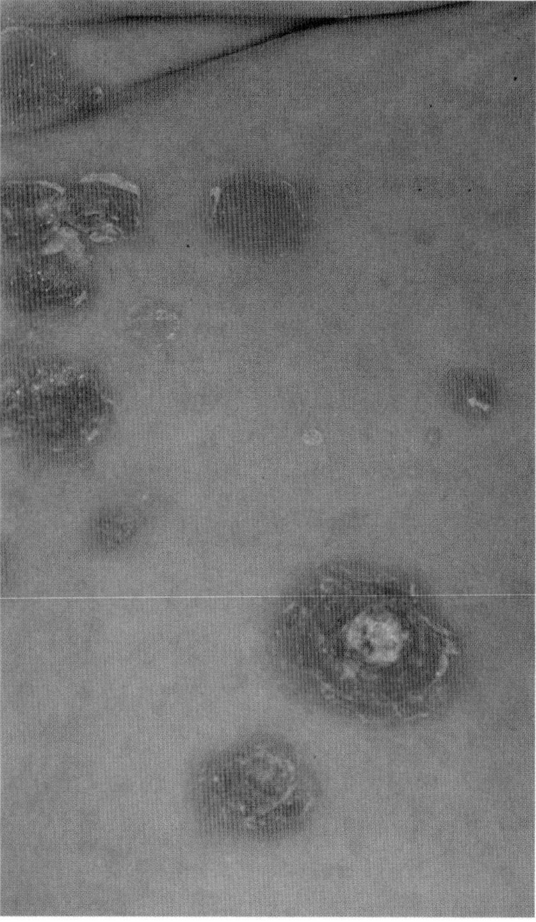

Figure 27.2. Bullous impetigo. A clear or pustular superficial bulla ruptures to form a round, very erythematous erosion, often with a surrounding collarette of scale (remnant of the blister roof).

Look-alikes

Disorder	Differentiating Features
Herpes simplex virus infection	• Clustered vesicles with surrounding erythema (ie, appear as on an erythematous base). • After vesicles rupture, ulcers form (deeper than the erosions observed in impetigo). • May occur inside the mouth or on other mucous membranes and usually painful.
Varicella-zoster virus infection	**Varicella** • Individual vesicles with surrounding erythema. • Rash begins on the trunk and then spreads to the extremities. • Rash tends to have symmetric distribution. • Mucous membranes often involved.
	Zoster • Clustered vesicles with surrounding erythema located in a dermatomal distribution • History of past acute varicella or varicella vaccination
Folliculitis	• Small follicular-centered pustules (1–2 mm) with rim of surrounding erythema. • Hair may be seen protruding from center of pustule (most easily visualized with side lighting).
Ecthyma	• Indurated, painful papules that have surrounding erythema • Often presents as punched-out, crusted, ulcerated papules • Usually caused by *Streptococcus pyogenes*
Contact dermatitis	• May be vesicles or bullae. • Itching commonly reported (not typical in impetigo). • Location of lesions corresponds to exposure to the contact allergen. • Configuration of lesions may be unusual (eg, linear in plant dermatitis).
Inflicted cigarette burns	• Uniform lesion size (around 8 mm) • Often located on the hands and feet • Usually heal with scarring • Often deeper in depth than impetigo

How to Make the Diagnosis

- The diagnosis is most often made based on the clinical findings.
- Gram stain of the contents of a vesicle or bulla demonstrates gram-positive cocci.
- Bacterial culture can assist in identifying the specific etiologic agent and antibiotic sensitivities.

Treatment

- For milder, localized cases of nonbullous impetigo, topical mupirocin or retapamulin can be applied 3 times daily for 5 to 7 days.
- When bullous impetigo is present or there is more widespread involvement in nonbullous impetigo, a 7- to 10-day course of a systemic antibiotic (eg, cephalexin) may be necessary, with attention to resistance patterns for each geographic location.
- Failure of response in 48 hours may be due to infection by methicillin-resistant *S aureus* and suggests the need for culture and a potential change of therapy to clindamycin, doxycycline (in children >8 years), trimethoprim-sulfamethoxazole, or another appropriate agent (as determined by results of antibiotic susceptibility testing).
- Warm water compresses can facilitate gentle debridement of the crusts.

Treating Associated Conditions

- Although uncommon, it is important to remember that if the impetigo is due to a nephritogenic strain of *S pyogenes*, acute glomerulonephritis can be a sequela.

Prognosis

- The prognosis for children with simple impetigo is good, and complete resolution is typical.

When to Worry or Refer

- Consider referral to a dermatologist for patients who have severe or extensive disease in whom the diagnosis is in question or for those who do not respond to standard treatment.

Resources for Families

- American Academy of Pediatrics: HealthyChildren.org.
  www.HealthyChildren.org/impetigo
- MedlinePlus: Information for patients and families (in English and Spanish) sponsored by the National Library of Medicine and National Institutes of Health.
  www.nlm.nih.gov/medlineplus/impetigo.html
- WebMD: Information for families is contained in the Health A-Z topics.
  www.webmd.com/skin-problems-and-treatments/guide/understanding-impetigo-basics

CHAPTER 28

Perianal Bacterial Dermatitis

Introduction/Etiology/Epidemiology

- Perianal bacterial dermatitis (formerly known as perianal streptococcal dermatitis) is a distinctive superficial cellulitis caused by group A ß-hemolytic streptococcus (GABHS) or *Staphylococcus aureus*.
- There is a male predominance, and the condition has a peak incidence of 3 to 4 years of age.
- Other family members may be similarly affected (especially if there is a history of co-bathing), or patient may have concomitant streptococcal pharyngitis.

Signs and Symptoms

- The typical presentation is that of intense perianal erythema (Figure 28.1), often with associated pruritus or burning.
- Maceration, exudate, fissuring, or desquamation may also be present.
- The border between affected and unaffected skin is usually distinct.
- Balanoposthitis or vulvovaginitis may also be present.
- Parents may report that the child has pain with defecation, stool-holding, blood-tinged stools, or increased irritability.
- Fever is rare.

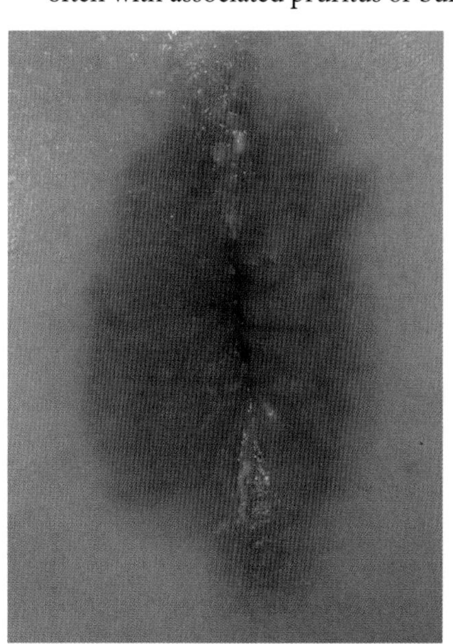

Figure 28.1. Perianal bacterial dermatitis is characterized by marked perianal erythema and purulent drainage.

Look-alikes

In each of the conditions listed herein, a bacterial culture would fail to demonstrate group A ß-hemolytic streptococcus.

Disorder	Differentiating Features
Candidiasis	• Erythema primarily involves the fold areas. • Satellite papules or papulopustules often present. • Exudate is white, often "cheesy" rather than purulent. • Typically painless and associated symptoms (eg, painful defecation) usually absent.
Psoriasis	• Sharply demarcated plaques. • Psoriasis lesions may be seen elsewhere (eg, umbilicus, scalp). • Family history may be positive for psoriasis. • Pitting of the nails may be present.
Seborrheic dermatitis	• Erythematous patches with greasy yellow scale • Other sites (eg, scalp, umbilicus, anterior diaper area) often affected without localization to just the perianal area
Irritant contact dermatitis	• May see lichenification from chronic scratching • Not usually as intensely red as perianal bacterial dermatitis • Usually lacks purulent drainage
Pinworm infestation (*Enterobius vermicularis*)	• Pruritus is the prominent symptom, especially at night. • May see worms with flashlight after child is sleeping. • May coexist with perianal bacterial dermatitis.
Lichen sclerosus et atrophicus	• Presents as hypopigmentation with atrophy of genital area, primarily in females. • "Cigarette-paper" wrinkling of the affected skin often present. • Tends to be distributed in an hourglass configuration (involving vulva, perineum, and perianal area). • Early disease may present with erythema, occasional bullae, or hemorrhage. • Dysuria may be reported.
Sexual abuse	• Lacerations may be evident, especially if the abuse was recent. • Bruising of the surrounding areas may be present. • Vulvovaginitis from gonococcal infection reveals drainage which is more greenish in color, usually malodorous.

How to Make the Diagnosis

- The diagnosis is suspected clinically and confirmed with bacterial skin culture.
- A specific request to the laboratory is usually necessary because routine processing of perianal swabs may involve inhibitors to the growth of GABHS.
- *Staphylococcus aureus* is becoming more frequent as the etiologic agent.

Treatment

- Oral penicillin or amoxicillin (erythromycin may be used if penicillin allergy) for 10 days, combined with topical antibiotics.
- Antistaphylococcal antibiotic may be necessary if caused by *S aureus;* the antibiotic selected should be guided by sensitivity testing results.

Treating Associated Conditions

- Vulvovaginitis or balanoposthitis, if present, usually responds to the same therapy.
- Guttate psoriasis may be associated with the condition and is treated with therapies typical for psoriasis. (See Papulosquamous Diseases [chapters 46–52].)

Prognosis

- The prognosis is excellent, usually with complete healing following therapy.
- More than one course of treatment is occasionally required.

When to Worry or Refer

- Consider referral to a dermatologist when the diagnosis is in doubt or when disease is severe or extensive or does not respond to standard treatment.
- If the history or examination findings are concerning for abuse, appropriate evaluation and reporting to child protective services is indicated.

Resource for Families

- MedlinePlus: Information for patients and families (in English and Spanish) sponsored by the National Library of Medicine and National Institutes of Health.
  www.nlm.nih.gov/medlineplus/ency/article/001346.htm

Skin Infections

Systemic Bacterial, Rickettsial, or Spirochetal Infections With Skin Manifestations

Lyme Disease

Introduction/Etiology/Epidemiology

- Caused by the spirochete *Borrelia burgdorferi.*
- Most common vector-borne disease in the United States.
- Three clinical stages
  - Early localized
  - Early disseminated
  - Late
- The infection occurs following a bite from a nymph tick. The most common tick vectors in the United States are
  - *Ixodes scapularis* (deer tick) in the East and Midwest
  - *Ixodes pacificus* (Western black-legged tick) in the West
- Incubation from tick bite to the appearance of erythema migrans ranges from 1 to 32 days (median 11 days).

Signs and Symptoms

- Early localized stage begins 7 to 14 days after the tick bite (range 1–32 days).
  - Erythema migrans is the first clinical manifestation of Lyme disease.
    - Appears at the site of the tick bite as an erythematous macule or papule.
    - Lesion expands rapidly to form a large (>5 cm), round erythematous patch often showing central clearing (ie, forming a ring) (Figure 29.1).
    - Bull's-eye appearance with concentric rings appears in a minority of cases.
  - Accompanying features include fever, malaise, headache, mild meningismus, myalgias, lymphadenopathy, and arthralgias.
- Early disseminated stage begins 3 to 5 weeks after the tick bite.
  - Multiple erythema migrans lesions are characteristic.
  - Intermittent migratory arthralgias and myalgias, headache (often severe), fatigue, conjunctivitis.

  - Neurologic manifestations, including peripheral and cranial neuropathy (most commonly seventh nerve or Bell palsy), lymphocytic meningitis.
  - Ophthalmologic manifestations, including uveitis, conjunctivitis, and optic neuritis, may occur.
  - Carditis leading to atrioventricular conduction defects occurs rarely in children.
- Late disease begins weeks to months after the tick bite.
  - Arthritis, usually monoarticular or oligoarticular, particularly in large joints. Joint swelling often is out of proportion to the degree of pain or disability.
  - Encephalopathy, encephalomyelitis, peripheral neuropathy.
  - Skin manifestations may include lymphocytoma cutis and acrodermatitis chronica atrophicans.

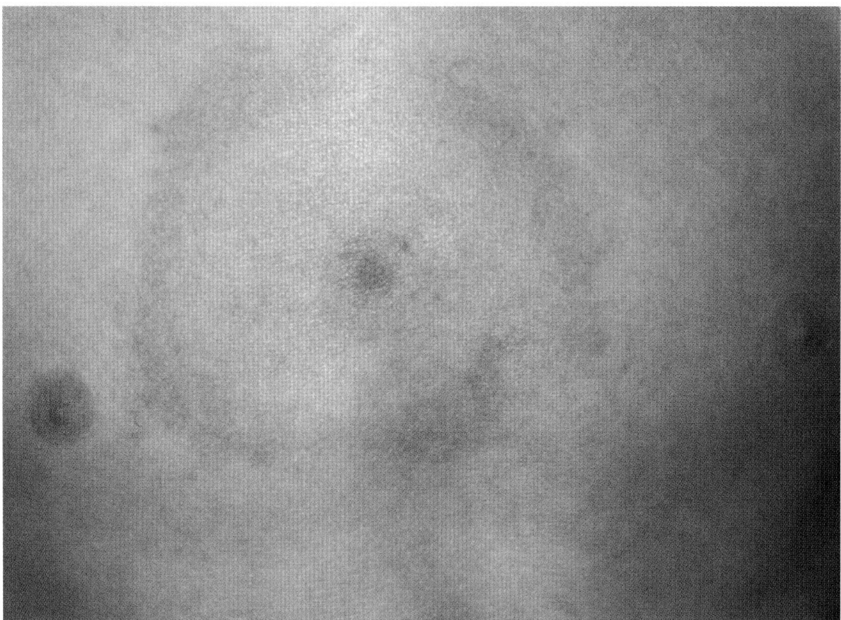

Figure 29.1. Annular erythema migrans lesion of Lyme disease.

Look-alikes (Differential Diagnosis of Erythema Migrans)

Disorder	Differentiating Features
Erythema multiforme	• Lesions are smaller than erythema migrans and multiple target lesions present, especially on the extremities, palms, and soles. • Lesions may develop a vesicular center.
Fixed drug eruption	• Often dusky purple to hyperpigmented patch or plaque. • Central erosion may be present. • Recur in same location with each exposure to offending agent.
Tinea corporis	• Presents as an annular red plaque (palpable), not patch • Scale usually present
Urticaria	• Multiple lesions nearly always present. • Lesions come and go quickly (usually within hours). • Presents as erythematous wheals, often arcuate or annular in appearance. • Usually pruritic.
Arthropod bites	• Multiple lesions often present. • Pruritus very common, often severe. • Edematous papules or papulovesicles, not rings. • Papules may be clustered in linear groupings ("breakfast, lunch, and dinner" sign).

How to Make the Diagnosis

- The diagnosis of Lyme disease is usually suggested clinically based on the appearance of erythema migrans, especially when history of a tick bite is present.
- Recognition that a tick bite occurred is very uncommon because the nymphs are tiny.
- Antibody testing using enzyme immunoassay or immunofluorescent antibody assay with confirmation of equivocal or positive results by Western immunoblotting (IgG and IgM) can establish the diagnosis.
  - However, antibody tests may be falsely negative in early localized disease and, for this reason, testing is not recommended for children who have erythema migrans.

Treatment

- Early localized disease is treated with doxycycline (if the patient is ≥8 years) for 14 days. In children younger than 8 years, amoxicillin or cefuroxime are the agents of choice; response is often slow, over several weeks.
- Early disseminated or late disease is treated with the same oral regimen as early localized disease. Treatment duration ranges from 14 to 28 days depending on the clinical manifestation (eg, 14 days for multiple erythema migrans; 28 days for arthritis). If persistent or recurrent arthritis, carditis, or meningitis is present, oral or intravenous therapy may be used, including ceftriaxone (alternatives: penicillin and cefotaxime) with treatment lengths varying based on specific clinical manifestations. Encephalitis and other neurologic manifestations require intravenous therapy for 14 to 28 days. (Consult an infectious disease specialist or the most recent edition of *Red Book: Report of the Committee on Infectious Diseases,* **www.aapredbook.org,** for assistance in management of these complications.)
- Tick avoidance is important for prevention.

Treating Associated Conditions

- A subset of treated patients may continue to have arthralgia and fatigue, a condition known as posttreatment Lyme disease syndrome. The cause of this condition is unknown but has not been linked to ongoing infection, and long-term antibiotic therapy has not been shown to be effective.

Prognosis

- The prognosis for children with Lyme disease is excellent when it is diagnosed early and treated promptly.

When to Worry or Refer

- Consider referral to a dermatologist or infectious disease specialist for patients who have atypical or persistent findings or who do not respond to standard treatment.

Resources for Families

- American Academy of Pediatrics: HealthyChildren.org.
  www.HealthyChildren.org/lymedisease
- American Lyme Disease Foundation: Provides information about Lyme disease (in English and Spanish) and supports research into the disease.
  www.aldf.com
- Centers for Disease Control and Prevention: Learn about Lyme disease.
  www.cdc.gov/lyme
- LymeNet (Lyme Disease Network): Nonprofit organization that provides information about Lyme disease and links to support groups.
  www.lyme.net
- MedlinePlus: Information for patients and families (in English and Spanish) sponsored by the National Library of Medicine and National Institutes of Health.
  www.nlm.nih.gov/medlineplus/lymedisease.html

Meningococcemia

Introduction/Etiology/Epidemiology

- Caused by *Neisseria meningitidis.*
- Leading cause of bacterial meningitis in children aged 11 to 17 years in the United States.
- Transmission via respiratory droplets or direct/indirect oral contact.
- Approximately two-thirds of patients with meningococcemia will develop cutaneous manifestations.
- Incubation period is 1 to 10 days.

Signs and Symptoms

- Symptoms
  - At the outset, symptoms may mimic a viral illness (eg, fever, myalgias, headache, malaise). Early findings in young children may include leg pain, cold hands and feet, and abnormal skin color.
  - May have associated meningitis with headache, photophobia, vomiting, and nuchal rigidity.
- Cutaneous findings
  - Early on there are erythematous, urticarial, or morbilliform macules and papules.
  - Petechiae, pustules, and vesicles often develop.
  - Purpuric lesions with jagged edges (Figure 30.1) may occur; may progress to necrosis, ulcers, and eschar.
  - Conjunctivae and retinae may reveal petechiae.
- Patients may develop profound hypotension and shock with overwhelming meningococcemia.
- Disseminated intravascular coagulation (DIC) (Figure 30.2) may occur and, when present along with purpuric and necrotic plaques, is termed purpura fulminans.

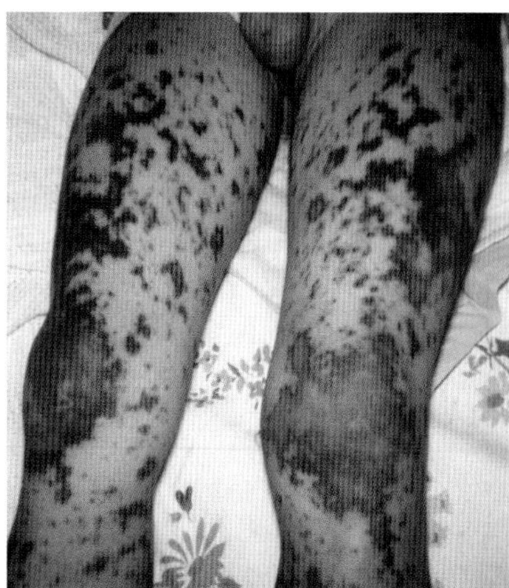

Figure 30.1. Meningococcemia. Purpuric plaques with jagged borders and early necrosis.

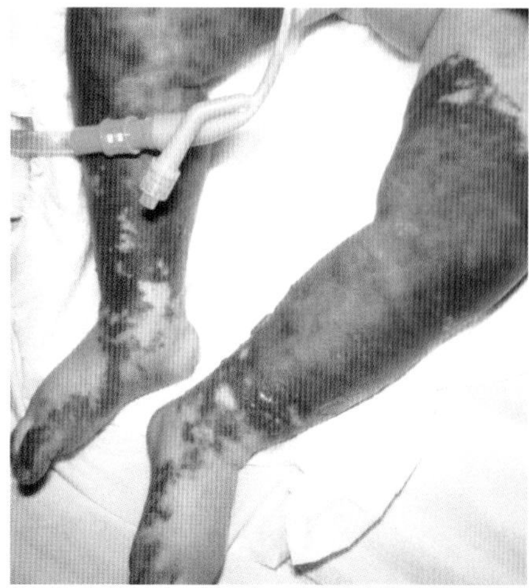

Figure 30.2. Meningococcemia. Disseminated intravascular coagulation.

Look-alikes

In each of the disorders listed herein, bacterial cultures will be negative or will not reveal *Neisseria meningitidis.*

Disorder	Differentiating Features
Gonococcemia	• May have petechiae or pustules, but they tend to be fewer in number than in meningococcemia. • Arthritis or arthralgias are present. • Patients usually appear less ill.
Rocky Mountain spotted fever	• History of tick bite may be elicited. • Patients initially appear less toxic than those who have meningococcemia. • Rash characteristically begins on the palms and soles as petechial macules and papules and then spreads centrally. • Severe headache common.
Henoch-Schönlein purpura	• Petechiae or palpable purpura most pronounced in dependent areas. • Edema common. • If fever present, usually low grade. • Gastrointestinal and joint complaints common. • Nephritis may be present.
Other bacteremias (eg, *Streptococcus pneumoniae, Haemophilus influenzae* type b, gram-negative)	• Organisms seen on Gram stain of petechiae, buffy coat, or cerebrospinal fluid • Blood culture results

How to Make the Diagnosis

- Culture of the blood and cerebrospinal fluid (CSF) are confirmatory.
- Antigen detection tests performed on CSF can be helpful but are not recommended for use with serum or urine specimens.

Treatment

- Supportive therapy, including fluids and vasoactive agents, as needed.
- Empiric therapy with ceftriaxone or cefotaxime is recommended. Once a microbiological diagnosis is established, intravenous penicillin G is recommended at a dose of 300,000 U/kg per day up to a maximum of 12 million units per day divided every 4 to 6 hours. Cefotaxime, ceftriaxone, and ampicillin are acceptable alternatives. In a patient with anaphylactic penicillin allergy, chloramphenicol is recommended if available. If chloramphenicol is not available, meropenem can be used, recognizing that the rate of cross-reactivity in penicillin-allergic adults is 2% to 3%. Consultation with a pediatric infectious disease specialist or the most recent *Red Book: Report of the Committee on Infectious Diseases* (**www.aapredbook.org**) is recommended.
- Intermediate penicillin resistance is an increasing concern (especially in travelers from areas where penicillin resistance has been reported); as a result, some recommend using ceftriaxone, cefotaxime, or chloramphenicol until susceptibilities are available.
- A quadrivalent conjugate meningococcal vaccine immunization is now routinely recommended at age 11 years. It can be used to prevent infection in high-risk groups from age 9 months to 55 years.

Treating Associated Conditions

- If the patient develops DIC, appropriate therapeutic measures should be instituted.
- Close contacts within 7 days prior to onset of illness (eg, household, child care, slept or ate in same dwelling) should receive chemoprophylaxis.

Prognosis

- The mortality for invasive meningococcemia is approximately 8% to 10%.

When to Worry or Refer

- Patients with a presumed or confirmed diagnosis of meningococcemia should be evaluated in conjunction with an infectious disease specialist.

Resources for Families

- Centers for Disease Control and Prevention. Meningococcal disease.
  www.cdc.gov/meningococcal
- MedlinePlus: Information for patients and families (in English and Spanish) sponsored by the National Library of Medicine and National Institutes of Health.
  www.nlm.nih.gov/medlineplus/ency/article/001349.htm
- National Meningitis Association: Site established by parents of children who died of meningitis. Provides information about meningitis.
  www.nmaus.org

CHAPTER
31

Rocky Mountain Spotted Fever (RMSF)

Introduction/Etiology/Epidemiology

- The most common rickettsial infection in the United States.
- Caused by *Rickettsia rickettsii,* transmitted to humans by a tick bite.
- Tick vectors are dog ticks and wood ticks in different geographic areas of the United States.
- Typically, there is a history of tick exposure (no history of tick bite in about half of pediatric cases), and transmission parallels the tick season (highest incidence April–September).
- Although it occurs in children, it is more common in adults due to occupational exposure (eg, forest rangers, outdoor workers).
- Incubation period is 2 to 14 days.
- Rapidly progressive (and potentially fatal) if not recognized, diagnosed, and treated early.

Signs and Symptoms

- Prodromal symptoms include
  - Malaise, myalgias
  - Headache (may be severe)
  - Nausea and vomiting
  - Photophobia
- Subsequently, fever and rash develop.
- May present with prolonged capillary refill, weak pulses, or frank shock.

- Exanthem is present in approximately 80% to 90% of patients.
  - Lesions are initially non-pruritic erythematous macules and papules occurring on the wrists and ankles (Figure 31.1).
  - Lesions then spread centripetally (Figure 31.2) and distally to the palms and soles (see Figure 31.1).
  - The lesions evolve into petechial or purpuric macules and papules.
  - Larger areas of purpura or necrosis may occur.
- Patients may develop multisystem disease (central nervous system, cardiac, pulmonary, renal) and disseminated intravascular coagulation (DIC).

Look-alikes

Note: history of tick bite absent in each of the following diagnoses:

Disorder	Differentiating Features
Meningococcemia	• Disease typically has abrupt onset with fever, myalgia, limb pain, prostration. • Papular, petechial, and purpuric lesions. • Meningeal signs may be present. • Hypotension, shock, DIC may develop rapidly.
Henoch-Schönlein purpura	• Petechiae or palpable purpura most pronounced in dependent areas. • Lesions tend to be larger than those seen in RMSF. • Edema common. • If fever present, usually low grade. • Gastrointestinal and joint complaints common. • Nephritis may be present.
Other bacteremias (eg, *Streptococcus pneumoniae*, *Haemophilus influenzae* type b, gram-negative)	• Organisms seen on Gram stain of petechiae, buffy coat, or cerebrospinal fluid. • Culture of organisms from a normally sterile site establishes the diagnosis.
Gonococcemia	• May have petechiae, but they tend to be fewer in number than in RMSF. • Arthritis or arthralgias are present. • Patients usually appear less ill.
Atypical measles	• Seen in individuals exposed to natural measles after receiving killed virus vaccinations. • High fever, headache, and myalgias; pneumonia and pleural effusions may also be present. • Hemorrhagic exanthem, which may be similar to RMSF.

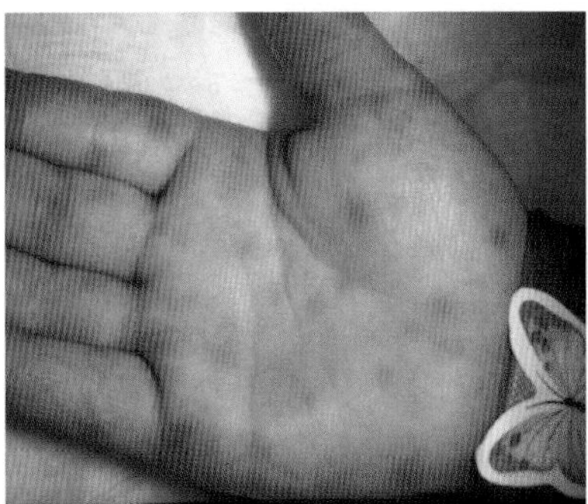

Figure 31.1. Rocky Mountain spotted fever. Note erythematous petechial macules on the palm.

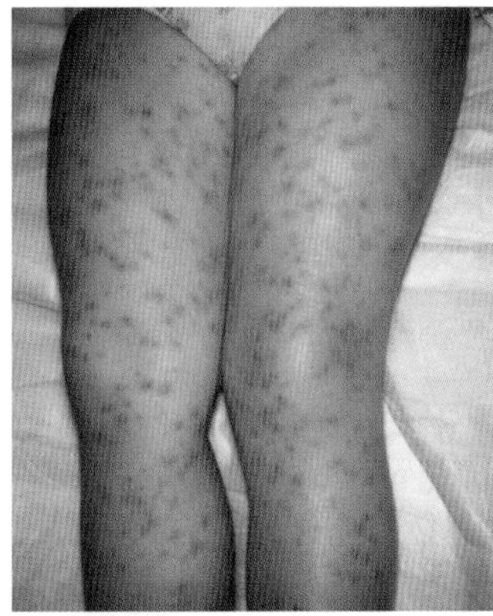

Figure 31.2. Rocky Mountain spotted fever with petechial lesions of the legs.

How to Make the Diagnosis

- The diagnosis is made clinically (and treatment initiated based on clinical information) and then confirmed by diagnostic testing.
  - A negative serologic test result from the acute phase of the disease does not exclude RMSF because IgM and IgG antibodies begin to rise 7 to 10 days after the onset of symptoms.
  - A 4-fold or greater change in IgG titer between acute- and convalescent-phase titers (obtained 2–6 weeks apart) is diagnostic when determined by immunofluorescent antibody assay, enzyme immunoassay, complement fixation, latex agglutination, indirect hemagglutination, or microagglutination tests.
  - Immunofluorescent antibody assay is the gold-standard serologic test.
- Biopsy shows a mononuclear infiltrate with fibrin and thrombi; immunohistochemical stains may reveal the organism
- Early laboratory findings may include thrombocytopenia, increased number of band forms (with normal or only slightly elevated white blood cell count), elevated liver transaminases, or hyponatremia.

Treatment

- Supportive therapy may be necessary, including fluids and vasoactive agents.
- Treatment should be started as soon as the diagnosis is suspected (prior to diagnostic confirmation).
- Doxycycline is the drug of choice for children of any age. The risk of dental staining from doxycycline (which may be less than the risk with other tetracyclines) in children younger than 8 years is outweighed by the risks of morbidity without treatment.
- Treatment is given until the patient has been afebrile for 3 days and has shown clinical improvement. The usual duration of therapy is 7 to 10 days.

Prognosis

- The prognosis for children with RMSF is good when diagnosed and treated early.
- Mortality rates are highest in males, people older than 50 years, children 5 to 9 years of age, and those with no history of a tick bite.

When to Worry or Refer

- Consultation with an infectious disease specialist is warranted for any patient with a presumed or confirmed diagnosis of RMSF.

Resources for Families

- Centers for Disease Control and Prevention: Patient information. **www.cdc.gov/rmsf**
- MedlinePlus: Information for patients and families (in English and Spanish) sponsored by the National Library of Medicine and National Institutes of Health. **www.nlm.nih.gov/medlineplus/ency/article/000654.htm**
- WebMD: Information for families is contained in the Health A-Z topics. **www.webmd.com/skin-problems-and-treatments/rocky-mountain-spotted-fever**

Scarlet Fever

Introduction/Etiology/Epidemiology

- The association of an exanthem (toxin-mediated) and group A ß-hemolytic streptococcal (ie, *Streptococcus pyogenes*) pharyngitis.
- Rarely, the eruption can be associated with a group A ß-hemolytic streptococcal infection of a surgical wound, termed surgical scarlet fever.
- The eruption is also known as scarlatina.
- Etiology is pyrogenic A, B, C, and F exotoxin-producing *S pyogenes.*
- Age group most affected is 4 to 8 years.

Signs and Symptoms

- Fever.
- Pharyngitis, including erythema of the posterior pharynx, tonsillar exudates, and soft palate petechiae.
- Tender cervical lymphadenopathy.
- Headache and malaise are common.
- Skin eruption presents as discrete pinpoint erythematous papules, sometimes likened to the consistency of sandpaper (sandpaper rash) (Figure 32.1).
- Occasionally, small vesicles (miliary sudamina) may be seen on the abdomen, hands, and feet.
- Skin eruption is accentuated in fold areas (Pastia lines with confluent petechiae in folds may also be present) (Figure 32.2) and circumoral pallor is commonly present.
- The tongue initially has a white coating ("white strawberry tongue") and later reveals prominent papillae and hyperemia ("red strawberry tongue") (Figure 32.3).

- Desquamation is often noted in the perineal area during the acute infection, and peripheral desquamation (eg, affecting the hands and fingers) is seen 2 to 3 weeks after the onset of illness (Figure 32.4).
- A mild form of staphylococcal scalded skin syndrome (staphylococcal scarlet fever) may present with an identical rash, but the strawberry tongue and palatal enanthem of streptococcal scarlet fever are absent.

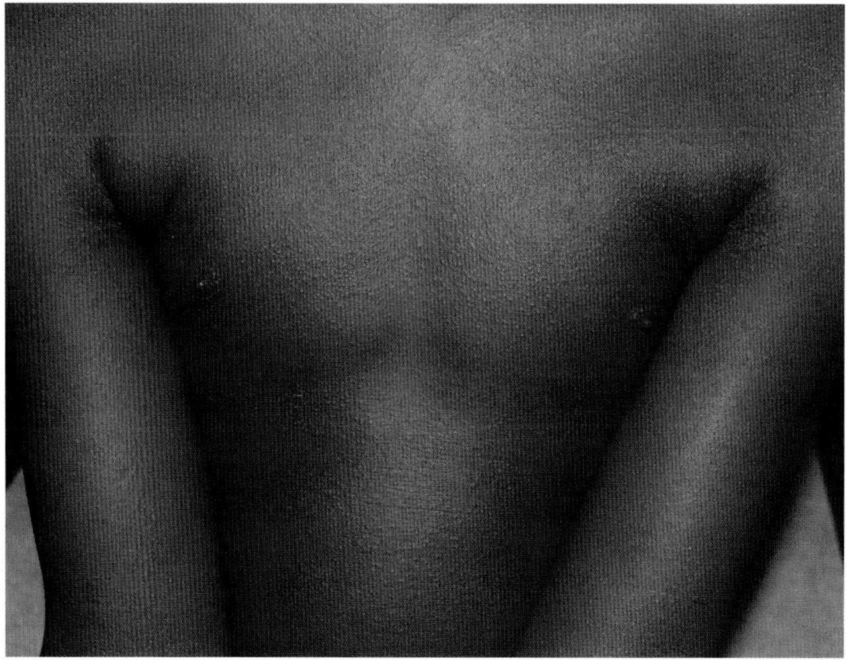

Figure 32.1. The rash of scarlet fever is composed of tiny papules.

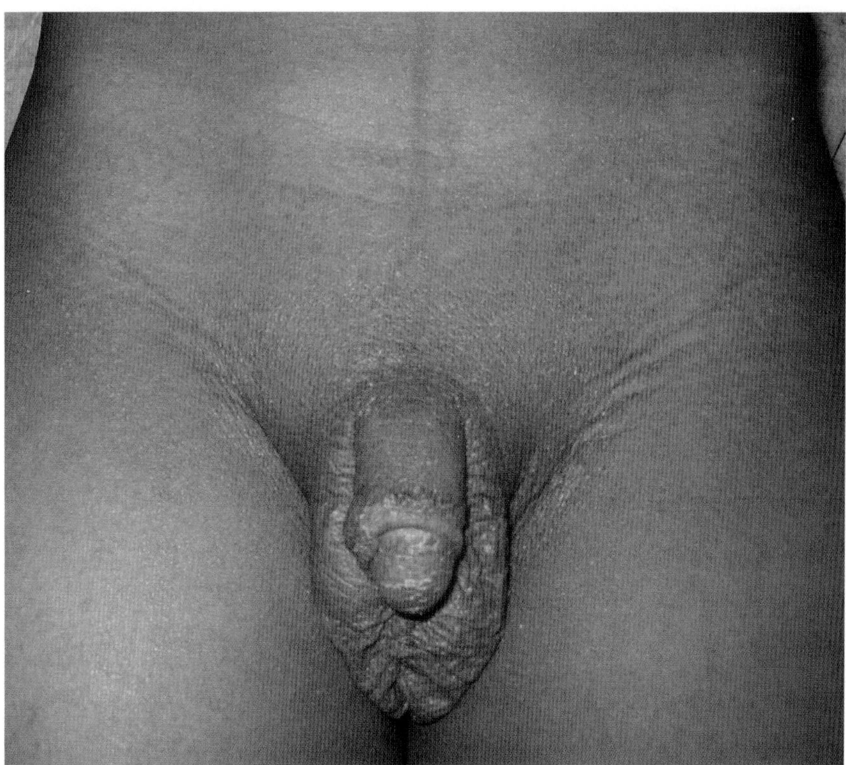

Figure 32.2. In scarlet fever, the rash often is accentuated in skinfolds.

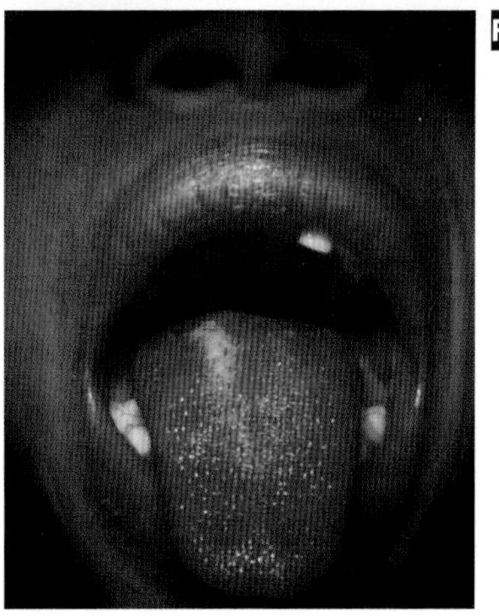

Figure 32.3. Scarlet fever. Red strawberry tongue.

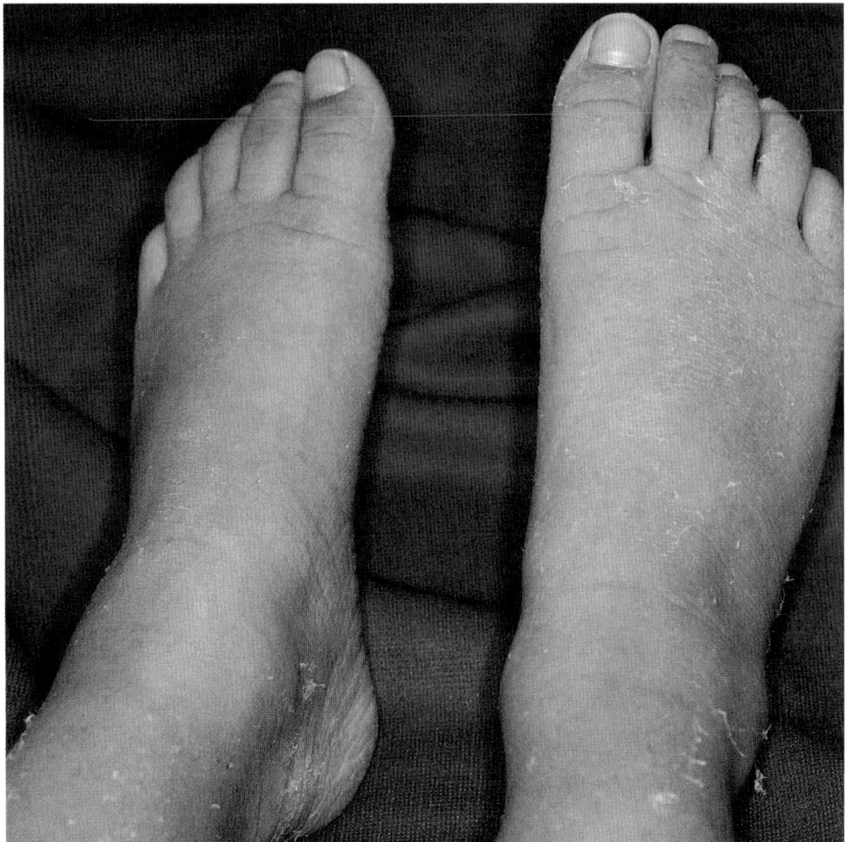

Figure 32.4. Scarlet fever, with desquamation of the ankles and feet in a 5-year-old girl receiving antibiotic therapy.

Look-alikes

In each of the disorders listed below, testing for pharyngeal infection with *S pyogenes* would be negative.

Disorder	Differentiating Features
Staphylococcal scarlet fever	• Rash identical to that of streptococcal scarlet fever • Strawberry tongue and palatal petechiae absent
Staphylococcal scalded skin syndrome	• Erythema more widespread • Bullae form, with subsequent rupture, peeling, and moist, denuded painful areas • Oral mucous membranes usually spared
Toxic shock syndrome (TSS)	• Patients appear more ill. • Hypotension and multiorgan involvement present. • Conjunctival injection seen in TSS, usually absent in scarlet fever.
Kawasaki disease	• Associated with prolonged high fever and classic constellation of clinical signs. • Skin eruption polymorphous but not typically sandpaper-like. • Oral changes consist primarily of hyperemia with lip fissuring; pharyngitis and pharyngeal symptoms absent. • Nonpurulent conjunctival injection usually seen.
Infectious mononucleosis	• May be clinically similar to scarlet fever. • Reactive lymphocytosis often present. • Hepatosplenomegaly may be present. • Exanthem may appear or accentuate following administration of amoxicillin or ampicillin.
Arcanobacterium haemolyticum infection	• Similar clinical presentation to scarlet fever, but palatal petechiae and strawberry tongue are usually absent. • Typically affects teenagers or young adults. • If seeking diagnostic confirmation, laboratory should be notified to ensure throat swab specimen is plated on appropriate media.
Parvovirus B19 infection	• May mimic early scarlet fever. • Slapped cheek eruption may mimic circumoral pallor. • Pharyngitis mild or absent. • Eruption lacy and reticulated, not sandpaper-like.

How to Make the Diagnosis

- The diagnosis of scarlet fever is most often made clinically.
- A rapid streptococcal test or pharyngeal culture will confirm the diagnosis.
- When both are negative with a typical clinical picture, consider staphylococcal scarlet fever, infectious mononucleosis, or *Arcanobacterium haemolyticum* infection (especially if adolescent).

Treatment

- The treatment of scarlet fever is the same as that for streptococcal pharyngitis (ie, penicillin V or amoxicillin divided 2 to 3 times daily for 10 days). However, oral amoxicillin given as a single daily dose for 10 days is as effective as penicillin V given 3 times daily for 10 days.
- Azithromycin, clarithromycin, erythromycin, or clindamycin may be used in penicillin-allergic patients.
- Intramuscular penicillin G benzathine, given in a single dose, is an appropriate alternative, particularly in children who are vomiting or in whom compliance is uncertain.

Treating Associated Conditions

- Acute rheumatic fever and acute glomerulonephritis are possible non-suppurative sequelae of *S pyogenes* infections; the former is usually prevented with adequate treatment of the antecedent streptococcal infection.
- If a streptococcal strain associated with rheumatic fever has been detected in a community, patients should be observed for rheumatic fever symptoms.

Prognosis

- The prognosis is excellent, and most children recover fully without any long-term sequelae.

When to Worry or Refer

- Consider referral to a dermatologist for patients who have an exanthem with atypical features or who do not respond to standard treatment.

Resources for Families

- American Academy of Pediatrics: HealthyChildren.org.
www.HealthyChildren.org/GroupAStrept
- MedlinePlus: Information for patients and families (in English and Spanish) sponsored by the National Library of Medicine and National Institutes of Health.
www.nlm.nih.gov/medlineplus/streptococcalinfections.html
- WebMD: Information for families is contained in the Health A-Z topics.
www.webmd.com/a-to-z-guides/understanding-scarlet-fever-basics

Staphylococcal Scalded Skin Syndrome (SSSS)

Introduction/Etiology/Epidemiology

- Caused by an exfoliative toxin A and B produced by *Staphylococcus aureus*, most often from phage group 2.
- The toxin is spread hematogenously from the primary site of infection; it causes a cleavage in the granular layer of the epidermis that leads to bullae formation.
- Most often seen in children younger than 5 years.
- When seen in older children, it is more often mild unless occurring in the setting of renal insufficiency or immunocompromise.

Signs and Symptoms

- Patients present with generalized erythema (often described as scarlatiniform), tender skin, and irritability.
- Fever is occasionally, but not always, present.
- Flaccid bullae form, especially in intertriginous areas (Figure 33.1).
- Bullae rupture easily and produce large eroded areas surrounded by collarettes of skin (that represent the remnants of the blister roof).
- Nikolsky sign is present (lateral pressure on the skin causes a bulla to enlarge or an erosion to form).
- Crusting is present around the mouth, often with radial fissuring (ie, a "sunburst" appearance) (Figure 33.2).
- Common initial sites of infection include conjunctivae, nares, perioral area, and (in neonates) the umbilical region or an infected circumcision site.
- Oral mucous membrane changes are classically absent, but purulent conjunctivitis often is present.
- With healing, there is widespread desquamation.

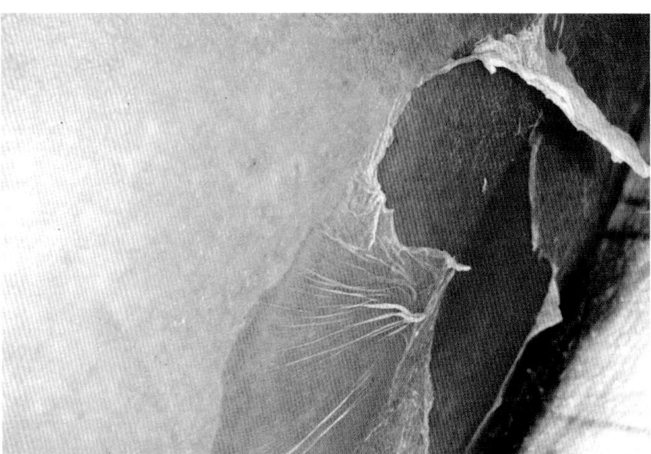

Figure 33.1. Staphylococcal scalded skin syndrome. Flaccid bullae form and rupture rapidly.

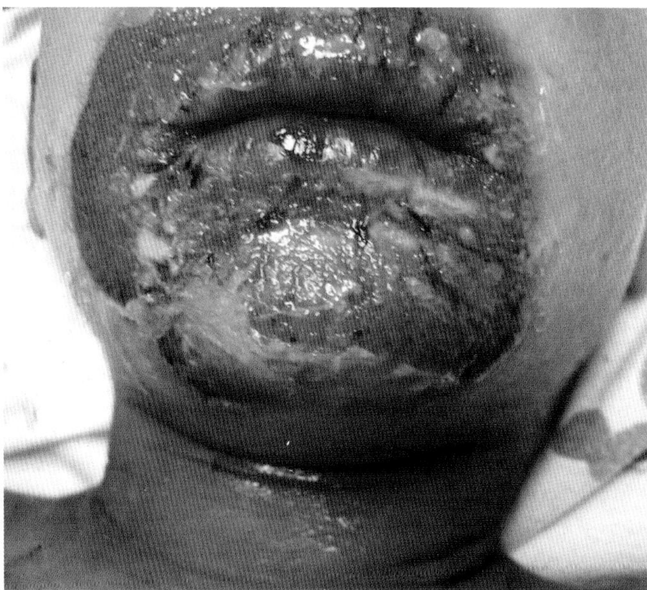

Figure 33.2. In staphylococcal scalded skin syndrome, erosions around the mouth often take on a "sunburst" appearance.

Look-alikes

Disorder	Differentiating Features
Streptococcal scarlet fever	• Eruption composed of fine papules (not diffuse macular erythema) • Blisters and erosions not present
Bullous impetigo	• Discrete and localized bullae. • Widespread erythema not present. • Patients appear well. • Fever usually absent.
Cellulitis	• Typically presents as ill-defined localized indurated plaque (The remainder of the skin looks normal.) • May be edematous, but blister formation rarely occurs
Stevens-Johnson syndrome	• Blisters more tense and more discrete. • Typical target lesions may be present, with involvement of the palms and soles. • Erosions of the mucous membranes are present. • Widespread erosions unusual. • Frozen section of blister roof reveals full-thickness epidermis (only a few cell layers in SSSS). • History of herpes simplex virus or mycoplasma infection may be present.
Toxic shock syndrome	• Patients appear quite ill. • Hypotension and multiorgan involvement. • Skin blistering and denudation not typically seen. • Conjunctival injection present.
Kawasaki disease	• Associated with a prolonged high fever and classic constellation of clinical signs • Erythema not usually as widespread • Skin eruption polymorphous but not typically bullous or denuded • Oral changes common, including hyperemia with lip fissuring • Nonpurulent conjunctival bulbar injection usually seen
Immersion burn	• Not generalized; buttocks or lower extremities usually involved • Intertriginous areas spared • History incompatible with child's development or examination findings

How to Make the Diagnosis

- A history of contact with a staphylococcus-infected individual, especially in the setting of a community epidemic, may be present.
- Bullae are sterile, but culture from an initial site of infection or colonization may be positive for *S aureus*.
- Frozen section of a blister roof will confirm skin separation at the granular layer.

Treatment

- Oral systemic antistaphylococcal antibiotic for mild cases.
- Neonates and children with severe disease or who are toxic in appearance should receive parenteral therapy with antibiotics adequate to cover methicillin-resistant *S aureus* (eg, often a bactericidal agent like vancomycin or nafcillin combined with clindamycin [to reduce toxin production]).
- For those with severe disease and widespread erosions, closely monitor fluid and electrolyte status.

Treating Associated Conditions

- In patients with widespread denudation, fluid and electrolyte status should be closely monitored.
- If concomitant staphylococcal bacteremia is present, hospitalization with intravenous therapy is necessary. (See Treatment for details.)

Prognosis

- The prognosis for children with SSSS is generally good.
- Skin generally heals without scarring within 2 weeks.
- Neonates have an increased risk of morbidity and mortality.

When to Worry or Refer

- Consider referral to a dermatologist or infectious disease specialist for patients who have an atypical presentation or who do not respond to standard treatment.
- Patients with severe or widespread disease and neonates with SSSS should be hospitalized for observation, parenteral fluid administration, and antimicrobial therapy.

Resources for Families

- American Academy of Pediatrics: HealthyChildren.org. **https://www.healthychildren.org/English/health-issues/conditions/infections/Pages/Staphylococcal-Infections.aspx**
- Mayo Clinic: Staph infections. **www.mayoclinic.org/diseases-conditions/staph-infections/basics/definition/CON-20031418?p=1**

CHAPTER 34

Toxic Shock Syndrome (TSS)

Introduction/Etiology/Epidemiology

- A constellation of symptoms including fever, rash, hypotension (or orthostatic hypotension or syncope), and multiorgan dysfunction.
- Caused by toxin-producing *Staphylococcus aureus* or *Streptococcus pyogenes.*
- Staphylococcal TSS is most often caused by TSS toxin 1, a superantigen that stimulates production of tumor necrosis factor and other inflammatory mediators.
- Streptococcal TSS is caused by one of several exotoxins. (See Look-alikes for discussion of streptococcal TSS.)
- Toxin is produced by organisms particularly in suppurative sites, such as surgical wound infections or skin and soft tissue infections. Classically, staphylococcal TSS was associated with the use of superabsorbent tampons. The site of primary infection may not be immediately evident.

Signs and Symptoms

- The case definitions for staphylococcal and streptococcal TSS are presented in Table 34.1.
- Mucocutaneous findings in TSS
  - Generalized macular erythema (Figure 34.1)
  - Conjunctival injection
  - Necrolysis (necrosis with exfoliation)
  - Multiple pustules
  - Desquamation (seen 1–2 weeks following the onset of disease)

Table 34.1. Diagnostic Criteria for Staphylococcal and Streptococcal Toxic Shock Syndrome

Staphylococcal Toxic Shock Syndrome	Streptococcal Toxic Shock Syndrome
Clinical Findings • Fever: temperature ≥38.9°C • Rash: diffuse macular erythroderma • Desquamation: 1 to 2 weeks after onset (especially palms, soles, fingers, toes) • Hypotension: systolic blood pressure ≤90 for adults and <5th percentile for age for children <16 years, or orthostatic changes (blood pressure decline, syncope, dizziness) • Involvement of 3 or more of the following systems: – Gastrointestinal: vomiting or diarrhea – Muscular: severe myalgia or creatine kinase greater than twice the upper limit of normal – Mucous membrane hyperemia – Renal: sterile pyuria; blood urea nitrogen or creatinine greater than twice the upper limit of normal – Hepatic: total bilirubin, aspartate aminotransferase, or alanine aminotransferase greater than twice the upper limit of normal – Hematologic: platelet count ≤100,000/mm^3 – Central nervous system: disorientation, altered consciousness without focal neurologic signs	**I. Isolation of group A streptococcus** A. From a normally sterile site (eg, blood, cerebrospinal fluid, peritoneal fluid, tissue biopsy specimen) B. From a nonsterile site (eg, throat, sputum, vagina, open surgical wound, skin lesion) **II. Clinical signs of severity** A. Hypotension: systolic blood pressure ≤90 for adults and <5th percentile for age for children AND B. Two or more of the following signs: • Renal impairment: creatinine concentration ≥2 mg/dL for adults or at least 2 times the upper limit of normal for age • Coagulopathy: platelet count ≤100,000/mm^3 or disseminated intravascular coagulation • Hepatic involvement: total bilirubin, aspartate aminotransferase, or alanine aminotransferase greater than twice the upper limit of normal for age • Adult respiratory distress syndrome • A generalized erythematous macular rash that may desquamate • Soft tissue necrosis, including necrotizing fasciitis or myositis, or gangrene

Table 34.1. Diagnostic Criteria for Staphylococcal and Streptococcal Toxic Shock Syndrome *(continued)*

Staphylococcal Toxic Shock Syndrome	Streptococcal Toxic Shock Syndrome
Laboratory Criteria • Negative results on the following tests if performed: – Blood, throat, or cerebrospinal fluid cultures; however, blood culture may be positive in select cases for *Staphylococcus aureus.* – Serologic tests for Rocky Mountain spotted fever, leptospirosis, or measles.	**Laboratory Criteria:** as previous
Case Classification • Probable: A case meets laboratory criteria and 4 of 5 clinical findings are present. • Confirmed: A case meets laboratory criteria and all 5 clinical findings, including desquamation (unless the patient dies before desquamation appears).	**Case Classification** • Definite: Case fulfills criteria IA, IIA, and IIB. • Probable: Case fulfills criteria IB, IIA, and IIB (if no other cause for the illness is identified).

Adapted from American Academy of Pediatrics. *Red Book: 2015 Report of the Committee on Infectious Diseases.* Kimberlin DW, Brady MT, Jackson MA, Long SS, eds. Elk Grove Village, IL: American Academy of Pediatrics; 2015.

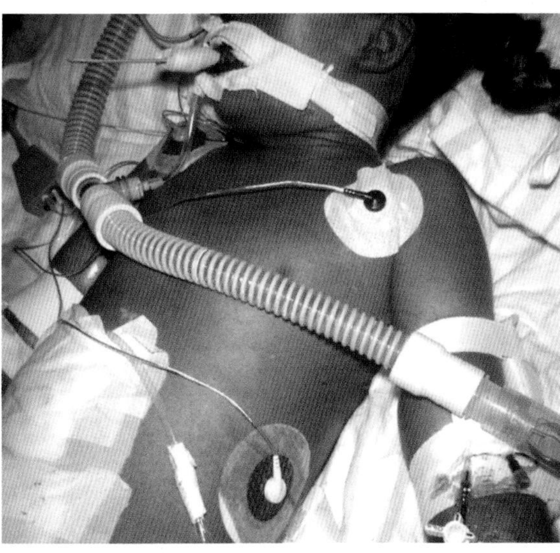

Figure 34.1. Toxic shock syndrome. This patient had widespread erythema, adult respiratory distress–like syndrome, and renal failure.

Look-alikes

Disorder	Differentiating Features
Staphylococcal scalded skin syndrome	• Crusting may be noted in perioral, perinasal regions. • Hypotension not typically present. • Bullae form, with subsequent rupture, peeling, and appearance of moist denuded painful areas. • Multiorgan involvement usually absent.
Streptococcal scarlet fever	• Eruption composed of fine papules (not diffuse macular erythema). • Multiorgan involvement absent.
Staphylococcal scarlet fever	• Eruption composed of fine papules (not diffuse macular erythema). • Multiorgan involvement absent.
Stevens-Johnson syndrome	• Presents with tense discrete blisters. • Typical target lesions may be present. • Erosions of the mucous membranes present. • Hypotension absent. • Multiorgan involvement not typically present.
Kawasaki disease	• Associated with prolonged high fever and classic constellation of clinical signs • Diffuse erythroderma not typical • Hypotension not typically present • Prominent cervical lymphadenopathy often present

How to Make the Diagnosis

- Diagnosis is confirmed by meeting the diagnostic criteria as detailed (or referenced) previously.
- In staphylococcal TSS, a positive culture is not required to make the diagnosis.
- In streptococcal TSS, isolation of group A streptococci may be from blood, cerebrospinal fluid, tissue biopsy, or peritoneal fluid ("definite" case when other criteria present) or throat, sputum, or vagina ("probable" case when other criteria present).

Treatment

- Supportive therapy, including maintaining fluid status and use of vasoactive agents as necessary. Anticipate multiple-system organ failure.
- Perform a thorough search for and adequate drainage of suppurative sites. For streptococcal TSS with necrotizing fasciitis, emergent surgical debridement is needed.
- Specific therapy with antistaphylococcal antibiotic with activity against methicillin-resistant *S aureus* (eg, vancomycin).
- Addition of clindamycin (which inhibits toxin synthesis in susceptible isolates of *S aureus* and *S pyogenes*) often is recommended. The use of clindamycin alone is not recommended.
- Use of intravenous immunoglobulin should be considered.

Treating Associated Conditions

- Because multiorgan involvement is the norm, affected patients need appropriate monitoring and supportive care in a critical care setting.

Prognosis

- Mortality associated with staphylococcal TSS is approximately 3%. Pediatric mortality associated with streptococcal TSS is higher, especially when necrotizing fasciitis is present.
- Recovery time is shortened and mortality is lowered with use of appropriate antibiotics and eradication of the toxin-producing organisms from the colonized site(s).

When to Worry or Refer

- Consider referral to an infectious disease specialist for patients who have an atypical presentation or who do not respond to standard treatment. Most or all patients with suspected or confirmed TSS require intensive care.
- Early consultation with surgical services for drainage or debridement of identified suppurative foci may be lifesaving.

Resources for Families

- American Academy of Pediatrics: HealthyChildren.org.
  www.HealthyChildren.org/toxicshock
- MedlinePlus: Information for patients and families (in English and Spanish) sponsored by the National Library of Medicine and National Institutes of Health.
  https://www.nlm.nih.gov/medlineplus/ency/article/000653.htm
- Toxic Shock Syndrome Information Service: An industry-sponsored site in the United Kingdom that provides information about TSS.
  www.toxicshock.com
- WebMD: Information for families is contained in the Health A-Z topics.
  www.webmd.com/women/guide/understanding-toxic-shock-syndrome-basics

Skin Infections

Fungal and Yeast Infections

CHAPTER 35

Candida

Introduction/Etiology/Epidemiology

- *Candida* species are ubiquitous and normally are noninvasive.
- *Candida albicans* exists as normal flora in the gastrointestinal tract and mucocutaneous surfaces of humans.
- In immunocompromised hosts, *C albicans* may invade mucous membranes or moist or macerated cutaneous surfaces.
- Note: The next 5 chapters (34A–34E) outline various *Candida* disorders.

Resources for Families

- American Academy of Pediatrics: HealthyChildren.org. **www.HealthyChildren.org/candida**
- MedlinePlus: Information for patients and families (in English and Spanish) sponsored by the National Library of Medicine and National Institutes of Health. **https://www.nlm.nih.gov/medlineplus/ency/article/000880.htm**

CHAPTER 35A

Angular Cheilitis/Perlèche

Introduction/Etiology/Epidemiology

- Inflammation and maceration of the angles of the mouth (ie, angular cheilitis or perlèche) can result from repeated licking, excessive salivation, or drooling.
- *Candida* species may then secondarily infect the areas directly or by extension of oral thrush.
- Perlèche is frequently observed in children with neurologic deficits who have difficulty managing oral secretions. It may also be seen with increased frequency in children who have increased drooling related to the presence of orthodontic appliances.

Signs and Symptoms

- Erythema and fissuring of the angles of the mouth (Figure 35A.1).
- Exudate may be present.

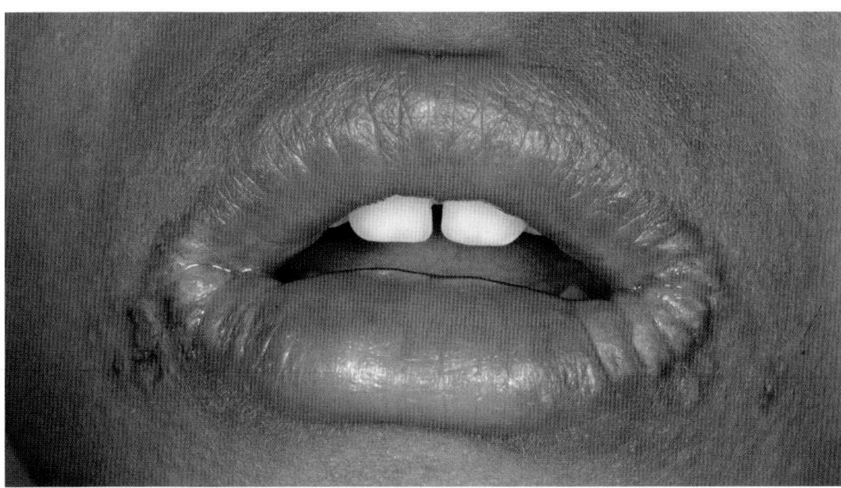

Figure 35A.1. Erythema, maceration, and fissuring of the corners of the mouth are observed in angular cheilitis.

Look-alikes

Disorder	Differentiating Features
Localized trauma	• Historical information suggesting trauma (eg, frequent and aggressive dental flossing)
Contact dermatitis	• Historical information suggesting exposure to an allergen
Lip-licking dermatitis	• Historical information suggesting lip licking • Well-defined erythematous patch surrounding mouth • Occasionally may have associated angular cheilitis
Secondary syphilis (mucous patch)	• Patients generally have rash elsewhere. • Patients often have systemic symptoms, including fever, malaise, or arthralgias, and generalized lymphadenopathy.

How to Make the Diagnosis

- The diagnosis is usually made clinically.
- If uncertainty exists, the diagnosis may be confirmed by microscopic observation of budding yeast or pseudohyphae in a potassium hydroxide preparation performed on scrapings of lesions (Figure 35A.2).

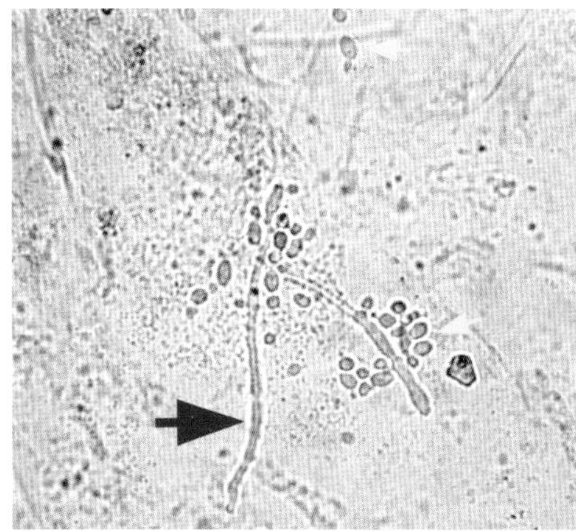

Figure 35A.2. A potassium hydroxide preparation reveals pseudohyphae (red arrow) and spores (yellow arrows) of *Candida* species.

Treatment

- Treatment focuses on the control or elimination of the inflammatory component with a topical steroid or topical calcineurin inhibitor, often in combination with the application of a topical antifungal agent (eg, nystatin, an imidazole antifungal) if secondary *Candida* infection is suspected.
- A combination antifungal-corticosteroid preparation (eg, nystatin in 0.1% triamcinolone ointment) is also usually quite effective, applied twice daily to the mouth angles until improved.
- Minimize predisposing factors such as lip licking, thumb sucking, and vigorous flossing.
- Persistent or repeated infection suggests a need for consideration of immunodeficiency.

Treating Associated Conditions

- Identify and eliminate exposure to contactants responsible for allergic contact dermatitis.

Prognosis

- The prognosis for patients with angular cheilitis is excellent, but underlying predisposing conditions may lead to recurrences.

When to Worry or Refer

- Consider consultation with a dermatologist when the diagnosis is in doubt or lesions fail to respond to appropriate therapy.
- When confronting treatment-resistant cases, consider contact dermatitis, diabetes mellitus, or other immunosuppression.

Candidal Diaper Dermatitis

Introduction/Etiology/Epidemiology

- Common infection often precipitated by compromise of the cutaneous barrier (eg, by irritant diaper dermatitis)

Signs and Symptoms

- Confluent, beefy red patch that involves the creases; satellite lesions (eg, papules, pustules) are present beyond the advancing border (Figure 35B.1).
- Often complicates noninfectious forms of diaper dermatitis (eg, irritant diaper dermatitis) and may occur as an adverse effect of oral antibiotic treatment.

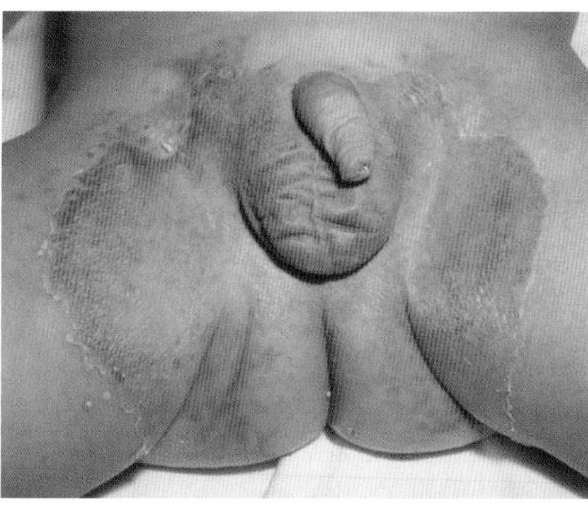

Figure 35B.1. Bright red patches that involve the creases and convexities are observed in candidal diaper dermatitis. Satellite lesions and scale are present.

Look-alikes (See also Chapter 91, Diaper Dermatitis.)

Disorder	Differentiating Features
Irritant dermatitis	• Erythematous patches involve the lower abdomen, buttocks, and thighs. • Convex surfaces involved. • Inguinal folds often spared.
Seborrheic dermatitis	• Salmon-pink patches with greasy scale that involve convexities and inguinal creases. • Involvement of scalp, face, retroauricular creases, umbilicus, or chest may be present.
Intertrigo	• Erythema and superficial erosions located in the inguinal creases • May become secondarily infected with *Candida* species or *Streptococcus pyogenes*
Psoriasis	• Erythematous scaling papules or plaques (scaling of the scalp and umbilicus may be present). • Lesions in the diaper area often lack scale characteristic of lesions elsewhere.
Acrodermatitis enteropathica	• Often begins when infants are weaned from human to cow milk formula. • Scaling erythematous eruption located around mouth and in diaper area. • Infants may have sparse hair, diarrhea, or failure to gain weight.
Langerhans cell histiocytosis	• Vesicles or pustules (often with a hemorrhagic crust); erythematous, orange, or yellow-brown papules or nodules; petechiae; erosions (especially in the diaper area, axillae, neck folds) • May have associated lymphadenopathy, bone swelling, diabetes insipidus • Resistant to standard therapies

How to Make the Diagnosis

- The diagnosis is usually made clinically.
- If diagnostic uncertainty exists, a potassium hydroxide preparation examination performed on scale will reveal pseudohyphae or spores (see Figure 35A.2).

Treatment

- Topical anti-candidal agent (eg, nystatin, an imidazole)

Treating Associated Conditions

- If thrush is present, treat with oral nystatin or fluconazole.

Prognosis

- The prognosis for infants is excellent.

When to Worry or Refer

- Failure to respond to appropriate anti-candidal therapy warrants careful reconsideration of the diagnosis. However, repeated episodes are not uncommon in healthy infants.
- Persistent or recurrent episodes of candidal infection may suggest immunodeficiency, including HIV infection. However, repeated episodes without additional symptoms are not uncommon in healthy infants.

Chronic Paronychia

Introduction/Etiology/Epidemiology

- Chronic paronychia is common among children who are thumb suckers, nail biters, or nail pickers.
- *Candida* species usually are responsible.

Signs and Symptoms

- Non-tender erythematous swelling of the skin surrounding the nail (Figure 35C.1).
- Loss of the cuticle in affected digits is common.
- Associated nail dystrophy may be present, most often presenting as pits or transverse ridges; yellow debris and separation of the nail plate from the nail bed may be present.

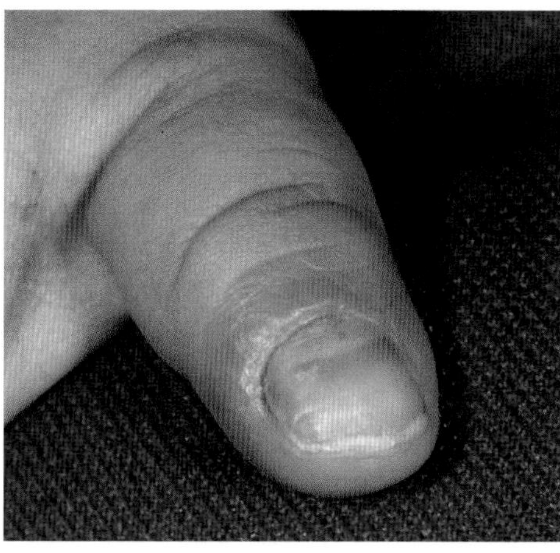

Figure 35C.1. Chronic paronychia due to *Candida*. There is periungual erythema and loss of the cuticle.

Look-alikes

Disorder	Differentiating Features
Acute paronychia	• Acute onset with painful swelling, erythema, and purulent exudate • Culture often positive for *Staphylococcus aureus*
Tinea unguium (onychomycosis)	• Skin surrounding nail usually normal • When toenails infected, usually evidence of associated tinea pedis (eg, fissuring, scaling, maceration between the digits) • Nail usually thickened and white to yellow, with debris under the nail plate
Herpetic whitlow	• Acute onset of painful clustered vesicles or a bulla on an erythematous base • May be located on a digit but seldom limited to proximal and lateral nail folds
Blistering dactylitis	• Acute onset of a bulla affecting distal portion of a digit • Located on digit but not limited to proximal or lateral nail folds
Chronic mucocutaneous candidiasis	• Multiple digits involved • Associated recurrent candidal mucosal or other skin surface infections • May have associated immunologic or endocrinologic abnormalities

How to Make the Diagnosis

- The diagnosis is usually made clinically.
- If uncertainty exists, the diagnosis may be confirmed by microscopic observation of budding yeast or pseudohyphae in a potassium hydroxide preparation performed on scrapings of the affected area (see Figure 35A.2).

Treatment

- Treatment is complicated by predisposing behaviors that cause trauma or moisture (eg, nail biting, thumb sucking). When possible, these factors should be addressed.
- Topical nystatin or an imidazole antifungal agent applied during the day and under occlusion at night (care must be taken to secure occlusive dressings to prevent aspiration by young patients).
- Oral fluconazole may be indicated in severe or persistent cases.

Treating Associated Conditions

Thumb sucking

- Provide positive feedback for substitute behaviors.
- Use of noxious agents to control thumb sucking should be considered second-line therapy.

Prognosis

- Long-term prognosis is excellent (once predisposing factors have been eliminated).

When to Worry or Refer

- Involvement of multiple nails along with recurrent mucosal or skin infection may indicate the presence of chronic mucocutaneous candidiasis.

CHAPTER 35D

Neonatal/Congenital Candidiasis

Introduction/Etiology/Epidemiology

- Uncommon infection that may be observed at birth or within a week of delivery.
- *Candida albicans* is acquired during passage through a colonized birth canal or by ascending infection before delivery.

Signs and Symptoms

- Eruption presents as papules and pustules superimposed on an erythematous base (Figure 35D.1) or as diffuse erythema with scaling.
- Presence of papules and pustules on the palms and soles is characteristic.
- Nail dystrophy with yellow discoloration may be present.
- Any body surface may be involved.
- Most full-term infants experience a benign course, but very low birth weight infants are at higher risk for invasive disease.

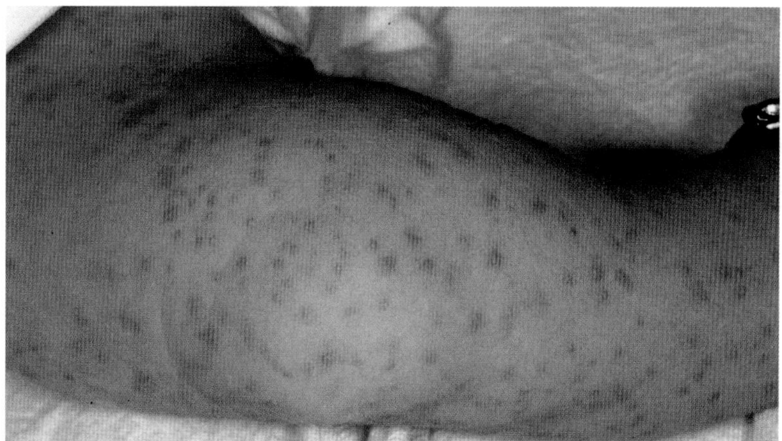

Figure 35D.1. Congenital candidiasis is characterized by erythematous papules, pustules, and scaling.

Look-alikes

In each of the disorders listed herein, a potassium hydroxide preparation would fail to demonstrate the pseudohyphae and spores that would be observed in candidal infection.

Disorder	Differentiating Features
Erythema toxicum	• Discrete, blotchy, erythematous macules or patches, each with a central papule, vesicle, or pustule. • Typically not present at birth. • Vesicular/pustular fluid contains eosinophils.
Transient neonatal pustular melanosis	• Pustules (without erythema) or ruptured pustules, which appear as small freckle-like hyperpigmented macules surrounded by a rim of scale. • Pustular fluid contains neutrophils.
Miliaria rubra	• Erythematous papules and papulopustules, often located in occluded areas and skinfolds
Neonatal cephalic pustulosis (neonatal acne)	• Papules and pustules typically limited to face
Staphylococcal folliculitis	• White to slightly yellow pustules with surrounding rim of erythema. • Gram stain or bacterial culture will reveal *Staphylococcus aureus.*
Scabies	• Occurs rarely during first month of life. • Generalized eruption; may have vesicles but usually will be accompanied by erythematous papules or nodules and burrows. • Mineral oil preparation of scrapings of lesions will reveal mites, eggs, or fecal material.
Neonatal herpes simplex virus infection	• Typically clustered vesicles on an erythematous base (although solitary vesicles occasionally occur). • Lesions concentrated on head, particularly at sites of trauma (eg, those caused by a scalp electrode). • Infants may have signs of sepsis (in disseminated disease), or seizures or coma (in central nervous system [CNS] disease). • Direct fluorescent examination, viral culture, or polymerase chain reaction (skin lesions, cerebrospinal fluid) will confirm diagnosis.
Infantile acropustulosis	• Usually begins in first months of life (not in first days). • Vesicles or pustules that are limited to the hands and feet, including the palms and soles, wrists and ankles. • Eruption lasts for 5 to 10 days and reappears every 2 to 4 weeks.
Incontinentia pigmenti	• Vesicles on an erythematous base appear at birth or within the first 2 weeks. • Lesions arranged in a linear fashion on the extremities or in a swirled pattern on the trunk (along the lines of Blaschko).
Eosinophilic pustular folliculitis	• Papules and pustules typically located on the scalp. • Exhibits a chronic, intermittent course. • Severe pruritus is usually present.

How to Make the Diagnosis

- The diagnosis is made by performing a potassium hydroxide preparation (see Figure 35A.2) and skin culture.

Treatment

- Topical application of an antifungal agent such as nystatin or clotrimazole.
- In neonates with diffuse skin involvement, oral fluconazole may accelerate resolution.
- In the rare patient who has evidence of (or risk factors for) systemic infection, complete evaluation for this possibility and parenteral antifungal therapy are required.

Prognosis

- The prognosis for infants with cutaneous congenital candidiasis is excellent.
- Low birth weight infants (or those born to mothers with a history of an indwelling device, eg, cervical cerclage, intrauterine device) are at increased risk for systemic involvement (eg, infection of blood, lungs, CNS, urinary tract).

When to Worry or Refer

- Consider consultation by a dermatologist when the diagnosis is in doubt or lesions fail to respond to appropriate therapy.
- When systemic disease is likely, immediate consultation with a pediatric infectious disease specialist is warranted.

CHAPTER 35E

Thrush

Introduction/Etiology/Epidemiology

- Common condition among young infants.
- Antibiotic therapy that disrupts the normal oral flora may be a predisposing factor.
- Recurrent or persistent thrush, especially in an infant with other signs or symptoms, should raise concern about immunocompromise (eg, HIV infection, another immunodeficiency disorder).

Signs and Symptoms

- Presents with discrete white plaques overlying an erythematous base that involve the buccal mucosa or tongue (Figures 35E.1 and 35E.2).
- Infants with oral thrush may be irritable and feed poorly.

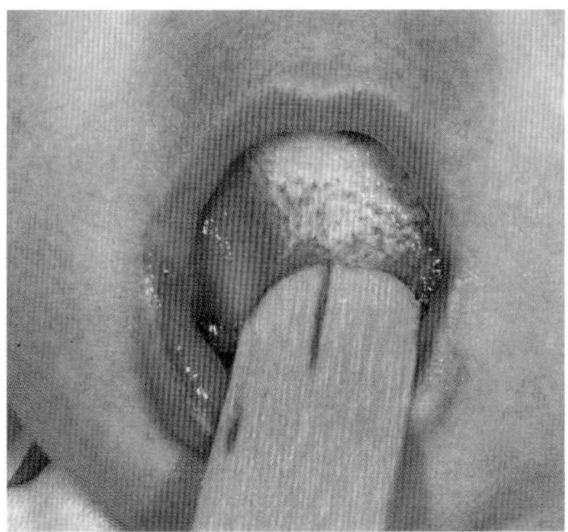

Figure 35E.1. White patches on the tongue or buccal mucosa are characteristic of thrush.

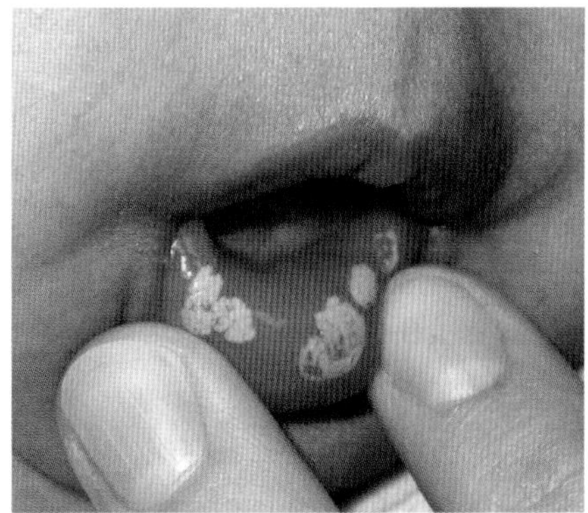

Figure 35E.2. White plaques on the lips of an infant who has thrush.

Look-alikes

Disorder	Differentiating Features
Retained food or formula	• White patches easily removed with a tongue depressor or gauze
Geographic tongue	• Well-defined, sometimes annular patches that may appear to be erosions located on tongue. • Pattern of involvement changes daily.
Herpetic gingivostomatitis	• Multiple painful vesicles and ulcers located on buccal mucosa, tongue, or gingivae. • Perioral skin often reveals similar lesions. • Children febrile, appear ill, and at risk for dehydration.
Herpangina	• Small vesicles or shallow ulcers typically located on tonsillar pillars, soft palate, tonsils, and uvula • Associated with fever, sore throat, or dysphagia
Koplik spots of measles	• Gray-white dots often with surrounding erythema. • Typically located on buccal mucosa adjacent to mandibular molars. • Patients generally appear ill with fever, cough, coryza, and conjunctivitis.

How to Make the Diagnosis

- The diagnosis usually is made based on clinical findings.
- If uncertainty exists, a potassium hydroxide preparation performed on a sample obtained from the mouth (by scraping the affected area with a tongue depressor) will demonstrate pseudohyphae or budding yeast (see Figure 35A.2).

Treatment

- Oral nystatin or fluconazole for the infant.
- Minimize predisposing factors such as contaminated pacifiers and nipples.
- If the infant is breastfeeding, assess for possible maternal candidal infection of the breast and treat accordingly.
- Persistent or frequently recurrent infections, especially in the presence of other signs and symptoms of systemic illness, should prompt consideration of an immunodeficiency.

Prognosis

- The prognosis for infants who have thrush is excellent, and the course is usually benign.

When to Worry or Refer

- When the diagnosis is in doubt or lesions fail to respond to appropriate therapy, consultation with an immunologist or pediatric infectious disease specialist is warranted.

CHAPTER 36

Onychomycosis

Introduction/Etiology/Epidemiology

- Dermatophyte infection of nails usually caused by *Trichophyton rubrum, Trichophyton mentagrophytes*, or *Epidermophyton floccosum* (occasionally, molds may cause onychomycosis).
- Common in adolescents and adults; less common in children.
- In most pediatric cases, there is a family history of tinea pedis or onychomycosis.

Signs and Symptoms

- Toenails are more frequently involved than fingernails.
- Two forms are recognized.
  - Subungual onychomycosis: thickening of the nail with yellow discoloration distally or laterally that indicates separation of the nail from the nail bed (ie, distal and lateral subungual onychomycosis, respectively) (Figure 36.1)
  - Superficial white onychomycosis: white discoloration with a fine, powdery scale (Figure 36.2)
- One or multiple nails may be involved, but "skip nails" (with no involvement) commonly seen.
- Most patients have evidence of coexisting tinea pedis.

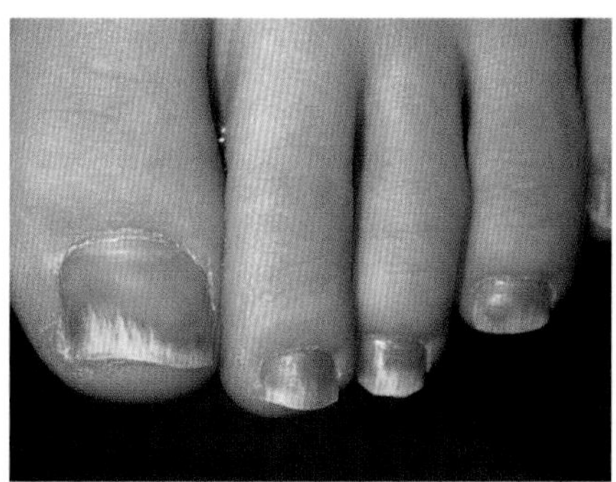

Figure 36.1. Thickening and yellowing of the nail and separation of the nail plate from the bed occur in subungual onychomycosis.

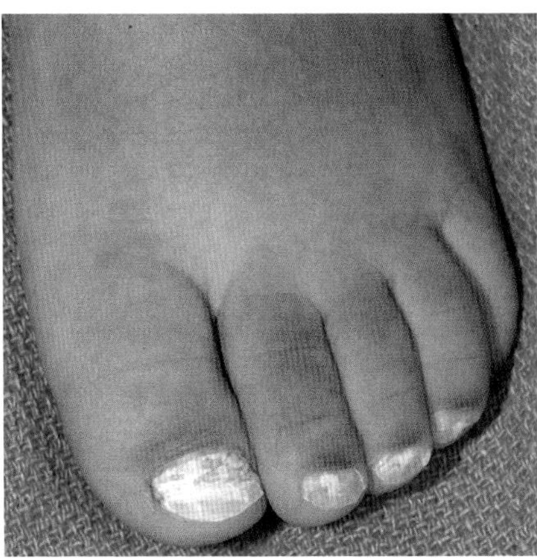

Figure 36.2. In superficial white onychomycosis, the surface of the nail appears white and has fine scale.

Look-alikes

In each of the conditions listed herein, a potassium hydroxide preparation or fungal culture would fail to confirm the presence of dermatophyte infection. Performance of these procedures often is necessary to assist in differential diagnosis.

Disorder	Differentiating Features
Psoriasis	• Nail pitting often present. • Typical psoriatic skin lesions may be present elsewhere.
Trachyonychia (20-nail dystrophy)	• Nails appear rough due to longitudinal ridging and are thin rather than thickened. • Pitting also commonly present.
Candidiasis	• Usually involves fingernails • Erythema and edema of proximal nail fold present • Loss of cuticle • Typically occurs in young children who suck their fingers
Pachyonychia congenita	• May be difficult to differentiate clinically from onychomycosis. • Thickening, tenting, and discoloration of fingernails and toenails. • Yellow or brown material accumulates beneath nail. • May have associated thickening of skin on palms and soles (keratoderma). • Positive family history for similar changes is common.
Lichen planus	• Typical skin lesions usually present (purple, polygonal papules and plaques). • Nails thin, have longitudinal striations or ridges, may split.

How to Make the Diagnosis

- The diagnosis usually is suspected clinically and may be confirmed by performing a potassium hydroxide preparation or fungal culture (eg, dermatophyte test medium, other fungal culture medium) on debris scraped from beneath the distal nail or nail clipping (distal or lateral subungual onychomycosis) or from the surface of the nail (superficial white onychomycosis).

Treatment

- Distal or lateral subungual onychomycosis (toenails)
  - Adolescents and adults: Oral therapy generally is required. (Be aware of potential drug interactions, adverse effects, and need for laboratory monitoring.)
    - Terbinafine 250 mg daily for 3 to 4 months
    - Itraconazole 200 mg daily for 12 weeks, or 200 mg twice daily for 7 days once monthly for 3 to 4 months (Courses should be separated by 21 days.)
    - Fluconazole: preferred by some but not US Food and Drug Administration (FDA) approved for the treatment of onychomycosis
    - Griseofulvin: poor cure rate, requires prolonged treatment course
  - Children: May respond to topical therapy (eg, ciclopirox, amorolfine). If oral therapy is prescribed, select dose based on weight. (Note: Itraconazole and fluconazole are not specifically FDA approved for use in the treatment of onychomycosis in children, so treatment with these agents for this indication is considered off-label.)
- Superficial white onychomycosis: may respond to topical therapy (eg, ciclopirox, amorolfine), but may also require systemic therapy.

Prognosis

- The prognosis for successful eradication and cure is guarded. Cure rates as high as 80% have been reported with oral therapy, but recurrences are common.
- To prevent recurrences, advise the patient to dry feet carefully after bathing or showering, wear protective footwear in public showers, wear absorbent socks, and apply an absorbent powder containing an antifungal agent (eg, Zeasorb AF, Tinactin, Desenex, Lotrimin AF).

When to Worry or Refer

- Consider consultation when the diagnosis is in doubt or when the patient fails to respond to appropriate therapy.

Resources for Families

- WebMD: Information for families is contained in the Health A-Z topics. **www.webmd.com/skin-problems-and-treatments/guide/fungal-nail-infections-topic-overview**

CHAPTER 37

Tinea Capitis

Introduction/Etiology/Epidemiology

- Common dermatophyte infection of the scalp; in the United States, *Trichophyton tonsurans*, *Microsporum canis*, and *Microsporum audouinii* are responsible for most cases.
- *T tonsurans* is responsible for more than 90% of US infections.
- For reasons unknown, African American children are disproportionately affected.

Signs and Symptoms

Three patterns of infection may be observed.

- Alopecia
  - One or more round or oval patches of partial to complete alopecia with associated scaling (Figure 37.1).
  - Infections caused by *T tonsurans* cause hairs to break at the scalp, resulting in black dot hairs (the remnants of hairs remaining within the follicle) (see Figure 37.1).
  - Infections caused by *Microsporum* species cause hairs to break further from the scalp, resulting in incomplete alopecia; black dot hairs are absent.
- Seborrheic
  - Mimics seborrheic dermatitis (ie, dandruff) with patchy or diffuse whitish to gray scale (Figure 37.2).
  - Alopecia may be subtle.
- Inflammatory: When an inflammatory response to the infecting agent occurs, patients may develop
  - Papules, pustules, and crusting that may mimic bacterial folliculitis
  - A tender, boggy mass known as a kerion (Figure 37.3)
- All forms of tinea capitis, but particularly inflammatory forms, may produce suboccipital or posterior cervical lymphadenopathy.

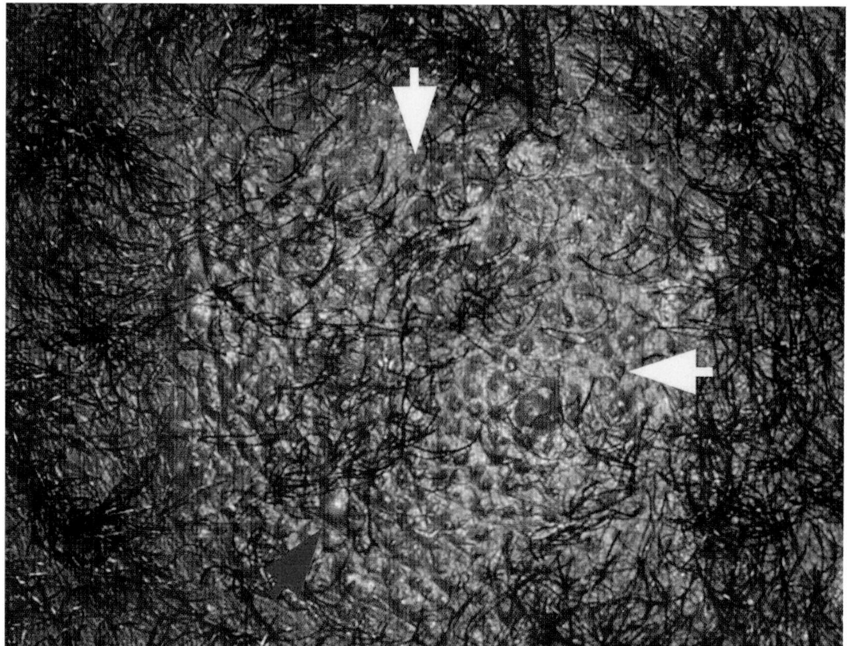

Figure 37.1. Tinea capitis. A well-defined patch of alopecia within which are scale, black dot hairs (yellow arrows) and pustules (red arrow).

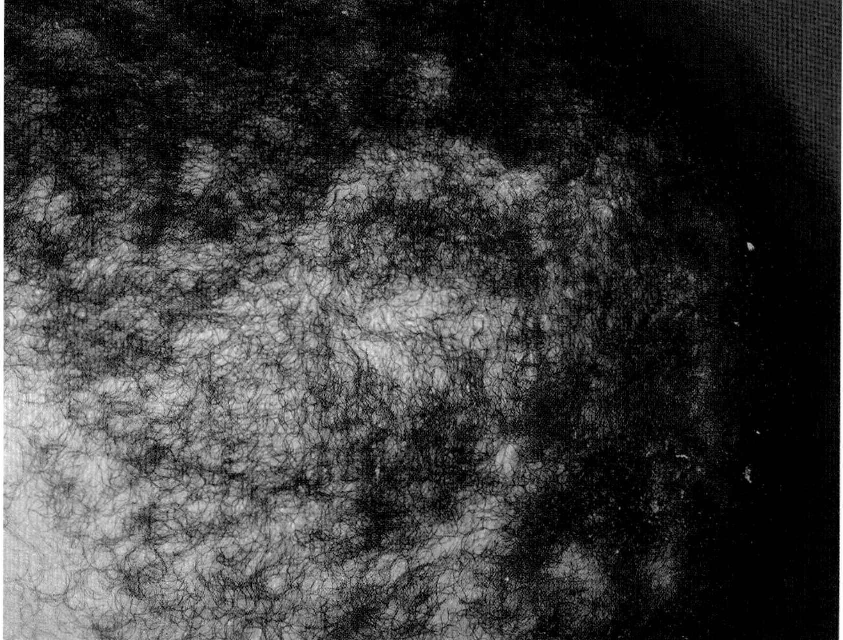

Figure 37.2. Diffuse scaling of the scalp is observed in the seborrheic form of tinea capitis.

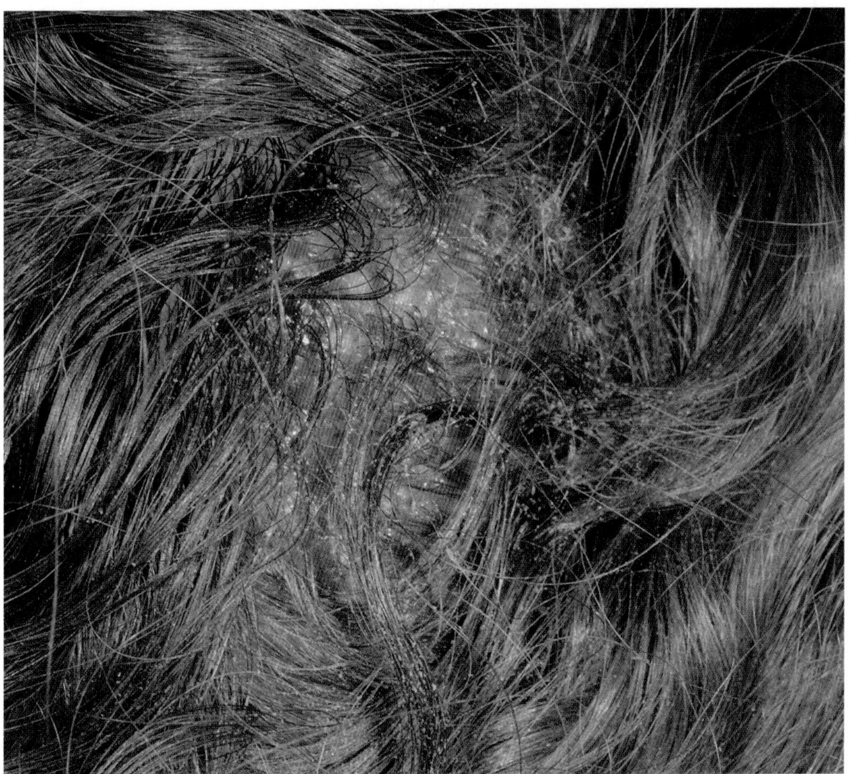

Figure 37.3. A kerion is a tender, boggy mass located on the scalp.

Look-alikes

In each of the conditions listed herein, a potassium hydroxide preparation or fungal culture would fail to confirm the presence of fungal infection.

Disorder	Differentiating Features
Alopecia areata	• Round or oval patches of alopecia that lack scaling, inflammation, or black dot hairs • Nail pitting often present
Trichotillomania	• Often ill-defined patches of alopecia within which hairs are of differing lengths. • Petechiae or hemorrhagic crusts may be present (if hairs pulled from the scalp). • Scaling and black dot hairs absent. • History of hair manipulation may be offered by family (but not always).
Bacterial folliculitis	• Alopecia and scaling absent • Culture positive for *Staphylococcus aureus* • Note: In patients who have tinea capitis, *S aureus* often can be cultured from the scalp (although the pustules themselves may be sterile).
Bacterial abscess	• Less likely to produce alopecia than a kerion. • Scaling absent. • Culture of contents usually reveals *S aureus* or other bacterial organisms • Note: In patients who have tinea capitis, *S aureus* often can be cultured from the scalp (although the pustules themselves may be sterile).
Traction alopecia	• Traction on hair may produce alopecia localized to areas where hair is parted. • Folliculitis may occur, but scaling and black dot hairs absent. • History of tight braids or ponytails often present, with hair thinning in peripheral zones.
Seborrheic dermatitis	• Typically does not produce alopecia • Unlikely to occur in children (most often affects infants and those at or beyond puberty)

How to Make the Diagnosis

- The diagnosis usually is made clinically and supported by laboratory testing.
  - The presence of occipital lymphadenopathy and alopecia, or lymphadenopathy and scaling, are highly predictive of tinea capitis.
- A potassium hydroxide preparation performed on infected hairs will reveal spores within the hair shaft (ie, endothrix infection as caused by *T tonsurans*) (Figure 37.4) or on the surface of hairs (ie, ectothrix infection as caused by *Microsporum* species).
- Culture (the gold standard for diagnosis) of scale or hair fragments on dermatophyte test medium (or other suitable medium) confirms the diagnosis (Figure 37.5). Consider performing a culture when diagnostic uncertainty exists; some also use culture to confirm a mycologic cure prior to discontinuation of therapy.
  - Specimens for culture may be obtained with a Cytobrush, toothbrush, or premoistened cotton-tipped applicator.
  - Sensitivity of culture is high, even with delay in inoculation of medium due to transportation of specimen to laboratory.
- Wood light examination is useful only in ectothrix infections (ie, those caused by *Microsporum* species). In such cases, infected hairs will fluoresce. Infections caused by *T tonsurans* (>90% of infections) do not fluoresce.

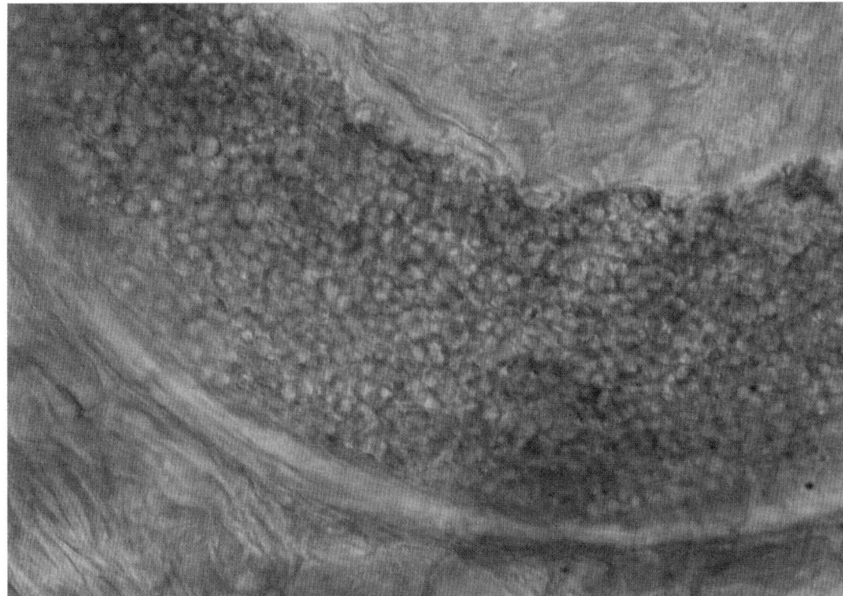

Figure 37.4. Tinea capitis caused by *Trichophyton tonsurans* produces an endothrix infection. The infected black dot hair is filled with arthrospores, the spherical objects shown here.

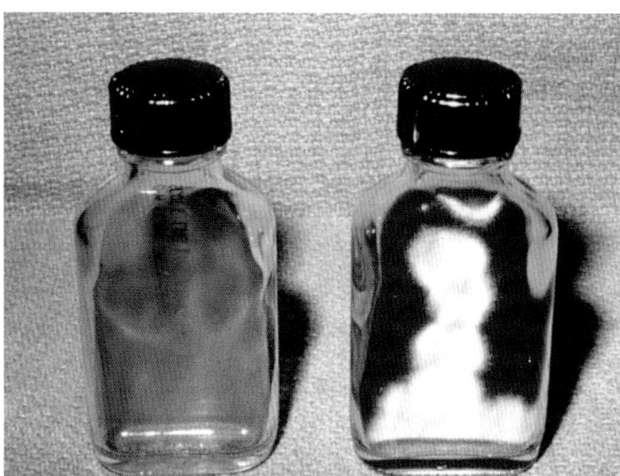

Figure 37.5. The diagnosis of tinea capitis may be confirmed by performing a fungal culture. Uninoculated medium is yellow (left). Within 2 weeks of inoculation with scale or black dot hairs scraped from the scalp, there is fungal growth and the medium turns red.

Treatment

- Oral therapy is required. A summary of treatment options is provided in Table 37.1.
  - The drug of choice remains griseofulvin at a dose of 20 to 25 mg/kg per day of the microsize preparation or 15 mg/kg per day of the ultramicrosize preparation. Patients should be treated for 6 to 8 weeks minimum. Laboratory monitoring is not necessary.
  - Terbinafine, fluconazole, and itraconazole have proven effective in treating tinea capitis (terbinafine and fluconazole have received specific US Food and Drug Administration approval for use in this infection).
    - These agents (particularly terbinafine) often are used to treat patients who fail to respond to griseofulvin. Some experts now use terbinafine as first-line therapy, given the shorter treatment course (compared with griseofulvin), high efficacy, and favorable cost profile (when tablets used).
    - Terbinafine is less effective than griseofulvin in the treatment of tinea capitis caused by *Microsporum* species.
    - Fluconazole is the only agent approved for use in those younger than 2 years, although others are used off-label.
- The use of an adjunctive antifungal shampoo containing selenium sulfide (1% or 2.5%) or ketoconazole 2% twice weekly will kill surface spores and, possibly, reduce spread of infection to others. The agent should be used for at least 2 weeks.
- Some authors recommend the addition of oral prednisone (eg, for 1–3 weeks) to the treatment regimen in patients who have severe inflammatory tinea capitis (ie, a kerion).

- Incision and drainage of a kerion is not indicated.
- Patients should be seen in follow-up 1 to 2 months after beginning therapy to assess response.
- Children should not be excluded from school once therapy is begun. Some experts recommend that asymptomatic family members use an antifungal shampoo, although evidence is lacking regarding the efficacy of this strategy. If a dog or cat is suspected to be the source of infection, the animal should be evaluated and treated if appropriate.

Table 37.1. Recommended Therapy for Tinea Capitis

Drug	Dosage	Duration
Griseofulvin microsize (liquid 125 mg/5 mL)	20–25 mg/kg/d	≥6 wk; continue until clinically clear
Griseofulvin ultramicrosize (tablets of varying size)	10–15 mg/kg/d	≥6 wk; continue until clinically clear
Terbinafine tablets (250 mg)	4–6 mg/kg/d 10–20 kg: 62.5 mg 20–40 kg: 125 mg >40 kg: 250 mg	*T tonsurans:* 2–6 wk *M canis:* 8–12 wk
Terbinafine granules (125 mg and 187.5 mg)	<25 kg: 125 mg 25–35 kg: 187.5 mg >35 kg: 250 mg	FDA approved for children ≥4 y 6-wk duration for all species
Fluconazole	6 mg/kg/d	3–6 wk FDA approved for the treatment of oral candidiasis in children ≥6 mo but not approved for the treatment of tinea capitis

Abbreviation: FDA, US Food and Drug Administration.
From American Academy of Pediatrics. Tinea capitis. In: Kimberlin DW, Brady MT, Jackson MA, Long SS, eds. *Red Book: 2015 Report of the Committee on Infectious Diseases.* Elk Grove Village, IL: American Academy of Pediatrics; 2015:778–781.

Treating Associated Conditions

- Although *S aureus* may be cultured from the scalp of children who have tinea capitis, antibiotic treatment usually is unnecessary.
- If clinical evidence of secondary bacterial infection is present, an antistaphylococcal antibiotic should be prescribed.

Prognosis

- The prognosis is excellent. With treatment, alopecia resolves in nearly all patients (those who have a large kerion occasionally will experience permanent alopecia).
- Reinfection is common in children who share potential fomites (eg, hats, scarves, headgear, earphones, combs, brushes) or those who are reexposed to infection (from children or pets).

When to Worry or Refer

- Refer patients if the diagnosis is in doubt or there is a failure to respond to therapy.

Resources for Families

- American Academy of Pediatrics: HealthyChildren.org.
  www.HealthyChildren.org/tinea
- MedlinePlus: Information for patients and families (in English and Spanish) sponsored by the National Library of Medicine and National Institutes of Health.
  https://www.nlm.nih.gov/medlineplus/ency/article/000878.htm

Tinea Corporis

Introduction/Etiology/Epidemiology

- Common fungal infection caused by the dermatophytes *Trichophyton tonsurans, Microsporum canis, Trichophyton mentagrophytes*, and *Trichophyton rubrum*

Signs and Symptoms

- Small lesions appear as erythematous scaling plaques.
  - As a lesion enlarges, it becomes annular (ie, ringlike) with a raised, advancing, erythematous border and central clearing (Figure 38.1).
  - Atypical lesions may be present (eg, large rings, incomplete rings) (Figure 38.2).
- Lesions are variably pruritic and may be single or multiple (Figure 38.3).
- Application of a topical corticosteroid (due to misdiagnosis) may alter the typical appearance of lesions (eg, lesions may lack scale or an annular appearance).
- Multiple or disseminated lesions often present in athletes with prolonged skin-to-skin contact (ie, wrestlers, when it has been termed tinea gladiatorum) or in immunocompromised patients.
- Especially in hair-bearing areas (eg, in young women who shave their legs), tinea corporis can manifest as a deep-seated infection referred to as Majocchi granuloma. This variant represents a granulomatous folliculitis or perifolliculitis. Majocchi granuloma may also occur when tinea corporis is inadvertently treated with a topical corticosteroid (Figure 38.4).

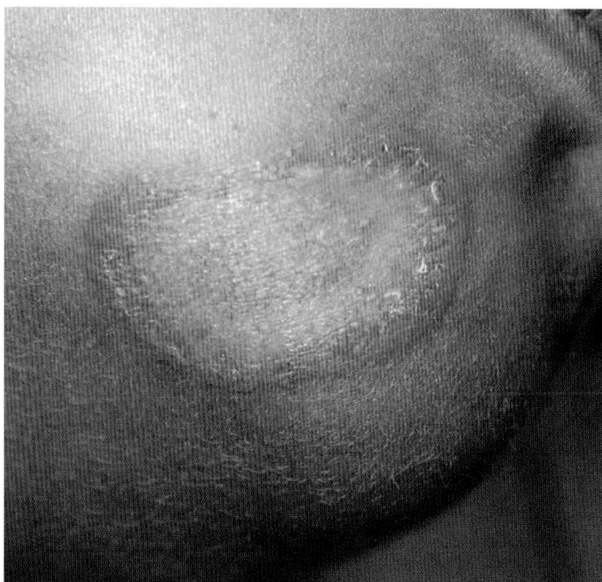

Figure 38.1. Lesions of tinea corporis are rings (ie, annuli) that have an elevated, erythematous, scaling border and central clearing.

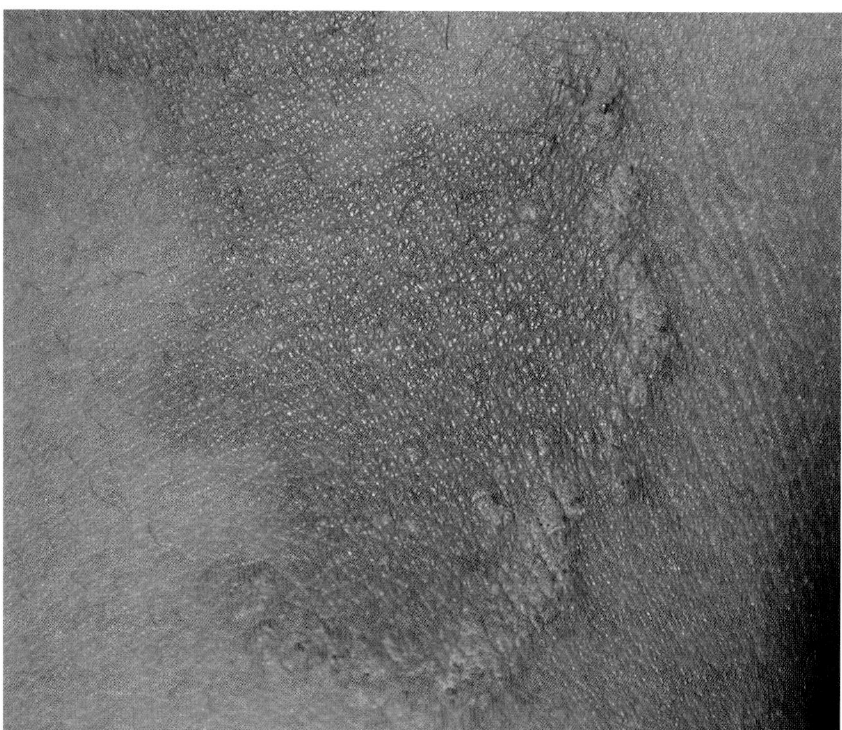

Figure 38.2. Occasionally, the lesions of tinea corporis may be atypical in their appearance. In this patient, there is an incomplete ring; however, the border is erythematous, elevated, and scaling.

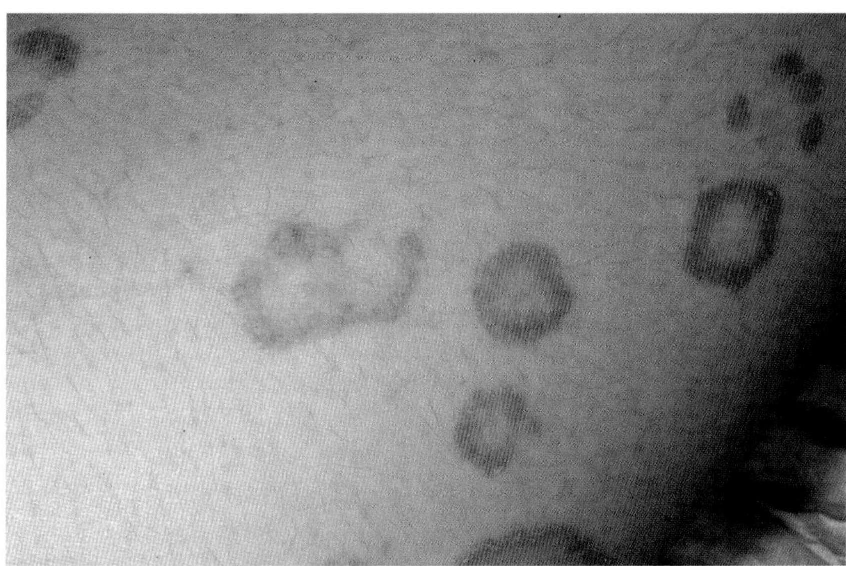

Figure 38.3. Lesions of tinea corporis may be multiple.

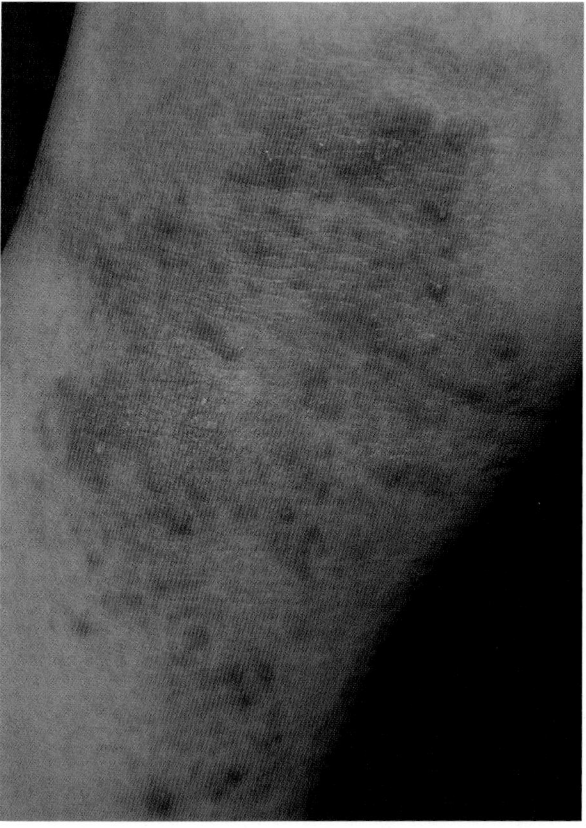

Figure 38.4. This child developed Majocchi granuloma after a lesion of tinea corporis (initially thought to represent nummular eczema) was treated with a topical corticosteroid. Note the presence of follicular-based papules and pustules.

Look-alikes

In each of the conditions listed herein, a potassium hydroxide preparation or fungal culture would fail to confirm the presence of fungal infection.

Disorder	Differentiating Features
Pityriasis rosea	• Herald patch of pityriasis rosea may be confused with tinea corporis; however, often lacks elevated border. • Later appearance of the generalized eruption assists in diagnosis of pityriasis rosea. • Scaling lags behind the red border and has its free edge pointing inward ("trailing scale"), as opposed to leading edge scale seen in tinea.
Granuloma annulare	• Papules or nodules coalesce to form rings or incomplete rings. • Lesions often have violaceous, not erythematous, color. • Scaling absent.
Nummular eczema	• Lesions are round but lack central clearing. • Crust (not scale) usually present; lesions lack an elevated border. • History of atopic dermatitis may be present.
Psoriasis	• Erythematous papules or plaques that typically lack central clearing. • Scale of psoriatic lesions thick, unlike finer scale of tinea corporis. • Removal of scale causes pinpoint bleeding (Auspitz sign).
Ecthyma	• Lesions have thick crust, not scale, with surrounding erythema and induration. • Central clearing absent.

How to Make the Diagnosis

- The diagnosis usually is made clinically but can be confirmed by a potassium hydroxide preparation performed on scale obtained from the border of the lesion (that demonstrates branching hyphae) (Figure 38.5) or culture (rarely necessary).

Treatment

- Apply a topical antifungal agent, such as an imidazole (eg, clotrimazole, miconazole, ketoconazole), allylamine (eg, terbinafine, naftifine), or tolnaftate. The agent is applied until the lesion resolves, typically within 2 weeks.
- Oral antifungal agents (eg, griseofulvin, fluconazole, terbinafine) are reserved for patients with multiple or very large lesions (eg, as might occur in immunosuppressed individuals). Longer courses with oral antifungal agents may be required for deeper-seated tinea infections, such as Majocchi granuloma.

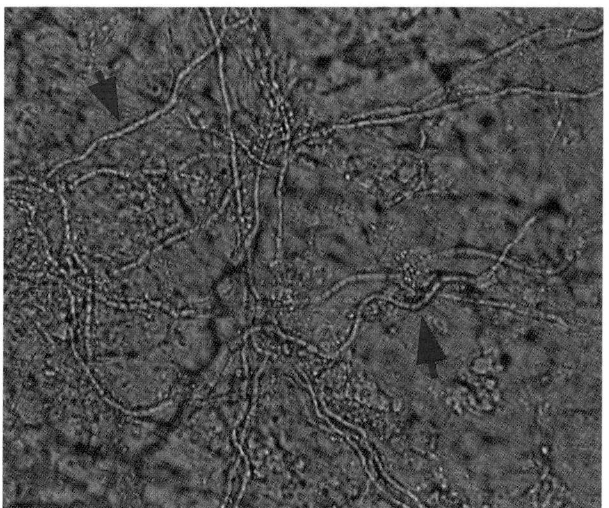

Figure 38.5. A potassium hydroxide preparation in tinea corporis; branching hyphae are seen (arrows).

Prognosis

- Prognosis is excellent, although recurrences are common when children are continually exposed to infected pets or farm animals.

When to Worry or Refer

- Refer patients in whom the diagnosis is in doubt or the lesion(s) fails to respond to appropriate therapy.

Resources for Families

- American Academy of Pediatrics: HealthyChildren.org. **www.HealthyChildren.org/tinea**
- MedlinePlus: Information for patients and families (in English and Spanish) sponsored by the National Library of Medicine and National Institutes of Health. **https://www.nlm.nih.gov/medlineplus/ency/article/000877.htm**
- WebMD: Information for families is contained in the Health A-Z topics. **www.webmd.com/skin-problems-and-treatments/guide/understanding-ring-worm-basics**

Tinea Cruris

Introduction/Etiology/Epidemiology

- Dermatophyte infection of the skin of the groin; usually caused by *Trichophyton mentagrophytes* or *Epidermophyton floccosum*.
- More common in men; rare before puberty.
- Especially prevalent in warm, humid conditions.
- May occur in epidemics among athletic teams or military recruits.
- Infection may be transmitted via fomites (eg, athletic gear, clothing, towels).

Signs and Symptoms

- Characterized by an erythematous patch on the inner thigh and inguinal crease (may be unilateral or bilateral) (Figure 39.1).
- Borders of lesions are elevated and exhibit scale.
- May be intensely pruritic; scratching leads to erosions, inflammation, and lichenification.
- Scrotum is usually spared, although scratching may produce lichenification.

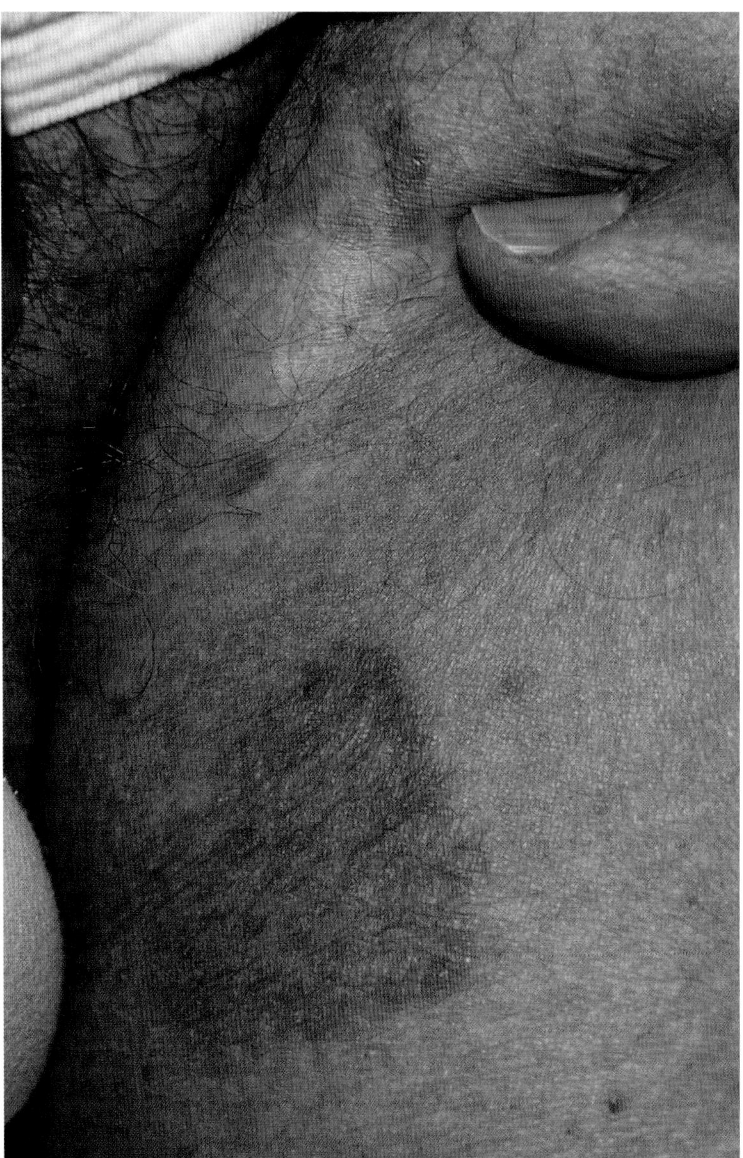

Figure 39.1. Tinea cruris is characterized by an erythematous or hyperpigmented patch with an elevated scaling border.

Look-alikes

In each of the conditions listed herein, a potassium hydroxide preparation or fungal culture would fail to confirm the presence of dermatophyte infection.

Disorder	Differentiating Features
Intertrigo	• Maceration caused by rubbing of apposing skin surfaces • Borders poorly defined; scaling absent
Candidiasis	• "Beefy" red patch • Satellite lesions (papules, papulopustules) present • Scrotum often involved
Erythrasma	• Often red-brown or brown. • Elevated border and scaling absent. • Wood light examination will reveal coral red fluorescence.

How to Make the Diagnosis

- The diagnosis is made clinically and may be confirmed by performing a potassium hydroxide preparation on scale obtained from the border of the lesion (that will reveal branching hyphae).

Treatment

- Topical application of an antifungal agent, such as an imidazole (eg, clotrimazole, miconazole, ketoconazole), allylamine (eg, terbinafine, naftifine), or tolnaftate. The agent is applied until the eruption resolves, typically within 3 to 4 weeks.
- Advise patients to avoid tight-fitting clothing, dry carefully after bathing or showering, and apply an absorbent powder.
- If patients experience frequent recurrences, recommend the regular use of an absorbent powder containing an antifungal agent (eg, Zeasorb AF, Tinactin, Desenex, Lotrimin AF).
- Oral antifungal therapy rarely is necessary and is reserved for patients who have severe or recalcitrant disease.

Prognosis

- The prognosis is excellent.
- Reinfection may occur unless the predisposing environmental conditions are altered.

When to Worry or Refer

- Consider consultation when the diagnosis is in doubt or when the patient fails to respond to appropriate therapy.

Resources for Families

- American Academy of Pediatrics: HealthyChildren.org. **www.HealthyChildren.org/tinea**
- WebMD: Information for families is contained in the Health A-Z topics. **www.webmd.com/men/tc/jock-itch-topic-overview**

Tinea Pedis

Introduction/Etiology/Epidemiology

- Dermatophyte infection of the feet; organisms responsible are *Trichophyton rubrum, Trichophyton mentagrophytes,* and *Epidermophyton floccosum.*
- Common in adolescents and adults; uncommon in childhood.
- Warm, moist environment of occlusive footwear predisposes to fungal infection.

Signs and Symptoms

Three forms of infection are recognized: interdigital, vesicular, and moccasin.

- Interdigital
  - Caused by *T rubrum* or *E floccosum.*
  - Pruritus, erythema, fissuring, scaling, and maceration occur in the interdigital spaces (Figure 40.1).
- Vesicular
  - Caused by *T mentagrophytes.*
  - Vesicles, bullae, and erosions appear on the instep of the foot (Figure 40.2).
- Moccasin
  - Caused by *T rubrum* or *E floccosum.*
  - Erythema and scaling involve much or all of the plantar surface and sides of the feet.
- Rarely, a dermatophytid (id) or autosensitization reaction occurs that produces a widespread eczematous-appearing eruption composed of papules or deep-seated vesicles.

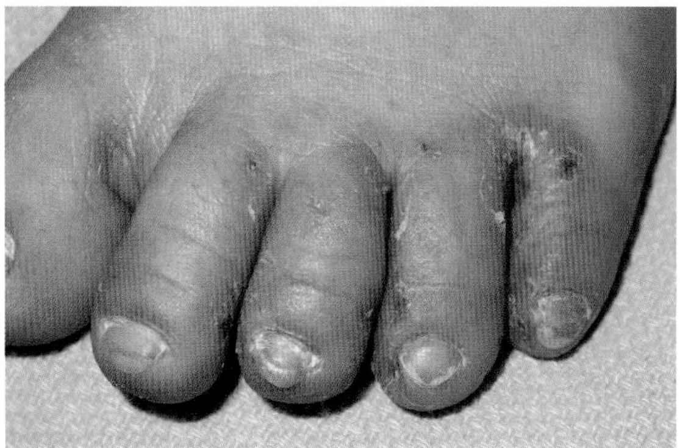

Figure 40.1. Scaling, fissuring, and erosions between the toes are seen in the interdigital form of tinea pedis.

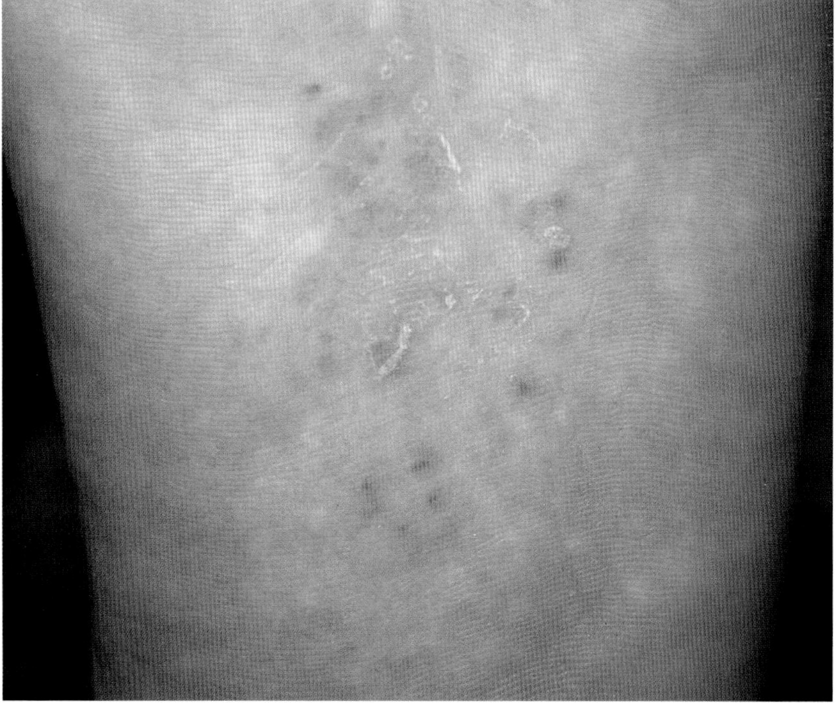

Figure 40.2. Erythematous papules and ruptured vesicles on the midfoot in vesicular tinea pedis.

Look-alikes

In each of the conditions listed herein, a potassium hydroxide preparation or fungal culture would fail to confirm the presence of fungal infection.

Disorder	Differentiating Features
Contact dermatitis	• Involves dorsum of feet; interdigital spaces spared
Juvenile plantar dermatosis	• Intense erythema with fissuring and pruritus occur on plantar foot, often with sparing of arch. • History of hyperhidrosis common. • Interdigital spaces spared. • History of atopic dermatitis often present.
Pitted keratolysis	• Small pits that may coalesce into larger, very superficial erosions present on plantar surface of foot • Hyperhidrosis and malodor often present • Interdigital spaces spared

How to Make the Diagnosis

- The diagnosis is made clinically.
- If uncertainty exists, a potassium hydroxide preparation (revealing branching hyphae) or fungal culture (eg, dermatophyte test medium) may be performed. (See Figure 37.5.)

Treatment

- For typical infections, application of a topical antifungal agent, such as an imidazole (eg, clotrimazole, miconazole, ketoconazole), allylamine (eg, terbinafine, naftifine), or tolnaftate, is appropriate. The agent is applied until the eruption clears, typically within 3 to 4 weeks.
- Widespread, resistant, or severe infections may require oral therapy with griseofulvin or another agent.
- Advise patients to keep their feet dry and, if possible, to wear well-ventilated shoes or sandals.
- For patients who experience recurrences, recommend the regular use of an absorbent powder containing an antifungal agent (eg, Zeasorb AF, Tinactin, Desenex, Lotrimin AF).

Treating Associated Conditions

- If treatment of concomitant nail infection (ie, onychomycosis) is desired, oral therapy with terbinafine or itraconazole will be required.

Prognosis

- The prognosis is excellent.
- To prevent recurrences, advise patients to dry carefully after bathing or showering, wear protective footwear in public showers, wear well-ventilated shoes or sandals, and regularly apply an absorbent powder containing an antifungal agent (eg, Zeasorb AF, Micatin, Tinactin).

When to Worry or Refer

- Consider consultation with a dermatologist when the diagnosis is in doubt or when the patient fails to respond to appropriate therapy.

Resources for Families

- American Academy of Pediatrics: HealthyChildren.org.
  www.HealthyChildren.org/tinea
- MedlinePlus: Information for patients and families (in English and Spanish) sponsored by the National Library of Medicine and National Institutes of Health.
  https://www.nlm.nih.gov/medlineplus/athletesfoot.html
- WebMD: Information for families is contained in the Health A-Z topics.
  www.webmd.com/skin-problems-and-treatments/tc/athletes-foot-topic-overview

CHAPTER 41

Tinea Versicolor

Introduction/Etiology/Epidemiology

- Tinea versicolor is a common fungal infection that occurs in adolescents and adults; it occurs rarely in children.
- Causative organism is *Malassezia* species (formerly *Pityrosporum* species), which invades the stratum corneum.
  - The organism is a common inhabitant of the skin. When it enters a mycelial phase, clinical disease results.
  - The organism thrives in hot, humid environments and is lipophilic, thriving on skin with available lipid.

Signs and Symptoms

- Characteristic lesions are small, hypopigmented or hyperpigmented, round or oval macules located on the trunk, proximal extremities, and neck (Figures 41.1 and 41.2).
  - Lesions have well-defined borders.
  - Individual lesions may coalesce into large patches.
- In fair-complexioned individuals who have hypopigmented lesions, sun exposure accentuates the appearance of the disorder, as surrounding normal skin darkens while infected skin does not.
- Lesions are generally asymptomatic (although pruritus may be present) but may cause considerable concern due to their appearance.

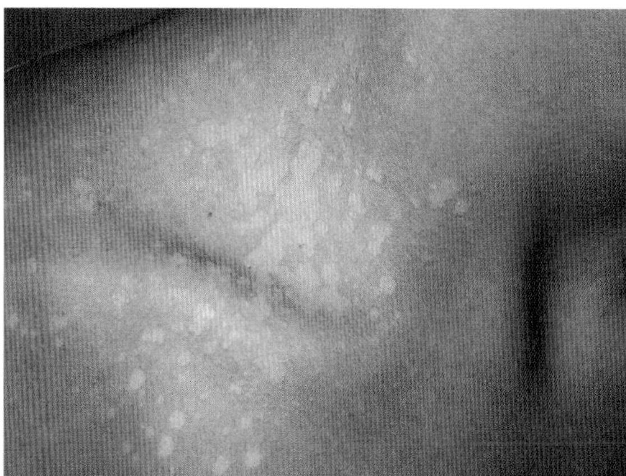

Figure 41.1. Well-defined hypopigmented scaling macules in tinea versicolor.

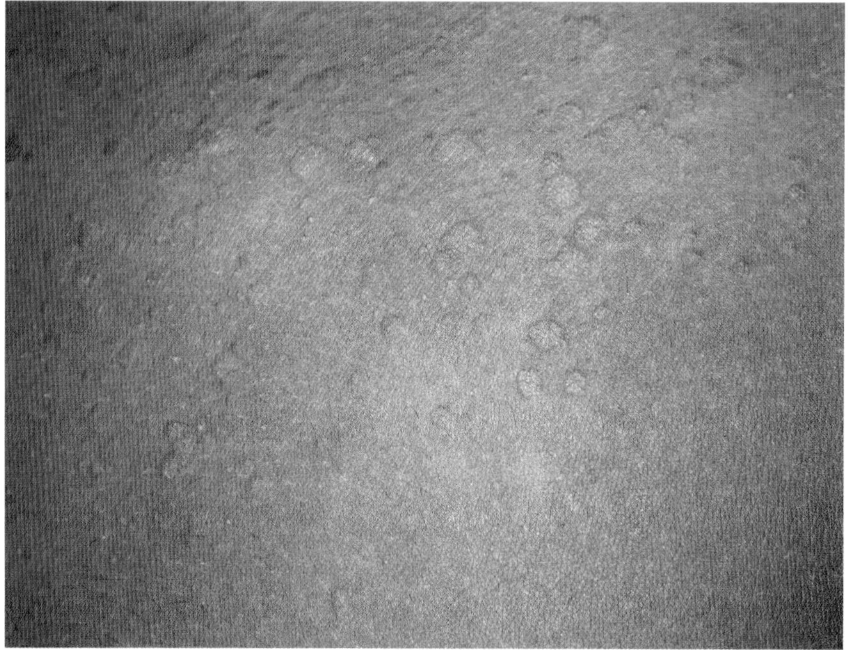

Figure 41.2. Well-defined hyperpigmented scaling macules in tinea versicolor.

Look-alikes

In each of the conditions listed herein, a potassium hydroxide preparation would fail to confirm the presence of spores and hyphae observed in tinea versicolor.

Disorder	Differentiating Features
Vitiligo	• Lesions of vitiligo depigmented so appear completely white. • Wood light examination reveals marked accentuation of depigmentation.
Pityriasis alba	• Lesions with indistinct borders • Most often occurs on the face
Pityriasis rosea	• Lesions elevated and inflammatory • Lesions arranged with long axes parallel to lines of skin tension

How to Make the Diagnosis

- The diagnosis usually is made clinically.
- If uncertainty exists, a potassium hydroxide preparation performed on scale from lesions will reveal short hyphae and spores (ie, "spaghetti and meatballs") (Figure 41.3).
- Examination of the skin with a Wood light in a darkened room may reveal a yellow-orange or blue-white fluorescence of affected areas.

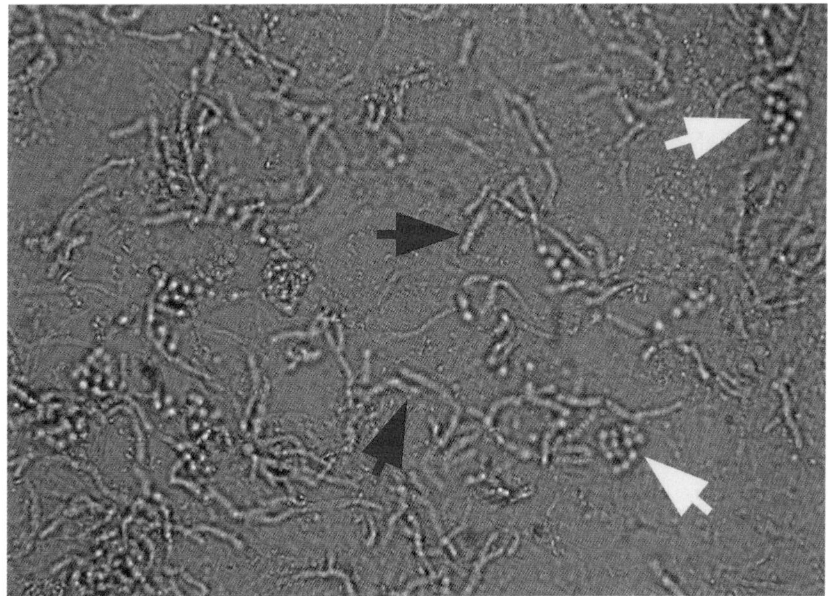

Figure 41.3. In tinea versicolor, potassium hydroxide preparation on scale obtained from a lesion demonstrates short hyphae (red arrows) and spores (yellow arrows) (ie, "spaghetti and meatballs").

Treatment

- Topical
  - If infection is very localized, topical antifungal agents (eg, imidazoles) are effective.
  - If infection is widespread (most patients), options include
    - Selenium sulfide 1% shampoo or 2.5% lotion
      - Apply to entire affected area 10 minutes daily for 7 days.
      - Apply for 8 to 12 hours once each month for 3 months thereafter (to prevent recurrence).
    - Ketoconazole shampoo
      - Apply for 5 minutes daily for 1 to 3 days (will need to use this agent or selenium sulfide for prophylaxis as described previously).
    - Terbinafine 1% spray
      - Apply 1 to 2 times daily for 2 to 4 weeks.
- Systemic (off-label)
  - Usually reserved for persistent or recurrent infections or for patients who cannot use topical therapy.
  - Options include fluconazole (400 mg once, or 300 mg once and repeated in 1 week) or itraconazole (400 mg once or 200 mg/d for 7 days). More recent recommendations suggest complete avoidance of ketoconazole (an agent which was classically recommended) due to rare, but possible, severe liver injury.
  - Advising physical activity following a dose promotes delivery of the drug to the skin surface via sweat and may enhance efficacy.
  - Prophylactic therapy with selenium sulfide (as previously described) should be advised.

Prognosis

- The prognosis is excellent, but recurrences are common.
- Advise patients that months may be required for normalization of pigmentation following effective treatment.

When to Worry or Refer

- Consider consultation when the diagnosis is in doubt or when the patient fails to respond to appropriate therapy.

Resources for Families

- American Academy of Pediatrics: HealthyChildren.org.
  www.HealthyChildren.org/tinea
- American Academy of Dermatology: Tinea versicolor.
  https://www.aad.org/public/diseases/color-problems/tinea-versicolor
- MedlinePlus: Information for patients and families (in English and Spanish) sponsored by the National Library of Medicine and National Institutes of Health.
  https://www.nlm.nih.gov/medlineplus/ency/article/001465.htm
- WebMD: Information for families is contained in the Health A-Z topics.
  www.webmd.com/skin-problems-and-treatments/tc/tinea-versicolor-topic-overview

Infestations

CHAPTER
42

Cutaneous Larva Migrans

Introduction/Etiology/Epidemiology

- Also known as creeping eruption, larva migrans.
- A self-limited skin eruption caused by accidental penetration of the human host by the dog hookworm (*Ancylostoma caninum*) and cat hookworm (*Ancylostoma braziliensis*). *Uncinaria stenocephala,* a hookworm that affects dogs and cats, has also been implicated in some cases. Other skin-penetrating nematodes may occasionally cause disease.
- Usually noted after travel to tropical regions, including southeastern United States (especially Florida and Georgia), Central and South America, Africa, and the Caribbean.
- May occur in epidemics in high-income countries and in tourists.
- Adult hookworms release eggs in host animal's intestines, and eggs pass with feces into soil.
- Eggs hatch, releasing larvae that penetrate human skin and wander aimlessly, producing serpiginous tracts.

Signs and Symptoms

- Erythematous, serpiginous plaques develop on skin.
- Incubation period may last for several weeks in some patients.
- Lesions may "advance" up to 2 mm per day.
- Most common locations include feet (Figure 42.1), buttocks, and genitalia.
- May be intensely pruritic.
- Blisters may rarely occur.
- Eosinophilic pneumonitis (Löffler syndrome) may rarely occur, but peripheral blood eosinophilia is common.
- Rarely, the larvae travel to the intestines, causing eosinophilic enteritis.

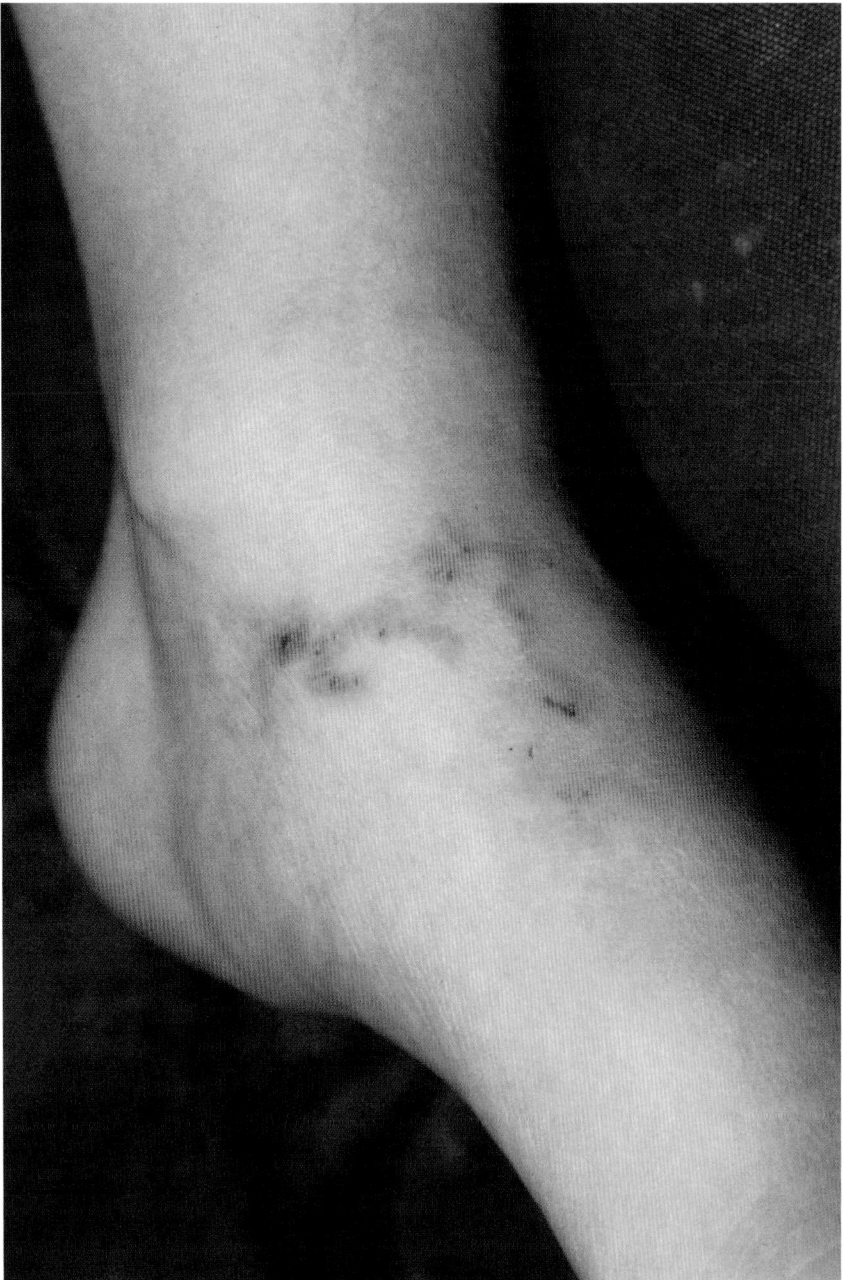

Figure 42.1. Cutaneous larva migrans. Note the serpiginous erythematous tracts.

Look-alikes

Disorder	Differentiating Features
Scabies	• Burrows short (up to a few millimeters), do not migrate • Widespread distribution, favoring folds, wrists, ankles, genitals, palms, and soles
Tinea corporis	• Annular plaques enlarge in a centrifugal pattern. • Scale commonly present. • Pruritus less significant than in cutaneous larva migrans.
Other nematode infestations	• Variety of systemic manifestations depending on nematode; may include *Strongyloides stercoralis* and *Gnathostoma spinigerum*
Allergic contact dermatitis	• Bizarre patterning may be present. • Vesicles and bullae common. • History may be useful.
Phytophotodermatitis	• Erythematous eruption, which also usually follows outdoor activities. • Patches correspond to sites of contact with offending photosensitizer (including lime or lemon juice, dill, parsley, parsnips, figs, celery); may present as linear streaks and "drip marks." • In addition to erythematous patches, vesicles and bullae are often present. • Heals with marked hyperpigmentation.

How to Make the Diagnosis

- Clinical examination findings combined with extreme pruritus and exposure history are usually confirmatory.
- Skin biopsy (rarely necessary) typically reveals intense eosinophilic infiltrate.

Treatment

- Process is self-limited, but symptoms usually necessitate therapy.
- Oral albendazole, ivermectin, or thiabendazole is effective.
  - Albendazole: 15 mg/kg per day (maximum 400 mg/d) for 3 days
  - Ivermectin: 200 mcg/kg given orally once daily for 1 to 2 days
  - Thiabendazole: 25 mg/kg per day, divided into 2 doses, for 2 to 5 days (rarely used now)
- Topical thiabendazole (500 mg/5 mL) applied 4 times daily is also effective.
- Cryotherapy (traditional treatment) is rarely effective and is traumatic for young children; it should be avoided.

Treating Associated Conditions

- Secondary bacterial infection should be treated with an appropriate systemic antibiotic.

Prognosis

- Cutaneous larva migrans resolves completely without permanent sequelae.

When to Worry or Refer

- Referral to a dermatologist should be considered for patients in whom the diagnosis is in question or for whom conventional therapy is unsuccessful.

Resources for Families

- Centers for Disease Control and Prevention: Parasites – Zoonotic Hookworm. **www.cdc.gov/parasites/zoonotichookworm/gen_info/faqs.html**
- DermNet NZ: Site sponsored by the New Zealand Dermatological Society, Inc.
  www.dermnetnz.org/arthropods/larva-migrans.html

Head Lice

Introduction/Etiology/Epidemiology

- Infestation occurs commonly in children attending child care or school.
- Caused by *Pediculus humanus capitis,* the human head louse.
- Less commonly seen in African American children.
- Transmission mainly via head-to-head contact; less commonly through fomites (eg, combs, hairbrushes, hats, towels, hooded jackets); prevention of spread is best focused on reducing active infestations and minimizing direct head-to-head contact.
- Affects all socioeconomic groups.
- Head louse (unlike body louse) does not transmit disease.

Signs and Symptoms

- Pruritus is the most common symptom, although many children may be asymptomatic, especially during the first weeks of a primary infestation.
- Secondary excoriation and bacterial infection may be present.
- Evidence of infestation (live lice, nits, excoriations) is often most apparent behind the ears and at the nape of the neck.
- Regional (cervical, suboccipital) lymphadenopathy is common if there is secondary bacterial infection.
- Live lice may be seen and are 2 to 4 mm in length.
- Nits (eggs) present as 0.5- to 0.8-mm, tan-brown concretions firmly affixed to hair shafts (Figure 43.1).
- Hatched (nonviable) nits are usually white in color.

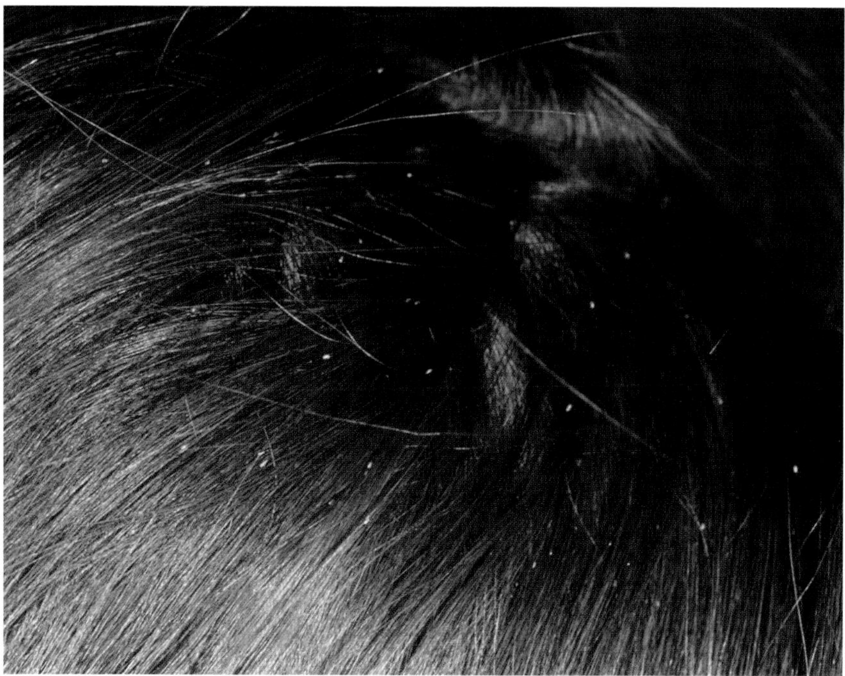

Figure 43.1. Head lice. Note numerous nits attached to hair shafts.

Look-alikes

Disorder	Differentiating Features
Seborrheic dermatitis	• Erythematous patches with greasy yellow scale • Absence of live lice or nits • White "dandruff" easily removed from hair shaft, unlike firmly affixed nits
Psoriasis	• Well-demarcated, erythematous, scaly papules and plaques • May note involvement in other regions (eg, elbows, knees, sacrum) • Absence of live lice or nits
Hair casts	• Easily removed from hair shaft
Piedra	• Loosely adherent, soft nodules of hair shaft • Causes hair breakage • May be black or white • May also involve axillary, pubic hair
Hair products	• Topically applied products (eg, hair spray, gel, mousse) may leave debris in hair that may mimic nits.

How to Make the Diagnosis

- Clinical examination: Identification of live lice is the gold standard for diagnosis but can be difficult. The presence of viable nits on hairs (within 1 cm of the scalp) is highly suggestive of active infestation.
- Viability of nits can be assessed by mounting affected hairs on a glass slide and performing low-power microscopic examination; viable nits have an intact operculum (cap) at the nonattached end.

Treatment

- Pediculicides are the treatment of choice and include
  - Permethrin 1% cream rinse, available over the counter; first-line therapy; applied to hair that has been shampooed and towel dried; left on for 10 minutes and then rinsed; approved in infants 2 months and older.
  - Synergized pyrethrins (pyrethrin + piperonyl butoxide), available in a variety of over-the-counter products; applied to dry hair; also used for 10 minutes; should not be used in individuals with allergy to chrysanthemums.
  - Benzyl alcohol 5% lotion, available by prescription, is a suffocation-based pediculicide that contains no neurotoxic pesticide; applied to dry hair, left on for 10 minutes, and then rinsed; benzyl alcohol "stuns" open respiratory spiracles , and mineral oil vehicle suffocates louse; approved in infants 6 months and older.
  - Malathion 0.5% lotion, available by prescription; applied to dry hair and rinsed in 8 to 12 hours; approved in children 6 years and older; product is flammable.
  - Spinosad 0.9% suspension, a fermentation product of the soil bacterium *Saccharopolyspora spinosa,* is applied to dry hair and rinsed in 10 minutes; approved in children 4 years and older.
  - Ivermectin 0.5% lotion is applied to dry hair and rinsed in 10 minutes; approved in infants 6 months and older.
  - Lindane shampoo 1% (left on for 4 minutes); available by prescription; reserved for those who have failed several other safer treatments; potentially neurotoxic and should be used with caution in children weighing less than 50 kg, pregnant or nursing women, and patients with traumatized or abraded skin; lindane has been banned for use in California and is no longer recommended by most experts for the treatment of lice.

- Repeat topical therapy (7–10 days after the initial treatment) is usually recommended to ensure killing of any eggs that hatch after first treatment but may vary by product.
- Oral ivermectin (200 mcg/kg single dose) has been used off-label for children older than 2 years who weigh 15 kg or more with resistant disease.
- Alternative off-label therapies include trimethoprim-sulfamethoxazole and "suffocation" therapies (eg, petroleum jelly, mayonnaise, olive oil); problem with latter is ability of human head louse to close respiratory spiracles temporarily, reopening them after removal of the occlusive agent.
- Before pediculicidal resistance is suggested, consider other causes of therapeutic failure, like misdiagnosis, repeat infestation, or treatment noncompliance.
- Manual removal of lice and nits with nit combing of wet hair is possible for those who prefer not to use a pediculicide. Professional "nit-removal salons" are available in some regions.
- Close contacts should be examined and treated (if necessary), and bedding and clothing should be machine washed and dried on a high-heat setting. Necessary shared headgear (eg, batting helmets, computer headphones) can be wiped with a damp cloth between uses.
- "No nit" policies, which prevent children with nits from attending child care or school, are not effective and can lead to academic and social struggles for children. No healthy child should be excluded from or allowed to miss school time because of head lice.

Treating Associated Conditions

- Secondary bacterial infection should be treated with an appropriate systemic antibiotic.
- Scalp dermatitis can be treated with topical corticosteroid solution (eg, fluocinolone 0.01% scalp solution, mometasone 0.1% solution).
- Severe pruritus may necessitate oral antihistamine therapy.

Prognosis

- Most patients with head lice respond well to therapy, and there are no permanent sequelae.

When to Worry or Refer

- Consider referral to a dermatologist for patients with disease that seems to be resistant to standard therapy (after considering misdiagnosis, reinfestation, or treatment noncompliance).

Resources for Families

- American Academy of Pediatrics: HealthyChildren.org.
www.HealthyChildren.org/lice
www.HealthyChildren.org/licenews
- Centers for Disease Control and Prevention: Parasites – lice – head lice.
www.cdc.gov/parasites/lice/head
- The National Pediculosis Association, Inc.: Welcome to HeadLice.org.
www.headlice.org
- MedlinePlus: Information for patients and families (in English and Spanish) sponsored by the National Library of Medicine and National Institutes of Health.
https://www.nlm.nih.gov/medlineplus/ency/article/000840.htm

CHAPTER 44

Insect Bites and Papular Urticaria

Introduction/Etiology/Epidemiology

- Insect and arachnid bites occur throughout the world and may show seasonal variation.
- Some of dermatologic significance include 8-legged arachnids (mites, ticks, spiders, scorpions) and 6-legged insects (lice, flies, mosquitoes, fleas, bugs, bees, wasps, ants, caterpillars, and beetles).
- Some of these arthropods may be vectors for significant diseases.
- Protection against bites is a vital step in prevention of these reactions.
- Host reaction represents immune response against proteins found in arthropod saliva.
- This discussion includes mosquitoes, fleas, mites, bedbugs, ticks, and papular urticaria.

Signs and Symptoms

- Mosquitoes
  - Most common bite reactions in infants and children in the United States.
  - May serve worldwide as vectors for disease (eg, encephalitis [including West Nile encephalitis], yellow fever, malaria, dengue, filariasis).
  - Classically present as edematous, erythematous papules and urticarial wheals (Figure 44.1).
  - Small central crust or punctum may be visible at site of bite.
  - Vesicles, bullae, or hemorrhage may occur.
  - Excoriation may lead to secondary eczematous changes and impetiginization.
  - Systemic hypersensitivity reactions/anaphylaxis rarely are present.

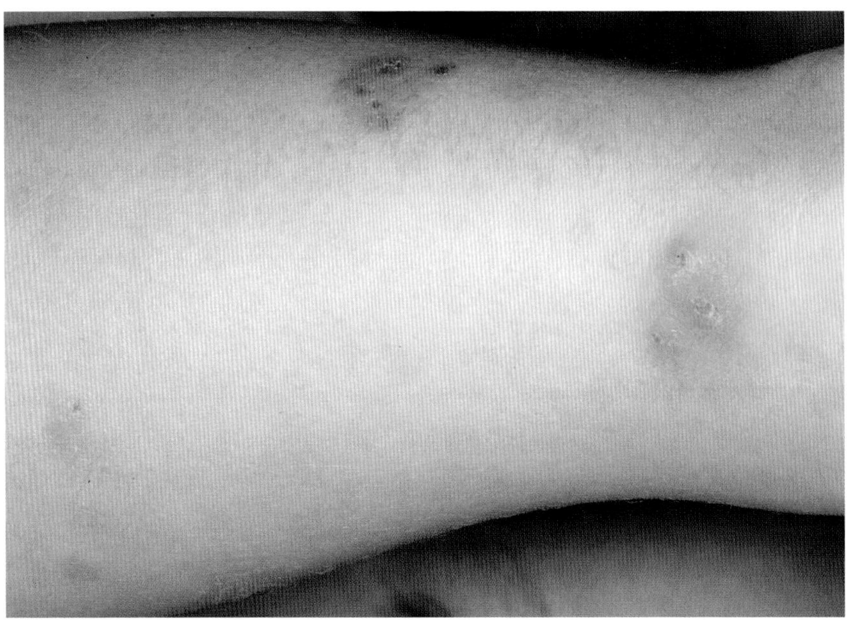

Figure 44.1. Mosquito bites.

- Fleas
  - Ubiquitous insects with little host specificity.
  - Common fleas in the United States include human flea (*Pulex irritans*), cat flea (*Ctenocephalides felis*), and dog flea (*Ctenocephalides canis*).
  - May be vectors for cat-scratch disease, endemic typhus, and plague.
  - In addition to animal (pet) carriers, fleas may be found in carpets, floors, sandboxes, beaches, and grassy areas.
  - Bites result in extremely pruritic papules or urticarial wheals, often with a central punctum.
  - Reactions may evolve into large bullae (Figure 44.2).
  - Most common location is the lower extremities; upper extremities and areas covered by tight clothing also common.
  - Because fleas jump but cannot fly, bite reactions are often clustered in a linear configuration ("breakfast, lunch, and dinner" sign; Figure 44.3).

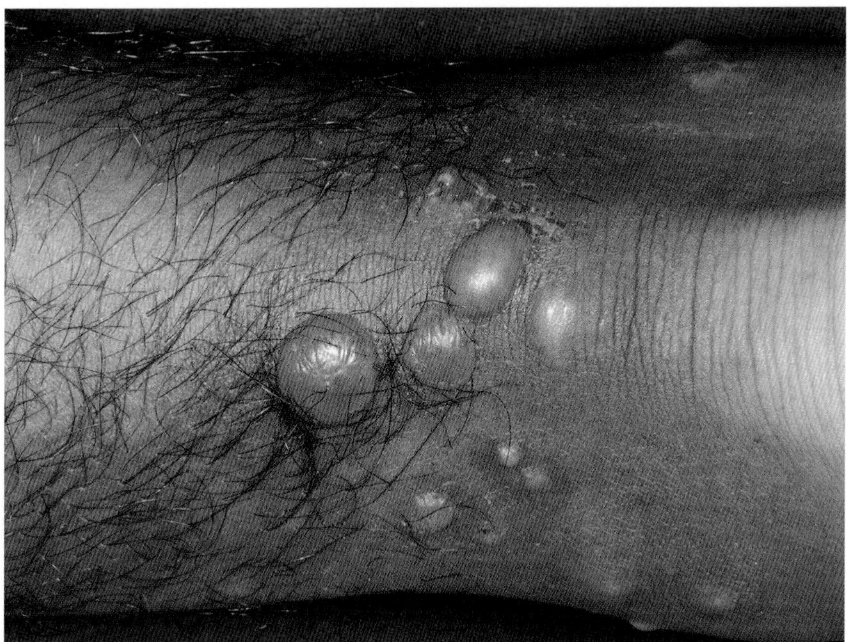

Figure 44.2. Bullous flea bite reaction.

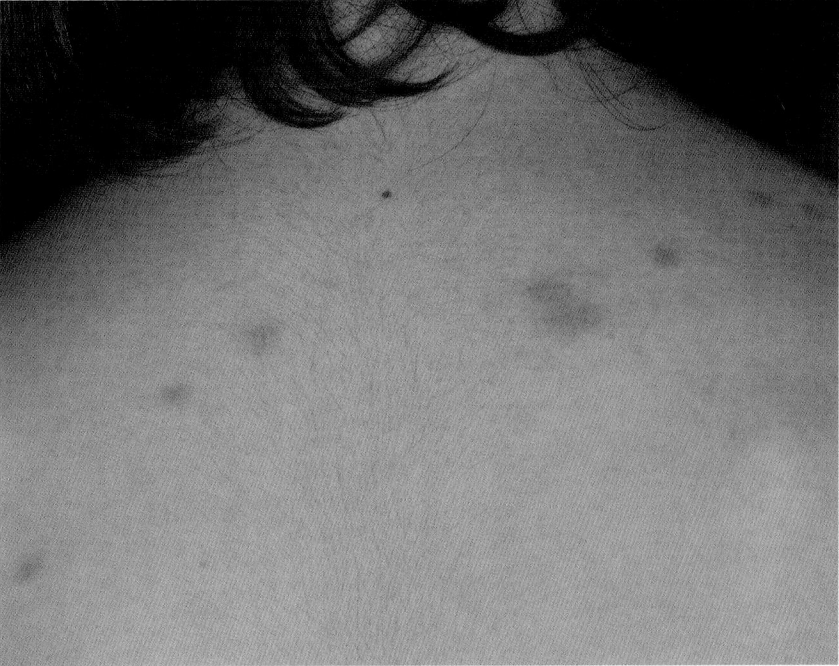

Figure 44.3. Flea bites. Note the "breakfast, lunch, and dinner" sign.

- Mites
  - Small (0.1–2.0 mm) arachnids with numerous species, many of which live as parasites on animals or plants.
  - Bites result in local reactions, and some may serve as vectors for disease.
  - Mites of significance to humans include harvest mite (chiggers), grain mite, house mouse mite (vector for rickettsialpox), wheat mite, avian mite, dust mite, snake mite, rat/fowl mites, scrub mite (vector for scrub typhus), and mold mite.
  - Clinically present as pruritic, erythematous urticarial 1- to 2-mm papules, occasionally with a visible central punctum or hemorrhage; lesions often are multiple (Figure 44.4).
  - "Summer penile syndrome" is an acute hypersensitivity to chigger bites, presenting with intense penile swelling and pruritus.
  - *Cheyletiella,* which are non-burrowing animal-specific mites (cats, dogs, rabbits), may bite humans, resulting in grouped, pruritic papules. In infested pets, patches of fine powdery scale ("walking dandruff") are present.

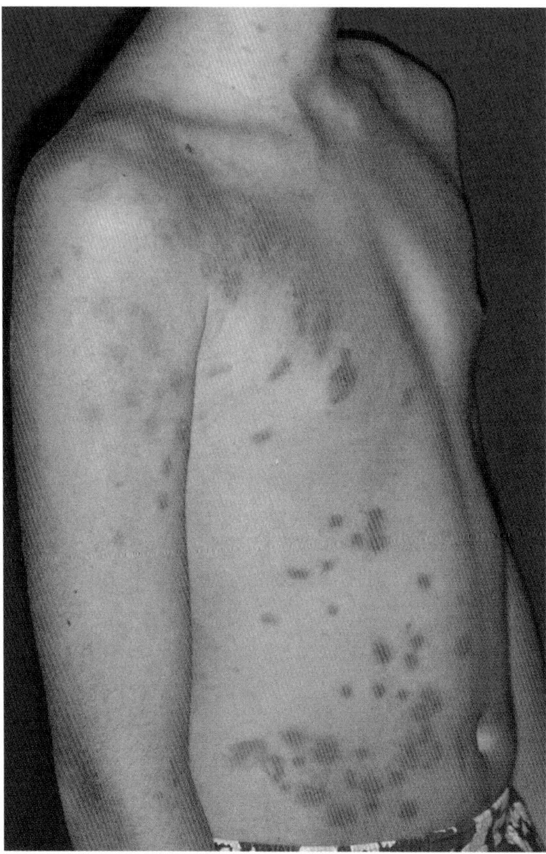

Figure 44.4. Mite bites. Multiple, clustered, edematous red papules and plaques.

- Bedbugs
  - *Cimex lectularius* most common species to parasitize humans.
  - Nocturnal insects that reside in cracks and crevices, coming out to feed at night.
  - Three to 7 mm in size, with flattened oval bodies (Figure 44.5).
  - Bite reactions are erythematous papules with occasional bullous component.
  - Linear clustering of reactions may be present (similar to "breakfast, lunch, and dinner" sign seen with flea bites).
  - Potential vectors for blood-borne pathogens; methicillin-resistant *Staphylococcus aureus* and vancomycin-resistant *Enterococcus faecium* have also been recovered from some bedbugs.
  - Resurgence in bedbugs has been noted in recent years, especially in hotels, hostels, and travel vessels (aircraft, trains, cruise ships).
- Ticks
  - See Systemic Bacterial, Rickettsial, or Spirochetal Infections With Skin Manifestations (chapters 29–34) for a discussion of Lyme disease.
  - Important vectors for disease, including Lyme disease, relapsing fever, Rocky Mountain spotted fever, Mediterranean spotted fever, Q fever, ehrlichiosis, babesiosis, Colorado tick fever, and tularemia.
  - Acute and chronic dermatoses may result from bites.
  - Acute reaction may include erythematous, papular, nodular, bullous, or necrotic lesions.
  - Chronic changes include persistent nodules (may have lymphoma-like characteristics on histologic examination), granulomas ("tick bite granuloma"), alopecia.
  - Tick paralysis consists of ascending motor weakness and paralysis, resulting from neurotoxin that is injected while tick is engorged; reversible on removal of tick. It has been noted more commonly in young girls, possibly owing to longer hair, which may make tick identification more challenging.
  - Tick removal is best accomplished by grasping the tick close to the skin with forceps and using gentle but steady traction, with care to avoid twisting, crushing, or severing the arachnid. Several commercial devices are available.

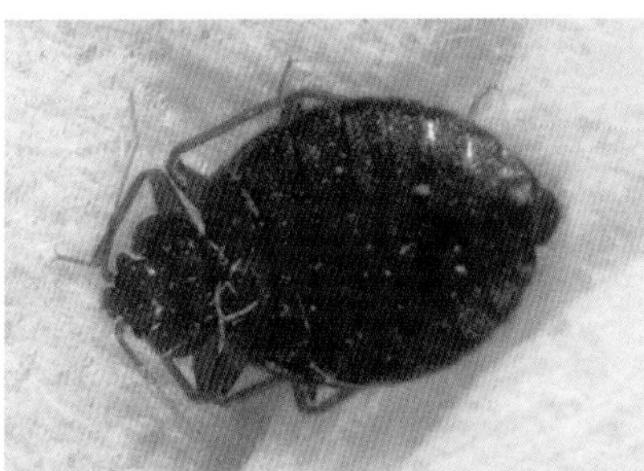

Figure 44.5. Bedbug. Note the flattened, oval body of this bug, which was brought in to the clinic by the patient's mother.

- Papular urticaria
  - Common, chronic condition of recurrent papules as a result of hypersensitivity to arthropod bites.
  - Flea bites are the most common cause.
  - Most common in late spring and summer.
  - Lesions are erythematous, urticarial pruritic papules (Figure 44.6).
  - May be generalized or erupt only at sites of past bite reactions.
  - Excoriation and secondary bacterial superinfection are common.
  - Lesions often heal with postinflammatory hyperpigmentation; recurrence is common.

Look-alikes

Disorder	Differentiating Features
Pityriasis lichenoides	• Scaly or necrotic papules and plaques • Diffuse distribution • Usually nonpruritic • Erupt in recurrent, cyclical fashion
Lymphomatoid papulosis	• Red-brown papules and nodules. • Usually nonpruritic. • Histologic evaluation reveals lymphoma-like changes.
Bullous pemphigoid	• Unusual in children • Widespread, tense bullae and vesicles • Occasional mucosal involvement
Urticaria	• Transient, with individual lesions resolving over hours • Puncta, crusting vesicles, bullae absent
Bullous impetigo	• Fragile bullae that rupture easily • Moist, erosive surface with peripheral collarette of scale • Painful rather than pruritic
Gianotti-Crosti syndrome	• Edematous, erythematous papules lacking central puncta • Symmetric distribution on extensor upper and lower extremities, cheeks, and buttocks

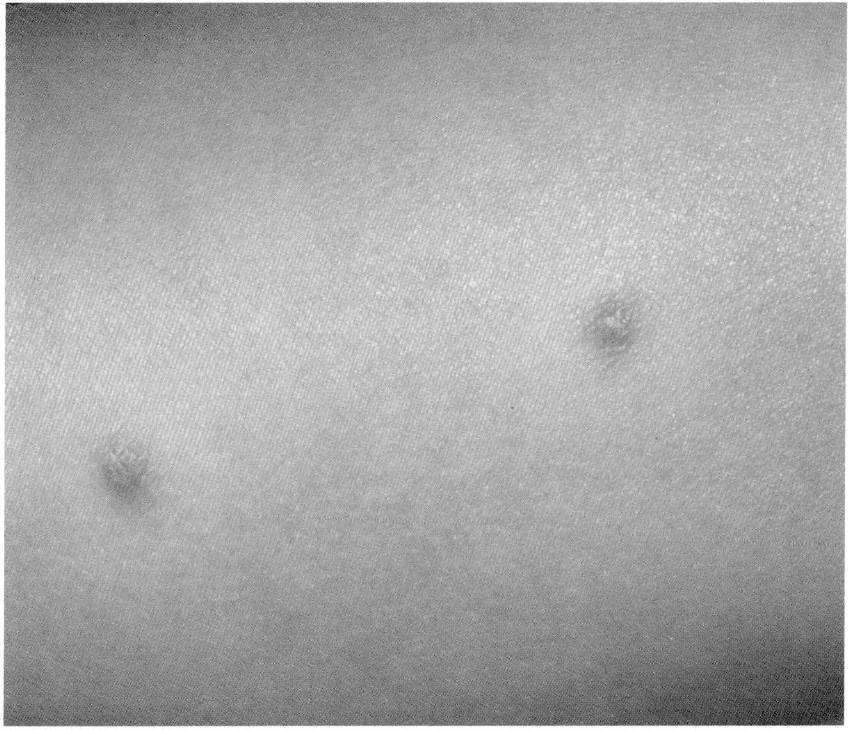

Figure 44.6. Papular urticaria. These edematous, pruritic red papules intermittently flared at sites of prior flea bites.

How to Make the Diagnosis

- Clinical examination, revealing edematous, pruritic papules and plaques with central puncta, crusting, vesicles, hemorrhage, or bullae.
- Skin biopsy (rarely necessary) reveals dermal and epidermal edema and numerous eosinophils.

Treatment

- Oral antihistamines.
- Cool compresses.
- Topical antipruritic agents, including calamine lotion, camphor, and menthol lotions. Parents should be cautioned to secure camphor-containing agents to avoid inadvertent ingestion, which could be dangerous.

- For severe or more symptomatic lesions, use topical corticosteroid ointments or creams.
  - In younger children: mild- to mid-strength preparations.
  - In older children, teens, and adults: class I through II products often necessary (for non-facial, non-fold, nongenital regions only).
  - Applied once to twice daily.
  - Consider occlusion for severe reactions.
- Prevention includes avoidance of high-risk activities or exposure times, use of protective clothing, and use of insect repellents.
  - Most effective repellent is N,N-diethyl-3-methylbenzamide or DEET.
    - DEET is a broad-spectrum repellent with activity against mosquitoes, fleas, biting flies, and ticks.
    - Available in a variety of concentrations and vehicles.
    - Products with 10% to 30% concentration of DEET will provide adequate protection in most circumstances (around 2–5 hours of protection, depending on the concentration used).
    - DEET should not be used in infants younger than 2 months.
    - Repellent should be applied lightly and evenly (avoid skin saturation) on exposed skin, with caution not to apply near the eyes, mouth, or hands of young children.
    - DEET should not be applied to open wounds or inflamed areas.
    - Combination DEET and sunscreen preparations are not recommended because the need for frequent sunscreen application will result in unnecessary DEET exposure and potential toxicity.
    - Once indoors, all areas of application should be washed with soap and water.
  - Other options for most insects (excluding ticks) include picaridin, oil of lemon eucalyptus, and soybean oil; picaridin has a reported efficacy similar to that for DEET.
  - Citronella, the active ingredient is many "natural" repellents, including oils, torch fuels, and candles, is not as effective as DEET or picaridin and should not be relied on as sole repellent in high-risk settings.
  - Permethrin 0.5% spray is useful when applied to clothing, tents, and sleeping bags; it has activity against ticks, mosquitoes, flies, and chiggers.
- For mosquitoes: Efforts to reduce insect populations (individual and community) are helpful.
- For fleas: Treatment of suspected animal hosts and cleaning of fomites (carpets, floors, furniture) should be considered.

- For bedbugs: Consultation with a professional pest control service or cooperative extension is recommended. Although a variety of eradication strategies may be employed (eg, insecticides, steam treatment), heat treatment has become increasingly popular and is effective. In this procedure, conducted by professional pest control services, the air temperature in a room or house is raised to greater than 120°F for several hours, killing bedbugs and their eggs. Clothing and bedding should be washed in hot water and dried at high temperature.

Treating Associated Conditions

- Secondary bacterial infection of bite reactions should be treated with an appropriate systemic antibiotic.
- Tick bite granulomas may require treatment with intralesional corticosteroid injection or surgical excision.

Prognosis

- Typical, uncomplicated bite reactions resolve completely without permanent sequelae.
- Papular urticaria may persist for months, rarely years, requiring intermittent therapy as necessary.

When to Worry or Refer

- Referral to a dermatologist should be considered for "bite reactions" that do not resolve or have atypical features.

Resources for Families

- MedicineNet.com: Bug bites and stings.
  www.medicinenet.com/bug_bites_and_stings/article.htm
- WebMD: Information for families is contained in the Health A-Z topics.
  www.webmd.com/allergies/urticaria-papular

Scabies

Introduction/Etiology/Epidemiology

- A worldwide problem affecting all ages, races, and socioeconomic strata.
- Caused by *Sarcoptes scabiei* variety *hominis*, the human scabies mite.
- Higher incidence in situations of overcrowding.
- Transmission via direct skin-to-skin contact; acquisition from fomites (bedding, clothing) is less common.
- Incubation period is approximately 3 weeks but shorter with reinfestation.
- Female mite lays eggs in skin burrows, which propagates the infestation.

Signs and Symptoms

- Pruritus (often most intense at night) may be severe and present before clinical lesions are apparent.
- Papules, burrows (white-gray threadlike lines), vesiculopustules common (Figures 45.1 and 45.2).
- Nodules, which are seen primarily in infants, may persist for months and represent a vigorous host immune response (Figure 45.3).
- Common locations include interdigital spaces, wrists, ankles, axillae, waist, groin, palms, and soles.
- Scalp involvement may be seen in infants.
- Secondary superinfection (usually *Staphylococcus aureus* or *Streptococcus pyogenes*) may occur.

- Crusted (Norwegian) scabies
  - Occurs in immunocompromised patients, especially those infected with HIV, or debilitated individuals
  - Presents as scaly, erythematous, hyperkeratotic plaques with excoriation
  - May mimic eczema, psoriasis, or warts
  - Frequently misdiagnosed and mismanaged given nondescript presentation
  - Extremely contagious given the high number of mites that are present

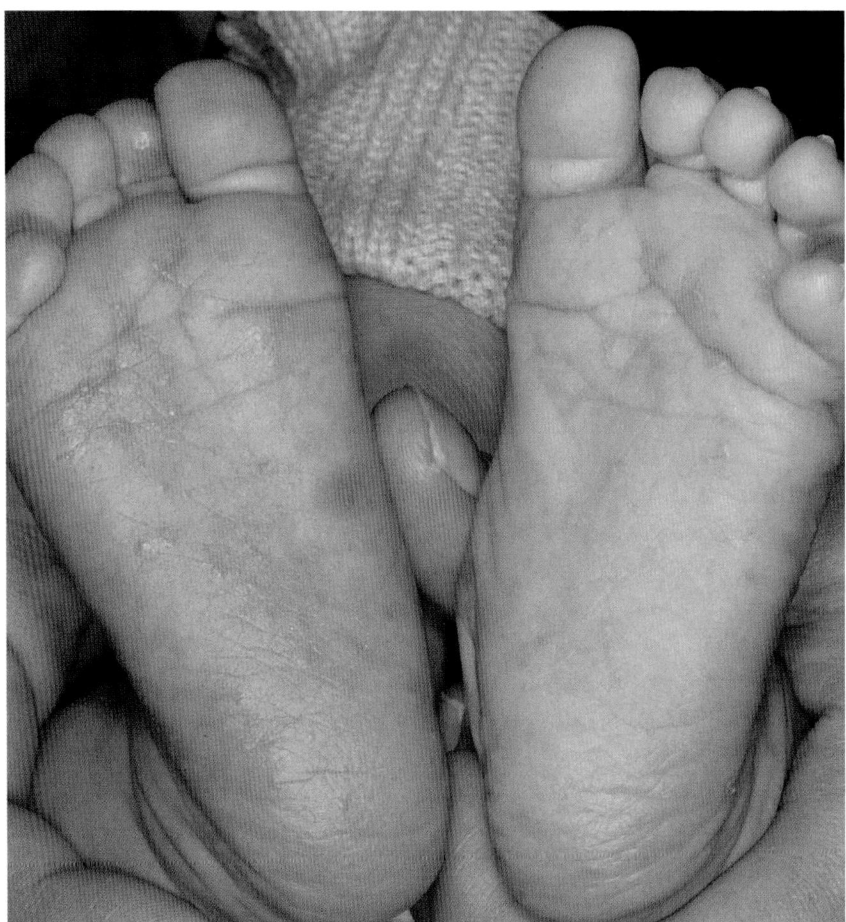

Figure 45.1. Scabies.

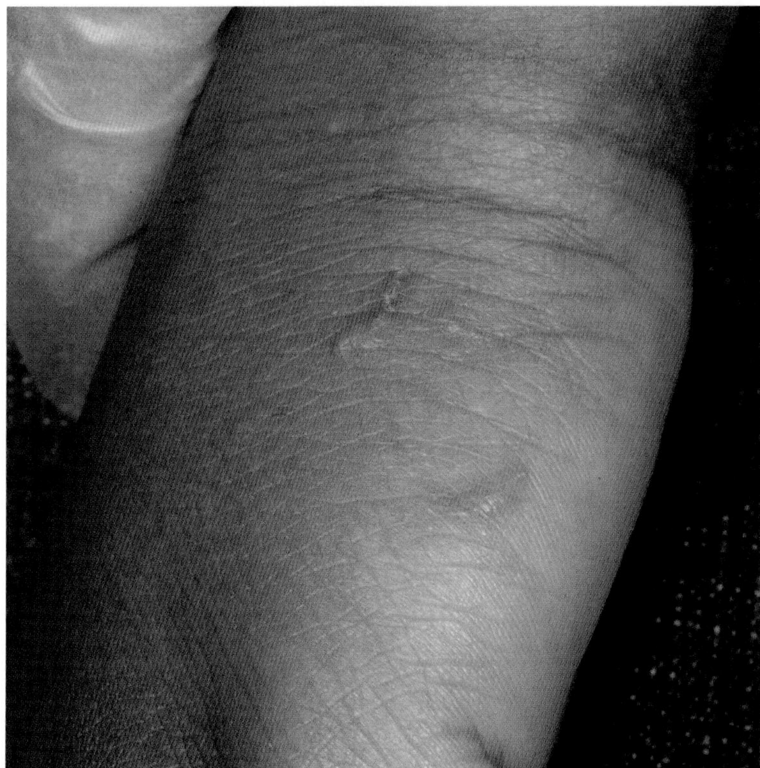

Figure 45.2. Scabies. Note linear burrows.

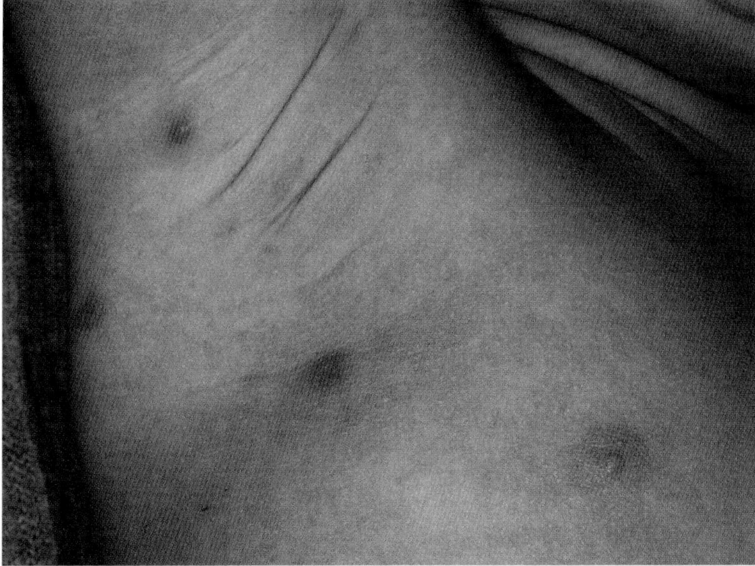

Figure 45.3. Scabies nodules in an infant.

Look-alikes

Disorder	Differentiating Features
Acropustulosis of infancy	• Vesicopustules of wrists, palms, ankles, and plantar feet occur in cyclical fashion, every 2–4 weeks. • Does not respond to permethrin therapy. • May represent a post-scabies hypersensitivity response.
Arthropod bites	• Tend to be more discrete and fewer in number • Palms and soles usually spared • May be clustered in linear fashion
Atopic dermatitis	• Atopic history common • Characteristic distribution by age • Diaper area/genitals usually spared in infants • Lichenification often present
Contact dermatitis	• Discrete patterning may be evident at sites of contact. • Less often papular, burrows absent. • Vesicles or bullae may be present.
Impetigo (crusted)	• Usually more focal • Most common on the face, especially areas around the nose and mouth
Langerhans cell histiocytosis	• Prominence of erythema and erosions in folds • Lymphadenopathy common • May have petechial or purpuric component • Associated bone lesions or other organ involvement
Papular urticaria	• Recurrent erythematous urticarial papules • Burrows, vesicopustules absent
Psoriasis	• Characteristic distribution, including scalp, elbows, knees, and sacral area • Sharply demarcated papulosquamous lesions (scaling papules and plaques)
Seborrheic dermatitis	• Erythema with greasy scaling • Favors scalp, postauricular creases, skinfolds, groin, and umbilicus • Lacks burrows, papules
Viral exanthem	• Erythematous macules and papules. • Vesicopustules, burrows typically absent. • Associated symptoms/signs of viral illness may be present.

How to Make the Diagnosis

- Clinical features usually suggest the diagnosis.
- Confirmation made by mineral oil examination (see Chapter 2, Diagnostic Techniques), with microscopic identification of mites, eggs, or feces (scybala) (Figure 45.4).
- Skin biopsy rarely is necessary.

Treatment

- Treatment of choice is 5% permethrin cream, applied from neck to feet (head to feet in infants) and left on for 8 to 14 hours prior to rinsing.
- Permethrin should be thoroughly applied in a thin, even coat; should include web spaces, umbilicus, genitals, and gluteal cleft.
- Second treatment with permethrin 1 week following the initial treatment is recommended by some experts.
- Signs and symptoms of scabies may persist for several weeks following therapy and may be treated with topical antipruritics/anti-inflammatories and oral antihistamines as necessary.

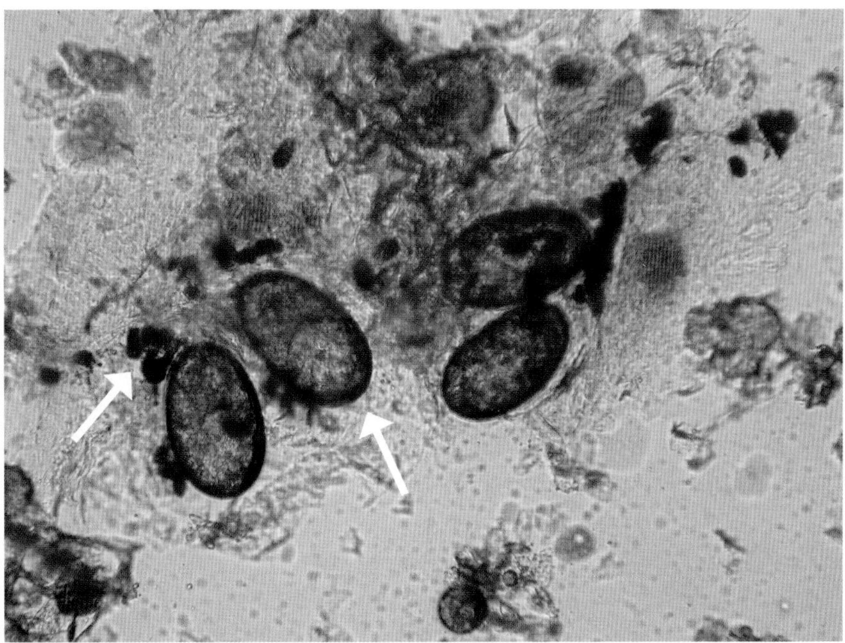

Figure 45.4. Mineral oil preparation in scabies (40x magnification). Note dark-brown fecal pellets (scybala) (small arrow) and larger, oval-shaped eggs (large arrow).

- Alternative therapies include
  - 5% to 10% sulfur in petrolatum.
  - Crotamiton 10% cream or lotion (high failure rate).
  - Lindane lotion 1%; used extensively in the past but should be reserved only for those who have failed several other safer treatments; potentially neurotoxic and should be used with caution in children weighing less than 50 kg, pregnant or nursing women, and patients with traumatized or abraded skin. Lindane has been banned in California and is no longer recommended by most experts for the treatment of scabies.
  - Single-dose ivermectin (200 mcg/kg per dose) has been used (off-label) for crusted scabies or disease in immunocompromised patients; topical ivermectin is reportedly effective.
- Environmental decontamination important: Machine wash clothing, bed linens, and towels in hot water and dry on high-heat setting.
- Prophylactic therapy of household members and other close contacts should be performed at the time the index case is treated initially.

Treating Associated Conditions

- Secondary bacterial infection: Treat with appropriate systemic antibiotic therapy.
- Scabies nodules: May be treated with topical or intralesional corticosteroids.

Prognosis

- Scabies usually responds well to therapy, and there are no permanent sequelae.
- Patients with Norwegian (crusted) scabies may be more resistant to treatment and may require multimodal or repeat therapy.

When to Worry or Refer

- Consider referral to a dermatologist if the diagnosis is in question, for patients who have severe or extensive disease, or for those who do not respond to standard treatment.

Resources for Families

- American Academy of Pediatrics: HealthyChildren.org.
  www.HealthyChildren.org/scabies
- American Academy of Dermatology: Scabies.
  https://www.aad.org/public/diseases/contagious-skin-diseases/scabies
- MedlinePlus: Information for patients and families (in English and Spanish) sponsored by the National Library of Medicine and National Institutes of Health.
  https://www.nlm.nih.gov/medlineplus/ency/article/000830.htm

Papulosquamous Diseases

CHAPTER 46

Lichen Nitidus

Introduction/Etiology/Epidemiology

- Lichen nitidus is a benign asymptomatic chronic eruption of unknown cause.
- Onset occurs in late childhood or adolescence.

Signs and Symptoms

- Patients present with an asymptomatic or mildly pruritic eruption composed of minute (1–2 mm), flat-topped skin-colored or white papules (Figure 46.1).
- Lesions often are clustered into circular plaques and may appear at any location.
- Papules may be arranged in a linear distribution at sites of trauma due to scratching (ie, the Koebner phenomenon) (see Figure 46.1).
- Lichen nitidus is a self-limited disorder.

Figure 46.1. White, flat-topped papules, some in a linear arrangement, are characteristic of lichen nitidus.

Look-alikes

Disorder	Differentiating Features
Molluscum contagiosum	• Papules often vary in size. • Larger lesions exhibit umbilication. • Lesions more pearly and translucent in quality.
Flat warts	• Variably sized verrucous, flat-topped papules • Clustering into circular plaques not usually seen
Papular atopic dermatitis	• Lesions are pruritic and skin-colored. • Evidence of atopic dermatitis elsewhere on the body. • Koebner phenomenon not observed.
Keratosis pilaris	• Skin-colored, keratotic (not flat-topped) papules centered about follicles • Koebner phenomenon not observed • Bilaterally symmetric distribution on cheeks, upper lateral arms and thighs
Lichen planus	• Papules larger • Papules pruritic, purple, polygonal (ie, have angulated borders), and often involve the penis
Lichen spinulosus	• Clustered, skin-colored, keratotic (not flat-topped) papules centered about follicles • Koebner phenomenon not observed

How to Make the Diagnosis

- The diagnosis is made clinically.

Treatment

- No therapy is required.
- For patients who experience pruritus, a topical corticosteroid or topical calcineurin inhibitor may be applied or an oral antihistamine prescribed.

Prognosis

- The prognosis is excellent, with spontaneous resolution usually occurring within 12 months.

When to Worry or Refer

- Consider consultation if the diagnosis is uncertain or if the disease is widespread and symptomatic (eg, there is severe pruritus).

CHAPTER 47

Lichen Planus (LP)

Introduction/Etiology/Epidemiology

- Lichen planus is a distinctive papulosquamous eruption.
- The cause of LP is unknown; however, there is inflammatory damage to the cells of the basal layer of the epidermis.
  - Lichen planus may occur in association with hepatitis C infection.
  - Reactions to drugs may cause an LP-like eruption.

Signs and Symptoms

- The lesions of LP are described as papules that are planar (flat-topped), pruritic, purple, and polygonal (angulated borders) and often involve the penis (the Ps of LP) (Figure 47.1).
  - Individual papules may coalesce into plaques, form rings, or be distributed in a linear fashion.
  - The surface of lesions may exhibit a network of fine white lines (ie, Wickham striae).
  - The flexor surfaces of the forearms and wrists, anterior legs, penis, and presacral areas most often are affected.
  - Papules may be distributed in a linear array at sites of trauma due to scratching (ie, the Koebner phenomenon).
- The oral mucosae often exhibit a white, lacy, or reticulated appearance (Figure 47.2); erosions may be present.
- Other findings include nail dystrophy or scarring alopecia.
- Pruritus typically is severe.
- Lesions range from asymptomatic to mildly pruritic.

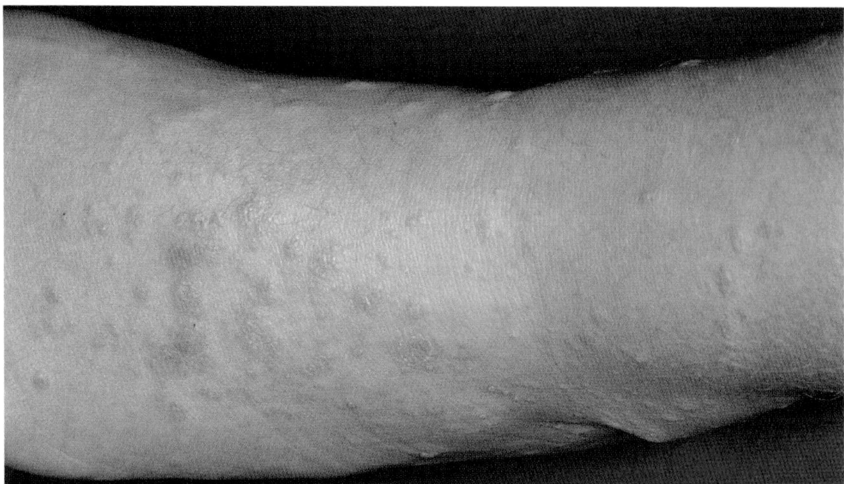

Figure 47.1. Violaceous, flat-topped papules are observed in lichen planus.

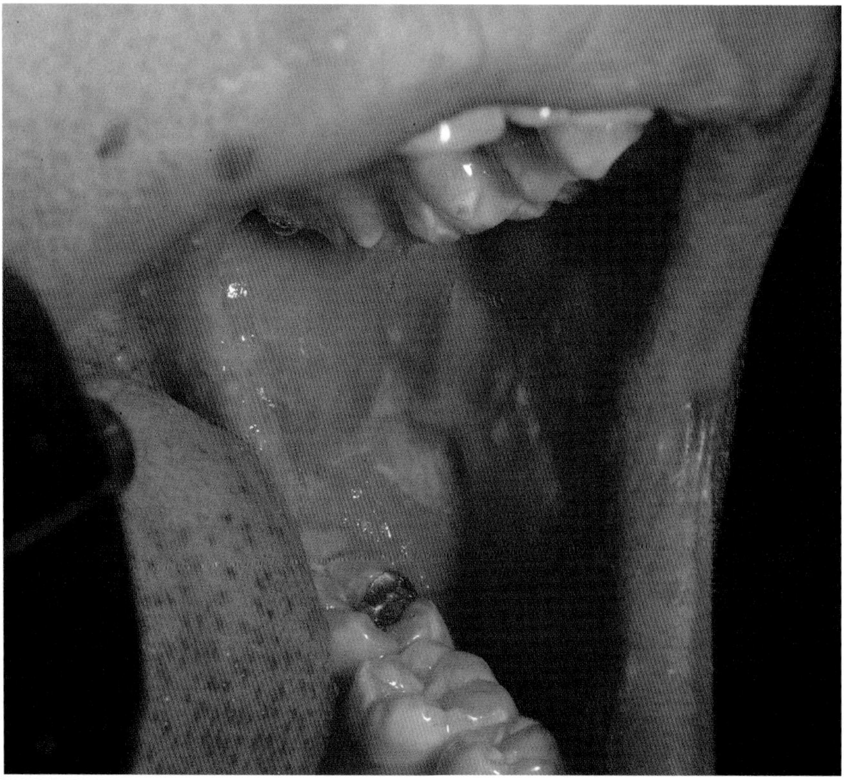

Figure 47.2. White, lacy, or reticulated lesions often are observed on the buccal mucosa of patients who have lichen planus.

Look-alikes

Disorder	Differentiating Features
Psoriasis	• Erythematous and covered by thick, adherent scale
Keratosis pilaris	• Rough, keratotic papules centered about follicles • Skin-colored or slightly erythematous • Bilaterally symmetric distribution on cheeks, upper lateral arms, and thighs
Lichen nitidus	• Small (1–2 mm), white, flat-topped papules
Lichen striatus	• May be difficult to distinguish from linear LP • Process localized (lesions in a linear arrangement) and not present elsewhere • Associated hypopigmentation common

How to Make the Diagnosis

- The diagnosis is suspected clinically and may be confirmed by cutaneous biopsy.

Treatment

- Mid-potency or stronger topical corticosteroids are used to control pruritus and hasten the resolution of lesions.
- Oral ulcers may be treated with a potent topical corticosteroid applied 3 to 4 times daily as needed.
- In children with severe, widespread, or recalcitrant disease, treatment options include an oral corticosteroid or an oral retinoid; ultraviolet B phototherapy occasionally is used for severe cases.

Prognosis

- The prognosis is good; most pediatric patients experience a resolution of disease within 6 to 12 months of beginning therapy.
- Recurrences of LP are uncommon.

When to Worry or Refer

- Most patients who have LP will benefit from consultation with a pediatric dermatologist.
- Refer patients if the diagnosis is in doubt, when therapy fails, or when the disease is severe or widespread.

Resources for Families

- American Academy of Dermatology: Lichen planus. **https://www.aad.org/public/diseases/rashes/lichen-planus**
- MedlinePlus: Information for patients and families (in English and Spanish) sponsored by the National Library of Medicine and National Institutes of Health. **https://www.nlm.nih.gov/medlineplus/ency/article/000867.htm**
- WebMD: Information for families is contained in the Health A-Z topics. **www.webmd.com/skin-problems-and-treatments/guide/common-rashes**

CHAPTER 48

Lichen Striatus

Introduction/Etiology/Epidemiology

- Lichen striatus is a self-limited papulosquamous inflammatory disease of unknown cause.
- It most often occurs in young children (median age of onset is 2–3 years); females are affected more often than males.

Signs and Symptoms

- Lesions are small, erythematous or violaceous papules that typically begin on a proximal extremity and then extend down the extremity (although lesions may appear on the trunk and, less commonly, the face) (Figures 48.1 and 48.2).
  - The lesions follow lines of Blaschko (the paths of embryonic neural crest cell migration).
  - Distal extension of lesions may involve a nail, creating dystrophy.
  - Within 1 to 2 years, the papules resolve, leaving hypopigmentation that ultimately resolves.
- Lesions range from asymptomatic to mildly pruritic.

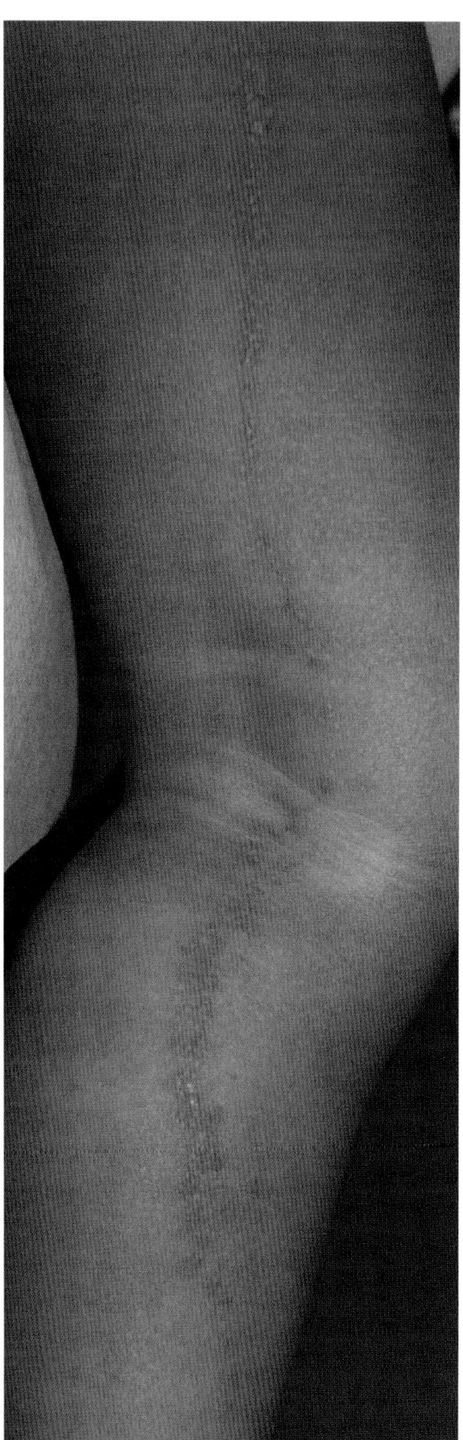

Figure 48.1. Linear arrangement of papules on the posterior thigh and leg in lichen striatus.

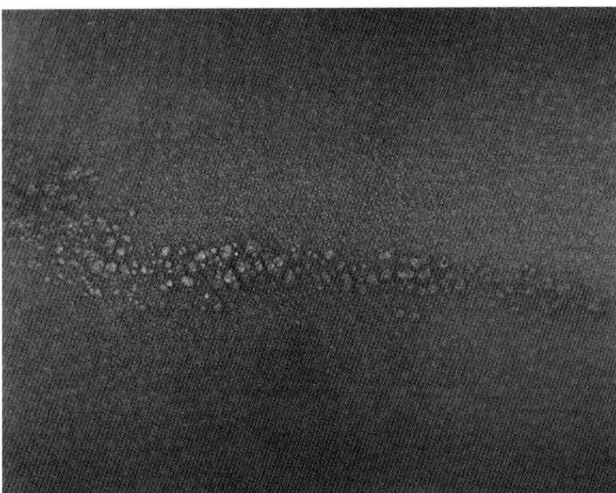

Figure 48.2. Close-up view of the patient in Figure 48.1. Note that in lichen striatus, the papules are flat-topped (ie, lichenoid).

Look-alikes

Disorder	Differentiating Features
Psoriasis	• Koebner phenomenon may cause some lesions to occur in linear arrangement, but typical lesions will be present elsewhere. • Lesions have thick adherent scale; if scale is removed, pinpoint bleeding may occur (Auspitz sign).
Lichen planus	• Koebner phenomenon may cause some lesions to occur in a linear arrangement, but typical lesions will be present elsewhere.
Lichen nitidus	• Koebner phenomenon may cause some lesions to occur in a linear arrangement, but typical lesions will be present elsewhere. • Small (1–2 mm), white papules.
Linear epidermal nevus	• Hyperpigmented plaque often with a rough surface • Often present at birth • Does not resolve spontaneously

How to Make the Diagnosis

- The diagnosis is made clinically.

Treatment

- No treatment is necessary.
- The application of a mid-potency topical corticosteroid may be of some benefit when inflammatory lesions (ie, erythematous papules) are present.

Prognosis

- The prognosis is excellent, with spontaneous resolution occurring within 1 to 3 years.
- Recurrences are uncommon.

When to Worry or Refer

- Refer patients in whom the diagnosis is uncertain.

Resources for Families

- American Osteopathic College of Dermatology: Patient information. **www.aocd.org/?page=LichenStriatus**

CHAPTER

49

Pityriasis Lichenoides

Introduction/Etiology/Epidemiology

- Pityriasis lichenoides is an uncommon papulosquamous eruption seen in children and young adults.
- Etiology is unclear and most cases are idiopathic.
  - Some consider this condition to be a self-limited, cutaneous lymphoproliferative disorder.
- Pityriasis lichenoides is often considered a disease spectrum with acute and chronic forms. Clinical overlap between the 2 types often exists.
  - Pityriasis lichenoides et varioliformis acuta (PLEVA)—characterized by the acute onset of crops of red or red-brown macules and papules that become vesicular or necrotic or form crust or scale.
  - Pityriasis lichenoides chronica (PLC)—characterized by the gradual onset of crops of scaling papules and small plaques that resolve and recur over a period of several months to years, often healing with postinflammatory dyspigmentation.
- Mucha-Habermann disease is an older term that has traditionally been applied to PLEVA, but many consider this term broadly within the entire spectrum of disease.

Signs and Symptoms

- Pityriasis lichenoides et varioliformis acuta
  - Abrupt onset of red to red-brown macules or papules (2–5 mm in diameter). Lesions may become vesicular, necrotic, hemorrhagic, or purpuric and may develop crust or scale (Figure 49.1).
  - An important clue is the presence of lesions in various stages of development.

- As the condition evolves, lesions may become hemorrhagic, crusted, and necrotic, sometimes resulting in varioliform (chickenpox-like) scars and dyspigmentation.
- Most patients with PLEVA are asymptomatic, but some experience pruritus or systemic symptoms, such as fever, lymphadenopathy, and malaise.
- A rare subtype of PLEVA (febrile ulceronecrotic Mucha-Habermann disease) causes more widespread involvement with large necrotic and ulcerative nodules and plaques. Constitutional symptoms and high fever are often present.

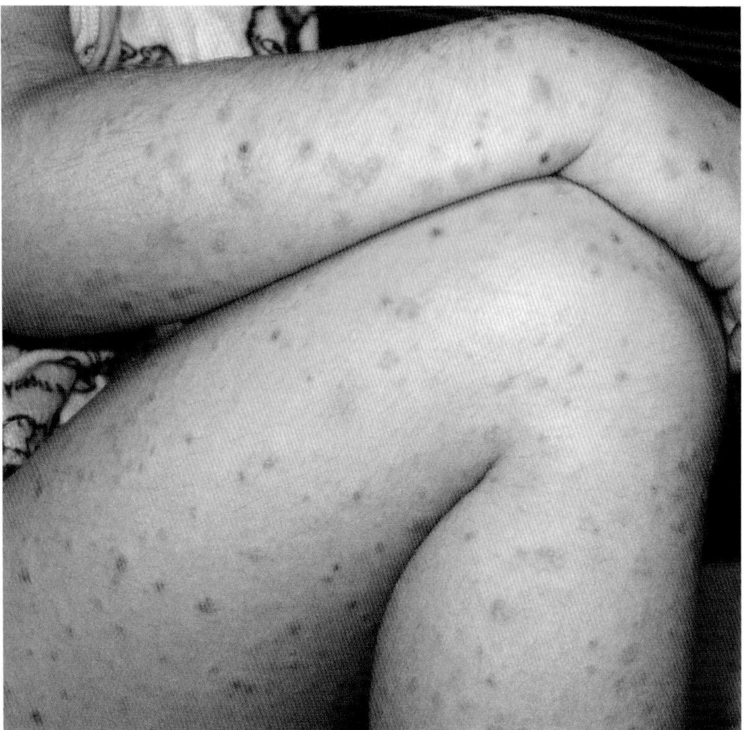

Figure 49.1. Erythematous-crusted papules of pityriasis lichenoides et varioliformis acuta are seen in this child.

- Pityriasis lichenoides chronica
  - Gradual onset of red-brown papules, often with an overlying scale or crust.
  - Lesions often appear, subside, and reappear in crops over weeks to months (sometimes years). Lesions are typically at various stages and morphologies (Figure 49.2). Postinflammatory dyspigmentation is often seen.
  - Constitutional symptoms are not typically seen in PLC, and lesions are usually asymptomatic.
- A widespread distribution is typically seen in PLEVA and PLC, with most lesions appearing on the trunk, buttocks, and extremities.
  - Involvement of the proximal extremities is typical; the palms and soles are usually spared.
  - Facial involvement is uncommon but may occur in darker skin types.
  - Clinical overlap often occurs between PLEVA, PLC, and pityriasis rosea.

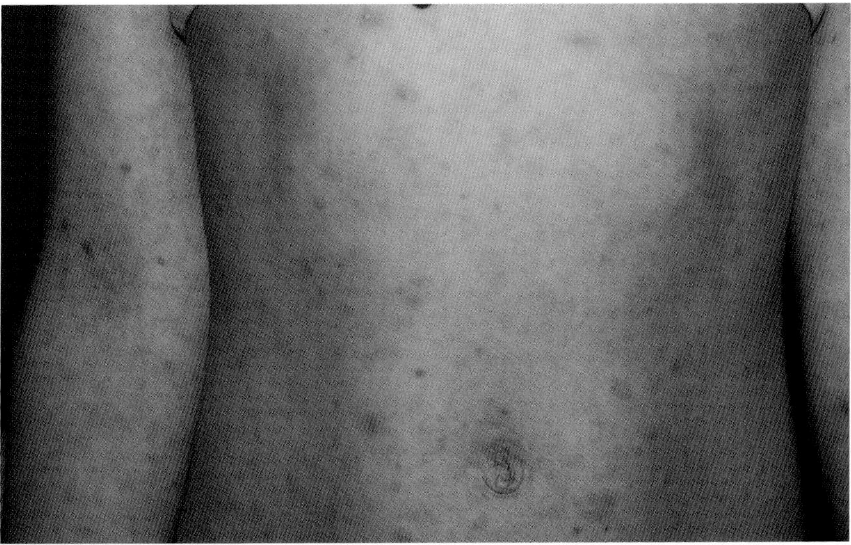

Figure 49.2. Crops of scaling papules are seen in this patient with pityriasis lichenoides chronica.

Look-alikes

Disorder	Differentiating Features
Pityriasis rosea	• Small, thin oval plaques with long axes parallel to lines of skin tension. • Typically lacks crusting, necrosis, blistering; hemorrhage only occasionally present. • Lesions covered by thin, fine "trailing scale" (lags behind advancing red border, and free edge of scale points inward toward center of plaque). • Course is typically less prolonged.
Guttate psoriasis	• Lesions covered with a thick, adherent silvery scale • Lesions not usually present in differing stages • Crusted, hemorrhagic, vesicular and necrotic lesions absent
Lichen planus	• Purple, polygonal papules and small plaques. • Fine scale (not thick adherent scale) is present. • Oral involvement common, with thin, white, elevated linear lesions forming a lacy, reticulated appearance. • Pruritus is common. • Crusted, hemorrhagic, vesicular, and necrotic lesions usually absent.
Varicella	• May resemble PLEVA (when PLEVA is characterized by papules and vesicles). • More rapid progression of lesions, with more extensive involvement of face, scalp, and mucous membranes. • Distribution is classically centripetal, with most lesions on the trunk and fewer on the distal extremities. • Patient more often ill with fever and other systemic symptoms. • Shorter duration of disease than pityriasis lichenoides. • Markedly decreased incidence in era of universal varicella vaccination.
Gianotti-Crosti syndrome	• Symmetric, predominantly facial, buttock and extensor extremity distribution with minimal involvement of the trunk. • Lesions are monomorphic, lack mica scale, and usually do not appear in recurrent crops. • Duration is typically less prolonged than pityriasis lichenoides.
Secondary syphilis	• Patients often ill with fever and lymphadenopathy. • Lesions often present on the palms and soles. • Lesions typically do not appear in recurrent crops.

How to Make the Diagnosis

- The diagnosis is usually made clinically based on the appearance and distribution of the lesions. If the diagnosis is in doubt, skin biopsy may be performed.

Treatment

- Treatment is often dependent on symptoms, and not all cases of pityriasis lichenoides require therapy.
- While topical steroids and oral antihistamines may be effective in cases associated with pruritus, neither have been shown to alter the disease course.
- Oral antibiotics (eg, erythromycin, azithromycin, tetracyclines [for those older than 8 years]), perhaps owing to their anti-inflammatory effect, have been shown to be effective in some patients. Patients typically are treated for several months. If a response is achieved, the dose may then be tapered and the drug ultimately discontinued.
- Ultraviolet therapy, particularly UV-B, has also been demonstrated to be an effective and safe treatment option.
- In rare instances, methotrexate has been used but only in the context of severe, refractory cases failing to respond to conservative measures.

Prognosis

- Prognosis is favorable, as pityriasis lichenoides is usually a self-limited disorder.
- The duration of pityriasis lichenoides is often unpredictable and variable, with some cases lasting weeks to months, while others may last for years.
- Pityriasis lichenoides et varioliformis acuta typically has a shorter duration, but some cases may evolve into PLC. Flares and remissions over a period of months to years is typically seen in patients with PLC.
- Generally, there is a tendency toward improvement during the summer months, which is most likely related to natural ultraviolet exposure.

When to Worry or Refer

- If the diagnosis is in doubt, consider dermatology consultation or possible histopathologic confirmation.

Resources for Families

- British Association of Dermatologists: Patient information leaflets. **www.bad.org.uk/for-the-public/patient-information-leaflets/pityriasis-lichenoides**
- Medscape: Background. **http://emedicine.medscape.com/article/1099078-overview**
- American Osteopathic College of Dermatology: Pityriasis lichenoides. **www.aocd.org/?PityriasisLichenoid**

CHAPTER 50

Pityriasis Rosea

Introduction/Etiology/Epidemiology

- Pityriasis rosea is a benign, self-limited, papulosquamous eruption of children and young adults.
- Etiology is unknown.
  - Seasonal incidence and clustering of cases suggest an infectious agent.
  - Some evidence supports a role for human herpesvirus 7.

Signs and Symptoms

- The initial lesion in as many as 80% of patients is the herald patch, a round or oval erythematous patch with a scaling border and central clearing that may be mistaken for tinea corporis or nummular eczema (Figure 50.1).
- Within 2 weeks, a generalized, sometimes pruritic, eruption appears; individual lesions are erythematous papules and small (5–10 mm), thin, oval plaques with scale.
  - The plaques are oriented with their long axes parallel to lines of skin tension.
  - Lesions are concentrated on the trunk; on the back, the alignment of lesions may mimic the boughs of a fir tree (ie, the Christmas tree distribution) (Figure 50.2).
  - "Trailing scale" is present: Scale lags behind the advancing red border, with free edge pointing inward toward the center of the plaque.

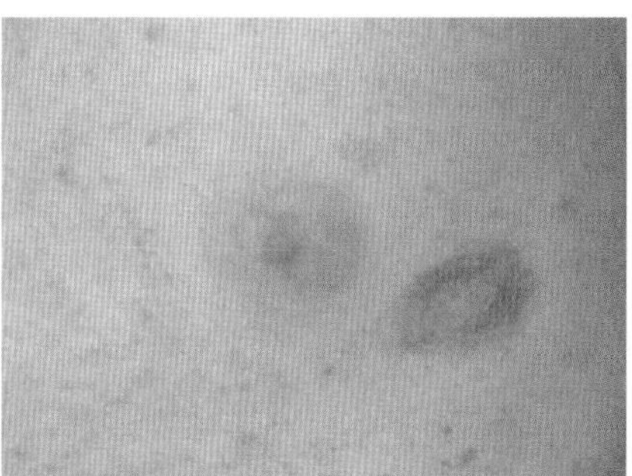

Figure 50.1. The herald patch is a round or oval erythematous patch that may be mistaken for tinea corporis.

- In persons with skin of color, the appearance of the eruption may differ.
  - The eruption may appear papular with few plaques (Figure 50.3).
  - The eruption may have an inverse distribution with lesions concentrated on the neck, proximal extremities, groin, and axillae; there may be relative sparing of the trunk.
- New lesions appear for 2 to 3 weeks, and the eruption resolves typically over several weeks to months.

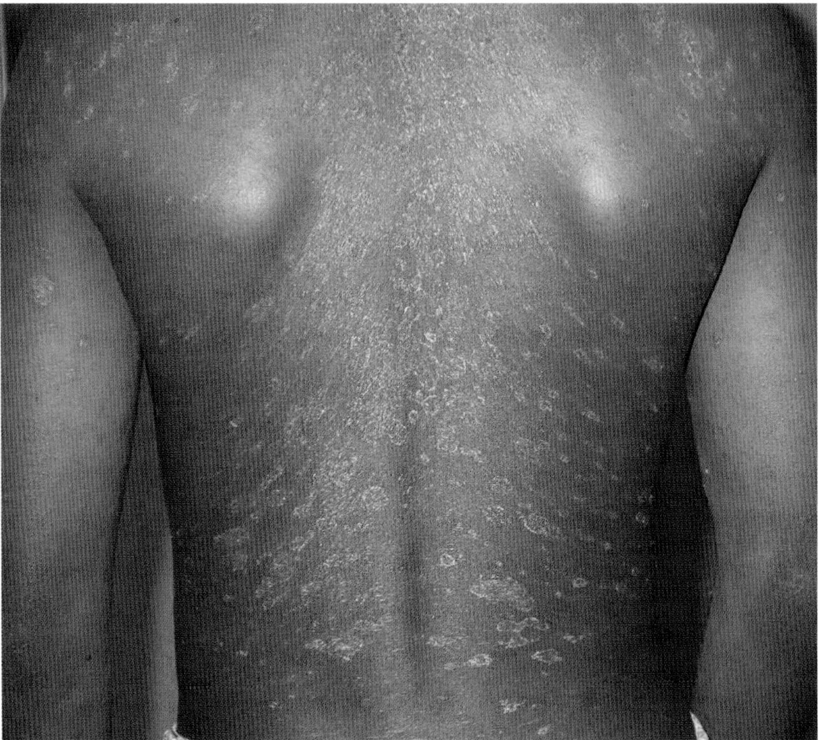

Figure 50.2. On the back, the alignment of lesions along lines of skin stress may mimic the appearance of the boughs of a fir tree (ie, the Christmas tree appearance).

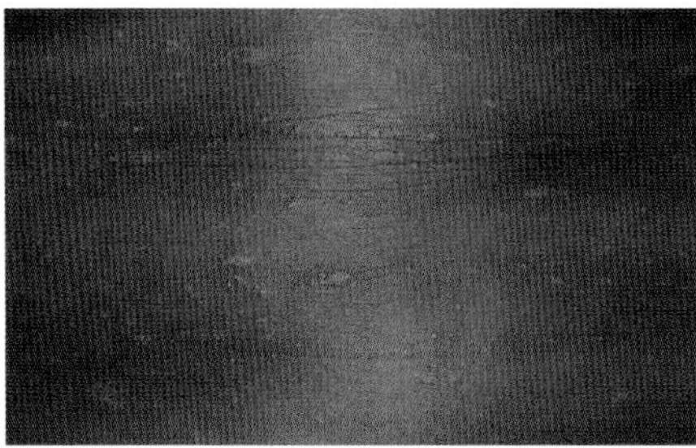

Figure 50.3. Papules and plaques in an African American child who has pityriasis rosea.

Look-alikes

Disorder	Differentiating Features
Tinea corporis	• May be confused with herald patch of pityriasis rosea. • Border often more elevated. • Potassium hydroxide preparation performed on scale from lesion reveals hyphae. • Generalized eruption not usually seen. • Trailing scale is absent.
Nummular eczema	• May be confused with herald patch of pityriasis rosea. • Covered with crust, as well as scale. • Pruritus very common. • Generalized eruption would not be seen. • Trailing scale is absent.
Secondary syphilis	• Patients often ill with fever and lymphadenopathy. • Lesions often present on the palms and soles.
Guttate psoriasis	• Lesions not oriented along lines of skin stress. • Lesions covered with a thick, adherent scale.
Pityriasis lichenoides chronica	• Often involves the extremities as well as the trunk • Buttock involvement common • Lesions not classically oriented along lines of skin tension • Course more prolonged than that of pityriasis rosea

How to Make the Diagnosis

- The diagnosis is made clinically.

Treatment

- Most children with pityriasis rosea require no therapy.
- If pruritus is present, an emollient containing menthol or phenol may be applied as needed (acts as a counterirritant that masks the sensation of pruritus) or a sedating antihistamine prescribed.
- Judicious sun exposure may reduce pruritus and hasten the resolution of the eruption; ultraviolet phototherapy occasionally is used for severe cases.
- Counsel the patient and family about the prolonged course of the eruption.

Prognosis

- Prognosis is excellent, although the prolonged time required for resolution may be frustrating to patients and families.

When to Worry or Refer

- Consider consultation when the diagnosis is in doubt.
- If patient exhibits signs of secondary syphilis (eg, oral or genital mucosal lesions, lesions on the palms or soles), perform appropriate testing (ie, rapid plasma reagin or Venereal Disease Research Laboratory test).
- If lesions persist for more than 3 months, consider referral to a pediatric dermatologist to assess for pityriasis lichenoides chronica, a disorder that (in its early stages) may mimic pityriasis rosea.

Resources for Families

- American Academy of Pediatrics: HealthyChildren.org. **www.HealthyChildren.org/pityriasisrosea**
- American Academy of Dermatology: Pityriasis rosea. **https://www.aad.org/public/diseases/rashes/pityriasis-rosea**
- MedlinePlus: Information for patients and families (in English and Spanish) sponsored by the National Library of Medicine and National Institutes of Health. **https://www.nlm.nih.gov/medlineplus/ency/article/000871.htm**

Psoriasis

Introduction/Etiology/Epidemiology

- Papulosquamous (ie, elevated lesions with scale) condition with a tendency o persist or recur for years.
- Characterized by inflammation and hyperproliferation of the epidermis.
- Likely results from a genetic predisposition (family history often is positive) and an environmental trigger (eg, infection, trauma).
- Recent literature links psoriasis to other systemic comorbidities, in particular a higher prevalence of metabolic syndrome (ie, obesity, dyslipidemia, hypertension, and elevated blood glucose) and cardiovascular disease, in children and adults. Psoriasis may occur in some children with juvenile idiopathic arthritis (JIA). Typically, this occurs within 2 years of diagnosis of JIA.

Signs and Symptoms

- Appearance of lesions
  - Lesions are well-defined papules and plaques that are pink to deep red and have an adherent white to silvery "micaceous" scale (Figure 51.1).
    - Removal of scale produces bleeding points (Auspitz sign) (Figure 51.2).
    - Scale may be absent or less prominent in occluded areas (eg, diaper area, axillae) (Figure 51.3).
  - Variants
    - Infantile psoriasis: may appear as generalized erythroderma or as sharply demarcated erythema (with minimal scale) in diaper region, axillae, and umbilicus.
    - Guttate psoriasis: Often precipitated by pharyngeal or perianal *Streptococcus pyogenes* infection; begins as generalized erythematous macules and papules (that may mimic a viral exanthem); later, characteristic scale appears (Figure 51.4).
    - Pustular psoriasis: small pustules studded over the surface of deep red plaques.
    - Inverse psoriasis: Lesions located predominantly in the axillae and groin.

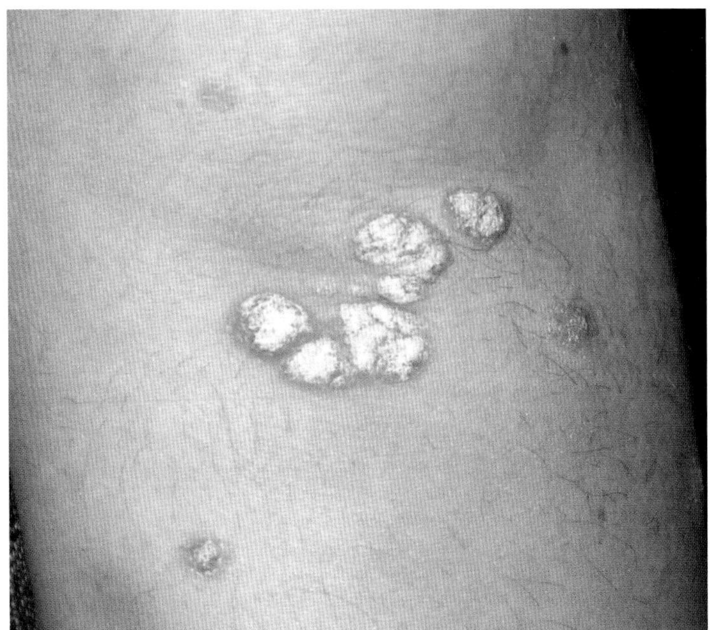

Figure 51.1. Typical lesions of psoriasis are erythematous papules and plaques that have a thick adherent scale.

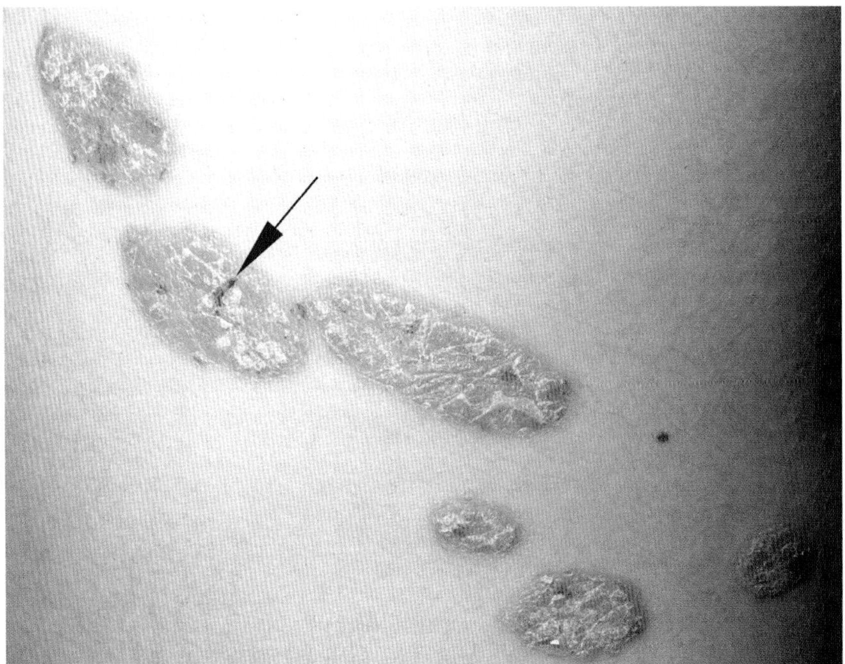

Figure 51.2. In psoriasis, removal of scale from a lesion causes pinpoint bleeding (arrow), the Auspitz sign.

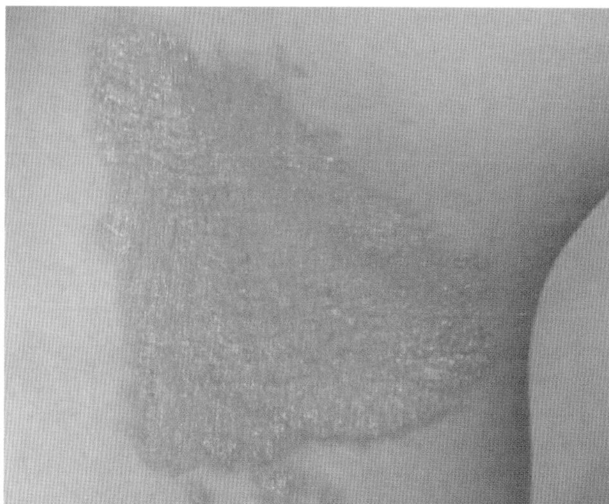

Figure 51.3. In occluded areas, such as the axilla, the lesions of psoriasis may lack scale.

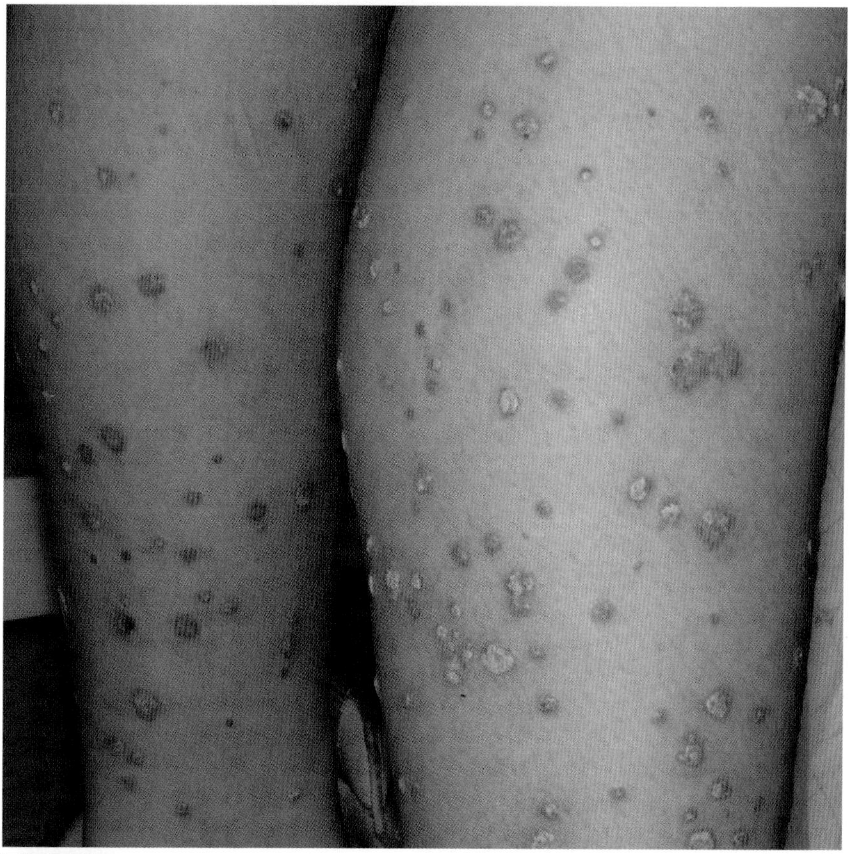

Figure 51.4. Guttate psoriasis is characterized by an eruption composed of widespread macules or papules that may mimic a viral exanthem. Over time, the lesions develop thick scale.

- Distribution
  - Scalp (scaling and erythema) (Figure 51.5), posterior auricular, elbows, knees, umbilicus, and gluteal cleft; however, any body region may be affected.
  - Lesions appear in areas of trauma (ie, Koebner phenomenon), explaining involvement of the extensor surfaces of the extremities.
  - Nail involvement is common, consisting of pitting or thickening and yellowing.

Look-alikes

Disorder	Differentiating Features
Lichen planus	• Purple, polygonal papules and small plaques. • Fine scale (not thick adherent scale) is present. • Oral involvement common, with thin, white, elevated linear lesions forming a lacy, reticulated appearance.
Dermatomyositis	• Patients may exhibit muscle weakness. • Characteristic cutaneous findings include heliotrope rash and Gottron papules (erythematous papules located over the dorsal surfaces of interphalangeal joints of the fingers).
Pityriasis rosea	• May be confused with guttate psoriasis • Small, thin oval plaques with long axes parallel to lines of skin tension • Lesions covered by thin, fine "trailing scale" (lags behind advancing red border, and free edge of scale points inward toward center of plaque)
Seborrheic dermatitis	• May be difficult to distinguish from psoriasis when only the scalp and face are involved. • Typical lesions have greasy scale. • Auspitz sign absent. • In infants, seborrheic dermatitis and psoriasis may be indistinguishable.

How to Make the Diagnosis

- The diagnosis is made clinically based on the appearance and distribution of lesions.
- Observation of Auspitz sign strongly suggests a diagnosis of psoriasis.

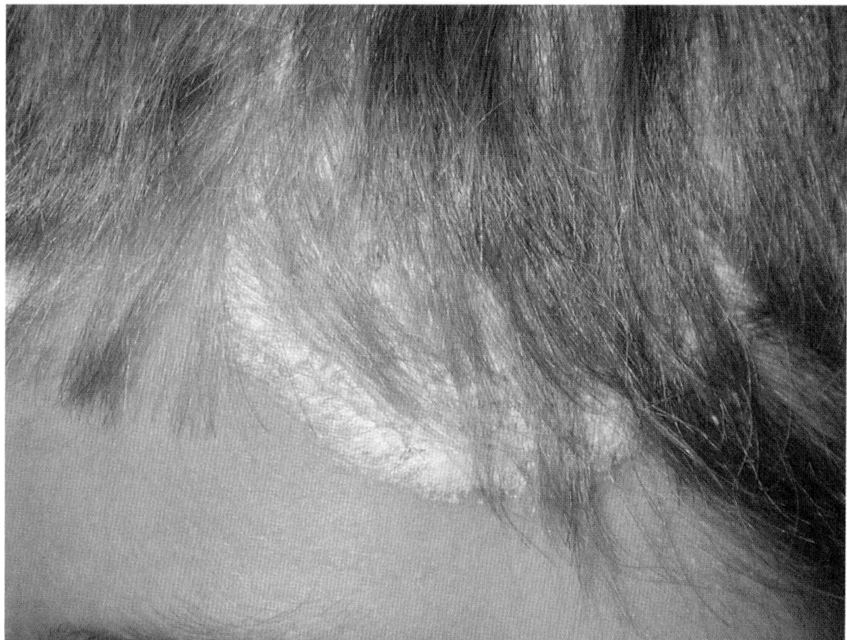

Figure 51.5. On the scalp, psoriasis causes erythema and thick scale.

Treatment

- Therapy is directed at reducing inflammation and normalizing epidermal proliferation.
- Topical therapy (first line): Treatment often employs more than one agent.
  - Mid-potency (or, occasionally, high-potency) topical glucocorticoids (often used in conjunction with calcipotriene)
  - Calcipotriene: normalizes epidermal proliferation; may be used as monotherapy or in conjunction with topical corticosteroids; may cause hypercalcemia in infants or small children who may require large surface area application
  - Others: anthralin or liquor carbonis detergens (tar derivatives) and topical retinoids occasionally used
- Photochemotherapy: Ultraviolet B or ultraviolet A therapy (alone or combined with psoralen, when known as PUVA) may be used for patients with severe disease who fail topical therapy.
- Systemic therapy: Methotrexate, cyclosporine A, or acitretin may be used for patients with severe disease who fail topical therapy. Biologic agents (that target TNF-α, IL-17 or IL-23) occasionally are used, but long-term safety in children remains unclear for IL-17 and IL-23 biologics.

Treating Associated Conditions

- When guttate psoriasis is suspected, test for pharyngeal (or perianal if the physical examination is suggestive) *S pyogenes* infection and treat if infection is confirmed.

Prognosis

- Psoriasis is a chronic disease, and recurrences may be anticipated.

When to Worry or Refer

- For patients with significant disease, consult with or refer to a pediatric dermatologist to optimize therapy.
- Refer patients in whom the diagnosis is uncertain, those who do not respond to appropriate therapy, or those who develop pustular disease.

Resources for Families

- American Academy of Dermatology: Psoriasis. **https://www.aad.org/public/diseases/scaly-skin/psoriasis**
- MedlinePlus: Information for patients and families (in English and Spanish) sponsored by the National Library of Medicine and National Institutes of Health. **https://www.nlm.nih.gov/medlineplus/ency/article/000434.htm**
- National Psoriasis Foundation: Provides extensive information (English and Spanish) about the disease and its treatment. **https://www.psoriasis.org**
- Society for Pediatric Dermatology: Patient handout on psoriasis. **http://pedsderm.net/for-patients-families/patient-handouts**

Seborrheic Dermatitis

Introduction/Etiology/Epidemiology

- Chronic dermatitis of unknown cause. May be related to an inflammatory response to the yeasts of the genus *Malassezia* (formerly *Pityrosporum*).
- Seborrheic dermatitis may be divided into 2 main variants.
  - Infantile: presents from soon after birth to about 1 year of age
  - Adolescent and adult: occurs primarily in older children (who have experienced adrenarche) or postpubertal individuals
- In addition to these variants, seborrheic dermatitis may also occasionally occur in toddlers and elementary school-aged children.

Signs and Symptoms

- Infantile
  - Characterized by yellowish greasy scale on the scalp (ie, cradle cap) (Figure 52.1) and erythematous patches with greasy scale that have a predilection for the face and flexural areas (eg, retroauricular region, axillae, groin) (Figures 52.2 and 52.3)
  - Occasionally may have near total skin involvement
  - Shares considerable clinical overlap with atopic dermatitis and infantile psoriasis
- Adolescent and adult
  - Most common presentation is scaling of the scalp (ie, dandruff).
  - Patients may exhibit erythematous poorly defined scaling patches on scalp, ears, eyebrows, nasolabial folds (Figure 52.4), central chest, and beard area in males.
  - Pruritus is variable.

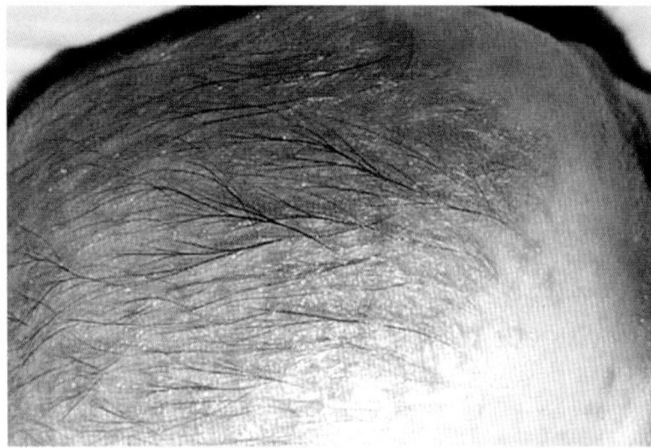

Figure 52.1. Greasy scale on the scalp of an infant (ie, cradle cap).

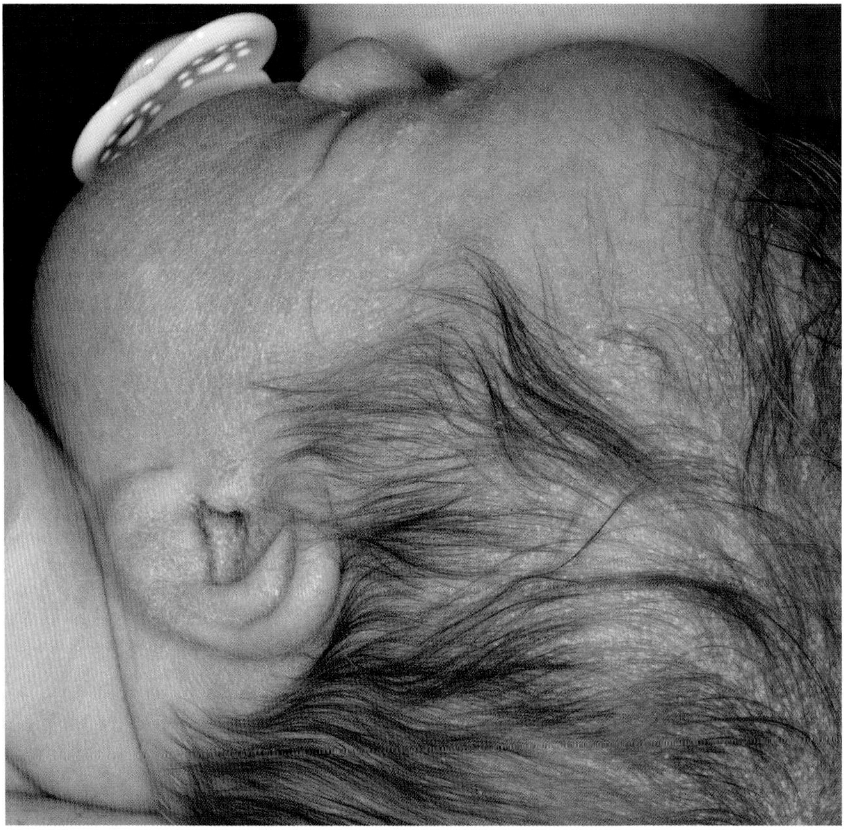

Figure 52.2. Erythematous patches with greasy scale on the face of an infant who has seborrheic dermatitis.

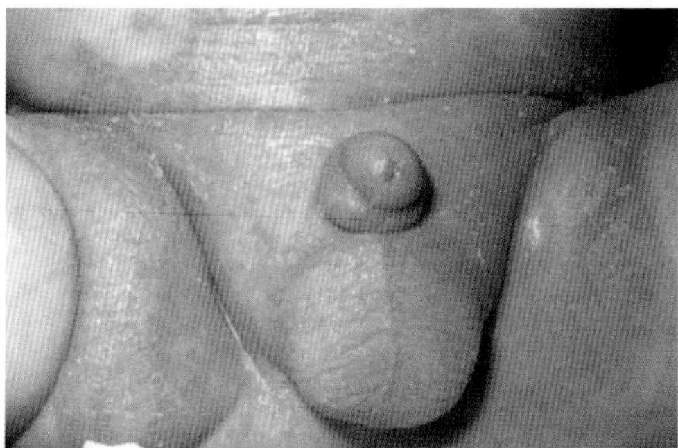

Figure 52.3. In the diaper area, seborrheic dermatitis produces salmon-colored patches with greasy scale that involve the creases and convexities.

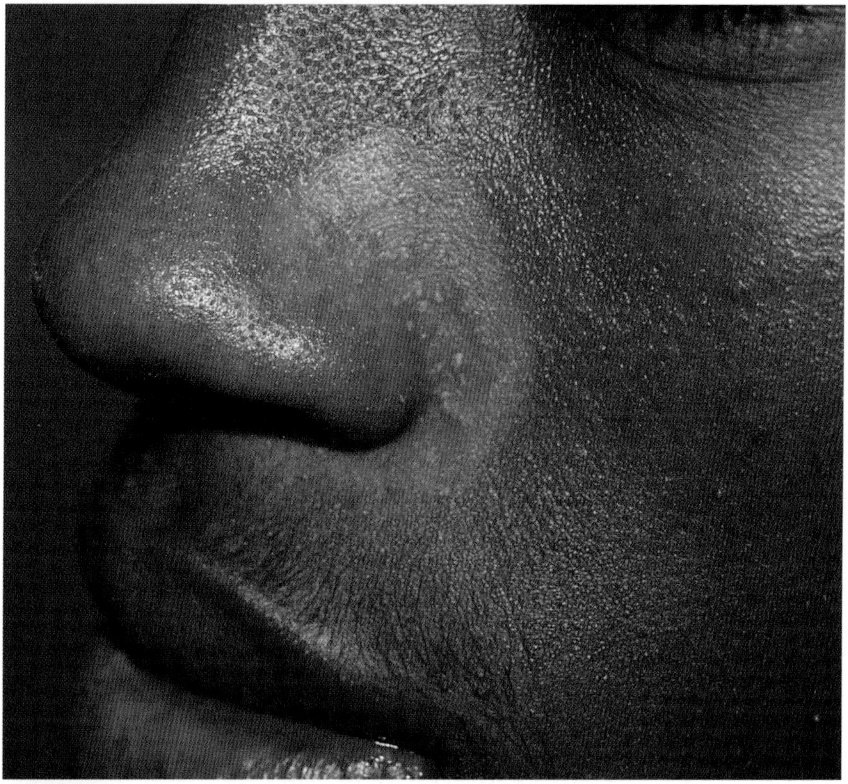

Figure 52.4. Seborrheic dermatitis involving the nasolabial folds has resulted in postinflammatory hypopigmentation.

Look-alikes

Disorder	Differentiating Features
Infantile	
Atopic dermatitis	• Often difficult to distinguish from seborrheic dermatitis. • In infancy, lesions tend to spare flexural areas, particularly diaper area and axillae. • Family history of atopic disease supports diagnosis.
Scabies	• Papules, pustules, burrows, and vesicles • Presence of lesions on palms, soles, and genitals • Marked pruritus usually present • Diagnosis confirmed by mineral oil preparation performed on scrapings from lesions
Langerhans cell histiocytosis	• Erythematous, yellow or brown scaling papules, with predilection for the scalp, axillae, inguinal creases, palms, and soles. • Petechiae often present. • Lymphadenopathy often present. • Biopsy of lesion will confirm the diagnosis.
Psoriasis	• Tend to be well-defined plaques with thick, adherent, dry scale
Neonatal lupus erythematosus	• Annular erythematous plaques on sun-exposed regions, especially forehead and periorbital areas. • Minimal scaling; atrophy may be present. • Positive anti–SS-A (anti-Ro), anti–SS-B (anti-La), or anti-U1RNP antibodies present. • Congenital heart block may be present.
Adolescent and Adult	
Psoriasis	• May be difficult to differentiate from seborrheic dermatitis when involvement limited to the scalp or face. • Well-defined papules or plaques with thick, adherent, dry scale. • Pitting of nails may be present.
Periorificial dermatitis	• Erythematous papules and pustules located around mouth, nose, or eyes. • History of corticosteroid use on affected areas may be present.

How to Make the Diagnosis

- The diagnosis is made clinically based on the appearance and location of lesions.

Treatment

- Infantile
  - Scalp
    - May be controlled by gentle brushing to remove scale during daily shampooing. (Baby oil or mineral oil may be applied to loosen scale before shampooing.)
    - If these measures fail, an antiseborrheic shampoo (eg, one containing pyrithione zinc or selenium sulfide) may be used as needed.
    - Topical steroid solution, lotion, or cream is occasionally necessary when significant inflammation is present.
  - Skin
    - Lesions may be treated with a low-potency topical corticosteroid (eg, hydrocortisone 1% or 2.5%, alclometasone 0.05% ointment, desonide 0.05% ointment) twice daily as needed.
- Adolescent and adult
  - Scalp
    - To control scaling: Use an antiseborrheic shampoo (eg, one containing pyrithione zinc, selenium sulfide, ketoconazole, tar, or salicylic acid) as needed.
    - To control areas of erythema: Apply a mid-potency topical corticosteroid (eg, fluocinolone, triamcinolone) at bedtime as needed; solution, foam, or lotion vehicle may be preferable to cream or ointment.
  - Skin
    - Lesions may be treated with hydrocortisone 1% or 2.5% or ketoconazole cream applied twice daily as needed.

Prognosis

- Infantile seborrheic dermatitis has a good prognosis, usually clearing rapidly with appropriate topical therapy.
- Adolescent/adult seborrheic dermatitis often is a chronic condition requiring ongoing therapy.

When to Worry or Refer

- When the diagnosis is uncertain or the patient fails to respond to appropriate therapy
- When petechiae, purpura, or erosions (especially in skinfolds) are present, suggesting possible Langerhans cell histiocytosis

Resources for Families

- American Academy of Pediatrics: HealthyChildren.org. **www.HealthyChildren.org/cradlecap**
- American Academy of Dermatology: Seborrheic dermatitis. **https://www.aad.org/public/diseases/scaly-skin/seborrheic-dermatitis**
- MedlinePlus: Information for patients and families (in English and Spanish) sponsored by the National Library of Medicine and National Institutes of Health. **https://www.nlm.nih.gov/medlineplus/ency/article/000963.htm**

Vascular Lesions

Cutis Marmorata

Introduction/Etiology/Epidemiology

- Cutis marmorata
  - May be present at birth as a benign transient mottling of skin color responsive to cutaneous temperature changes.
  - Caused by vasomotor instability.
  - Most infants exhibit cutis marmorata for a few months.
- Cutis marmorata telangiectatica congenita (CMTC) (congenital phlebectasia)
  - Uncommon congenital vascular process that persists for life
  - May have associated soft tissue hypoplasia underlying vascular changes or other developmental anomalies (See Chapter 54.)

Signs and Symptoms

- Cutis marmorata presents as a lacy, reticulated, blanching erythematous or violaceous mottled or marbled appearance that becomes more apparent in cooler temperatures (Figure 53.1).
- Usually disappears with rewarming.

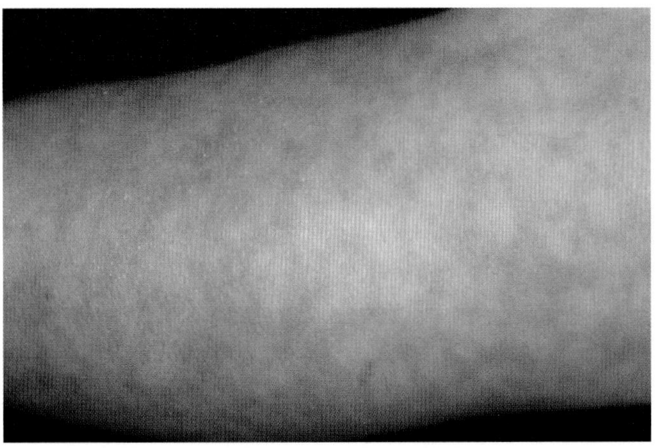

Figure 53.1. Cutis marmorata presents as a lacy, reticulated, or mottled erythema or violaceous appearance.

Look-alikes

Disorder	Differentiating Features
Erythema infectiosum	• Acquired, not congenital. • Erythematous, lacy, reticulated erythema. • After resolution, rash may reappear following activity or sun exposure.
Livedo reticularis	• Appearance may be identical to cutis marmorata. • Acquired form may be associated with many systemic disorders.
Port-wine stain	• Telangiectatic appearance may be present, but primary lesion erythematous patch. • Reticulated variant may be difficult to distinguish from CMTC early on; with time, features of port-wine stain may become more apparent.
Cutis marmorata telangiectatica congenita	• Reticular vascular pattern present at birth but shows no tendency to resolve with rewarming. – Usually is localized, involving one extremity (less likely to be generalized). – Less responsive to environmental temperature changes. – Affected areas may occasionally be slightly atrophic (depressed) or ulcerated.

How to Make the Diagnosis

- The diagnosis is made clinically.

Treatment

- Cutis marmorata requires no treatment.

Treating Associated Conditions

- Cutis marmorata is harmless and self-limited, so no treatment is needed.
- Persistent cutis marmorata may be seen in association with some chromosomal defects and Cornelia de Lange syndrome.

Prognosis

- Cutis marmorata resolves spontaneously.

When to Worry or Refer

- Consider referral if cutis marmorata persists.

CHAPTER 54

Cutis Marmorata Telangiectatica Congenita (CMTC)

Introduction/Etiology/Epidemiology

- Also known as congenital generalized phlebectasia
- Distinguished from cutis marmorata by failure of lesions to resolve with rewarming
- Etiology unknown
- Presents at or shortly after birth

Signs and Symptoms

- Reticulated mottling involving one or several limbs (Figures 54.1 and 54.2).
- Occasional truncal or facial involvement.
- May have associated skin atrophy, occasional deep purple color, or ulceration.
- Rewarming fails to lead to resolution.
- Ipsilateral limb hypoplasia common, usually of no functional significance.
- Less common associations include port-wine stain and ophthalmologic or neurologic abnormalities.
- Rare association of macrocephaly, craniofacial and skeletal anomalies, and developmental delay termed macrocephaly-capillary malformations; lesions may appear similar to CMTC but actually represent reticulate port-wine stains.
- Adams-Oliver syndrome characterized by CMTC in association with transverse limb defects and scalp aplasia cutis.

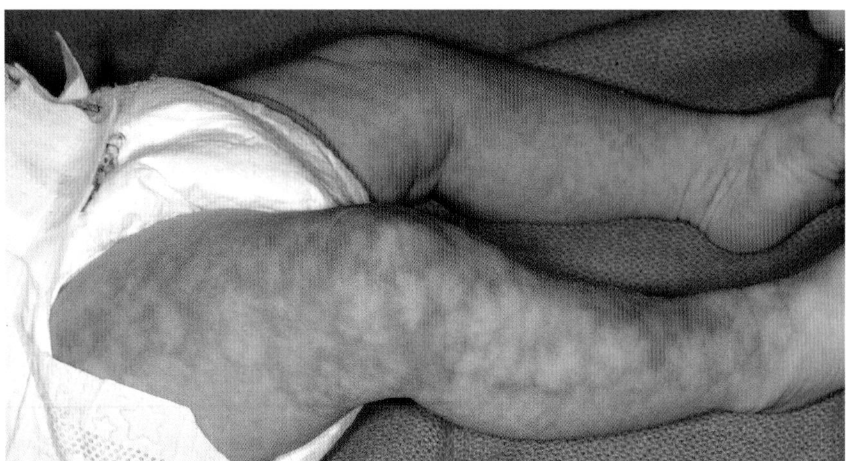

Figure 54.1. Cutis marmorata telangiectatica congenita. Reticulated mottling of the lower extremity.

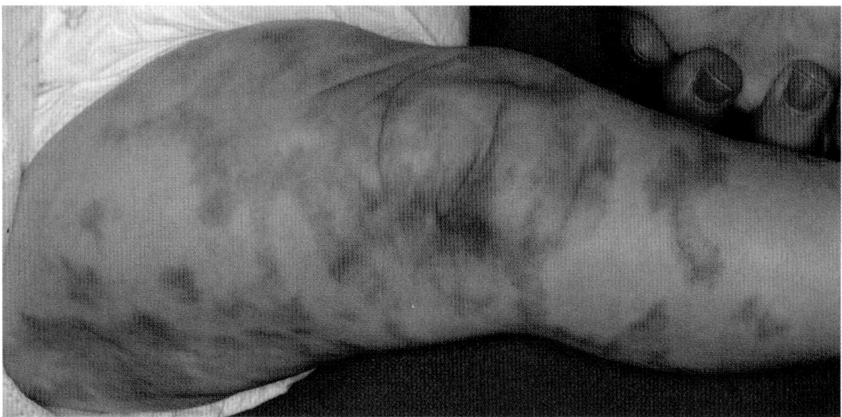

Figure 54.2. Cutis marmorata telangiectatica congenita. Mottling of the lower extremity was present in this infant, with some areas showing more accentuation.

Look-alikes

Disorder	Differentiating Features
Cutis marmorata	• Disappears with rewarming • Symmetrically distributed (not limited to one extremity) • Resolves rapidly over first months to 1 year of life
Reticulated port-wine stain	• Persists indefinitely • Less mottled in appearance • When more extensive, may be associated with macrocephaly and other malformations, developmental delay
Klippel-Trénaunay syndrome	• Associated venous varicosities. • Limb overgrowth, rather than hypoplasia. • Port-wine stains present. • Concomitant lymphedema may be present.
Persistent cutis marmorata	• Associated condition usually present (eg, Down syndrome, homocystinuria, de Lange syndrome) • Widespread skin involvement
Livedo reticularis	• Extremely rare in infants • Associated condition usually present (eg, hematologic disorder, coagulopathy, paraproteinemia, autoimmune disease)

How to Make the Diagnosis

- Clinical examination is usually sufficient.
- Skin biopsy (rarely performed) reveals dilated dermal capillaries and veins.

Treatment

- Usually unnecessary.
- Lesions fade over several years.

Treating Associated Conditions

- Limb hypoplasia requires no therapy.
- Limb length discrepancy extremely rare; if present, refer to orthopedic surgeon.

Prognosis

- The lesions of CMTC generally fade over time with no permanent sequelae.

When to Worry or Refer

- Consider referral to a pediatric dermatologist for patients in whom the diagnosis is in question.
- Consider referral to a pediatric ophthalmologist for patients with extensive or facial involvement; reported rare associations in this setting include glaucoma, retinal detachment, and retinal pigmentation.
- Consider referral to a pediatric neurologist for patients with neurodevelopmental symptoms or concerns.

Resources for Families

- Cincinnati Children's Hospital Medical Center: Patient information. **www.cincinnatichildrens.org/health/c/ctmc**
- WebMD: Information for families is contained in the Health A-Z topics. **www.webmd.com/children/cutis-marmorata-telangiectatica-congenita**

CHAPTER 55

Infantile Hemangioma

Introduction/Etiology/Epidemiology

- Most common benign tumor of infancy.
- Present in 4% to 5% of infants.
- Composed of benign proliferations of endothelial tissue.
- Most common in whites, females, and premature infants.
- Other risk factors include advanced maternal age, placenta previa, multiple gestation pregnancy, and maternal hypertension/preeclampsia.
- Pathogenesis remains speculative.
- Typically become evident around 1 to 2 weeks of age, with growth (proliferative) phase for first year, followed by phases of plateau and spontaneous involution.
- May be congenital.
- Most of growth phase occurs during first 5 months of life.
- Most lesions begin to involute between 6 and 12 months of age, and most involution occurs by age 4 years.
- Involution may not lead to complete resolution of all skin changes.

Signs and Symptoms

- Precursor lesions (sometimes called pre-hemangiomas) may present as an area of skin that is pale, ecchymotic, or ulcerated or that has telangiectasias.
- Superficial hemangiomas
  - Bright red, dome-shaped papules, plaques (Figure 55.1), and tumors
  - Rubbery; may compress with palpation
- Deep hemangiomas
  - Blue-purple subcutaneous nodules and tumors
  - May have prominent surface telangiectasias (Figure 55.2)
  - May be warm to palpation

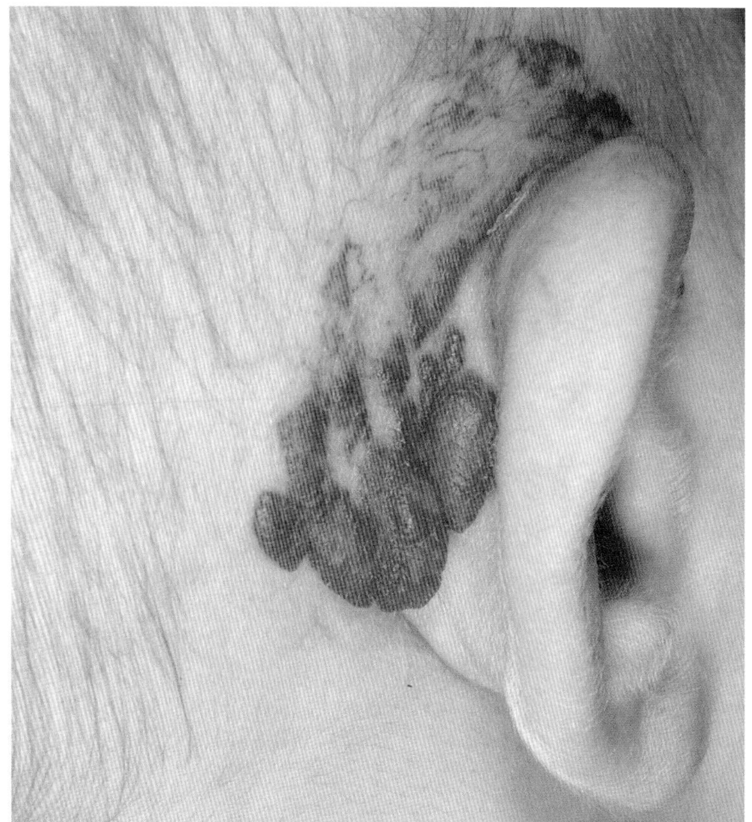

Figure 55.1. Superficial infantile hemangioma.

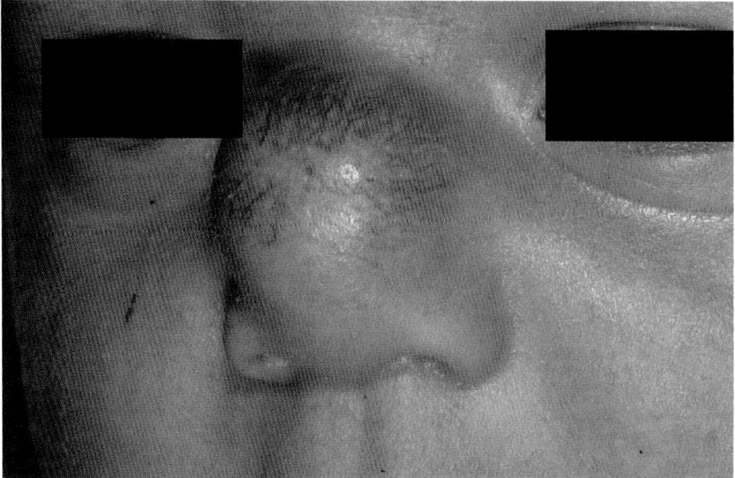

Figure 55.2. Deep infantile hemangioma of the nasal bridge. Note the surface telangiectasias.

- Combined hemangiomas
  - Superficial and deep components
  - Bright red surface component, deeper blue nodular component (Figures 55.3 and 55.4)
- Clinical variants
  - Segmental hemangioma
    - Involve broad anatomic region (Figure 55.5); may be determined by embryonic placodes
    - Often unilateral, with respect for the midline
    - Higher incidence of complications (rapid growth, ulceration) and associations (visceral hemangiomatosis, malformations [eg, urogenital anomalies], PHACES syndrome [See page 360.])
  - Non-involuting congenital hemangioma (NICH)
    - Well-circumscribed blue nodule with telangiectatic surface and peripheral pallor (Figure 55.6).
    - No spontaneous involution; persists indefinitely.
    - This lesion (and rapidly involuting congenital hemangioma) appears to be an entity distinct from typical infantile hemangioma.
  - Rapidly involuting congenital hemangioma
    - Variety of clinical presentations, including appearances similar to NICH or typical infantile hemangioma and appearance as firm, violaceous tumor
    - Rapid involution over first year of life

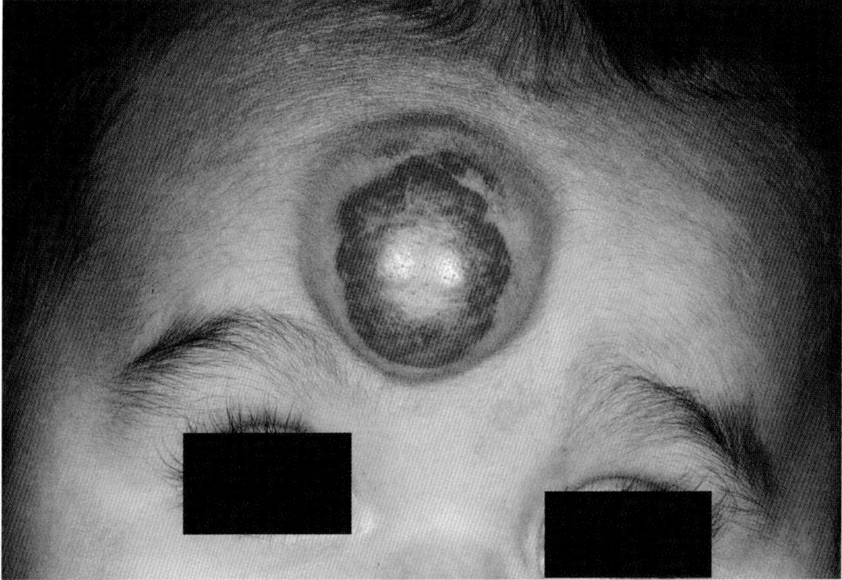

Figure 55.3. Combined infantile hemangioma.

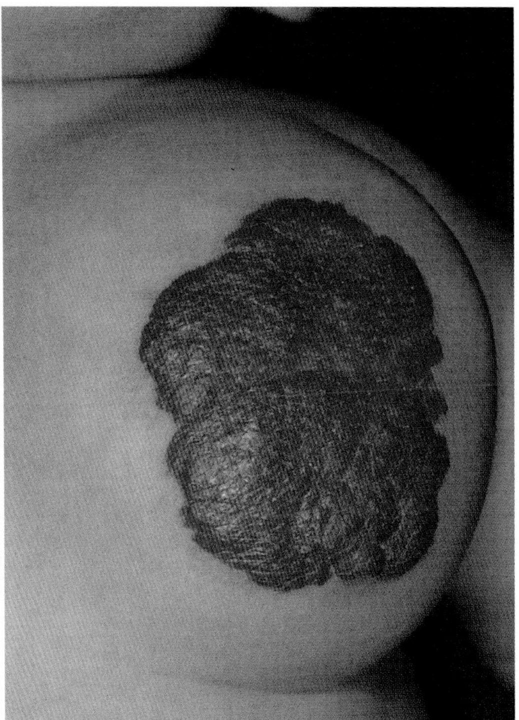

Figure 55.4. Combined infantile hemangioma of the breast.

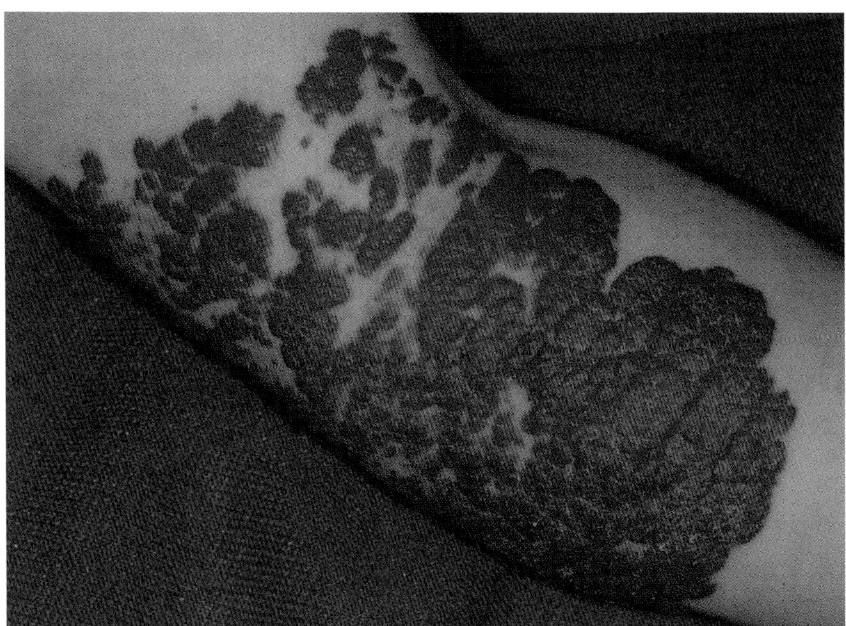

Figure 55.5. Segmental infantile hemangioma. Note the broad anatomic region involved.

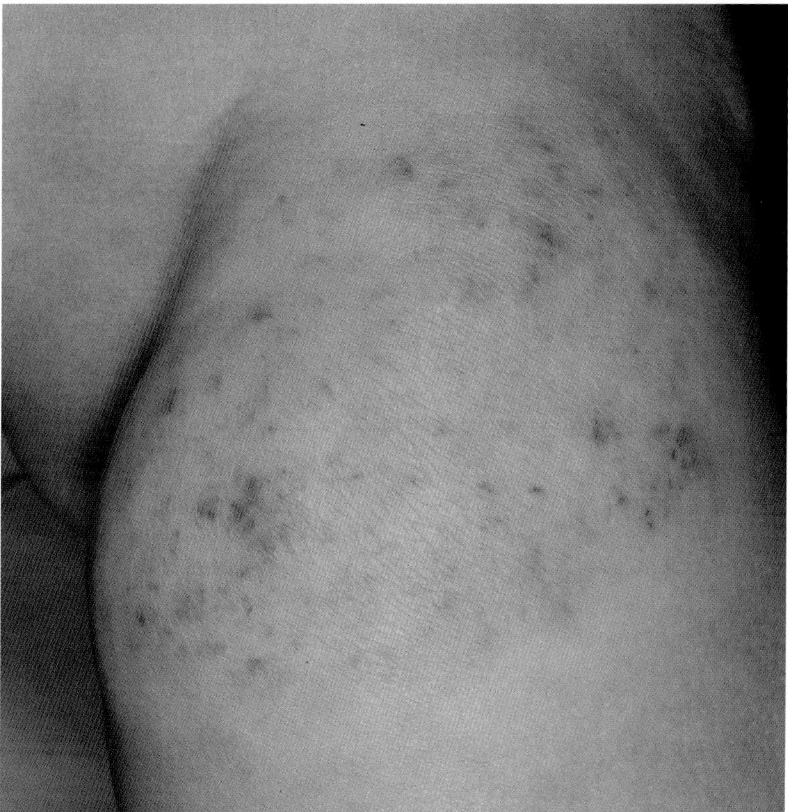

Figure 55.6. Non-involuting congenital hemangioma. Note the peripheral rim of pallor and coarse surface telangiectasias.

- Multiple hemangiomas
  - Multiple cutaneous hemangiomas with (diffuse neonatal hemangiomatosis) or without (benign neonatal hemangiomatosis) extracutaneous organ involvement.
  - May range from several (Figure 55.7) to hundreds of lesions.
  - Liver, gastrointestinal tract, and central nervous system most common sites of internal involvement.
  - Greater risk of hepatic involvement with 5 or more skin hemangiomas.
  - Complications include visceral hemorrhage, anemia, congestive cardiac failure.
  - Infants with liver hemangiomas (especially the diffuse form) may also have associated hypothyroidism.
  - Abdominal ultrasonography most useful screening examination; should be considered in young infants when 5 or more lesions present or in presence of hepatomegaly or signs/symptoms of congestive heart failure.

- Beard hemangiomas
  - Lesions involve lower lip, neck, chin, and mandibular regions (Figure 55.8).
  - Increased risk of airway hemangiomatosis.
  - May present with biphasic stridor, hoarseness.
  - If clinically suspected, direct laryngoscopy is indicated.
- PHACES syndrome
  - Large, segmental facial (or, occasionally, upper trunk or neck) hemangioma in association with other developmental defects.
  - Clinical findings include **p**osterior fossa defects (eg, Dandy-Walker malformation), **h**emangioma, **a**rterial anomalies (mainly of head and neck vasculature), **c**ardiac anomalies/aortic coarctation, **e**ye abnormalities, and **s**ternal clefting/supraumbilical abdominal raphe.
  - Infants are at risk for progressive cerebrovascular disease, including risk for arterial ischemic stroke.
- Lumbosacral hemangiomas
  - May be associated with occult spinal dysraphism, spinal cord defects.
  - Sacral and perineal lesions may also be associated with anorectal or urogenital anomalies.
  - Associated abnormalities most likely with extensive lesions or when other lumbosacral findings present (eg, lipoma, gluteal cleft deviation, prominent sacral dimple).
  - PELVIS syndrome has been used to describe infants with **p**erineal hemangioma, **e**xternal genitalia malformations, **l**ipomyelomeningocele, **v**esicorenal abnormalities, **i**mperforate anus, and **s**kin tag; this association is also known under the acronym LUMBAR syndrome and may also include arterial anomalies and bony deformities.
  - Hemangiomas in this setting may involve not only the perineum but also the lumbosacral region, genitalia, or lower extremity; they are usually of the segmental type.
  - Magnetic resonance imaging useful for screening, when indicated.

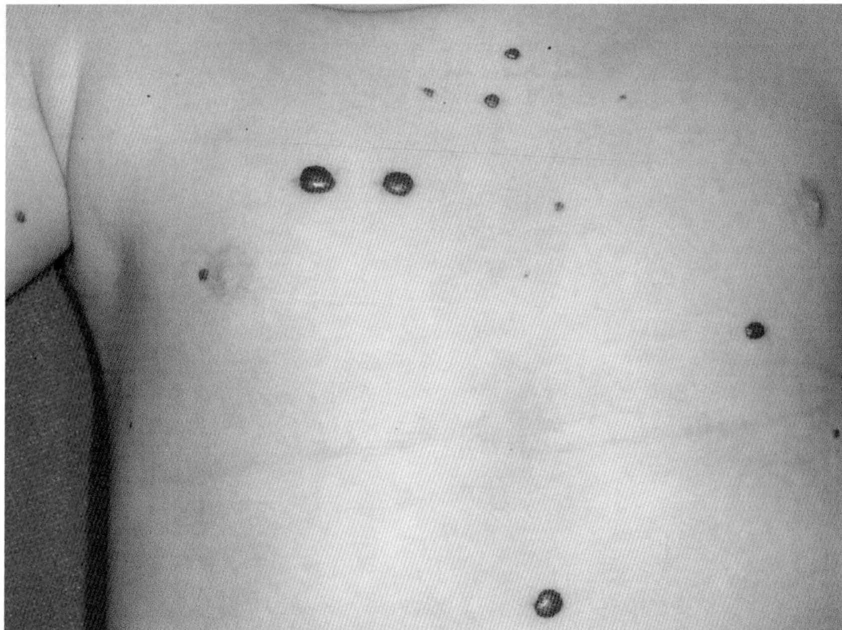

Figure 55.7. Neonatal hemangiomatosis. This infant had multiple small hemangiomas in the liver as well.

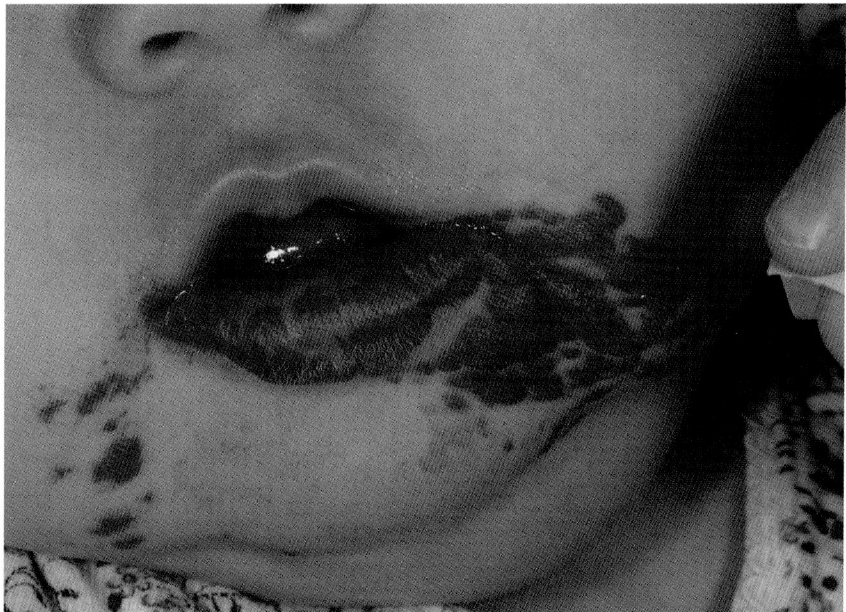

Figure 55.8. Beard distribution infantile hemangioma. This infant girl also had a subglottic hemangioma.

Look-alikes

Disorder	Differentiating Features
Port-wine stain	• May simulate early superficial hemangioma • Static lesion, remains flat without proliferation • Does not involute spontaneously
Venous malformation	• May simulate deep hemangioma • Static lesion, lacks natural history of hemangioma • Does not involute spontaneously • May develop thromboses, become painful
Lymphatic malformation	• May simulate deep hemangioma. • Lacks overlying blue hue. • Static lesion, lacks natural history of hemangioma. • Translucent flesh-colored to hemorrhagic papules may be present on overlying skin surface (microcystic component).
Arteriovenous malformation	• May simulate superficial or deep hemangioma. • Aggressive growth patterns. • Pulsatile with an audible bruit. • Spontaneous involution does not occur.
Kaposiform hemangioendothelioma	• Red-purple tumor • Infiltrative growth nature, may be nodular • May be associated with Kasabach-Merritt phenomenon (ie, thrombocytopenia, hemolytic anemia)
Pyogenic granuloma	• Small, red papule or nodule • Moist friable surface, narrow base • Typically appear only after several months of life (and usually after first year)
Soft tissue malignancy	• Rhabdomyosarcoma, fibrosarcoma, neuroblastoma. • Growth pattern may be more aggressive. • Usually less homogeneous in appearance. • If diagnosis in question, tissue biopsy indicated.

How to Make the Diagnosis

- Clinical examination and history usually suggest the diagnosis.
- Ultrasound, magnetic resonance imaging occasionally indicated/useful; ultrasound most useful in evaluating for liver involvement in patients with multiple skin hemangiomas; magnetic resonance plays most important role in evaluation for associated visceral or arterial anomalies in patients with more extensive lesions of the face, neck, and upper trunk (PHACES syndrome) or anogenital, lumbosacral regions (PELVIS syndrome).

- Tissue biopsy rarely necessary; when in question, diagnosis can be confirmed with immunostaining for glucose transporter 1 (GLUT1), FcγRII, merosin, and Lewis Y antigen; GLUT1 staining is typically negative for non-involuting congenital hemangioma and rapidly involuting congenital hemangioma.

Treatment

- Dictated by extent of involvement, location of lesion(s), age of the patient, and associated complications.
- Goals of therapy are to minimize pain, prevent long-term deformity, prevent life- or function-threatening complications, and minimize psychosocial distress.
- Therapeutic options
  - Active nonintervention
    - Emotional support, guidance, education
    - Referral to family support groups, educational resources
  - Local wound care
    - For ulcerated lesions: topical antibiotics (eg, bacitracin, mupirocin, metronidazole), nonstick wound dressings, compresses
    - Becaplermin (recombinant platelet-derived growth factor) gel; off-label, may be useful for ulcerated lesions
  - Systemic antibiotic therapy
    - For moderate or severe secondary infection
  - Pain control
    - For ulcerated lesions
    - Includes local wound care, oral analgesics, topical anesthetics (sparingly used), pulsed dye laser therapy, oral narcotic analgesics (rarely)
  - Topical corticosteroids
    - Potent formulations may be useful when applied nightly to localized, superficial lesions.
  - Intralesional corticosteroids
    - May be useful for localized lesions; caution with periocular hemangiomas
  - Oral corticosteroids
    - Traditional mainstay of therapy.
    - Usually prednisolone or prednisone, 2 to 4 mg/kg per day.
    - Toxicity profile predictable; most infants respond promptly to therapy.
    - Live virus vaccines must be avoided until off of therapy for 1 month.
    - Transient decrease in linear growth velocity common.
    - Concomitant administration of H_2-receptor antagonist (eg, ranitidine) useful for gastritis prophylaxis.

- Oral propranolol
  - Current gold-standard therapy for infantile hemangiomas.
  - Nonselective ß-blocker used traditionally for cardiac indications; US Food and Drug Administration approved for treatment of hemangiomas in infants 5 weeks to 5 months of age.
  - Useful for slowing growth/accelerating involution of hemangiomas.
  - Mechanisms of action unclear; may include vasoconstriction, apoptosis, inhibition of angiogenic growth factors.
  - Typically started at dose of 1 to 1.5 mg/kg/d and titrated up to 2 to 3 mg/kg/d, divided 2 to 3 times daily; always give concomitant with (or after) feeding.
  - Risks include hypoglycemia, hypotension, bradycardia, bronchospasm, hypothermia, and sleep disruption/night terrors.
  - Contraindicated with sinus bradycardia, hypotension, heart block, asthma; patients at risk for PHACES syndrome should complete head/neck imaging first and, if arterial abnormalities present, started on therapy only in consultation with a pediatric neurologist.
  - Baseline heart rate, blood pressure, and (especially in high-risk infants) electrocardiogram recommended; vitals repeated at 1 and 2 hours following initial dose.
- Topical timolol
  - Being used off-label by some clinicians for superficial, uncomplicated, and functionally insignificant hemangiomas
  - Typically, the gel-forming ophthalmic solution, in a 0.25% to 0.5% concentration; applied as one drop rubbed in well 2 to 3 times daily
- Pulsed dye laser therapy
  - Mainly useful for ulcerated lesions or early superficial hemangiomas; may also play a role in treating persistent telangiectasias following involution
- Recombinant interferon alfa
  - Reserved for life- and function-threatening hemangiomas, which are refractory to other medical therapies
  - Administered via daily subcutaneous injection, 1 to 3 million U/m^2 per day
  - Risk of spastic diplegia; serial neurologic examinations indicated
- Vincristine
  - Chemotherapeutic agent shown to be beneficial for life-threatening lesions.
  - Administered via central venous catheter.
  - Risks include peripheral neuropathy.

- Surgical excision
  - Useful in selected situations, including involuted lesions, residual scars, or fibrofatty redundant tissue
  - Use during proliferative phase controversial; usually reserved for function-threatening, medication-resistant lesions

Treating Associated Conditions

- Ulceration
  - See previous discussion.
  - Most common in lesions located on lips, genitals, and perineum and perianal region.
  - Topical antibiotics (eg, bacitracin, mupirocin, metronidazole) are useful.
  - Systemic antibiotics may be necessary.
  - Nonstick wound dressings (eg, petrolatum-impregnated gauze) may be useful.
  - Consider bacterial culture, pulsed dye laser, or becaplermin gel when resistant to previously described measures.
  - Pain control is an important aspect of management.
- Residual skin changes
  - Residual telangiectasias following involution may require pulsed dye laser therapy.
  - Fibrofatty residua or scars remaining after involution may require surgical removal.
- Kasabach-Merritt phenomenon
  - Not associated with infantile hemangioma but, rather, kaposiform hemangioendothelioma or tufted angioma.
  - See Chapter 56.

Prognosis

- Uncomplicated infantile hemangiomas that are not function- or life-endangering have an excellent prognosis, with spontaneous involution over 5 to 10 years.
- In patients with function- or life-endangering lesions, prognosis depends on multiple variables, including location, complications, associated findings, timeliness of therapy, and response to therapy.

When to Worry or Refer

- Referral to a pediatric dermatologist (or other appropriate specialist) should be considered for hemangiomas in the following settings:
  - High-risk location
    - Periocular (most notable potential complications include astigmatism and light-deprivation amblyopia)
    - Nasal tip
    - Ear (when extensive)
    - Lips
    - Genitals or perineum
    - Lumbosacral region
    - Airway
    - Hepatic
  - Function-threatening
  - Life-threatening
  - Ulceration present
  - Multiple lesions
  - Beard distribution
  - Extensive facial, anogenital involvement

Resources for Families

- American Academy of Pediatrics: HealthyChildren.org.
  www.HealthyChildren.org/hemangioma
- Hemangioma Investigator Group: Multicenter clinical research consortium and source of patient education and support.
  www.hemangiomaeducation.org
- Hemangioma Support System: Provides support for parents.
  c/o Cynthia Schumerth
  1484 Sand Acres Dr
  DePere, WI 54115
  920/336-9399 (after 8:00 pm CT)
- National Organization of Vascular Anomalies: Patient information, resources, and support.
  www.novanews.org
- Society for Pediatric Dermatology: Patient handout on hemangiomas.
  http://pedsderm.net/for-patients-families/patient-handouts
- Vascular Birthmarks Foundation: Provides referrals, financial assistance, newsletter, conference, resource list for advocacy, support, and counseling.
  www.birthmark.org

CHAPTER 56

Kasabach-Merritt Phenomenon

Introduction/Etiology/Epidemiology

- Association of a vascular tumor with thrombocytopenia, hemolytic anemia, and coagulopathy
- Not associated with infantile hemangioma, as traditionally believed
- Vascular tumor usually kaposiform hemangioendothelioma or tufted angioma
- May be life-threatening

Signs and Symptoms

- Usually presents within the first few weeks or months of life, with sudden enlargement of preexisting vascular lesion (Figure 56.1) and occasional petechiae or purpura.
- Laboratory evaluation reveals thrombocytopenia, anemia, hypofibrinogenemia, elevated D-dimers, and prolongation of coagulation studies.
- Ecchymoses, epistaxis, hematuria, and hematochezia may also be present.
- Appearance of preexisting lesions
    - Kaposiform hemangioendothelioma
        - Firm, violaceous plaque or tumor
        - May expand rapidly and tends to be locally aggressive
        - Tends to persist indefinitely
    - Tufted angioma
        - Brightly erythematous plaque with induration
        - May spontaneously involute or persist indefinitely

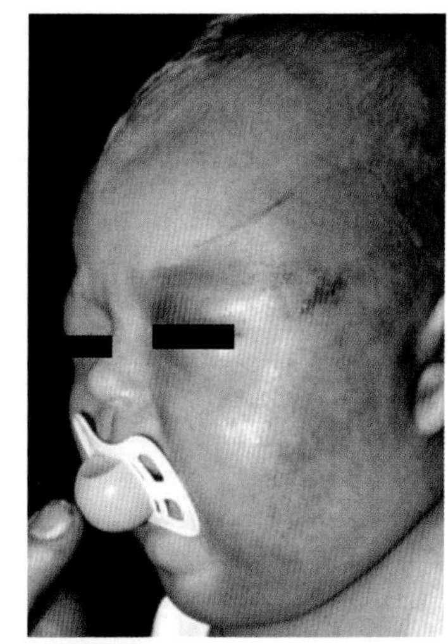

Figure 56.1. Kasabach-Merritt phenomenon. This congenital lesion of the lateral face and scalp enlarged in association with thrombocytopenia and coagulopathy.

Look-alikes

Disorder	Differentiating Features
Infantile hemangioma	• Follows course more typical of hemangioma • Not associated with thrombocytopenia or coagulopathy • Sudden enlargement (versus gradual) rare
Soft tissue malignancy (ie, rhabdomyosarcoma)	• Usually not associated with coagulopathy • Histologic features diagnostic

How to Make the Diagnosis

- Diagnosis is suggested by sudden enlargement of a vascular-appearing tumor.
- Laboratory findings of thrombocytopenia, hemolytic anemia, and coagulopathy are supportive.
- Tissue biopsy with histologic evaluation is confirmatory.

Treatment

- Challenging.
- Small lesions may be amenable to surgical excision.
- Medical therapy usually is necessary; options include high-dose corticosteroids, vincristine, cyclophosphamide, sirolimus, and antifibrinolytic therapy; vincristine in combination with corticosteroids is considered first-line by many experts. Interferon alfa has lost favor given the associated risk of spastic diplegia in young children.
- Red blood cell transfusions may be necessary.
- Platelet transfusions may lead to worsening and should be minimized.
- Embolization and radiation therapy occasionally are used.

Treating Associated Conditions

- Kaposiform hemangioendothelioma
  - Wide local excision, if localized and superficial.
  - Treatment otherwise is extremely difficult.
- Tufted angioma
  - Surgical excision, if lesions are small and localized.
  - Laser therapy shows inconsistent results.

Prognosis

- Mortality rate of 10% to 30%
- Prognosis poorer for patients with retroperitoneal involvement

When to Worry or Refer

- Consider referral in any patient with a
  - Rapidly expanding, vascular-appearing tumor
  - Vascular tumor in conjunction with cutaneous petechiae or purpura, thrombocytopenia, or coagulopathy

Resources for Families

- Cincinnati Children's Hospital Medical Center: Patient information. **www.cincinnatichildrens.org/health/info/vascular/diagnose/kasabach-merritt.htm**

CHAPTER 57

Pyogenic Granuloma

Introduction/Etiology/Epidemiology

- Also known as lobular capillary hemangioma
- Common in children and young adults
- Acquired vascular lesion of skin or mucous membranes
- Cause unknown, but appear to represent reactive neovascularization

Signs and Symptoms

- Solitary red papule or papulonodule, rarely larger than 1 cm.
- May be pedunculated (Figure 57.1).

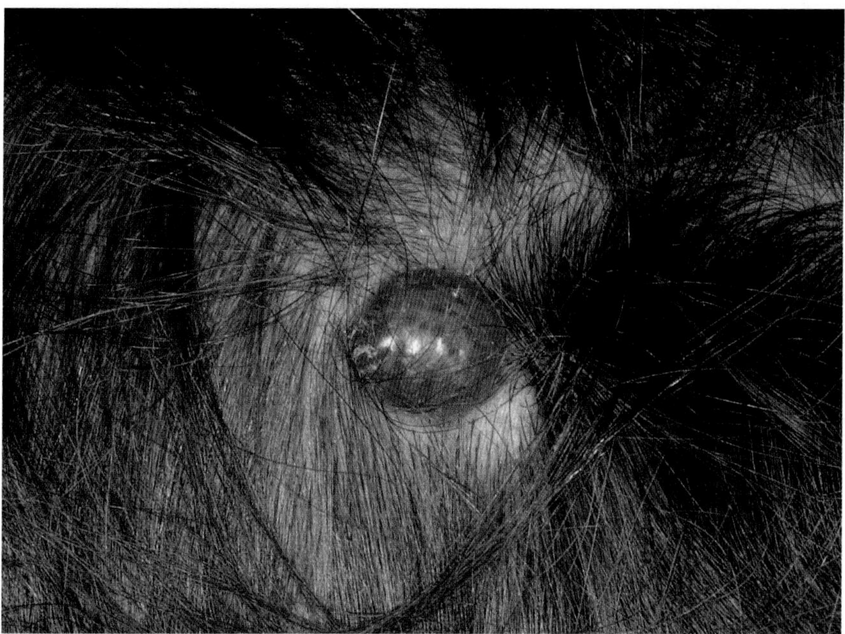

Figure 57.1. Pyogenic granuloma. A pedunculated, vascular papule on the scalp.

- Surface commonly bleeds or becomes erosive (Figure 57.2).
- Base of lesion may be surrounded by collarette of scale.
- May develop on surface of port-wine stain.
- Occasionally multiple.
- Common locations include hand, finger, face, and oral mucosa.

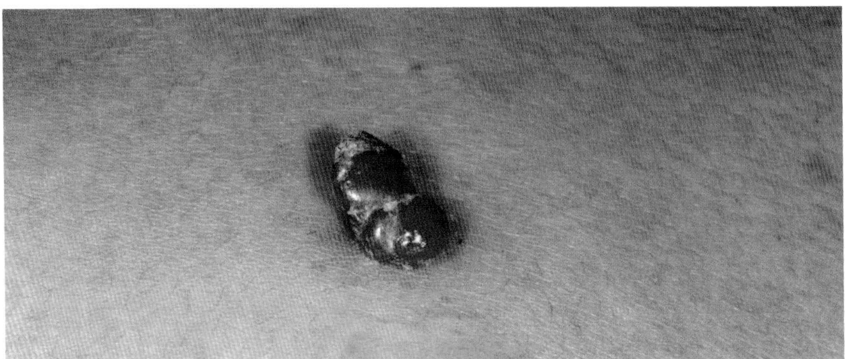

Figure 57.2. Pyogenic granuloma. This multilobulated, vascular papule was prone to recurrent bleeding and crusting (as noted at superior portion).

Look-alikes

Disorder	Differentiating Features
Infantile hemangioma	• Presents in early infancy • Rarely pedunculated • Often grows to >1 cm • History of proliferation followed by spontaneous involution
Juvenile xanthogranuloma	• Early lesion may appear vascular, but eventually yellow-orange hue becomes apparent. • Usually sessile (broad-based) rather than pedunculated. • Rarely becomes erosive on surface.
Spitz nevus	• Slowly growing papule. • Sessile (broad-based) rather than pedunculated. • Rarely becomes erosive on surface. • Diascopy (pressure with glass slide) may reveal brown pigment. • Dermoscopy (examination with a dermatoscope) may reveal characteristic pigment patterns.
Spider angioma	• May simulate early (small) pyogenic granuloma • Central papule remains <3 mm • Does not become erosive on surface • Peripheral telangiectatic vessels present

How to Make the Diagnosis

- Pyogenic granuloma is usually diagnosed based on the classic clinical features.
- Histologic evaluation is confirmatory following excision.

Treatment

- Shave excision followed by electrocautery of the base.
- Small lesions may be amenable to pulsed dye laser therapy, topical timolol gel.
- Very small lesions with eroded surface may respond to chemical cauterization with silver nitrate.
- Full-thickness excision occasionally indicated for larger lesions.

Prognosis

- The prognosis for an uncomplicated pyogenic granuloma is excellent.
- Recurrence is rare but may occur following excision.
- Patients with multiple, clustered (agminated) lesions are more prone to recurrence.

When to Worry or Refer

- Consider referral when the
  - Diagnosis is in question.
  - Patient or parent desires removal.
  - Lesion is erosive or bleeding.

Resources for Families

- American Osteopathic College of Dermatology: Patient information. **www.aocd.org/?page=PyogenicGranuloma**
- MedlinePlus: Information for patients and families (in English and Spanish) sponsored by the National Library of Medicine and National Institutes of Health. **https://www.nlm.nih.gov/medlineplus/ency/article/001464.htm**

CHAPTER 58

Telangiectasias

Introduction/Etiology/Epidemiology

- Telangiectasias represent dilatations of superficial capillaries.
- May be a manifestation of physical trauma, medications, hormonal abnormality, autoimmune disease, or genetic disorders.
- Often idiopathic in origin.
- Lesions disappear with diascopy (gentle downward pressure with a microscope slide).
- This discussion includes spider angioma, angioma serpiginosum, hereditary hemorrhagic telangiectasia (HHT), unilateral nevoid telangiectasia, generalized essential telangiectasia, and ataxia-telangiectasia.

Signs and Symptoms

- Spider angioma
  - Also known as nevus araneus.
  - Central red papule with peripheral, radiating telangiectatic vessels.
  - Occasionally, pulsation may be noted.
  - Most common on face, upper trunk, arms, and hands (Figure 58.1); multiple lesions are not unusual in children.
  - Occasionally associated with liver disease, estrogen therapy, pregnancy.

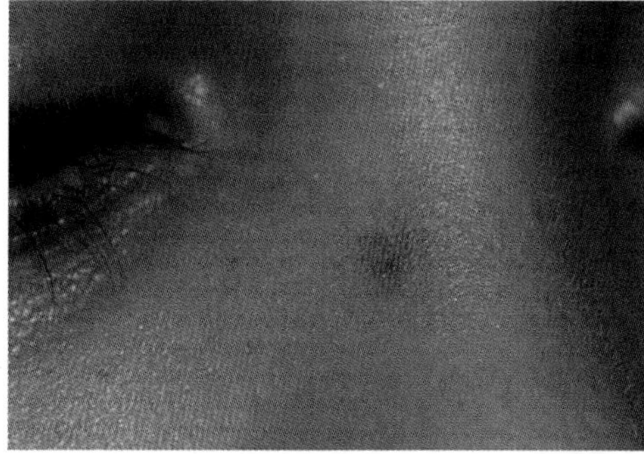

Figure 58.1. Spider angioma. Multiple lesions were also present on the hands of this young girl.

- Angioma serpiginosum
  - Rare; usually occurs in first 2 decades, mainly in girls
  - Punctate red to violaceous macules, usually in a linear or serpiginous pattern
  - Most common on the extremities
- Hereditary hemorrhagic telangiectasia (HHT)
  - Also known as Osler-Weber-Rendu syndrome.
  - Autosomal-dominant disorder characterized by mucocutaneous telangiectasias and bleeding diathesis.
  - Caused by mutations in *endoglin* gene (HHT1) or *activin receptor-like kinase 1* (ALK-1) gene (HHT2).
  - Mutations in *Smad4* result in HHT in association with juvenile polyposis.
  - Patients usually present with epistaxis and anemia secondary to gastrointestinal blood loss.
  - Papular or "mat-like" telangiectasias occur on mucous membranes (lips, tongue, nasal mucosa) and skin; usually first appearing during adolescence or later.
  - May develop arteriovenous malformations, especially in gastrointestinal tract, lungs, and brain.
- Unilateral nevoid telangiectasia
  - Segmental, unilateral distribution of skin telangiectasias (Figure 58.2)
  - May be dermatomal
  - May be congenital or acquired
  - May be associated with liver disease, puberty, pregnancy, or hormonal therapy
- Generalized essential telangiectasia
  - Widespread cutaneous telangiectasias with no bleeding diathesis.
  - More common in adult females, rare in children.
  - Most common site of involvement is the lower extremities.
- Ataxia-telangiectasia
  - Also known as Louis-Bar syndrome.
  - Autosomal-recessive disorder consisting of oculocutaneous telangiectasias, immunodeficiency, cerebellar ataxia, pulmonary infections, and predisposition toward hematologic malignancy.
  - Caused by mutation in the *ATM* (ataxia-telangiectasia mutated) gene.
  - Presents with truncal ataxia, other neurologic symptoms early in life.
  - Telangiectasias begin to appear at 3 to 5 years, characteristically involving the bulbar conjunctivae and sun-exposed skin; most common sites of skin involvement are the face, arms, and upper chest.

- May also have premature aging, pigmentary skin change, noninfectious skin granulomas (most common on the extremities), chronic sinopulmonary infections, bronchiectasis, and growth failure.
- Increased risk of Hodgkin disease, non-Hodgkin lymphoma, leukemia, and skin malignancy.

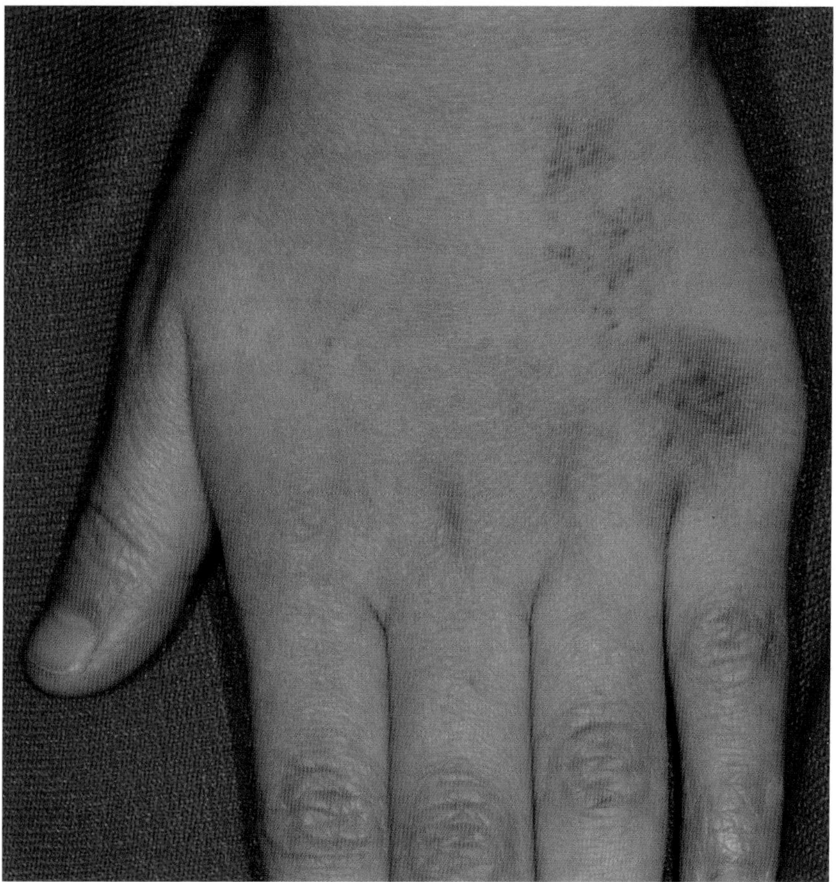

Figure 58.2. Unilateral nevoid telangiectasia. This girl had telangiectatic patches involving the dorsal hand and forearm, without any identified predisposing conditions.

Look-alikes

Disorder	Differentiating Features
Pyogenic granuloma, Spitz nevus	• Small lesions may simulate spider angioma. • Lack peripheral telangiectatic network. • With continued growth, both become larger than typical for spider angioma.
Cherry angioma	• Less common in children • Lacks peripheral telangiectatic network
Pigmented purpura	• May simulate angioma serpiginosum • More likely bilateral, with extravasated red blood cells noted on biopsy • Pink to tan or golden brown patches with petechiae present on diascopic examination

How to Make the Diagnosis

- Spider angioma, angioma serpiginosum, unilateral nevoid telangiectasia, and generalized essential telangiectasia usually are diagnosed based on clinical features.
- Skin biopsy may be useful for distinguishing angioma serpiginosum from pigmented purpura.
- Hereditary hemorrhagic telangiectasia suspected based on epistaxis history, family history, and examination findings; molecular-based diagnosis available.
- Ataxia-telangiectasia usually suspected based on history and clinical examination findings. Elevated α-fetoprotein and carcinoembryonic antigen and spontaneous chromosomal abnormalities support the diagnosis. Molecular-based diagnosis is available if familial mutation is known.

Treatment

- Spider angioma: electrocoagulation or pulsed dye laser if desired by the patient.
- Angioma serpiginosum, unilateral nevoid telangiectasia, generalized essential telangiectasia: usually not treated. If desired, pulsed dye laser therapy may be useful.
- Hereditary hemorrhagic telangiectasia: Treatment is dictated by extent of organ involvement; may include embolization, septal dermoplasty, desmopressin, antifibrinolytic agents, hormonal therapy, surgery, laser therapy, and transfusions.

- Ataxia-telangiectasia: Treatment is mainly supportive; aggressive surveillance for malignancy is vital, as is vigorous photoprotection (given increased risk of skin malignancy).

Treating Associated Conditions

- See Treatment.

Prognosis

- Patients with spider angioma, angioma serpiginosum, unilateral nevoid telangiectasia, or generalized essential telangiectasia, in the absence of associated systemic conditions, have an excellent prognosis with no long-term sequelae related to the skin lesions.
- The prognosis for patients with HHT depends on the extent of organ involvement and associated complications.
- Patients with ataxia-telangiectasia often die from chronic sinopulmonary disease or malignancy.

When to Worry or Refer

- Multiple spider angiomas may be associated with liver disease, pregnancy, or estrogen therapy.
- Consider referral for patients in whom the diagnosis is in question or when laser therapy is requested.
- In the child with a history of recurrent (especially nocturnal) epistaxis and mucocutaneous telangiectasias, consider referral to genetics, otolaryngology, and pediatric dermatology for possible HHT.
- In the child with ataxia, recurrent infections, and oculocutaneous telangiectasias, consider referral to pediatric neurology, genetics, and pediatric dermatology for possible ataxia-telangiectasia.

Resources for Families

- Cure HHT (HHT Foundation International): Provides support and information for individuals, families, and health care professionals.
  http://curehht.org
- A-T Society: Works to improve quality of life and care for people living with ataxia-telangiectasia while promoting research to lengthen lives and find a cure.
  www.atsociety.org.uk
- A-T Children's Project: Its mission is to encourage and support excellent laboratory research that will accelerate the discovery of a cure or possible therapies for ataxia-telangiectasia.
  www.atcp.org/page.aspx?pid=3371

CHAPTER 59

Vascular Malformations

Introduction/Etiology/Epidemiology

- Anomalous blood vessels without endothelial proliferation
- Usually present at birth
- Persist indefinitely
- Although nonproliferative, may gradually increase in size with growth of the individual
- Classified by the primary components
  - Capillary malformation
    - Salmon patch
    - Port-wine stain (PWS)
  - Venous malformation
  - Lymphatic malformation
    - Lymphedema
    - Microcystic lymphatic malformation
    - Macrocystic lymphatic malformation
  - Arteriovenous malformation
  - Combined malformations

Signs and Symptoms

- Capillary malformation
  - Salmon patch
    - Also known as nevus simplex, stork bite, angel kiss; present in 30% to 40% of newborns.
    - Dull pink macules and patches (Figure 59.1).
    - Posterior neck/scalp (stork bite), glabella (angel kiss), forehead, superior eyelids.
    - Occasional involvement of nose, nasolabial regions, philtrum.
    - No syndrome associations; usually fade by 2 years but may become more prominent with crying, straining, physical exertion.
    - Salmon patches on the posterior neck/scalp may occasionally develop overlying dermatitis, which responds to topical steroids or laser therapy.

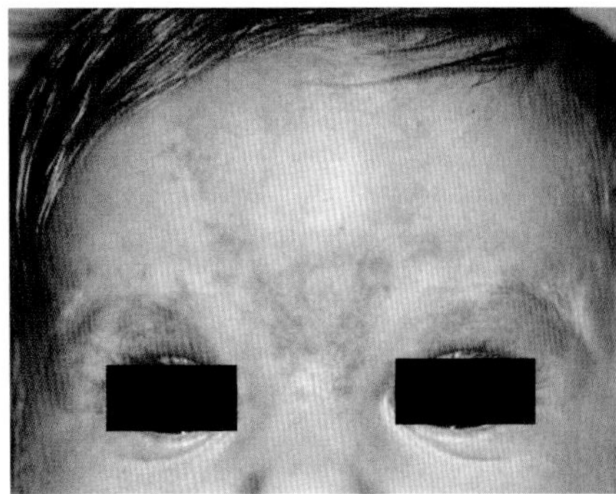

Figure 59.1. Salmon patch. Erythematous patches involving the glabella and eyelids.

- PWS
  - Also known as nevus flammeus.
  - May be isolated or associated with syndromes.
  - Caused by mutation in *GNAQ* in some patients (same mutation involved in Sturge-Weber syndrome).
  - Usually darker red, larger than salmon patch (Figures 59.2 and 59.3).
  - Early lesion may be indistinguishable from infantile hemangioma.
  - May darken and thicken with aging; occasionally develop pyogenic granulomas on surface.
  - Persists indefinitely; may pose psychosocial issue.
  - Syndrome associations outlined in Treating Associated Conditions.

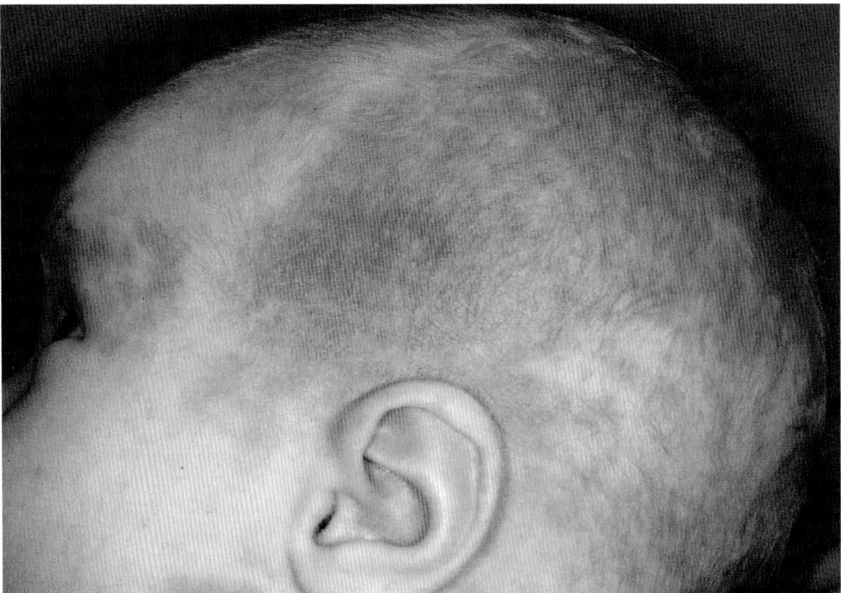

Figure 59.2. Port-wine stain. Dark red, vascular stain involving the scalp, with minimal extension onto the face.

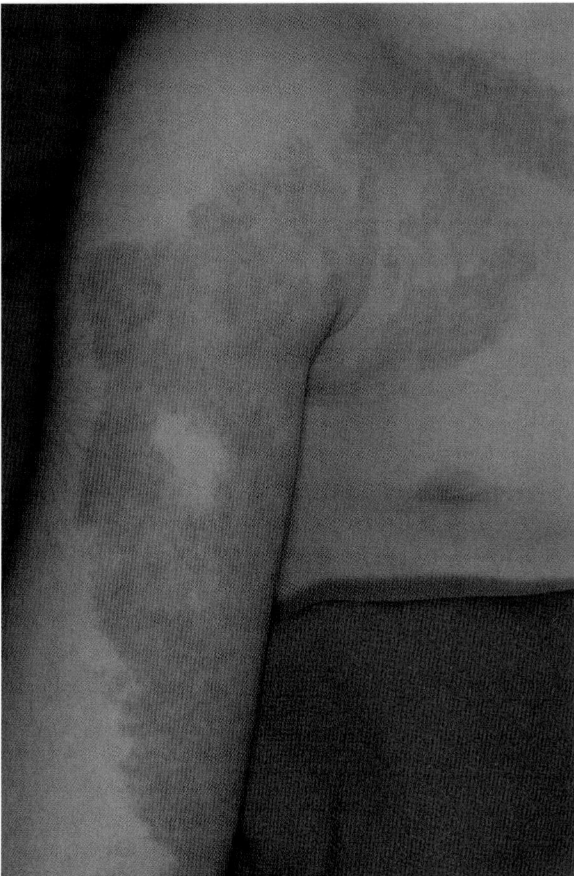

Figure 59.3. Port-wine stain. This lesion involves the lateral chest as well as upper arm.

- Venous malformation
  - Although present at birth, may not become obvious until later in life.
  - Blue or blue-purple in color.
  - Subcutaneous, compressible masses (Figure 59.4).
  - May be confused with deep infantile hemangioma in infants.
  - May occur on any part of the body.
  - May be associated with significant distortion, functional compromise.
  - Occasional thromboses, phleboliths may occur.
  - Rare associated syndromes include Maffucci syndrome and blue rubber bleb nevus syndrome.

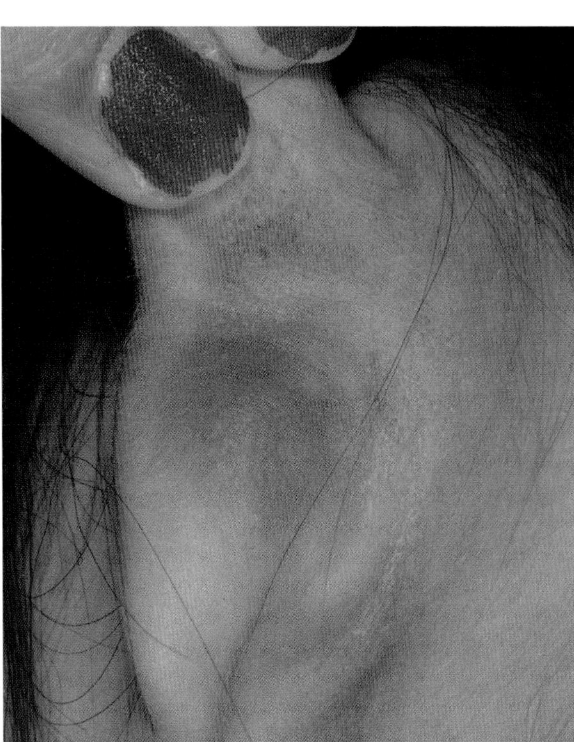

Figure 59.4. Venous malformation. This non-tender, compressible nodule on the posterior helix was present at birth.

- Lymphatic malformation
  - Lymphedema: may be congenital or acquired; lymph fluid collection in subcutaneous tissues, often extremities; may occur in setting of Turner and Noonan syndromes
  - Microcystic lymphatic malformation
    - Aggregates of microscopic lymphatic channels.
    - Present as plaques of clear or flesh-colored blebs; may be hemorrhagic (Figure 59.5).
    - Swelling and occasional bruising may occur.
  - Macrocystic lymphatic malformation
    - Large, interconnected lymphatic channels and cysts.
    - Old terminology: cystic hygroma, cavernous lymphangioma.
    - May be associated with Turner syndrome, Down syndrome, trisomy 18 or 13, Noonan syndrome.
    - Any location but favor head, neck, and chest.
    - Present as large, translucent masses (Figure 59.6).
    - Hemorrhage may present with swelling, tenderness, purple appearance.

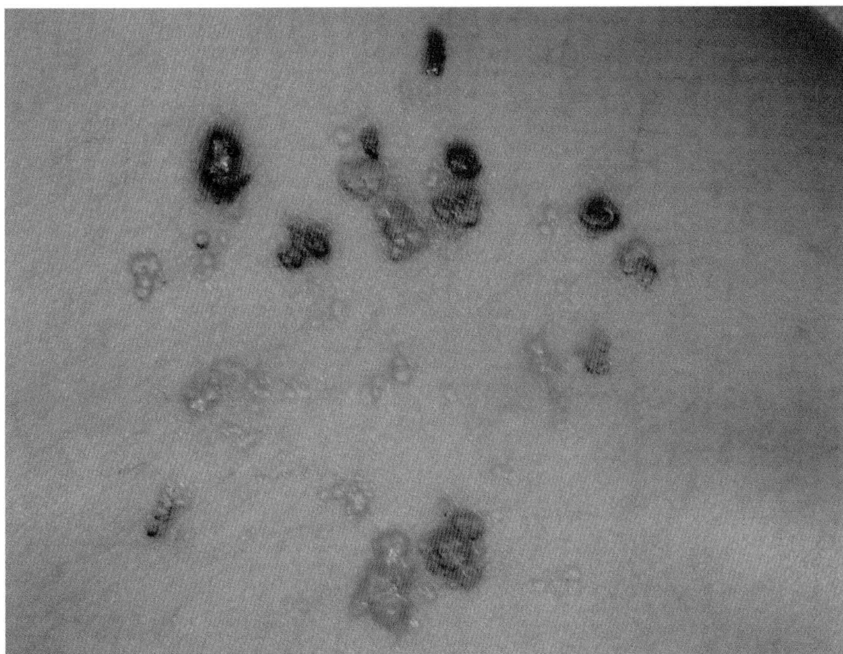

Figure 59.5. Microcystic lymphatic malformation. Translucent, grouped papules, some of which reveal a hemorrhagic component.

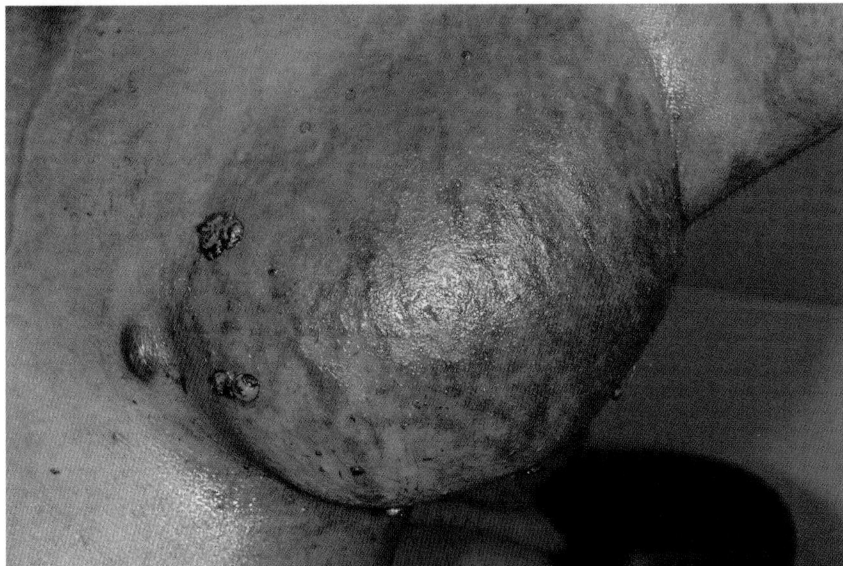

Figure 59.6. Macrocystic lymphatic malformation. A large mass of the lateral chest/anterior axillary region in a young girl. Note hemorrhagic lymphatic blebs on the medial surface.

- Arteriovenous malformation
  - Rare vascular malformation with arterial and venous components and arteriovenous shunting
  - May present as red patch simulating PWS, pulsating mass with thrills, or, occasionally, with necrosis and ulceration
  - May be classified from stage 1 (pink macules, which may mimic capillary malformation) to stage 4 (larger lesions associated with cardiac compromise)
- Combined malformations
  - Combination of 2 or more components (Figure 59.7)
  - Commonly capillary-lymphatic-venous or capillary-venous

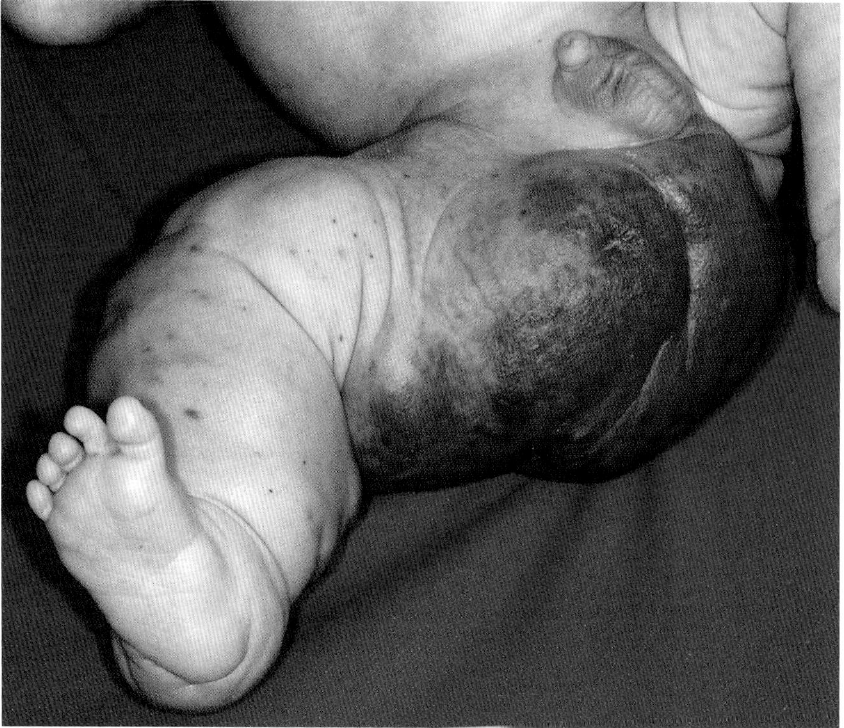

Figure 59.7. Combined vascular malformation. This extensive lesion of the buttock and lower extremity had capillary (red), venous (blue), and lymphatic (deeper aspect of the mass) components.

Look-alikes

Disorder	Differentiating Features
Infantile hemangioma	• Early (superficial) lesion may simulate salmon patch or PWS. • Proliferates, thickens with time. • May ulcerate, bleed. • Deep lesion may simulate venous malformation. • Natural history of growth during first year helps to distinguish hemangioma from vascular malformations. • Non-involuting congenital hemangioma distinguished by rim of pallor and telangiectatic surface network.
Bruising from birth trauma	• May simulate PWS • Resolves over first 1 to 2 weeks
Warts, molluscum	• May simulate microcystic lymphatic malformation. • Hemorrhage, intermittent swelling, and localization help to distinguish lymphatic malformation.
Herpes simplex virus (HSV) infection	• May simulate microcystic lymphatic malformation. • Pain, erosions, and rapid healing help to distinguish HSV.

How to Make the Diagnosis

- Clinical examination usually is sufficient for diagnosis.
- Venous malformation/macrocystic lymphatic malformation may be confirmed with computed tomography (CT), magnetic resonance imaging (MRI), or Doppler ultrasonography.
- Macrocystic lymphatic malformation may also be noted on prenatal ultrasonography.
- Arteriovenous malformation confirmed with ultrasonography; may require MRI/magnetic resonance angiography, CT, or arteriography.

Treatment

- Capillary malformation
  - Salmon patch
    - Education and reassurance.
    - Pulsed dye laser may be considered for persistent facial lesions.
  - PWS
    - Pulsed dye laser.
    - Cover-up cosmetics may need to be considered in older children.
- Venous malformation
  - Compression garments may minimize discomfort when lesions are painful.

- Percutaneous sclerosing therapy for select lesions.
- Surgical excision, occasionally.
- Low-dose aspirin (or other antiplatelet/anticoagulant medications) may be useful in patients with recurrent thromboses.
- Care should be multidisciplinary, when possible.

- Lymphatic malformation
  - Lymphedema
    - Massage, elevation
    - Compression garments
    - Intermittent pneumatic compression
    - Surgery reserved for severe deformity
  - Microcystic lymphatic malformation
    - Surgery, if necessary
  - Macrocystic lymphatic malformation
    - Percutaneous sclerosing therapy.
    - Surgery for select lesions.
    - Systemic sirolimus and sildenafil have been beneficial in some patients.

- Arteriovenous malformation
  - Surgical excision, embolization

Treating Associated Conditions

Associated Condition/ Syndrome	Comments/Treatment
Pyogenic granuloma located on a PWS	• Pulsed dye laser (if small) or excision with electrocautery
Sturge-Weber syndrome	• Caused by mutation in *GNAQ*. • PWS in first branch of the trigeminal nerve distribution may be associated with glaucoma and leptomeningeal angiomatosis (presents as seizures). • Multidisciplinary approach to evaluation/therapy; generally includes referral to neurology, ophthalmology, dermatology. • Pulsed dye laser for PWS.
Phakomatosis pigmentovascularis	• PWS in association with pigmented nevus (epidermal nevus, Mongolian spot, nevus spilus) or nevus anemicus. • Occasional systemic abnormalities. • Treatment of skin lesions usually unnecessary; pulsed dye laser may be used for PWS.

Associated Condition/ Syndrome	Comments/Treatment
Klippel-Trénaunay syndrome	• PWS with venous varicosity and tissue (bone and soft tissue) hyperplasia (Figure 59.8). • Most often involves an extremity. • Lymphedema is also often present. • Treatment may include compression, laser therapy, sclerosing therapy, vascular/orthopedic surgical procedures.
Proteus syndrome	• May be caused by mutation in AKT1 or PTEN in some patients • PWS in conjunction with tissue overgrowth • May include cerebriform hyperplasia of palms/soles, lipomas, epidermal nevi, lymphatic/venous malformations, disproportionate overgrowth, macrodactyly, macrocephaly • Multidisciplinary approach to evaluation/therapy; may include orthopedics, neurology, dermatology • CLOVES syndrome: similar to Proteus but consists of **c**ongenital **l**ipomatous **o**vergrowth, **v**ascular malformations, **e**pidermal nevi, **s**coliosis, other skeletal and spinal anomalies (including arteriovenous malformations, tethered spinal cord); lacks cerebriform palmoplantar hyperplasia characteristic of Proteus syndrome

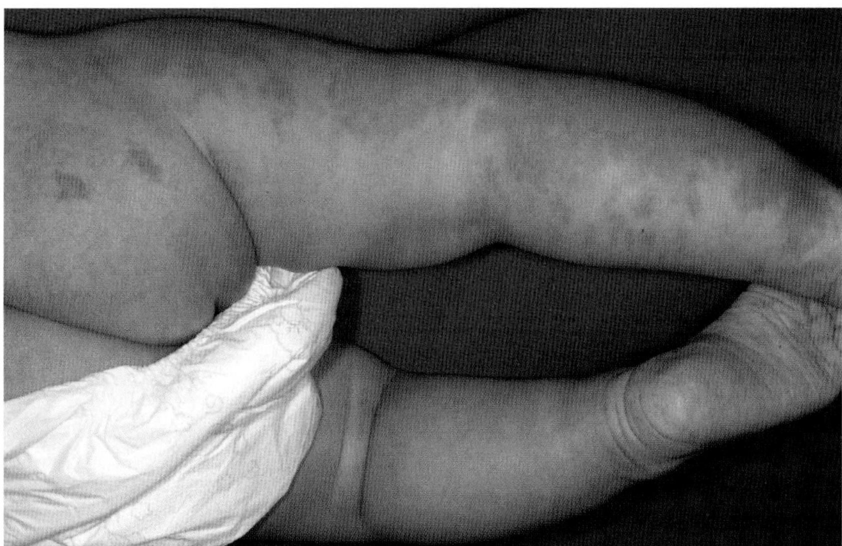

Figure 59.8. Klippel-Trénaunay syndrome. This infant with a port-wine stain and right lower extremity hypertrophy eventually developed venous varicosities.

Associated Condition/ Syndrome	Comments/Treatment
Macrocephaly-capillary malformation syndrome	• Macrocephaly and reticulate PWS. • Other features may include abnormal growth, craniofacial and skeletal anomalies, developmental delay, anatomic brain defects, connective tissue abnormalities. • Originally designated "macrocephaly-cutis marmorata telangiectatica congenita"; subsequently reclassified when stains noted to be more consistent with reticulate PWS. • Multidisciplinary approach to evaluation/therapy; may include neurology, neurosurgery, dermatology, orthopedics.
Capillary malformation-arteriovenous malformation syndrome	• Caused by mutation in *RASA1*. • Capillary malformations tend to be multiple and both congenital and acquired, with haphazard distribution; occasionally brown or gray in appearance. • Arteriovenous malformations may be cutaneous, subcutaneous, intramuscular, intraosseous, or cerebral; spinal arteriovenous malformations may also be present. • Multidisciplinary approach to evaluation/therapy; may include neurology, neurosurgery, dermatology, orthopedics. • Sturge-Weber syndrome is characterized by capillary malformations in conjunction with arteriovenous malformations and often extremity overgrowth; in some instances, these patients may have *RASA1* mutations.
Maffucci syndrome	• Venous malformations and enchondromas. • Risk of hemangioendothelioma, chondrosarcoma. • Treatment includes orthopedic monitoring/ care and malignancy surveillance.
Blue rubber bleb nevus syndrome	• Multiple venous malformations of skin and gastrointestinal tract. • Hemorrhage, iron deficiency anemia possible. • Occasional central nervous system involvement. • Treatment supportive; may include sclerosing therapy or band ligation of gastrointestinal tract lesions, bowel resection; systemic sirolimus has recently been reported.

Prognosis

- Variable
- Prognosis for salmon patch, nonsyndromic PWS, microcystic lymphatic malformation excellent
- Depends on multiple features, including size of lesion(s), location, complications, and any syndrome associations

When to Worry or Refer

- Referral should be considered for
  - Any facial PWS
  - PWS in association with other syndromic findings
  - Venous malformations that are larger, multiple, or associated with pain, bleeding, function impairment, or overgrowth
  - Lymphedema or macrocystic lymphatic malformation
  - Suspected arteriovenous malformation

Resources for Families

- AboutFace: Provides information, emotional support, and educational programs for individuals who have facial disfigurement.
  www.aboutfaceusa.org
- KT Foundation: Provides information for patients and families who have Klippel-Trénaunay syndrome.
  www.kt-foundation.org
- National Odd Shoe Exchange: A source of footwear for those requiring single shoes or pairs of differing sizes.
  www.oddshoe.org
- National Organization of Vascular Anomalies: Patient information, resources, and support.
  www.novanews.org
- Proteus Syndrome Foundation: Provides support and education for families living with and professionals caring for individuals who have Proteus syndrome.
  www.proteus-syndrome.org
- Sturge-Weber Foundation: Provides information and support for patients who have port-wine stains, Sturge-Weber syndrome, or Klippel-Trénaunay syndrome and their families.
  www.sturge-weber.org/medical-matters/sturge-weber-syndrome.html
- Vascular Birthmarks Foundation: Provides referrals, financial assistance, newsletter, biannual conference, resource list for clinics and doctors, advocacy, support, and counseling.
  www.birthmark.org

Disorders of Pigmentation

Hypopigmentation

Albinism

Introduction/Etiology/Epidemiology

- Albinism results from a generalized lack of production and distribution of melanin; several phenotypic variants exist.
  - It may be separated into forms that involve the skin, hair, and eyes (oculocutaneous albinism [OCA]) or only the eye (ocular albinism).
  - Nearly all forms of OCA are inherited in an autosomal-recessive manner.
- The most important biochemical distinction between the more common subtypes is the presence or absence of tyrosinase activity, although this has little clinical relevance. The genetic basis of most variants is now known and can be found in Online Mendelian Inheritance in Man (**www.ncbi.nlm.nih.gov/omim**).

Signs and Symptoms

There are 4 types of OCA; the 2 most common are discussed here.

- Oculocutaneous albinism type 1: separated into 2 forms depending on whether tyrosinase activity is absent (type A) or reduced (type B). In type 1A (ie, tyrosinase-negative OCA), patients exhibit
  - White hair and white skin (Figure 60.1)
  - Poor visual acuity, photophobia, nystagmus, and strabismus
  - Inability to tan or freckle and predisposition to skin cancer
  - Pale (often gray or blue) irides (see Figure 60.1)
  - Foveal hypoplasia
- Oculocutaneous albinism type 2 (ie, tyrosinase-positive OCA): most common form of OCA, particularly among individuals of African descent. In OCA2, patients exhibit
  - Yellow to red or light brown hair
  - White skin with minimal tanning ability
  - A tendency to develop freckles and nevi (often red) over time
  - Ocular findings that are less severe than in OCA type 1

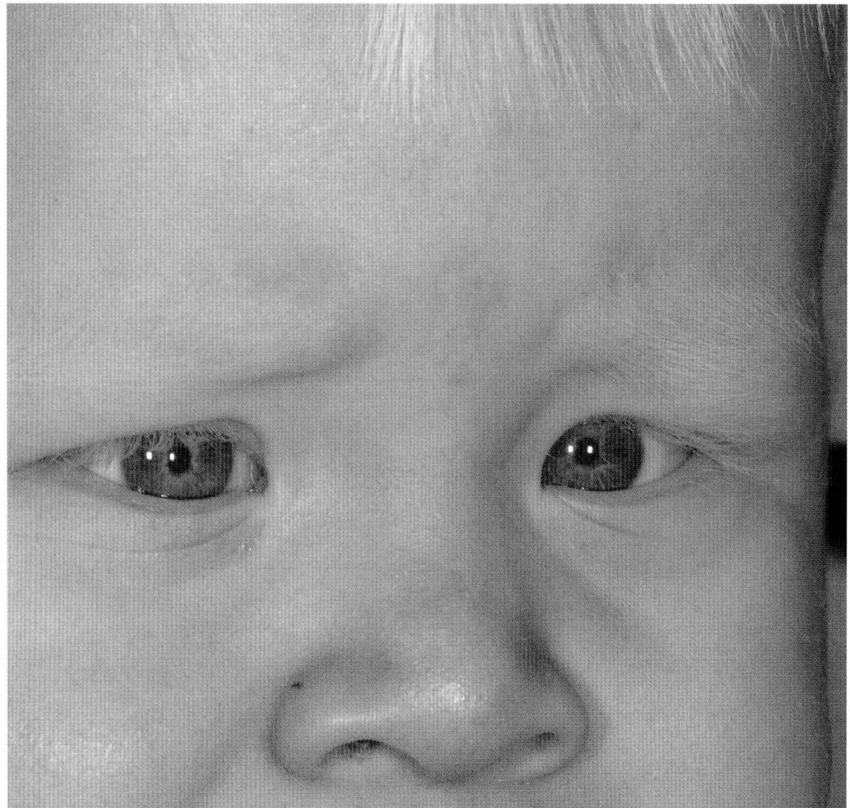

Figure 60.1. Oculocutaneous albinism. Absence of pigment in the skin, hair, and irides.

- Rare forms of albinism associated with systemic disease are
  - Hermansky-Pudlak syndrome: autosomal-recessive disorder characterized by OCA and bleeding diathesis
  - Chédiak-Higashi syndrome: autosomal-recessive disorder in which patients exhibit partial albinism, silvery hair, immune abnormalities, and eventual neurologic deterioration

Look-alikes

Disorder	Differentiating Features
Vitiligo	• Acquired (not congenital) localized pigment loss. • May be widespread but rarely affects total skin surface. • Ocular abnormalities are absent.
Piebaldism	• Congenital localized absence of pigment, often affecting the face or scalp • Most of the skin surface normal • May involve small adjacent area of depigmented hair (poliosis or "white forelock")
Waardenburg syndrome	• Pigmentary dilution of skin in conjunction with other characteristic features. • Sensorineural deafness common. • White forelock may be present. • Other abnormalities may include synophrys, heterochromia irides, pseudo-hypertelorism.

How to Make the Diagnosis

- Patients have very pale skin from birth with no ability to tan in early childhood.
- Distinguishing features include white or yellow hair, white skin, pale irides, photophobia, nystagmus, and poor visual acuity.
- Mutational analysis is available for diagnostic confirmation; mutations in the *TYR* gene cause type 1 OCA, while mutations in the *OCA2* gene result in type 2 OCA.

Treatment

- Strict photoprotection of skin and eyes is imperative from birth.
  - Use broad-spectrum sunscreens with a sun protection factor of 30 or higher.
  - Use product that provides UV-A and UV-B protection.
- Annual skin examination is recommended to observe for photodamage and premalignant or malignant lesions.
- Ophthalmologic consultation is indicated.

Treating Associated Conditions

- Bleeding tendency, neurologic symptoms, frequent infections, or other clinical features should prompt a search for associated syndromes.

Prognosis

- As a rule, most children do well. They require lifelong sun protection and surveillance for skin cancer.

When to Worry or Refer

- Changes in existing nevi or the sudden onset of a new lesion (eg, a red nodule) is worrisome and should be cause for concern. In patients who have albinism, melanoma is often amelanotic (ie, may appear red, pink, or white).
- Sudden changes in vision require immediate ophthalmologic consultation.

Resources for Families

- National Organization for Albinism and Hypopigmentation: Provides information and support for individuals who have albinism or hypopigmentation.
  www.albinism.org
- Vision for Tomorrow Foundation: Provides support and information on albinism and aniridia.
  www.visionfortomorrow.org
- Hermansky-Pudlak Syndrome Network Inc: Patient information.
  www.hpsnetwork.org

CHAPTER 61

Pigmentary Mosaicism, Hypopigmented

Introduction/Etiology/Epidemiology

- Pigmentary mosaicism is the term used to describe a group of disorders in which the skin has a patterned hypopigmentation or hyperpigmentation. In the hypopigmented form discussed in this chapter, affected skin is lighter than the background skin color but not completely depigmented (as would be the case in vitiligo).
- Pigmentary mosaicism is believed to be the result of genetic mutations that create a population of cells with more or less pigment potential than the surrounding normal skin. Mosaicism refers to the coexistence of 2 genetically distinct populations of cells within the same individual.
- Pigmentary mosaicism may be localized or generalized.
- Terminology used to describe hypopigmented pigmentary mosaicism is inconsistent. Terms such as nevus depigmentosus, segmental pigmentation disorder, nevoid hypomelanosis, and patterned pigmentation exist in the literature.
- In most cases, localized hypopigmented pigmentary mosaicism is a benign and isolated finding. When more generalized, it can be associated with skeletal, ocular, or neurologic (eg, seizures, developmental delay, macrocephaly) abnormalities, a condition also known as hypomelanosis of Ito.

Signs and Symptoms

- Hypopigmentation is present at birth but may be difficult to recognize in fair-skinned infants until background skin color develops and contrast between the 2 areas is appreciated.
- Common patterns of mosaic hypopigmentation include a large region or segment of the body (Figure 61.1) and whorled or linear bands (thin or broad) that follow the lines of Blaschko (Figure 61.2).
- Affected areas are typically sharply demarcated and usually respect the midline.

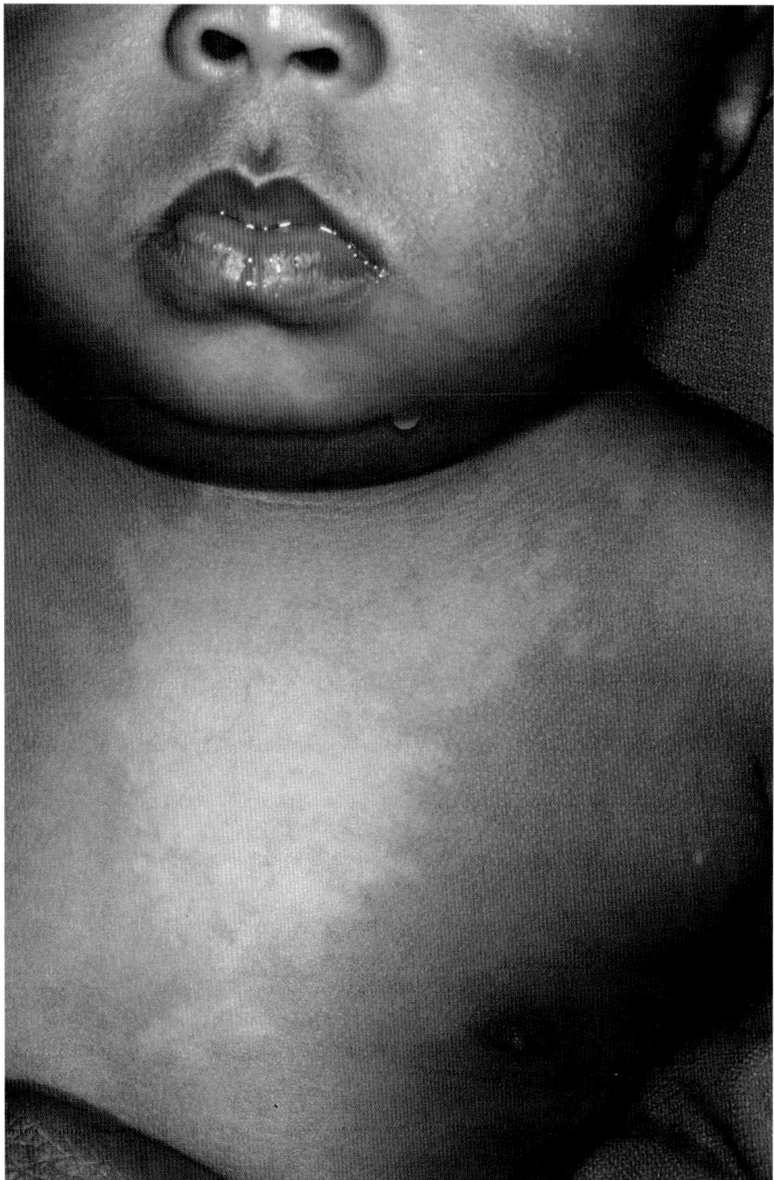

Figure 61.1. Pigmentary mosaicism, hypopigmented type. A large shaggy-bordered, hypopigmented patch on the chest that respects the midline. This lesion often is called a nevus depigmentosus, which is a misnomer, as the lesion is not depigmented.

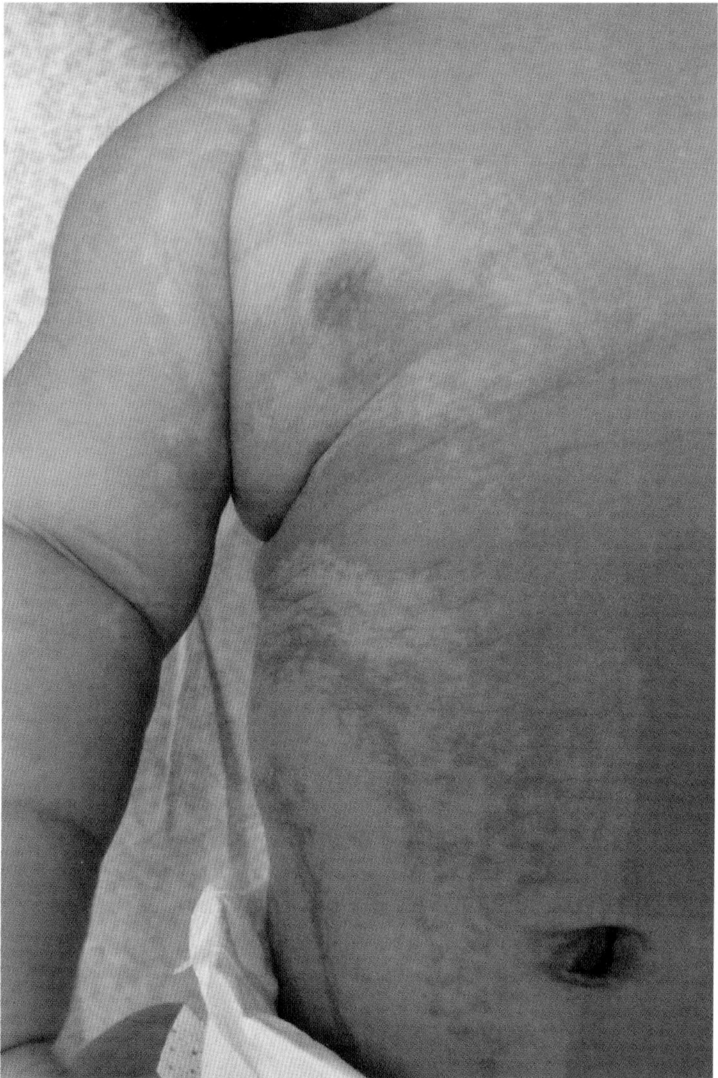

Figure 61.2. Pigmentary mosaicism, hypopigmented type. Whorled and curvilinear streaks of hypopigmentation that represent the lines of Blaschko and respect the midline.

Look-alikes

Disorder	Differentiating Features
Lichen striatus (hypopigmented phase)	• Usually begins in childhood; not present at birth. • Begins as pink to red papules (sometimes scaly). Typically lesions appear proximally on an extremity and extend distally. • Over time, papules resolve and linear hypopigmentation appears. • Eventual spontaneous resolution (unlike pigmentary mosaicism, which persists indefinitely).
Goltz syndrome (focal dermal hypoplasia)	• X-linked dominant inheritance. • Telangiectatic and atrophic streaks (along the lines of Blaschko) and soft papules due to fat herniation. • Associations may include dental, ophthalmologic, and skeletal anomalies.
Incontinentia pigmenti (fourth stage)	• X-linked dominant inheritance. • Vesicles are usually the initial presentation in newborn (first stage), distributed along the lines of Blaschko. • Warty lesions (second stage) give rise to hyperpigmentation (third stage) in a similar distribution pattern, followed by eventual hypopigmentation (fourth stage). • Hypopigmentation may be accompanied by atrophy and loss of hair. • Associations may include dental, ophthalmologic, neurologic, and skeletal anomalies.
Piebaldism	• Congenital depigmentation affecting the midline head or torso with focal and symmetric involvement of the extremities. • Associated poliosis ("white forelock") may be present. • May be an isolated cutaneous finding or associated with Waardenburg syndrome.
Vitiligo (segmental form)	• Usually begins in childhood or adolescence, not infancy. • Affected area is depigmented, not hypopigmented. • Borders tend to be more sharply demarcated, less shaggy.

How to Make the Diagnosis

- The diagnosis of hypopigmented pigmentary mosaicism is usually made based on the history and physical examination findings.
- Consider a formal ophthalmology examination to evaluate for ocular anomalies in children with the generalized type.
- If other malformations or neurodevelopmental abnormalities are absent, further workup is not indicated. If they are present, consultation with the appropriate specialist(s) is warranted.
- Rarely, karyotype analysis is performed (on blood or skin biopsy tissue) searching for chromosomal mosaicism.

Treatment

- There are no specific treatments for hypopigmented pigmentary mosaicism.

Prognosis

- In most cases, hypopigmented pigmentary mosaicism is a benign, isolated skin finding not associated with other medical concerns.
- In the rare patient who has generalized involvement, prognosis depends on the nature of any other organ abnormalities.

When to Worry or Refer

- Referral to dermatology is warranted when the diagnosis is uncertain.
- Referral to other specialists (eg, ophthalmology, neurology, genetics, orthopedics) is warranted when applicable.

Resources for Families

- National Organization for Rare Disorders: Hypomelanosis of Ito. **https://rarediseases.org/rare-diseases/hypomelanosis-of-ito**

CHAPTER 62

Pityriasis Alba

Introduction/Etiology/Epidemiology

- Pityriasis alba is thought to represent postinflammatory hypopigmentation.
- It is most often observed in children who have atopic dermatitis.

Signs and Symptoms

- Pityriasis alba appears as poorly defined macular areas of hypopigmentation (Figure 62.1), perhaps with very fine scale.
- Lesions are transient and may be located on face, trunk, or extremities.
- Lesions may become more apparent after sun exposure as normal skin tans but affected areas do not.

Look-alikes

Disorder	Differentiating Features
Vitiligo	• Lesions are depigmented (not hypopigmented) and well defined. • Hairs within affected areas depigmented. • Accentuation with Wood light examination.
Tinea versicolor	• Lesions well defined and typically concentrated on the trunk; individual lesions may coalesce into large patches. • Facial involvement less common. • Generally not seen in prepubertal patients. • Performance of a potassium hydroxide preparation on scale from lesions will reveal short hyphae and spores (ie, "spaghetti and meatballs").

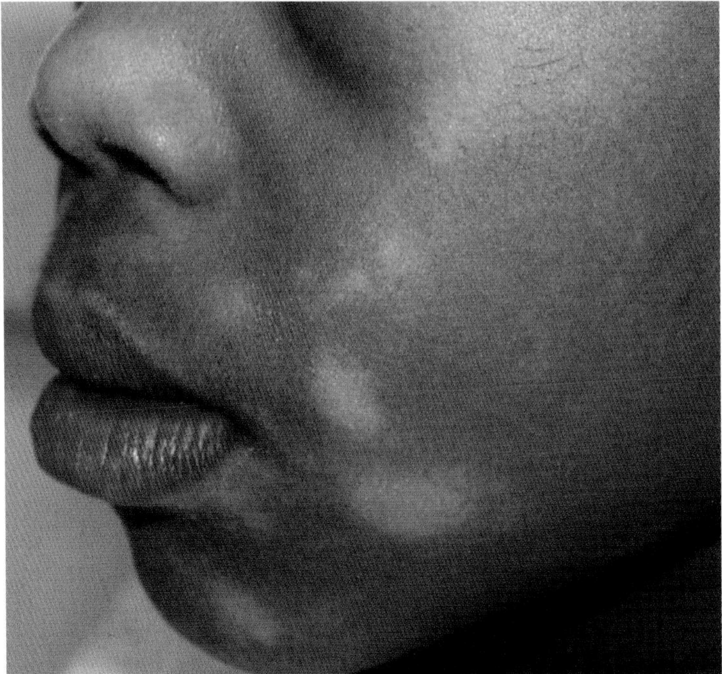

Figure 62.1. Pityriasis alba. Hypopigmented macules with indistinct borders.

How to Make the Diagnosis

- The diagnosis is made clinically based on the observation of poorly defined macules or patches of hypopigmentation that have fine scale.
- Atopic history (ie, presence of atopic dermatitis, asthma, or allergic rhinoconjunctivitis) common.

Treatment

- Application of an emollient is adequate for treatment in most cases.
- Some advise application of a topical corticosteroid or calcineurin inhibitor, particularly if the lesions are erythematous or pruritic. This will treat underlying inflammation and accelerate repigmentation.
- Counsel the patient and family that months will be required for return of normal pigmentation.

Treating Associated Conditions

- Treat associated atopic dermatitis if present.

Prognosis

- Lesions of pityriasis alba resolve with treatment, but new lesions may appear.
- The condition tends to resolve by mid-adolescence.

When to Worry or Refer

- Diagnostic uncertainty exists or lesions do not respond to therapy.

Resources for Families

- MedlinePlus: Information for patients and families (in English and Spanish) sponsored by the National Library of Medicine and National Institutes of Health.
  https://www.nlm.nih.gov/medlineplus/ency/article/001463.htm

CHAPTER 63

Postinflammatory Hypopigmentation

Introduction/Etiology/Epidemiology

- Hypopigmented macules and patches that result from inflammatory melanocyte damage
- Often a history of preceding inflammation, such as dermatitis, arthropod bite, or abrasion

Signs and Symptoms

- Hypopigmentation with indistinct margins and no surface change (Figure 63.1)
- No associated symptoms
- May have associated scar

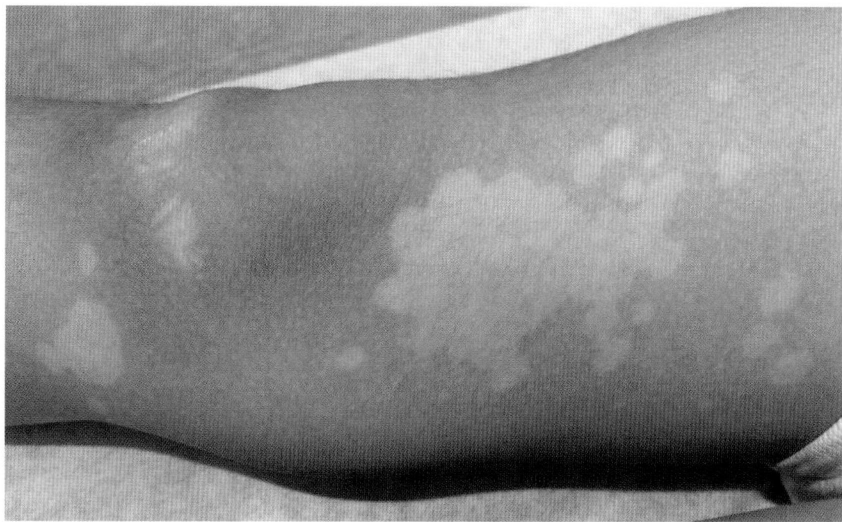

Figure 63.1. Postinflammatory hypopigmentation. Hypopigmented macules located at sites of prior bullous impetigo lesions.

Look-alikes

Disorder	Differentiating Features
Pityriasis alba	• Likely represents a form of postinflammatory hypopigmentation • Macules with indistinct borders and, occasionally, scale • Usually seen in the setting of atopic dermatitis • Most often occurs on the face
Vitiligo	• Well-defined depigmented (versus hypopigmented) macules or patches • Accentuation with Wood light examination
Tinea versicolor	• Well-defined hypopigmented macules and patches located on the trunk, proximal arms, and sides of neck. • Potassium hydroxide preparation of scale from lesions reveals short hyphae and spores (ie, "spaghetti and meatballs").
Piebaldism	• Congenital absence of pigment usually limited to one area • Well-defined depigmented (versus hypopigmented) macules or patches • May involve small adjacent area of depigmented hair (poliosis or white forelock)

How to Make the Diagnosis

- History of preceding inflammation is most useful clue.
- Lesions are hypopigmented (not depigmented).

Treatment

- No treatment necessary or available.
- Counsel the patient and family that months may be required for pigmentation to return to normal.
- Sun protection is vital (tanning of surrounding skin will make lesions more visible).

Treating Associated Conditions

- Manage the inflammatory condition (eg, atopic dermatitis) that precipitated the pigmentary change.

Prognosis

- If no associated scarring, repigmentation is typical, although months to years may be required for this to occur.

When to Worry or Refer

- Refer if uncertainty exists regarding the diagnosis.

Resources for Families

- National Organization for Albinism and Hypopigmentation: Provides information and support for individuals who have albinism or hypopigmentation.
  www.albinism.org

CHAPTER

64

Vitiligo

Introduction/Etiology/Epidemiology

- Vitiligo represents an acquired complete depigmentation of skin due to melanocyte destruction that is thought to be autoimmune in nature.
- Two main forms have been described: generalized and segmental (ie, involves one area of the body and typically does not cross the midline).
- Vitiligo develops in childhood or adolescence in about half of patients.

Signs and Symptoms

- Vitiligo presents as well-defined macules or patches of complete depigmentation (ie, the skin is completely white) with normal texture (Figure 64.1).
  - It may begin with speckled areas of hypopigmentation that continue to lose pigment and coalesce over time.
  - Lesions may be faintly erythematous early in the course.
  - Areas prone to trauma or pressure (eg, knees, elbows, small joints such as metacarpophalangeal joints, hips) are most frequently involved; this distribution may represent the Koebner phenomenon (appearance of lesions at sites of injury).
  - Other common locations include eyelids, perioral regions, axillae, and the groin.
- Generalized vitiligo often starts symmetrically on the arms, legs, or periorbital areas and may progress to involve large areas.
- Localized segmental vitiligo often follows a dermatomal distribution.
- Trichrome vitiligo is a variant seen in children; normal, hypopigmented, and depigmented patches are present simultaneously in an involved area.

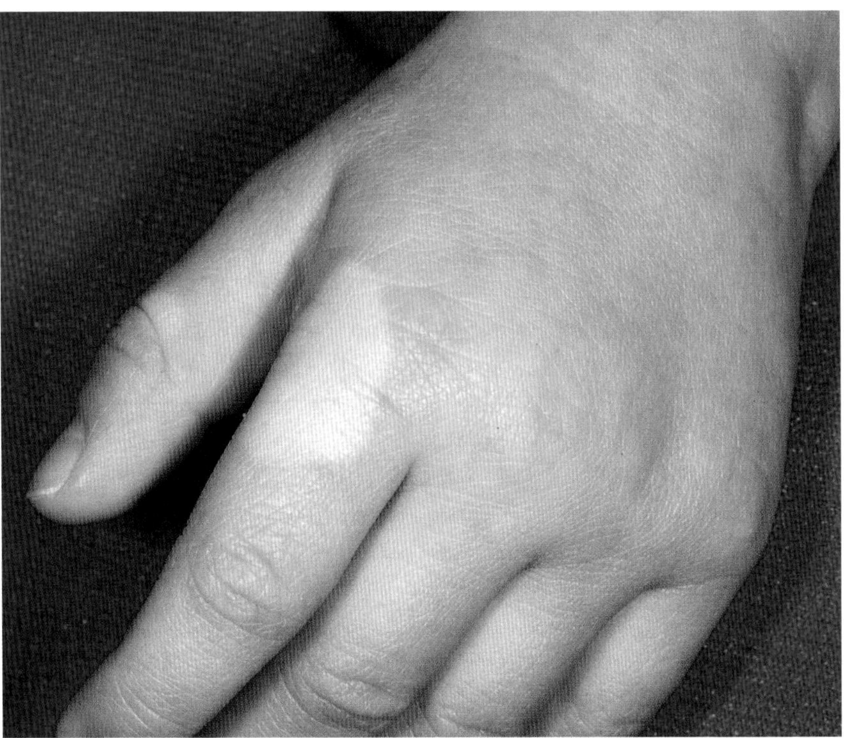

Figure 64.1. Vitiligo appears as well-defined areas of complete loss of pigmentation (ie, depigmentation).

Look-alikes

Disorder	Differentiating Features
Pityriasis alba	• Poorly defined areas of macular hypopigmentation (not depigmentation), often with associated scale • Atopic history common
Tinea versicolor	• Well-defined hypopigmented (not depigmented) macules and patches located on the trunk, upper arms, or neck. • Lesions often have associated fine scale and may be pruritic.
Piebaldism	• Congenital absence of pigmentation localized to one area • May involve small adjacent area of depigmented hair (poliosis or white forelock)
Waardenburg syndrome	• Pigmentary dilution of skin in conjunction with other characteristic features. • Sensorineural deafness common. • White forelock may be present. • Other abnormalities may include synophrys, heterochromia irides, pseudo-hypertelorism.

How to Make the Diagnosis

- The diagnosis of vitiligo is made clinically based on typical features (well-defined macules or patches of depigmentation).
- The distinction between hypopigmentation and depigmentation may be enhanced by examining the patient using a Wood light in a darkened room. Depigmented areas are well defined and strikingly prominent, while hypopigmented areas are less well defined.

Treatment

- Spontaneous repigmentation occurs in a few patients.
- Treatment is unsatisfactory, with numerous anecdotal topical and systemic agents having limited value.
- Patients who have vitiligo and desire therapy are best managed by or in consultation with a dermatologist. Some treatment options might include
  - Topical corticosteroids
  - Topical calcineurin inhibitors (eg, tacrolimus, pimecrolimus): most useful for facial lesions
  - Photochemotherapy employing psoralens plus UV-A: often used in children older than 12 years (rarely used in younger children)
  - Narrowband UV-B phototherapy
  - Excimer laser therapy
- For patients who do not desire specific medical therapy, options include application of a camouflage cream matched to the child's skin color and application of sunscreen (to protect depigmented skin and reduce tanning of normal skin).

Treating Associated Conditions

- Generalized (non-segmental) vitiligo is associated with an increased risk of autoimmune disease in the affected individual and first-degree relatives. While most children who have vitiligo have no associated conditions, it is important to gather a family history and be observant for the development of symptoms suggestive of inflammatory eye disease or autoimmune disease (eg, type 1 diabetes mellitus, pernicious anemia, hypothyroidism, hypoparathyroidism, celiac disease, Addison disease, autoimmune hepatitis).
- Most experts recommend thyroid function screening and antithyroid antibody levels for patients with vitiligo, with other testing performed only if indicated based on clinical signs or symptoms.

Prognosis

- Variable and unpredictable.
- Repigmentation, whether spontaneous or therapeutic, appears as perifollicular macules that coalesce to gradually fill in the area of depigmentation.

When to Worry or Refer

- Vitiligo is widespread or rapidly progressive, and phototherapy is being considered.
- Vitiligo develops along with inflammatory eye disease or another autoimmune disorder (in which case consultation with a pediatric endocrinologist is warranted). Consultation also may be of value if the patient has a first-degree relative with 2 autoimmune disorders. Rarely, vitiligo may be associated with autoimmune polyglandular syndromes, most notably type 1.

Resources for Families

- American Vitiligo Research Foundation: Provides education and support for persons who have vitiligo.
  www.avrf.org
- National Vitiligo Foundation Inc: Provides information and links to physicians for patients who have vitiligo.
  www.nvfi.org
- Society for Pediatric Dermatology: Patient handout on vitiligo.
  http://pedsderm.net/for-patients-families/patient-handouts
- Vitiligo Support International: Provides education and support for persons who have vitiligo.
  www.vitiligosupport.org

Disorders of Pigmentation

Hyperpigmentation

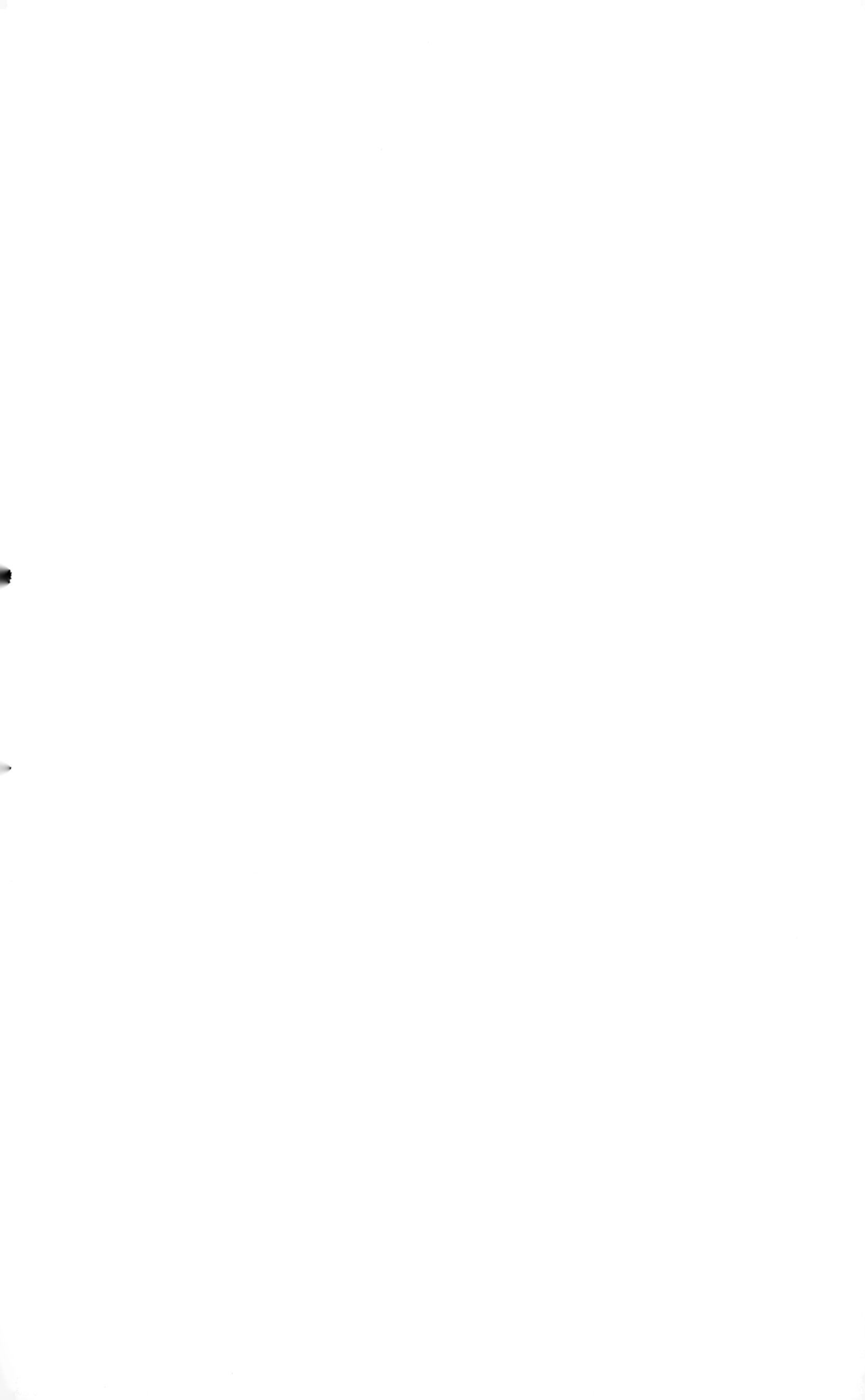

Acanthosis Nigricans

Introduction/Etiology/Epidemiology

- Represents epidermal proliferation process with minimal increase in melanin
- Believed to be due to insulin resistance and its effect on the skin
- May be seen in the following settings:
  - Obesity.
  - Insulin resistance syndromes.
  - Endocrinologic disorders (eg, diabetes mellitus, Addison disease, Cushing disease, hypothyroidism, hyperandrogenism, hypogonadism, polycystic ovary syndrome).
  - Medications (oral contraceptives, nicotinic acid).
- Malignancy: In adults, sudden onset of acanthosis nigricans may herald a malignant tumor, but no such association recognized in childhood.

Signs and Symptoms

- Velvety thickening of the skin creates a brown to gray-black color that may be mistaken by patients as dirt (Figure 65.1).
- Most commonly observed on the nape or sides of the neck, axillae, and groin (crural creases); some patients may exhibit lesions over the knuckles and around the mouth.

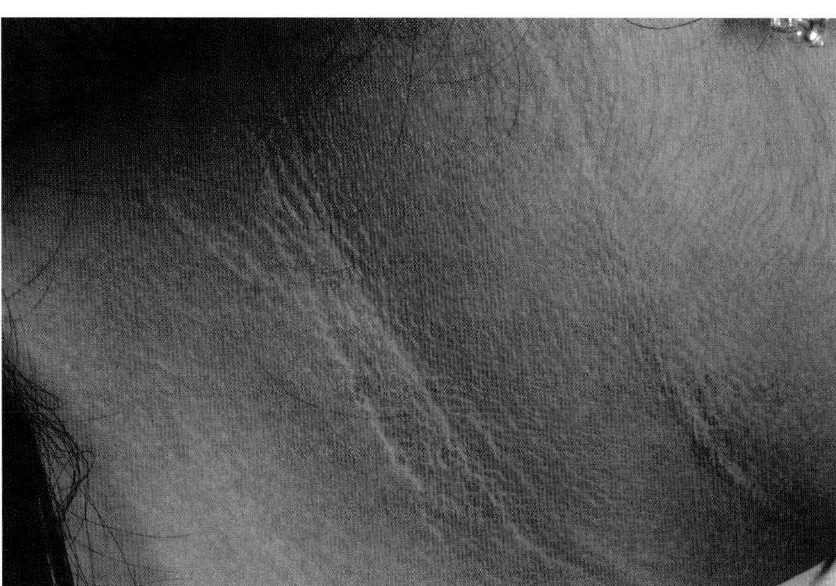

Figure 65.1. Velvety, hyperpigmented thickening of the skin characterizes acanthosis nigricans.

Look-alikes

Disorder	Differentiating Features
Postinflammatory hyperpigmentation	• Lacks the velvety texture of acanthosis nigricans
Lichenification (ie, thickening of the skin) associated with chronic atopic or contact dermatitis	• Lacks the velvety texture of acanthosis nigricans • Other features of atopic dermatitis often present • Pruritus common (acanthosis nigricans not pruritic)

How to Make the Diagnosis

- The diagnosis is made clinically based on the clinical appearance (ie, velvety thickening of skin) in typical locations.

Treatment

- Evaluate patient for underlying cause based on history and physical examination.
  - Consider obtaining a fasting glucose or glycated hemoglobin (A_{1c}) and lipid panel in patients who are obese, particularly those who have a family history of type 2 diabetes mellitus (some also recommend obtaining an insulin level).
  - Consider measuring an insulin level or obtaining other endocrinologic testing if the patient is not obese.
- Treatment of acanthosis nigricans is difficult and often unsatisfactory.
  - Consider application of keratolytic preparation (eg, one containing lactic or salicylic acid).
  - Extensive acanthosis nigricans may benefit from carbon dioxide laser resurfacing.
  - If otherwise indicated, metformin may improve acanthosis due to reduced insulin resistance.
  - Changes often (but not always) improve with weight loss (and resultant improved insulin sensitivity).

Treating Associated Conditions

- If an underlying disorder is identified in a patient who has acanthosis nigricans, it should be managed appropriately.
- Acanthosis nigricans is an important marker for insulin resistance, hyperlipidemia, and metabolic syndrome.

Prognosis

- Familial acanthosis nigricans has an excellent prognosis.
- If associated with other disorders, the prognosis depends on the other conditions.

When to Worry or Refer

- Consider referral or consultation for management of associated conditions.

Resources for Families

- MedlinePlus: Information for patients and families (in English and Spanish) sponsored by the National Library of Medicine and National Institutes of Health.
https://www.nlm.nih.gov/medlineplus/ency/article/000852.htm
- WebMD: Information for families is contained in the Health A-Z topics.
www.webmd.com/skin-problems-and-treatments/acanthosis-nigricans-overview

CHAPTER

66

Acquired Melanocytic Nevi

Introduction/Etiology/Epidemiology

- Acquired melanocytic nevi are common.
- Begin to appear after 2 to 3 years of age.
- Increase in number and reach a peak during the third decade.
- Often disappear with advancing age.

Signs and Symptoms

- Pigmented macules, papules, and plaques with variable surface changes
- Sometimes classified based on appearance
  - Junctional nevus: uniformly hyperpigmented (often brown) macule (Figure 66.1)
  - Compound nevus: uniformly hyperpigmented (often brown) slightly elevated papule (Figure 66.2)
  - Intradermal nevus: often light brown to flesh-colored and elevated (Figure 66.3)
- Variants of acquired nevi
  - Halo nevi
    - Acquired nevi that develop a surrounding ring of hypopigmentation or depigmentation (Figure 66.4).
    - Likely represents an immunologic response to melanocytes; often coexists with vitiligo (and may precede or follow this diagnosis).
    - Nearly always benign in children; refer for evaluation if the ring of hypopigmentation is incomplete or the nevus is abnormal using ABCDE criteria (see When to Worry or Refer).
    - Nevus and hypopigmentation ultimately resolve.

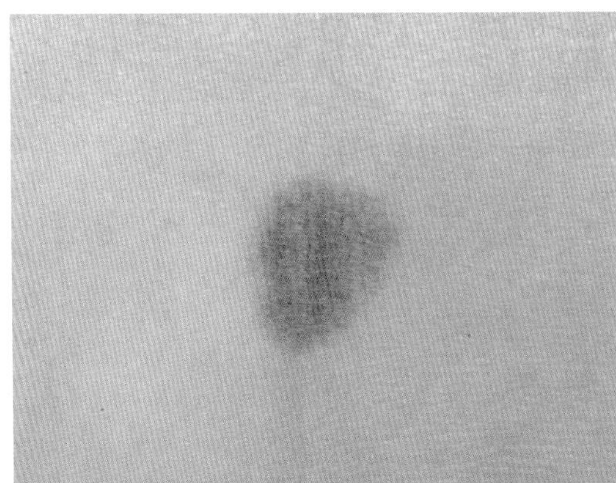

Figure 66.1. Junctional nevus.

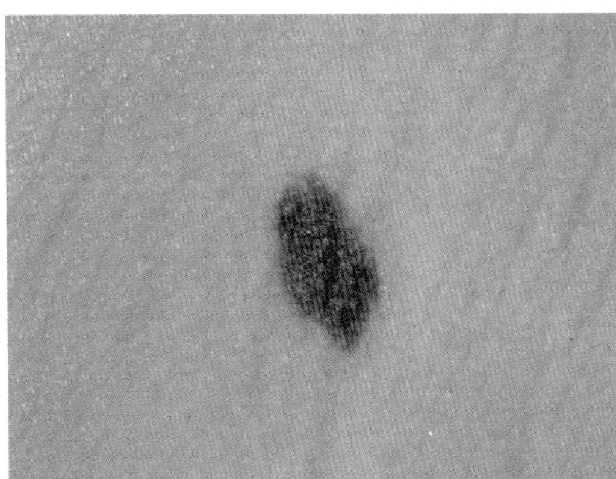

Figure 66.2. Compound nevus.

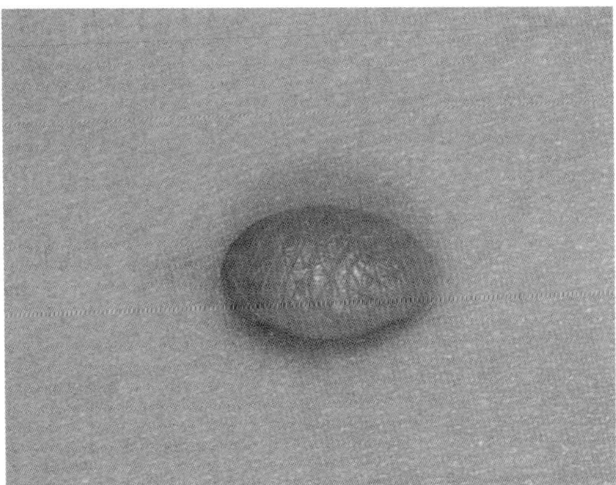

Figure 66.3. Intradermal nevus.

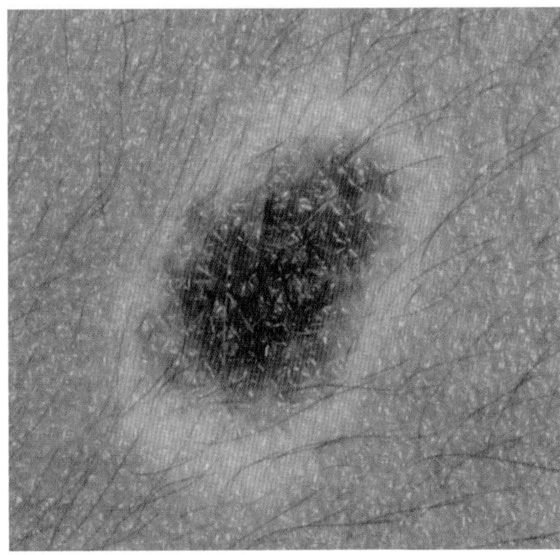

Figure 66.4. A halo nevus is an acquired nevus with a ring of surrounding hypopigmentation or depigmentation.

- Atypical nevi
  - Often larger (5–12 mm) than common acquired nevi; have irregular and ill-defined borders (Figure 66.5).
  - Color often is variegated with shades of brown, tan, or pink (Figure 66.6).
  - Individuals who have large numbers of atypical nevi or those who have a family history of melanoma in first-degree relatives have an increased risk of developing melanoma.
- "Eclipse" nevi
  - Nevus with central elevation simulating the appearance of a sunny-side up fried egg (see Figure 66.6).
  - Periphery often darker compared with the lighter central portions.
  - This phenotype is common on the scalps of older children and teenagers, and these nevi tend to behave in benign fashion.

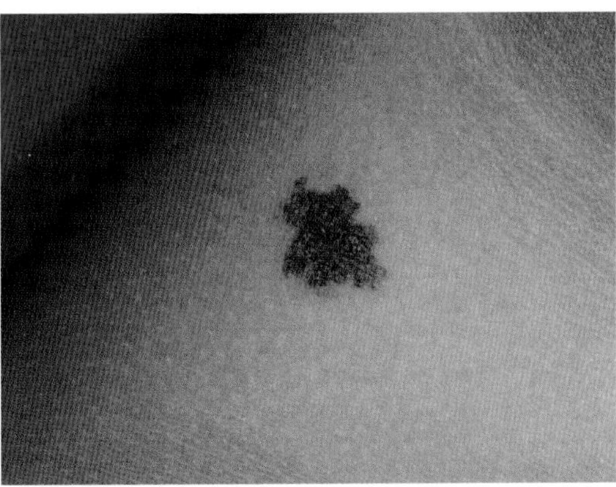

Figure 66.5. Atypical nevi are often larger (often 5–12 mm in diameter) and have irregular borders.

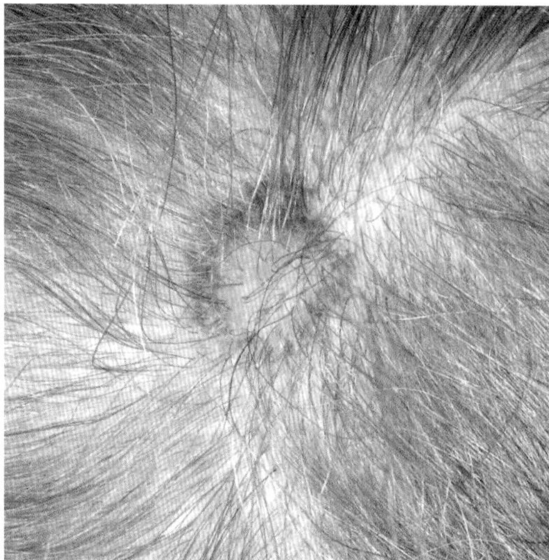

Figure 66.6. This benign "eclipse" nevus reveals pink and brown color; the lighter center is elevated, causing the lesion to have the appearance of a sunny-side up fried egg.

Look-alikes

Disorder	Differentiating Features
Ephelides	• Small, hyperpigmented macules located in sun-exposed areas such as the face, upper chest, and back • Become darker following sun exposure • Unlike melanocytic nevi, have no change in surface texture
Lentigines	• Small, hyperpigmented macules not limited to sun-exposed areas • Unlike melanocytic nevi, have no change in surface texture
Café au lait macules	• Hyperpigmented macules that are not elevated and have no change in surface texture; most often tan in color • Typically larger than acquired melanocytic nevi

How to Make the Diagnosis

- The diagnosis is made clinically based on the typical appearance of acquired nevi.

Treatment

- Benign-appearing nevi that are asymptomatic do not require removal.
- Rapidly changing or significantly atypical nevi must be assessed for possible malignant transformation.

Treating Associated Conditions

- Familial atypical mole/melanoma syndrome should be considered in a patient who has atypical (ie, dysplastic) moles and several family members with atypical (ie, dysplastic) nevi and at least one relative with melanoma. These patients require close surveillance to assess for the development of melanoma.

Prognosis

- Ordinary acquired nevi are inconsequential; however, all nevi should be monitored for ABCDE changes (see When to Worry or Refer).
- Atypical nevi may imply an increased risk for the development of melanoma.

When to Worry or Refer

- Melanoma is the malignant neoplasm of melanocytes that may arise de novo or from preexisting nevus. Consider the possibility of melanoma when a nevus exhibits any of the following ABCDE criteria:
  - **A**symmetry
  - **B**order irregularity
  - **C**olor variation (especially red, blue, black)
  - **D**iameter larger than about 6 mm
  - **E**volving lesion that is changing quickly
- Refer patients who have atypical nevi and a family history of atypical nevi or melanoma to a dermatologist.
- Refer patients who have atypical-appearing halo nevi (eg, those with an incomplete ring of hypopigmentation or an abnormal appearance using ABCDE criteria) to a dermatologist.

Resources for Families

- American Academy of Dermatology: Diseases and treatments (search options include "moles" and "melanoma")
  https://www.aad.org/public/diseases
- Society for Pediatric Dermatology: Patient handout on moles and melanoma.
  http://pedsderm.net/for-patients-families/patient-handouts

Café au Lait Macules

Introduction/Etiology/Epidemiology

- Isolated café au lait macules (also known as café au lait spots) may be seen in up to 2% of all infants and 10% of African American infants.
- The frequency of café au lait macules in older children is estimated at 13% for white and 27% for African American children.
- Small, solitary lesions are inconsequential, while multiple or large lesions may signal a syndromic association.

Signs and Symptoms

- Tan macules with well-defined borders (Figures 67.1 and 67.2)

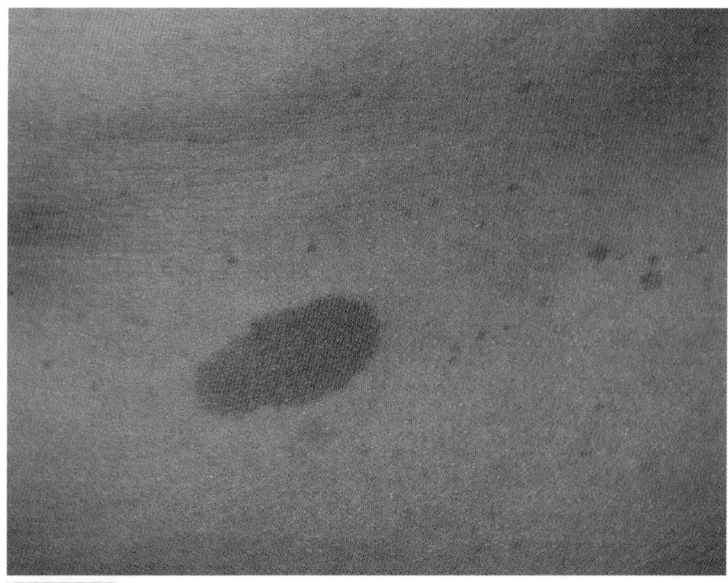

Figure 67.1. Multiple café au lait macules in a patient who has neurofibromatosis type 1.

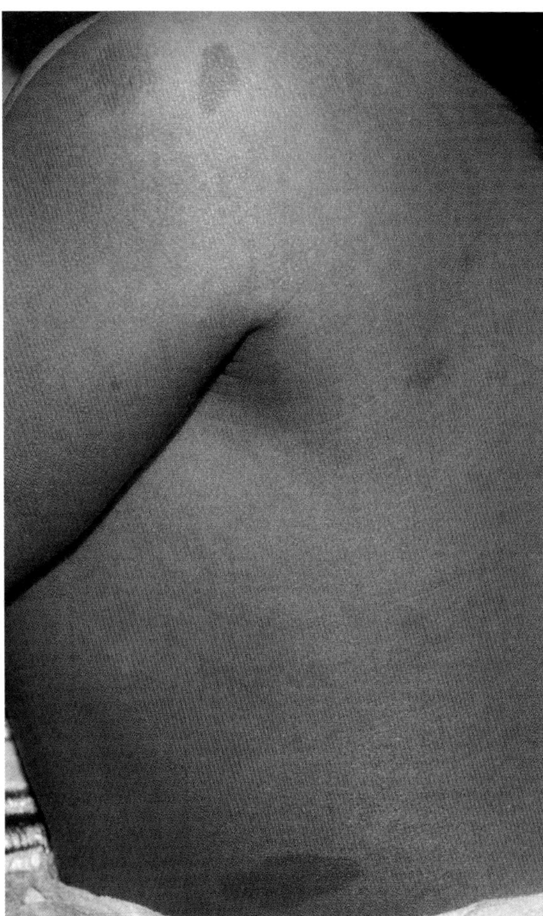

Figure 67.2. Multiple café au lait macules in an infant.

Look-alikes

Disorder	Differentiating Features
Ephelides (freckles)	• Small (typically smaller than café au lait macules), hyperpigmented macules in sun-exposed areas
Lentigines	• Small (typically smaller than café au lait macules), hyperpigmented macules that are not related to sun exposure
Congenital melanocytic nevus	• Typically more deeply pigmented than café au lait macules • Often slightly elevated and have a surface textural change • Hypertrichosis common
Postinflammatory hyperpigmentation	• History of preceding inflammatory process • Borders of lesions not well defined

How to Make the Diagnosis

- Diagnosis is made clinically based on the appearance of the macules.

Treatment

- No treatment is needed for café au lait macules.
- Multiple or very large lesions suggest the need to investigate for possible associated conditions.

Treating Associated Conditions

Numerous disorders may be associated with multiple café au lait macules. Some of the more common are summarized here.

- Neurofibromatosis type 1: See Chapter 83.
- McCune-Albright syndrome
  - Large segmental café au lait macule with very irregular (ie, "coast of Maine") borders; may be present at birth or develop later
  - Bony abnormalities
    - Polyostotic fibrous dysplasia: replacement of bone with fibrous tissue resulting in asymmetry and pathologic fractures.
    - Bony lesions often are ipsilateral to café au lait macule.
  - Endocrine abnormalities: precocious puberty (mainly in girls), hyperthyroidism, Cushing syndrome
- Silver-Russell syndrome: triangular face, short stature, skeletal asymmetry, and abnormal pubertal development
- Bloom syndrome: short stature, facial telangiectasias and erythema, and characteristic facies (ie, narrow face, prominent nose and ears)
- Watson syndrome: café au lait macules, mental retardation, axillary freckling, and pulmonic stenosis

Prognosis

- Isolated café au lait macules persist and are harmless (and have no malignant potential).

When to Worry or Refer

- Refer or obtain consultation for patients who have multiple or large lesions or when clinical features suggest an associated syndrome.

CHAPTER 68

Congenital Melanocytic Nevi (CMN)

Introduction/Etiology/Epidemiology

- Congenital melanocytic nevi (CMN) are found at birth in about 1% of newborns.
- Congenital melanocytic nevi have an increased risk of malignant transformation.
  - The risk for small lesions (<1.5 cm) is low.
  - The risk for large (20–40 cm) or "giant" lesions (>40 cm) is greater (perhaps as high as 4%–8% for giant lesions).

Signs and Symptoms

- Congenital melanocytic nevi usually are present at birth but may appear during the first 6 months.
- Most lesions are small (<1.5 cm in diameter).
  - Typically are larger than acquired nevi (Figure 68.1)
  - Usually are slightly elevated and have surface texture changes (Figure 68.2)
- Occasionally, lesions are large (ie, giant), measuring 20 cm or more, and have significant hair (Figure 68.3).

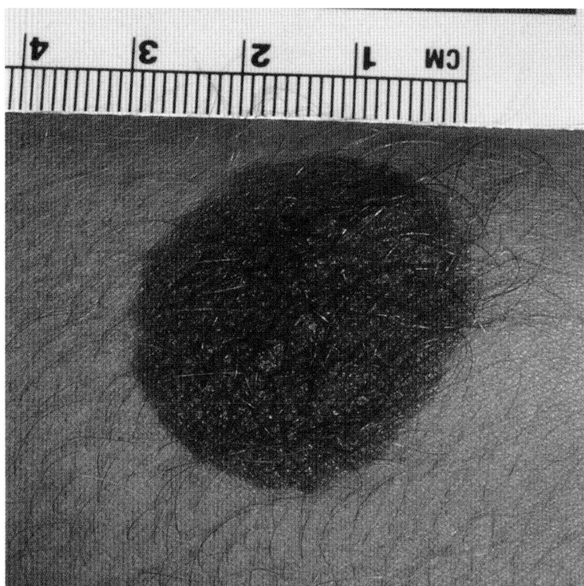

Figure 68.1. Congenital melanocytic nevus involving the scalp.

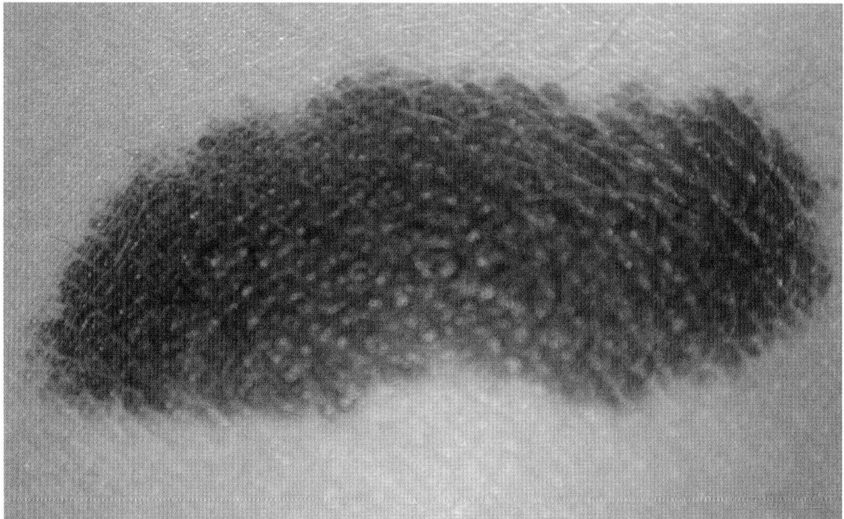

Figure 68.2. Congenital melanocytic nevus demonstrating surface textural change.

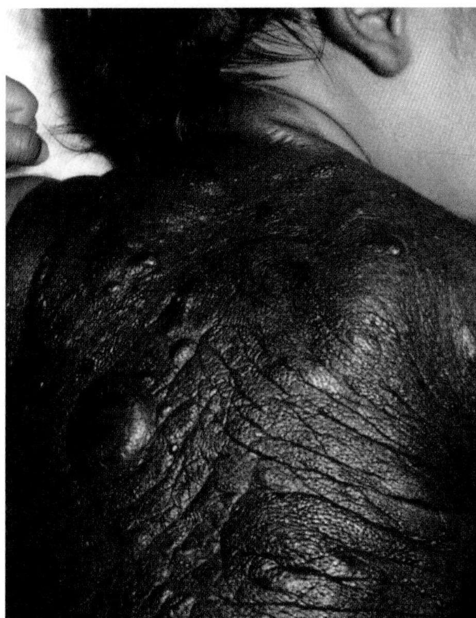

Figure 68.3. A large (ie, "giant") congenital melanocytic nevus involving the posterior trunk.

Look-alikes

Disorder	Differentiating Features
Ephelides	• Small, hyperpigmented macules located in sun-exposed areas such as the face, upper chest, and back. • Ephelides become darker following sun exposure. • Unlike CMN, have no change in surface texture.
Lentigines	• Small, hyperpigmented macules not limited to sun-exposed areas • Unlike CMN, have no change in surface texture
Café au lait macules	• Hyperpigmented macules that are not elevated and have no change in surface texture

How to Make the Diagnosis

- The diagnosis is made clinically based on the history and typical appearance of the lesion.

Treatment

- Small CMN that are asymptomatic and not changing may be observed or excised at puberty (malignant change before puberty is extraordinarily rare).
- Infants who have larger lesions should be referred to a plastic surgeon for possible excision.

Treating Associated Conditions

- Due to the risk of central nervous system involvement (neurocutaneous melanosis), in infants with extensive CMN on the head or overlying the midline of the back, and those with large numbers of satellite nevi, magnetic resonance imaging of the brain and spinal cord should be considered.

Prognosis

- Large congenital nevi are at significant risk for melanoma development and should be considered for removal.

When to Worry or Refer

- Melanoma is the malignant neoplasm of melanocytes that may arise de novo or from preexisting nevi. Consider the possibility of melanoma when a CMN exhibits any of the following ABCDE criteria:
  - **A**symmetry
  - **B**order irregularity
  - **C**olor variation (especially red, blue, black)
  - **D**iameter larger than about 6 mm (but this criterion is less useful for CMN, as they are often larger than this very early in life)
  - **E**volving lesion that is changing quickly
- Patients with CMN that are intermediate or large in size, or which show atypical features, should be referred for dermatologic evaluation.

Resources for Families

- Nevus Outreach (The Association for Large Nevi and Related Disorders): Provides support and information for patients who have large nevi or neurocutaneous melanosis.
  www.nevus.org
- The Nevus Network: Provides support and information for patients who have congenital nevi.
  www.nevusnetwork.org

CHAPTER 69

Ephelides

Introduction/Etiology/Epidemiology

- Ephelides (freckles) most often occur in white children and adults with fair skin and red hair.

Signs and Symptoms

- Small, red to tan (≤5 mm) macules without change in skin surface markings (Figure 69.1)
- Located on sun-exposed areas such as the face, upper chest, and back; do not occur on mucous membranes
- Darken in summer and lighten during winter

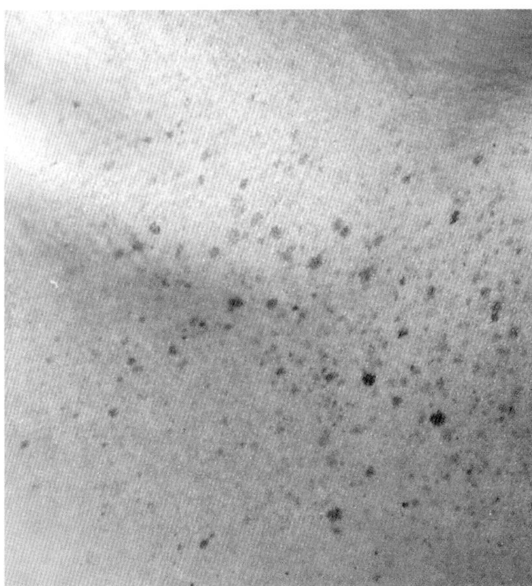

Figure 69.1. Ephelides (freckles) are small tan or red macules that appear in sun-exposed areas.

Look-alikes

Disorder	Differentiating Features
Café au lait macules	• Hyperpigmented macules typically larger than ephelides and not limited to sun-exposed areas
Lentigines	• Small, hyperpigmented macules not limited to sun-exposed areas
Melanocytic nevi	• Typically more deeply pigmented than ephelides • Often slightly elevated and have surface textural change

How to Make the Diagnosis

- The diagnosis is made clinically based on the appearance of the lesions.

Treatment

- If desired for cosmetic reasons, laser therapy may be considered.

Prognosis

- Lesions persist and darken with sun exposure.

When to Worry or Refer

- An ephelis that suddenly grows or turns black in color (may represent transforming junctional nevus rather than an ephelis)
- Numerous ephelides early in life following sun exposure (could represent xeroderma pigmentosum or other photosensitivity disorder)

CHAPTER 70

Lentigines

Introduction/Etiology/Epidemiology

- Lentigines are persistent macular areas of hyperpigmentation that can occur on any skin or mucosal surface, regardless of sun exposure.
- The incidence is unknown, but isolated lentigines appear to be very common.

Signs and Symptoms

- Lentigines are small (≤5 mm), hyperpigmented macules that mimic ephelides (ie, freckles).
  - Lentigines may be brown to black, are well-defined, and may be widely distributed (not limited to sun-exposed areas).
  - Lesions do not become more apparent following sun exposure.
  - Isolated lentigines have no clinical significance.
- Multiple lentigines may be associated with systemic disorders; the most common of these are
  - LEOPARD syndrome: LEOPARD is an acronym for the major defects in this autosomal dominantly inherited disorder: **l**entigines, **e**lectrocardiographic abnormalities, **o**cular hypertelorism, **p**ulmonic stenosis, **a**bnormal genitalia, **r**etarded growth, and sensorineural **d**eafness.
  - Peutz-Jeghers syndrome: autosomal-dominant disorder consisting of face, lip, and oral mucosa lentigines associated with benign intestinal polyposis (Figure 70.1).
  - Lentiginosis with cardiocutaneous myxomas consists of multiple lentigines associated with cardiac and subcutaneous myxomas. Disorders considered within this disease category include
    - Carney complex: lentigines, cardiac and other myxomas, and endocrine tumors
    - LAMB syndrome: **l**entigines, **a**trial myxomas, **m**ucocutaneous myxomas, and **b**lue nevi
    - NAME syndrome: **n**evi, **a**trial myxomas, **m**yxoid neurofibromas, **e**phelides, and **e**ndocrine neoplasia

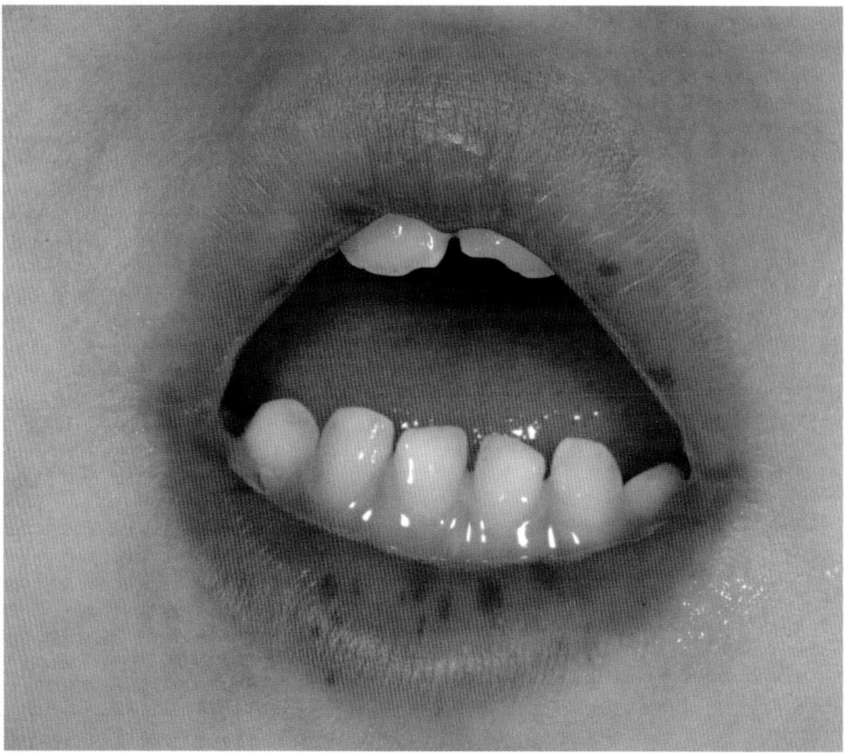

Figure 70.1. In Peutz-Jeghers syndrome, lentigines appear on the face, lips, and oral mucosa. They are associated with gastrointestinal polyposis.

Look-alikes

Disorder	Differentiating Features
Ephelides	• Small, hyperpigmented macules located in sun-exposed areas such as face, upper chest, and back. • Unlike lentigines, ephelides become darker following sun exposure and often fade in absence of sun (ie, winter months).
Café au lait macules	• Hyperpigmented macules typically larger than lentigines
Melanocytic nevi	• Typically more deeply pigmented than lentigines • Often slightly elevated and have surface textural change

How to Make the Diagnosis

- The diagnosis is made clinically based on the appearance and distribution (ie, not limited to sun-exposed areas) of lesions.

Treatment

- Lentigines do not require treatment unless desired for cosmetic reasons.
- Identification of multiple lentiginosis syndromes is of paramount importance.

Treating Associated Conditions

If multiple lentigines present, assess for clinical features of an associated syndrome (eg, LEOPARD, Peutz-Jeghers, lentiginosis with cardiocutaneous myxomas).

- If no mucosal lentigines, consider electrocardiography, echocardiography, hearing test.
- If mucosal lentigines, consider referral to gastroenterology.

Prognosis

- Excellent if isolated lentigines.
- Presence of an associated syndrome alters prognosis.

When to Worry or Refer

- Multiple or mucosal lentigines are observed (may indicate the presence of an associated disorder).

Mongolian Spots

Introduction/Etiology/Epidemiology

- The most common form of cutaneous hyperpigmentation seen in neonates.
- Common in infants of color; occurs in approximately 90% of African American and Native American, 80% of Asian, 70% of Hispanic, and 10% of white infants.
- Underlying pathology is dermal melanocytosis.

Signs and Symptoms

- Slate gray macular pigment present at birth (Figure 71.1).
- Common locations are the buttocks and mid-sacral area, but entire back, shoulders, and extremities may be involved (Figure 71.2).

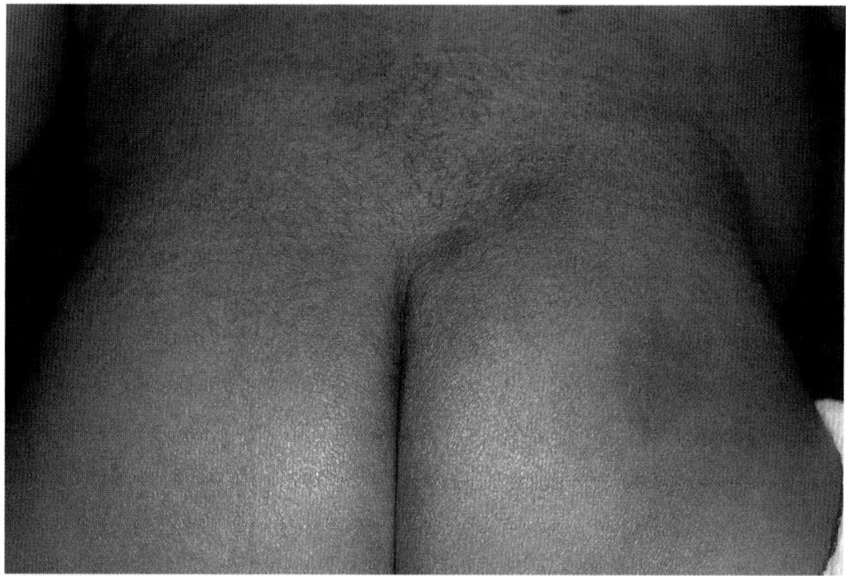

Figure 71.1. Mongolian spot. Blue-gray hyperpigmented macules over the buttocks.

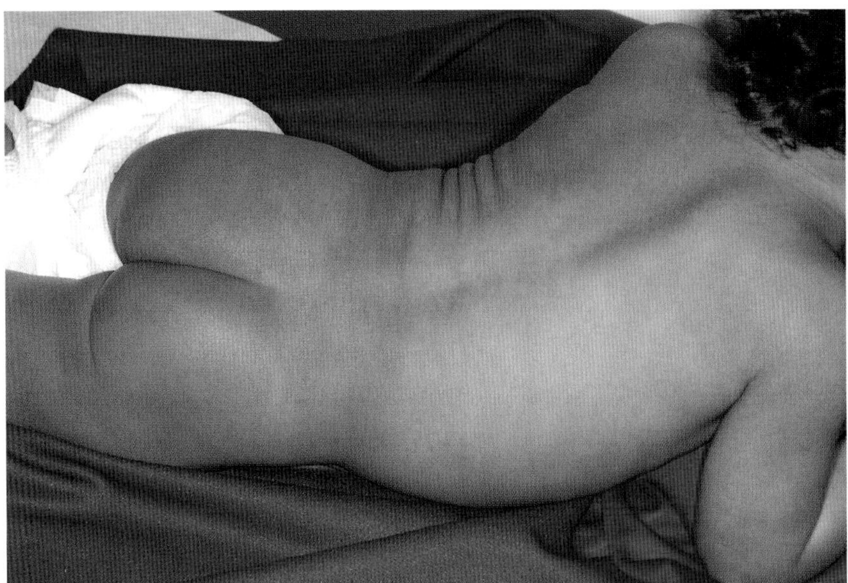

Figure 71.2. Mongolian spots. Blue-gray patches over the buttocks and upper back.

Look-alikes

Disorder	Differentiating Features
Nevus of Ota	• Blue-gray hyperpigmentation (due to dermal melanocytosis) of skin surrounding the eye; usually present at birth. • Scleral hyperpigmentation may be present. • Distinction from Mongolian spot based primarily on location and scleral involvement; histology of these 2 conditions may have overlapping features.
Nevus of Ito	• Blue-gray hyperpigmentation (due to dermal melanocytosis) that appears on shoulder. • Distinction from Mongolian spot based primarily on location; histology of these 2 conditions may have overlapping features.
Blue nevus	• Usually smaller than Mongolian spots • Usually solitary • Does not resolve spontaneously with time
Bruise	• History of trauma may be present. • Lesion evolves with typical color changes as erythrocytes degrade.
Minocycline hyperpigmentation	• History of minocycline use • Slate gray diffuse or focal hyperpigmentation • Often involves the pretibial regions or gingivae

How to Make the Diagnosis

- The diagnosis is made clinically. The presence of Mongolian spots should be documented in the medical record in the event concern is later raised that the lesions represent bruises.

Treatment

- No treatment is needed.

Prognosis

- Mongolian spots are harmless and often fade before adulthood.

When to Worry or Refer

- Multiple or extensive Mongolian spots occasionally have been observed with GM1 gangliosidosis or Hurler syndrome. Widespread Mongolian spots associated with cutaneous vascular lesions may suggest a mixed malformation syndrome.

Resources for Families

- American Academy of Pediatrics: HealthyChildren.org.
  www.HealthyChildren.org/birthmarks
- MedlinePlus: Information for patients and families (in English and Spanish) sponsored by the National Library of Medicine and National Institutes of Health.
  https://www.nlm.nih.gov/medlineplus/ency/article/001472.htm

Pigmentary Mosaicism, Hyperpigmented

Introduction/Etiology/Epidemiology

- Pigmentary mosaicism is the term used to describe a group of disorders in which the skin has a patterned hypopigmentation or hyperpigmentation. In the hyperpigmented form discussed in this chapter, affected skin is darker than the background skin color.
- Pigmentary mosaicism is believed to be the result of genetic mutations that create a population of cells with more or less pigment potential than the surrounding normal skin. Mosaicism refers to the coexistence of 2 genetically distinct populations of cells within the same individual.
- Pigmentary mosaicism may be localized or generalized.
- The terminology used to describe hyperpigmented pigmentary mosaicism is inconsistent. Terms such as giant café au lait macule, segmental pigmentation disorder, linear and whorled nevoid hypermelanosis, and patterned pigmentation are present in the literature.
- In most cases, localized hyperpigmented pigmentary mosaicism is a benign and isolated finding. When more generalized, it may be associated with skeletal, ocular, or neurologic abnormalities.

Signs and Symptoms

- Hyperpigmentation is noticed at birth or early in infancy, although its appreciation may be difficult to recognize in some young infants (who may initially present later, at 1–2 years of age). Affected areas are darker than the background skin color and may be more noticeable after sun exposure.
- One pattern of mosaic hyperpigmentation affects one or several large regions or segments of the body and has been termed, in some cases, segmental pigmentation disorder (Figure 72.1). Another typical pattern is whorled or linear bands (thin or broad) that follow the lines of Blaschko (Figure 72.2). In some cases, patients may have a mixture of hypopigmentation and hyperpigmentation, making it difficult to determine the "normal" background skin type.
- Affected areas are typically sharply demarcated and stop at the midline.

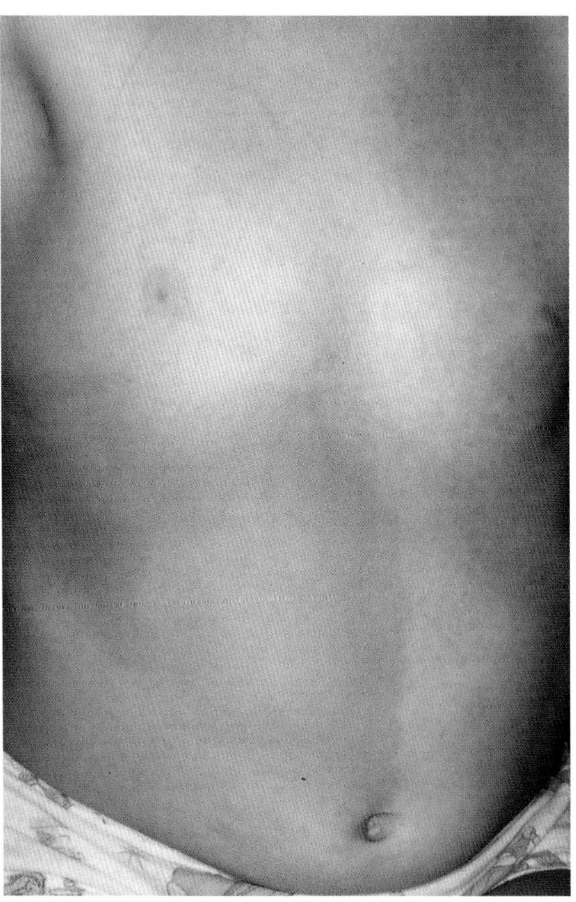

Figure 72.1. Pigmentary mosaicism, hyperpigmented type. This young girl has a large hyperpigmented patch involving a large region of the right abdomen (segmental pigmentation type).

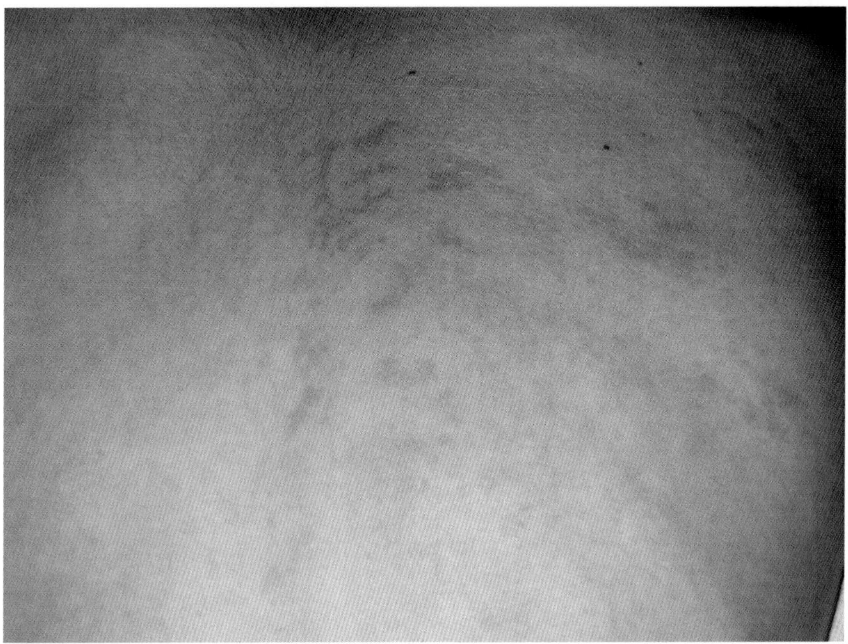

Figure 72.2. Pigmentary mosaicism, hyperpigmented type. This boy has linear and curvilinear hyperpigmented patches which follow the lines of Blaschko, limited to the right upper back.

Look-alikes

Disorder	Differentiating Features
McCune-Albright syndrome	• In addition to large café au lait macules (which may appear similar to segmental pigmentation type of pigmentary mosaicism), polyostotic fibrous dysplasia (often presenting as fractures) and endocrine hyperfunction (which may present as precocious puberty) are seen. • Skin and bone changes are typically unilateral (although this is also the case with localized pigmentary mosaicism).
Incontinentia pigmenti (third stage)	• X-linked dominant inheritance. • Vesicles are usually the initial presentation in newborn (first stage), distributed along the lines of Blaschko. • Warty lesions (second stage) give rise to eventual hyperpigmentation (third stage) in a similar distribution pattern. • Associations may include dental, ophthalmologic, neurologic, and skeletal anomalies.
Becker nevus (pilar and smooth muscle hamartoma)	• An irregular hyperpigmented patch or band occurring on the torso, often over the shoulder region. • Often presents or enlarges around the time of puberty. • Associated hypertrichosis and a pseudo-Darier sign (contraction of prominent arrector pili muscles) may be present.

How to Make the Diagnosis

- The diagnosis of hyperpigmented pigmentary mosaicism is usually made based on history and physical examination.
- Consider a formal ophthalmology examination to evaluate for ocular anomalies in children with the generalized type.
- If other malformations or neurodevelopmental abnormalities are absent, further workup is not indicated. If they are present, consultation with the appropriate specialist(s) is warranted.
- Rarely, karyotype analysis is performed (on blood or skin biopsy tissue) searching for chromosomal mosaicism.

Treatment

- There are no specific treatments for hyperpigmented pigmentary mosaicism.

Prognosis

- In most cases, hyperpigmented pigmentary mosaicism is a benign, isolated skin finding not associated with other medical concerns.
- In the rare patient who has generalized involvement, prognosis depends on the nature of any other organ abnormalities.

When to Worry or Refer

- Referral to dermatology is warranted when diagnosis is unclear.
- Referral to other specialists (eg, ophthalmology, neurology, genetics, orthopedics) is warranted when applicable.

Lumps and Bumps

CHAPTER 73

Cutaneous Mastocytosis

Introduction/Etiology/Epidemiology

- Three types of disease
  - Solitary mastocytoma
  - Urticaria pigmentosa (aka maculopapular cutaneous mastocytosis [MCM])
  - Diffuse cutaneous mastocytosis
- Increased number of mast cells present in the dermis in all forms.
- Most often occurs sporadically, although some reports of familial cases.
- In pediatric disease, most lesions appear prior to 2 years of age.

Signs and Symptoms

- Solitary mastocytoma (single lesion, Figures 73.1 and 73.2) and urticaria pigmentosa (multiple lesions, Figure 73.3) present as skin-colored, red to brown macules and papules.
- Some have a peau d'orange (orange peel–like) surface (see Figure 73.1).
- Children with diffuse cutaneous mastocytosis may have only a cobblestone or diffuse peau d'orange pattern noted on the skin.
- Lesions can occur on any part of the body.
- Darier sign is positive (the lesion urticates [becomes red and swollen] or blisters following stroking) (see Figure 73.2).
- As the lesions age, many will become just hyperpigmented macules.
- Macules can further resolve and leave normal-appearing skin.
- Systemic manifestations may include flushing, headache, abdominal cramping, diarrhea, nausea, bone pain, and pulmonary symptoms (less common in pediatric disease).

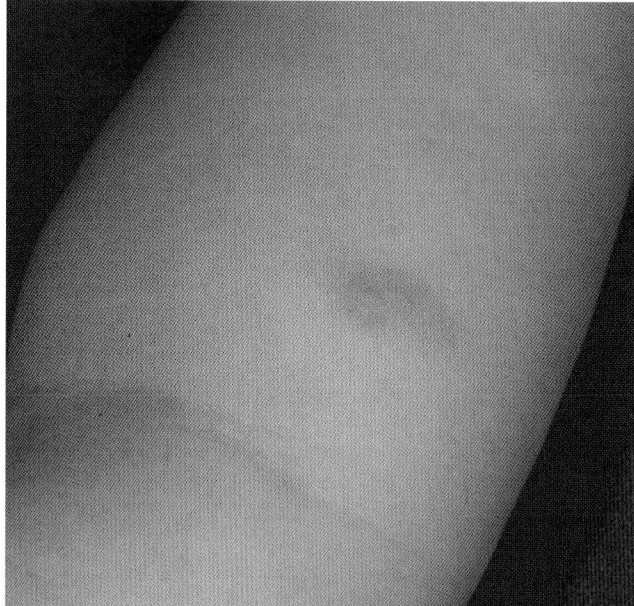

Figure 73.1. Solitary mastocytoma. A pink-orange plaque with a peau d'orange surface on the forearm of a male infant.

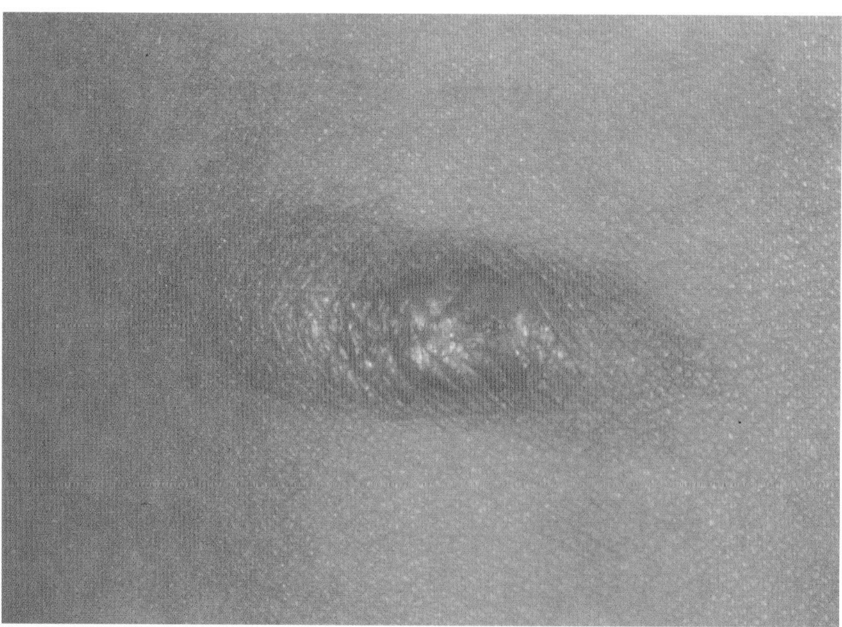

Figure 73.2. Mastocytoma with a positive Darier sign after stroking; the lesion has become red and more elevated.

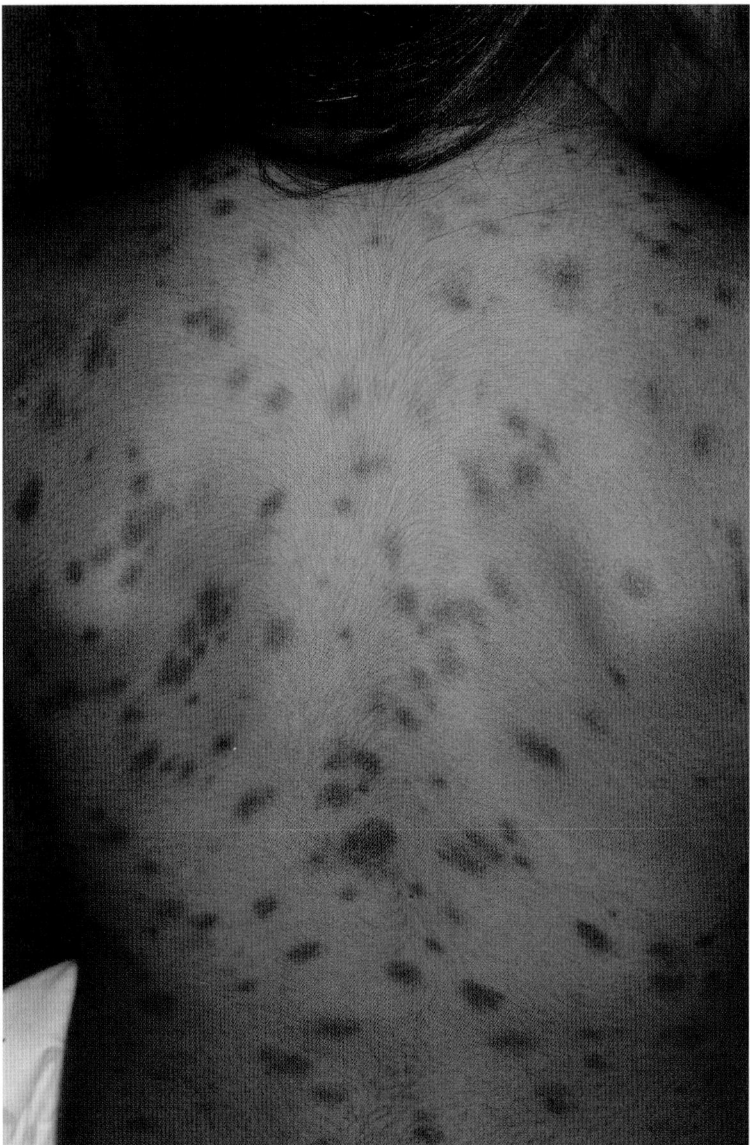

Figure 73.3. In urticaria pigmentosa, multiple hyperpigmented macules and papules are present. On close inspection, lesions have an orange peel–like (peau d'orange) appearance.

Look-alikes

Disorder	Differentiating Features
Solitary Mastocytoma	
Melanocytic nevus	• Negative Darier sign • No peau d'orange surface appearance • May reveal hypertrichosis • May reveal dark brown pigmentation
Nevus sebaceous	• Most often located on the scalp. • Negative Darier sign. • May have a linear patterning. • Most prominent color of appearance is yellow.
Juvenile xanthogranuloma	• Negative Darier sign. • Most prominent color of appearance is yellow, although early lesions may be erythematous. • Dome-shaped papule.
Bullous impetigo	• Recurrent blistering in same location unusual • Once resolved, no residual papule visible • Bacterial culture positive for *Staphylococcus aureus*
Cutaneous herpes simplex virus infection	• Recurrent blistering may occur in same location but appears as clustered vesicles on background of erythema. • Tingling or pain commonly present before blisters appear. • May leave residual scarring, but no papular lesion. • Viral culture positive for herpes simplex virus.
Urticaria Pigmentosa	
Urticaria	• Duration of lesions is hours, with frequent waxing and waning. • After resolution the skin looks normal, without residual hyperpigmentation or papules. • Blister formation does not usually occur.
Arthropod bites	• Often a central punctum is present on close inspection. • Pruritus common, often severe. • Lesions may be clustered in linear groupings. • Usually located on exposed areas of the body.
Nodular scabies	• Papules and nodules that persist after scabies infestation. • Darier sign only occasionally positive. • Lesions most common in flexures, on the penis and scrotum, or on the areolae. • Other family members may have a history of scabies infestation.
Café au lait macules/ neurofibromatosis	• Negative Darier sign. • Lesions are flat, non-palpable (and peau d'orange appearance is absent). • Axillary/inguinal freckling, neurofibromas may be present in those who have neurofibromatosis type 1.

How to Make the Diagnosis

- The diagnosis is usually based on clinical findings.
- Positive Darier sign (in appropriate clinical setting) is confirmatory.
- Skin biopsy reveals increased mast cells in the dermis (confirmed by special stains).

Treatment

- Avoid the following triggers (among others), which may cause mast cell degranulation (avoidance usually not necessary with solitary lesions):
  - Heat or overly hot baths
  - Aspirin
  - Alcohol
  - Ibuprofen
  - Codeine and morphine
  - Certain anesthetic agents
  - Radiocontrast dye
- Topical corticosteroids may occasionally be useful for solitary mastocytoma.
- Antihistamines may decrease urtication, minimize blister formation, and improve systemic symptoms.
  - A nonsedating histamine (H_1) antihistamine (eg, loratadine, cetirizine, levocetirizine, fexofenadine) is helpful as a first-line agent.
  - For those whose symptoms do not improve or are severe, consider adding one of the following:
    - Sedating H_1 antihistamine (eg, hydroxyzine, cyproheptadine): These may be administered at bedtime to avoid daytime sedation.
    - In severe disease, an H_2 receptor antagonist may also be useful in conjunction with H_1 blockers.
- Oral cromolyn sodium may be useful for associated gastrointestinal symptoms.
- Surgery can be considered for solitary lesions in an accessible location, when clinically indicated or requested.
- Pimecrolimus cream and biologic agents have also been reported.

Prognosis

- The prognosis for solitary mastocytoma and pediatric MCM/urticaria pigmentosa is excellent, with resolution occurring in most patients over several years.
- The resolution of diffuse cutaneous mastocytosis or familial mastocytosis is not as predictable.

When to Worry or Refer

- Consider referral to a dermatologist for patients who have severe or extensive disease, in whom the diagnosis is in question, or who do not respond to standard treatment.

Resources for Families

- Mastocytosis Society, Inc.: Provides information for patients, families, and medical providers.
  www.tmsforacure.org
- Mastokids.org: Provides information and support for patients who have pediatric mastocytosis and their families.
  www.mastokids.org

Dermoid Cysts

Introduction/Etiology/Epidemiology

- Develop from entrapment along the lines of embryonic closure.
- In contrast to epithelial cysts, dermoid cysts may have appendageal elements, including hair follicles, in addition to keratin.
- They are present at birth, although they may not become clinically apparent until later.
- These developmental remnants are distinct from dermoids of the ovary (ovarian teratomas) and do not contain multiple tissues such as teeth, bone, or thyroid.

Signs and Symptoms

- Dermoid cysts most commonly occur on the head or face; the most common location is on the orbital ridge, often the outer third of the eyebrow (Figures 74.1 and 74.2).
- They may also occur in the nasal midline (glabella, dorsal nose) and on the scalp.
- Midline lesions may be associated with deep extension and, occasionally, central nervous system communication.
- Some lesions reveal an overlying central punctum or sinus, and protruding hairs may be present; with midline lesions, the presence of an overlying pit may suggest a higher risk for intracranial extension.
- Dermoid cysts are most often solitary, non-tender, and mobile; the overlying epidermis is usually normal in appearance.

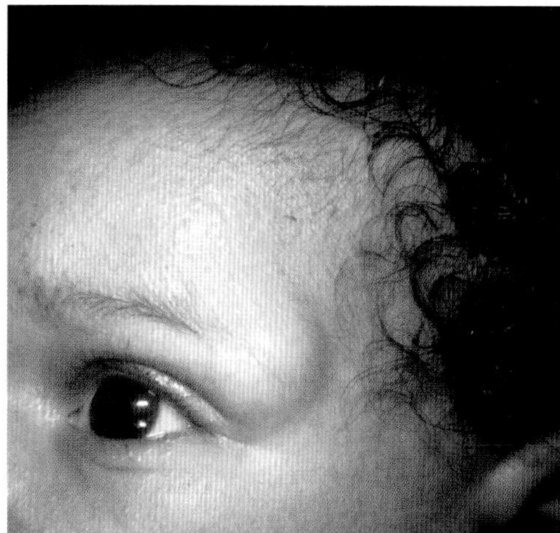

Figure 74.1. Dermoid cyst of the lateral eyebrow in a 3-week-old.

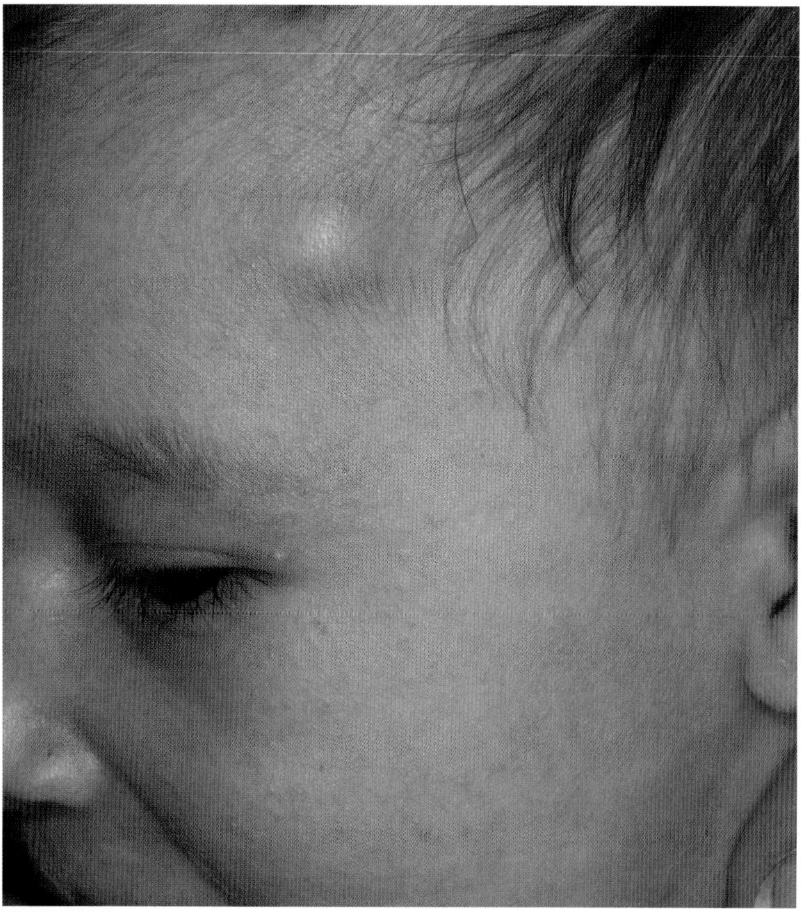

Figure 74.2. Dermoid cyst on the mid-lateral forehead in a 2-month-old boy.

Look-alikes

Disorder	Differentiating Features
Other epithelial cysts	• More common in adolescents and adults. • Usually acquired, rather than congenital. • Common locations include the scalp, face, neck, and upper trunk.
Milia	• Small (usually 1–2 mm) and more superficial • Often multiple • White in color
Cutaneous bronchogenic cyst	• Typically located on the midline chest, near the sternal notch • May be more firm • May have connection to underlying structures or a draining sinus
Pilomatricoma	• Usually acquired, rather than congenital • Often blue in appearance • Very firm to palpation

How to Make the Diagnosis

- The diagnosis is usually made clinically based on the characteristic presentation and location.

Treatment

- Clinical observation may be appropriate if small and uncomplicated and of no psychosocial concern.
- Surgical excision is the modality of choice for problematic or cosmetically displeasing lesions.
- Midline lesions should be imaged prior to any surgical procedure.

Prognosis

- The prognosis is excellent for uncomplicated dermoid cysts.

When to Worry or Refer

- Lesions that are inflamed, draining, rapidly growing in size, or symptomatic should be referred promptly for surgical excision.
- Midline cysts or sinuses should undergo magnetic resonance imaging or computed tomography to assess for a tract and intracranial connection.

Resources for Families

- Medscape: Provides a discussion of cutaneous dermoid cysts. **http://emedicine.medscape.com/article/1112963-overview**

Epidermal Nevi

Introduction/Etiology/Epidemiology

- Epidermal nevi are benign hamartomas derived from the ectoderm and are believed to be caused by mosaicism.
- They typically present at birth or during infancy; they often continue to expand during childhood.
- Several subtypes have been identified, including keratinocytic epidermal nevi (focus of this chapter), nevus comedonicus, and nevus sebaceous (of Jadassohn) (see Chapter 97).
- Mutations in fibroblast growth factor receptor 3 (*FGFR3*), *PIK3CA, HRAS, KRAS,* and *NRAS* have been identified in some patients.

Signs and Symptoms

- Usually asymptomatic.
- Epidermal nevi present as flesh-colored to tan/brown verrucous plaques (Figure 75.1).
- They are often linear or curvilinear in nature; larger lesions reveal distribution pattern along Blaschko lines.
- With time, they tend to become thicker and more verrucous.
- When more extensive lesions occur in a unilateral fashion (Figure 75.2), the term *nevus unius lateris* has been used.
- When diffuse, widespread lesions present, may be part of the *epidermal nevus syndrome,* which may include congenital anomalies and abnormalities in the central nervous system, eyes, and skeleton.

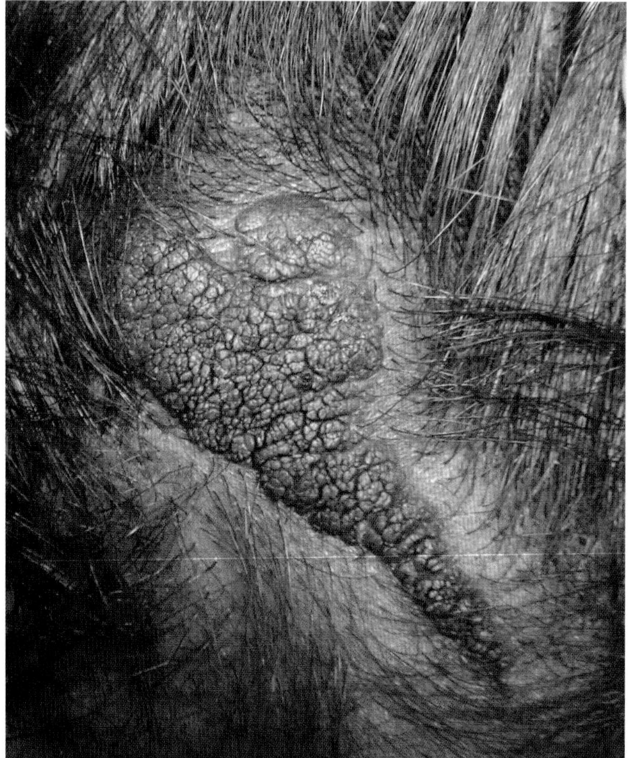

Figure 75.1. Epidermal nevus on the scalp. A verrucous, brown, linear plaque.

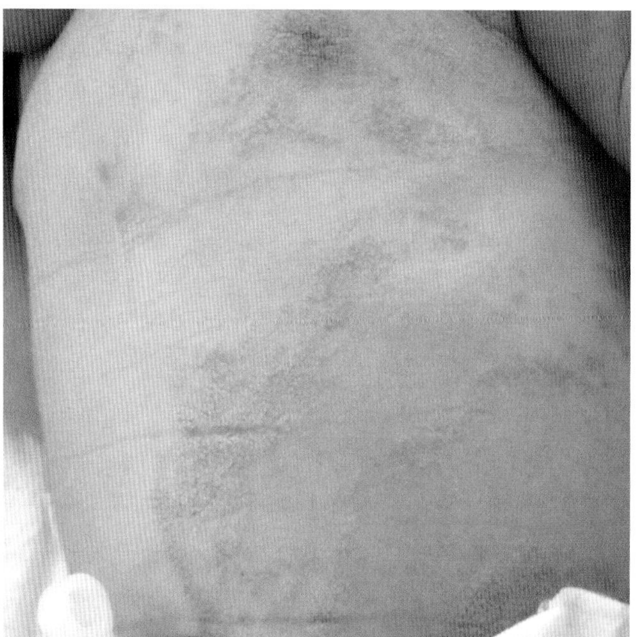

Figure 75.2. Extensive epidermal nevi on the left-sided trunk. This presentation has been termed *nevus unius lateris.*

Look-alikes

Disorder	Differentiating Features
Lichen striatus	• Also presents in a linear fashion but usually composed of erythematous scaly papules • Acquired, not congenital • Spontaneously resolves over 1 to 2 years with residual hypopigmentation
Incontinentia pigmenti	• Similar pattern of lesions (distributed in a linear or whorled pattern along lines of Blaschko) may be present. • In the neonate, usually presents with red papules and vesicles (stage 1). • Several subsequent phases of lesions may evolve with time, including verrucous (stage 2), hyperpigmented (stage 3), and hypopigmented (stage 4). • Most often diagnosed in girls because of X-linked dominant inheritance. • Other abnormalities may be present, including dental, ophthalmologic, neurologic, musculoskeletal.
Verruca vulgaris (wart)	• May be confused with smaller or more patchy epidermal nevi. • Although multiple warts may be linear (from koebnerization), they do not follow the distribution of Blaschko lines. • May resolve spontaneously.
Inflammatory linear verrucous epidermal nevus	• Linear distribution of erythematous, scaly papules coalescing into plaques; not typically as brown in color • Pruritus often severe • May mimic other inflammatory conditions such as psoriasis, lichen striatus, lichen planus

How to Make the Diagnosis

- The diagnosis of epidermal nevus is usually made clinically.
- If the diagnosis is in question, skin biopsy for histologic analysis can be performed and reveals acanthosis and papillomatosis.
- Some lesions may reveal histologic changes of epidermolytic hyperkeratosis.

Treatment

- Treatment is challenging and only necessary if requested by the patient or parents.
- Destructive therapies (ie, curettage or cryotherapy) usually followed by recurrence.
- Laser ablation may be effective, but response is unpredictable.
- Surgical excision is the most definitive treatment but may be limited by the resultant scarring.
- Topical therapies (eg, retinoids, topical chemotherapy) have been used with variable success; photodynamic therapy has been reported to be beneficial.

Prognosis

- The prognosis for epidermal nevi is excellent; most lesions are uncomplicated, the most significant concern being the potential for psychosocial ramifications.
- The prognosis for epidermal nevus syndrome is variable, depending on the extent of extracutaneous involvement.

When to Worry or Refer

- Referral to a dermatologist is appropriate for assistance with the diagnosis (if in question) and recommendations for further evaluation or therapy.
- Referral to other specialists, as appropriate, is indicated for patients with epidermal nevus syndrome.

Resources for Families

- Genetics Home Reference: Sponsored by US National Library of Medicine. **http://ghr.nlm.nih.gov/condition/epidermal-nevus**

CHAPTER 76

Granuloma Annulare

Introduction/Etiology/Epidemiology

- Granuloma annulare is a common skin disorder in children.
- Most commonly occurs in school-aged children; females are affected almost twice as often as males.
- Although a potential association with diabetes has been suggested in adults, this association has not been confirmed in children.

Signs and Symptoms

- Presents as annular, flesh-colored, erythematous or violaceous, non-scaling papules and plaques (Figure 76.1).
- Outer border often composed of numerous smaller papules.
- Common locations are areas of trauma (eg, dorsal feet and wrists).
- Subcutaneous lesions (most common in children) present as firm nodules with normal overlying skin; most often seen on anterior tibiae, fingers, and scalp.

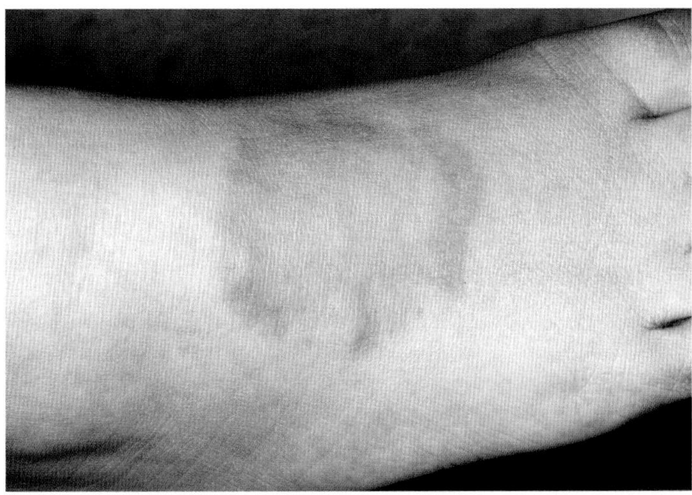

Figure 76.1. Annular plaque of granuloma annulare.

Look-alikes

Disorder	Differentiating Features
Tinea corporis	• Erythematous plaques with scale. • May spread in a pattern of autoinoculation. • Potassium hydroxide preparation of skin scrapings reveals hyphae. • Pruritus common.
Nummular eczema	• Scaly, often crusted, red papules and plaques • Central clearing less common • Pruritus very common
Soft tissue malignancy	• May be confused with subcutaneous granuloma annulare. • Other classic lesions of cutaneous granuloma annulare absent. • Biopsy may be necessary to rule out malignancy.
Rheumatoid nodules	• May be confused with subcutaneous granuloma annulare • Usually located overlying affected joints in patients with history of rheumatoid arthritis or other autoimmune condition
Sarcoidosis	• Cutaneous lesions may present as annular plaques. • Color tends to be more violaceous. • Face and nose most common locations. • Scarring possible. • May be associated with pulmonary symptoms, uveitis, hilar adenopathy.

How to Make the Diagnosis

- The diagnosis is usually made based on clinical findings.
- A biopsy shows focal collagen degeneration with reactive inflammation.

Treatment

- Reassurance and anticipatory guidance.
- Steroids used topically or intralesionally can sometimes decrease inflammation but must be used cautiously to prevent atrophy.

Treating Associated Conditions

- Not typically applicable.
- An association between granuloma annulare and other disorders (diabetes mellitus, hyperlipidemia, thyroid disease) has been suggested by some authors but remains controversial.

Prognosis

- The lesions of granuloma annulare tend to resolve after 2 to 4 years, leaving behind no permanent sequelae.
- Recurrence is common.

When to Worry or Refer

- Consider referral to a dermatologist for patients in whom the diagnosis is in question.

Resources for Families

- MedlinePlus: Information for patients and families (in English and Spanish) sponsored by the National Library of Medicine and National Institutes of Health.
  www.nlm.nih.gov/medlineplus/ency/article/000833.htm

Juvenile Xanthogranuloma

Introduction/Etiology/Epidemiology

- Juvenile xanthogranulomas are benign nodular lesions occurring particularly in infants and young children.
- They are collections of xanthomatous cells, but no association with systemic hyperlipidemia exists.
- Lesions may be present at birth.
- Iris lesions can mimic retinoblastomas and may result in hyphema.

Signs and Symptoms

- Characterized by orange or yellow-brown firm papules or papulonodular lesions (Figures 77.1 and 77.2).
- Early lesions erythematous; eventually become lipidized, with yellow color predominating clinically.
- Often located in the head and neck area, although can be on any area of the body.
- May be solitary or multiple.
- Extracutaneous sites of involvement include eye (most common); less commonly, soft tissues, muscle, lung, liver, spleen, central nervous system, kidneys, and adrenal glands.

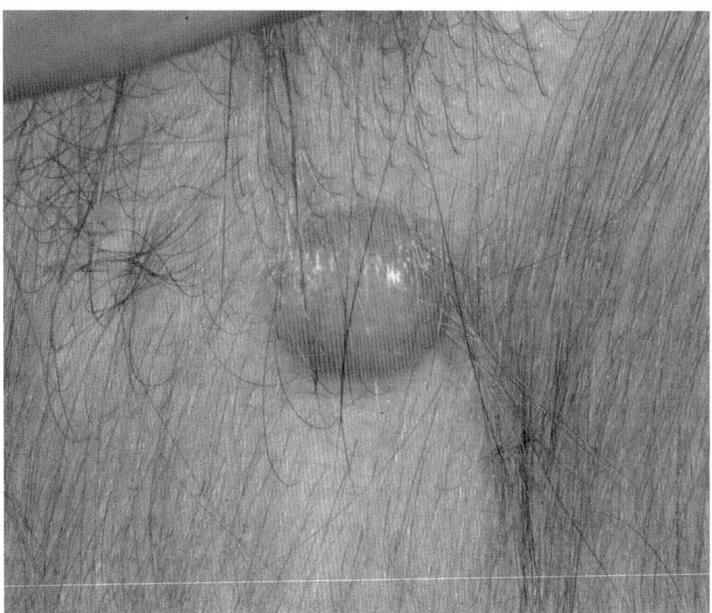

Figure 77.1. Juvenile xanthogranuloma of the scalp.

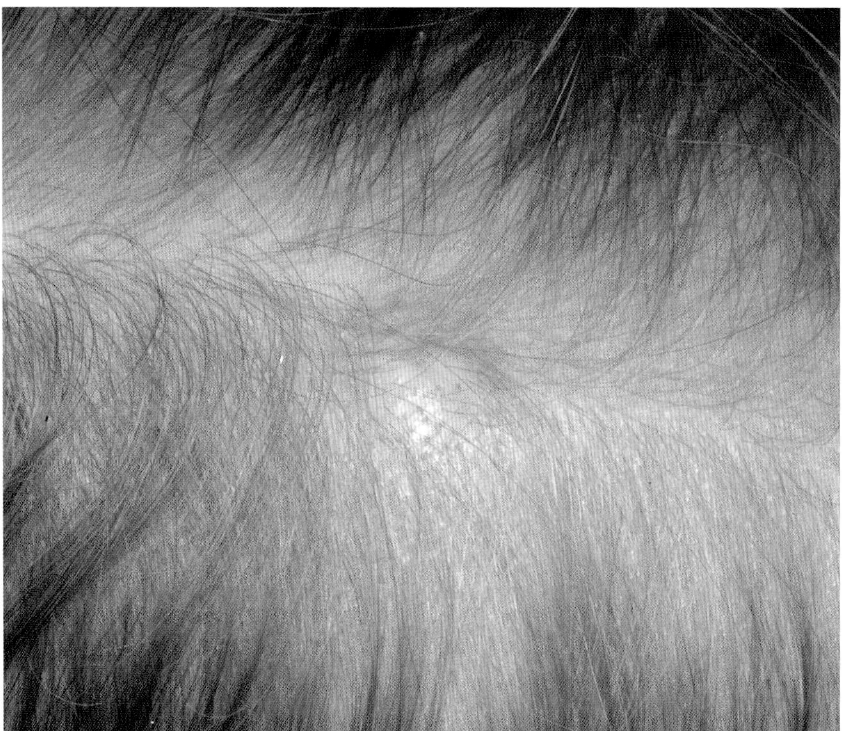

Figure 77.2. Juvenile xanthogranuloma of the scalp. A small yellow papule.

Look-alikes

Disorder	Differentiating Features
Spitz nevus	• Most often an intensely red papule • Does not undergo lipidization, so does not become yellow • May see brown pigment with diascopy (compressing lesion and viewing through a glass slide)
Solitary mastocytoma	• Red-brown papule with a peau d'orange surface • Urticates (becomes red and more elevated) with stroking (Darier sign)
Melanocytic nevus	• Usually tan to brown in color • May have associated hypertrichosis

How to Make the Diagnosis

- The diagnosis is usually made based on clinical findings.
- Biopsy of the lesion will show foamy, multinucleated histiocytic giant cells with scattered eosinophils.

Treatment

- Observation and reassurance.
- Most lesions resolve spontaneously over 10 years.
- Surgical excision, when requested or clinically indicated.

Treating Associated Conditions

- Children with multiple or facial lesions should be referred to ophthalmology for eye examination.
- Patients with neurofibromatosis type 1 and juvenile xanthogranulomas may have an increased risk of chronic leukemia and should be monitored closely.

Prognosis

- The prognosis for children with isolated cutaneous juvenile xanthogranulomas is excellent.

When to Worry or Refer

- See Treating Associated Conditions.
- Consider referral to a dermatologist when the diagnosis is in question.
- Neonates or infants with multiple lesions merit an evaluation for systemic involvement.

Resources for Families

- Medscape: Provides a discussion of juvenile xanthogranuloma. **http://emedicine.medscape.com/article/1111629-overview**

Bullous Diseases

CHAPTER 78

Childhood Dermatitis Herpetiformis

Introduction/Etiology/Epidemiology

- A rare immunobullous disorder in children.
- Associated with celiac disease (gluten-sensitive enteropathy) in 75% to 95% of affected patients.
- Typically seen between 2 and 7 years of age.
- Children diagnosed with celiac disease have circulating IgA antibodies to tissue transglutaminase and endomysium.

Signs and Symptoms

- Characterized by intensely pruritic papulovesicular lesions (Figure 78.1) with a bilateral, symmetric distribution
- Most often located on the extensor knees, elbows, sacrum, buttocks, posterior neck, scalp, and shoulders
- Mucous membrane involvement usually absent

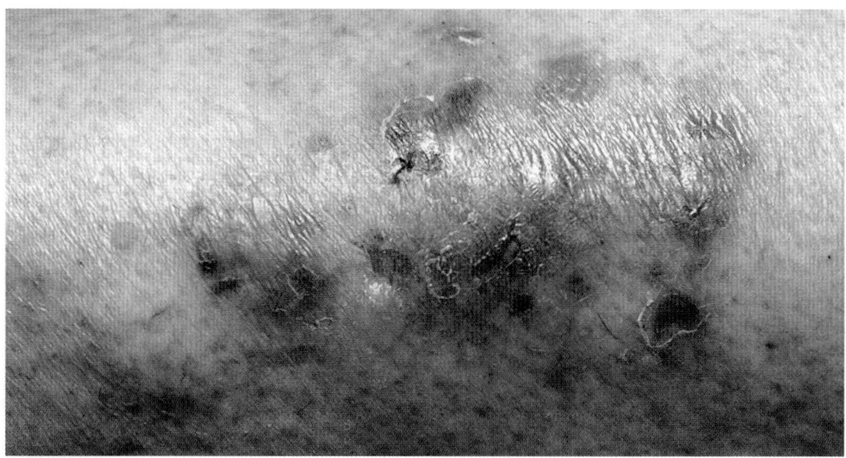

Figure 78.1. Dermatitis herpetiformis: vesicles and erosions are present.

Look-alikes

Disorder	Differentiating Features
Linear IgA dermatosis	• Bullae tend to be larger. • "Cluster of jewels" pattern (annular grouping of bullae) often noted. • Not as symmetric in distribution. • Direct immunofluorescence and immunoblotting studies help confirm diagnosis.
Bullous lupus erythematosus	• Other features of systemic lupus erythematosus (SLE) usually present. • Concentrated in sun-exposed areas. • Bullae tend to be larger. • Antinuclear antibody (and other serologic studies) will confirm diagnosis of SLE. • Direct immunofluorescence and immunoblotting studies help confirm the diagnosis.
Bullous pemphigoid	• Urticarial plaques present in addition to tense blisters. • Bullae tend to be larger. • Pruritus common with early lesions. • Direct immunofluorescence and immunoblotting studies help confirm the diagnosis.
Herpes simplex virus infection	• Most often clustered vesicles and erosions on an erythematous base • Often occur inside or around the mouth • Tend to be painful, less often pruritic • More often focal
Arthropod bites/papular urticaria	• Papules may have a central punctum on close inspection. • Usually concentrated on exposed areas of skin. • Linear groupings of papules may be observed.
Scabies	• Mixture of papules, linear burrows, and crusted papules. • Palm and sole lesions very common, as is involvement of the areolae and penis. • Other family members often report lesions or pruritus. • Mineral oil examination of skin scrapings confirms the diagnosis.
Pityriasis lichenoides et varioliformis acuta	• Scaly, red papules with necrotic surface changes. • Usually not pruritic. • Associated fever may be present. • Usually responds to treatment with oral erythromycin or tetracycline.

Look-alikes *(continued)*

Disorder	Differentiating Features
Epidermolysis bullosa	• Inherited (not acquired) mechanobullous disease. • Usually begins in neonatal period or during early infancy. • Blisters induced by trauma. • Blisters usually larger than those seen in dermatitis herpetiformis (with exception of some simplex forms of epidermolysis bullosa). • Certain subtypes may reveal nail dystrophy, milia, extensive scarring, mitten-hand deformities. • Immunomapping or electron microscopy of skin biopsy specimens confirms diagnosis.
Epidermolysis bullosa acquisita	• Acquired autoimmune blistering disease. • Blisters induced by trauma. • Scarring common. • Direct fluorescence and immunoblotting studies will help confirm diagnosis. • Blisters and erosions usually larger than those seen in dermatitis herpetiformis.

How to Make the Diagnosis

- The diagnosis is suggested clinically and confirmed by skin biopsy with immunofluorescence study, which reveals IgA at dermal papillary tips in a granular pattern.
- Circulating serum antibodies to tissue transglutaminase or endomysium may be present (in gluten-sensitive patients).

Treatment

- Dapsone at 1 to 2 mg/kg per day is usually very effective (must first confirm normal glucose-6-phosphate dehydrogenase level and follow complete blood cell counts and liver function tests).
- Sulfapyridine may be an effective alternative for therapy.
- Gluten-free diet may be effective in certain patients, although challenging for children and parents.

Treating Associated Conditions

- Patients with gluten sensitivity should be referred to an experienced gastroenterologist for baseline and follow-up care.

Prognosis

- The prognosis for children with dermatitis herpetiformis is unpredictable.
- Many recommend indefinite continuation of the gluten-free diet in gluten-sensitive individuals.

When to Worry or Refer

- Consider referral to a dermatologist for confirmation of diagnosis and comanagement.

Resources for Families

- Gluten Intolerance Group: Provides information about dermatitis herpetiformis.
  www.gluten.net
- National Institute of Diabetes and Digestive and Kidney Diseases: Health topics. Provides information about celiac disease.
  www.niddk.nih.gov/health-information/health-topics/digestive-diseases/celiac-disease/Pages/facts.aspx

CHAPTER 79

Epidermolysis Bullosa (EB)

Introduction/Etiology/Epidemiology

- A group of rare genetic skin disorders characterized by the formation of vesicles or bullae in response to frictional trauma
- Incidence of approximately 1 per 50,000 births
- Genders affected equally
- Classified into 3 general categories, based on the level of the cleavage plane within the dermal-epidermal junction
  - Epidermolysis bullosa simplex (EBS)
    - Autosomal dominant
    - Due to defects in keratin genes K5 or K14
    - Three major forms
      - Weber-Cockayne (EBS, localized)
      - Koebner (EBS, generalized intermediate)
      - Dowling-Meara (EBS, generalized severe)
    - Also, EBS with muscular dystrophy (autosomal recessive; caused by mutation in plectin) and some rarer forms due to mutations in transglutaminase 5, plakophilin-1, desmoplakin, plakoglobin
  - Junctional EB (JEB)
    - Autosomal recessive
    - Due to defects in
      - Laminin 332 (formerly laminin 5) (Herlitz; JEB, generalized severe)
      - Integrin $\alpha_6ß_4$ (JEB with pyloric atresia)
      - Collagen XVII (non-Herlitz; JEB, generalized intermediate)
  - Dystrophic EB (DEB)
    - Due to defects in collagen VII
    - Autosomal dominant (dominant dystrophic [DDEB])
    - Autosomal recessive (recessive dystrophic [RDEB])

Signs and Symptoms

- Epidermolysis bullosa simplex
  - Weber-Cockayne (EBS, localized)
    - Blisters primarily on the hands and feet (Figure 79.1)
    - May not present until adolescence or early adulthood in some patients
    - Hyperhidrosis common
  - Koebner (EBS, generalized intermediate)
    - Generalized blisters from birth or during infancy, especially on the arms and legs
    - Mild mucosal involvement
    - Occasional nail dystrophy
  - Dowling-Meara (EBS, generalized severe)
    - Vesicles arranged in a herpetiform pattern.
    - Blisters may be large during infancy, with significant oral mucosal involvement.
    - Blistering tends to become mild with age.
  - Epidermolysis bullosa simplex with muscular dystrophy
    - Resembles mild EBS.
    - Muscular dystrophy may develop anytime between infancy and third decade.

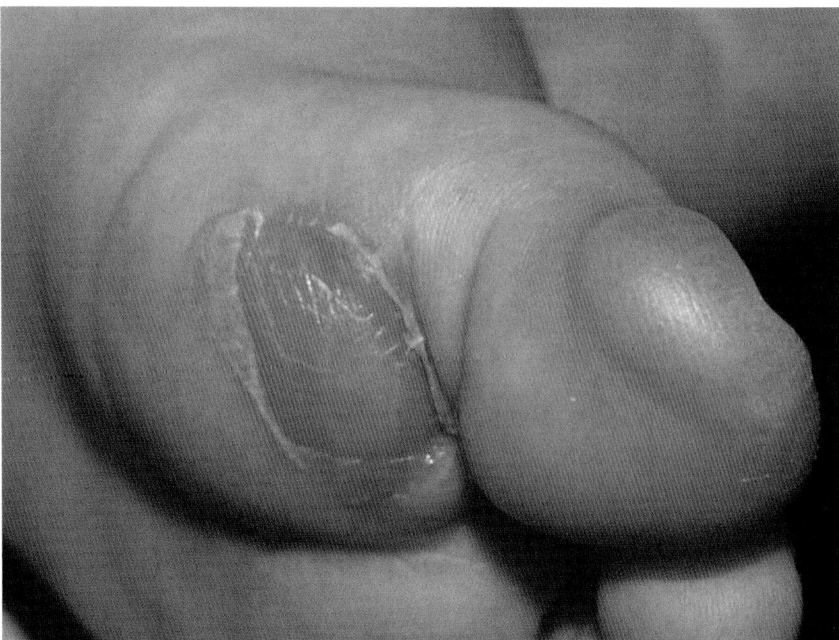

Figure 79.1. Epidermolysis bullosa simplex (Weber-Cockayne). This patient has a bulla involving the great toe and a healing bulla on the ball of the foot.

- Junctional EB
  - Herlitz (JEB, generalized severe)
    - 50% of affected children die in infancy, usually from sepsis, dehydration, or respiratory complications.
    - Lesions are typically seen at birth or soon after (Figure 79.2).
    - Blisters occur anywhere on the body, including mucous membranes.
    - Granulation tissue in perioral area is common.
    - Laryngeal involvement may be present, with hoarseness.
    - Growth retardation and anemia are common.
    - Nail dystrophy or anonychia often are present.
  - JEB with pyloric atresia (Figure 79.3)
    - Pyloric atresia and genitourinary anomalies are possible.
    - Prognosis is poor.
  - Non-Herlitz (JEB, generalized intermediate)
    - Similar to Herlitz form but milder.
    - Mucosal involvement is less severe.

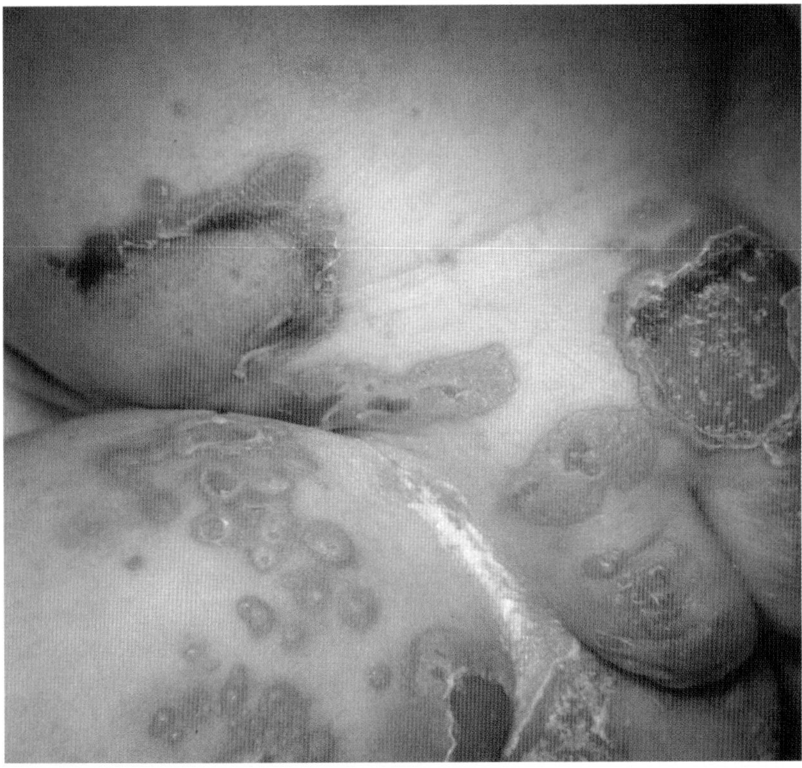

Figure 79.2. Numerous bullae and erosions in a patient with junctional epidermolysis bullosa (Herlitz, generalized severe).

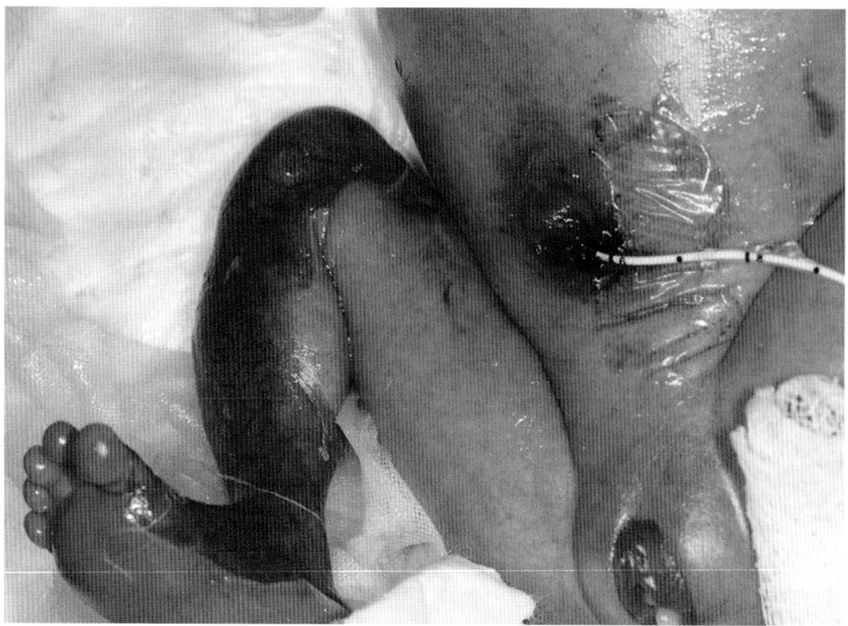

Figure 79.3. Denudation of the lower leg and foot in a newborn girl with junctional epidermolysis bullosa with pyloric atresia. She died shortly after birth from overwhelming infection.

- Dystrophic EB
  - Dominant DEB
    - Blistering most prominent on distal extremities, elbows, and knees.
    - Milia are common (Figure 79.4).
    - Scarring is present at prior blister sites.
    - Nail dystrophy is common.
  - Recessive DEB
    - Blisters are noted at birth and involve the skin and mucous membranes.
    - Widespread scarring is present.
    - Mitten deformities of hands and feet develop with digital fusion (Figure 79.5).
    - Teeth often are carious; delayed eruption may be noted.
    - Microstomia develops from scarring.
    - Other complications include difficulty swallowing (esophageal scarring), chronic anemia, growth failure, conjunctival scarring, and predisposition to squamous cell carcinoma.

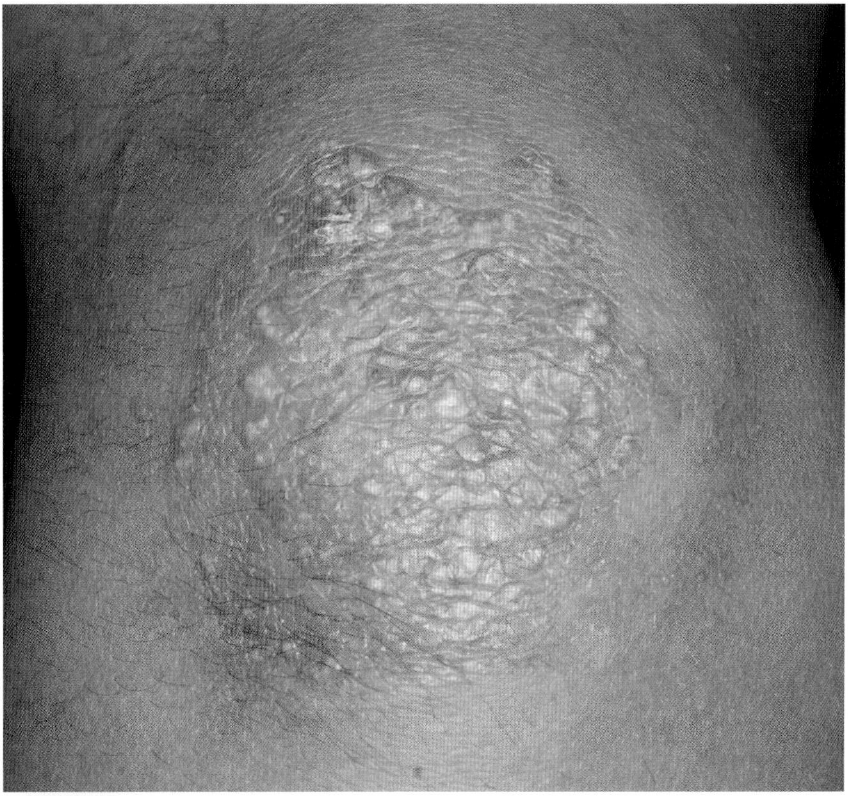

Figure 79.4. Scarring with milia formation on the knee of a young boy with dominant dystrophic epidermolysis bullosa.

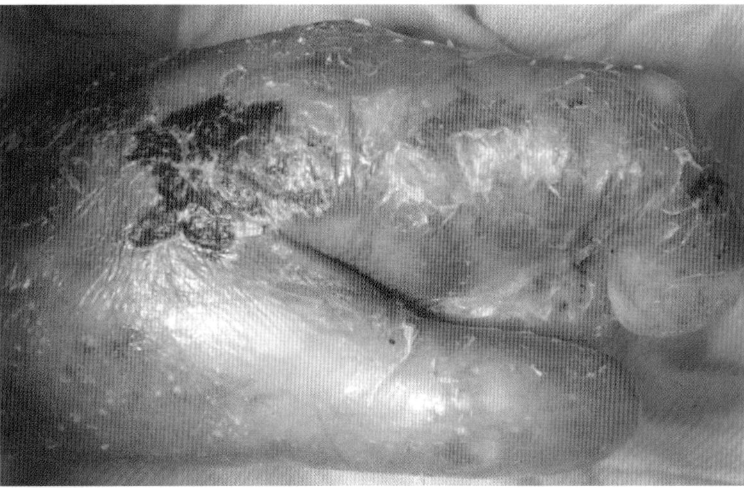

Figure 79.5. Mitten deformity of the hand of a patient with recessive dystrophic epidermolysis bullosa.

Look-alikes

Disorder	Differentiating Features
Bullous congenital ichthyosiform erythroderma	• Blisters may be present soon after birth, similar to EB. • Thickened areas of skin with ridging often present during infancy or develop with time. • Eventuates into an ichthyosis disorder (epidermolytic hyperkeratosis), with less propensity toward blistering.
Incontinentia pigmenti	• Small vesicles occur in clusters. • Blisters are arranged in a linear or whorled pattern, along lines of Blaschko. • Subsequent to blister stage, skin lesions appear verrucous or hyperpigmented. • Most patients are female (X-linked dominant). • Blisters not trauma-induced.
Bullous impetigo	• Does not usually present as a recurrent or chronic condition. • Involvement more focal. • Mucous membranes not involved. • Blisters rupture easily, leaving superficial erosions with peripheral collarettes of scale. • Blisters not trauma-induced.
Herpes simplex virus infection	• Most often clustered vesicles and erosions with an erythematous surround • Usually more focal • Blisters not trauma-induced
Bullous pemphigoid	• Urticarial plaques present in addition to tense blisters. • Blisters not trauma-induced. • Pruritus common with early lesions. • Direct fluorescence and immunoblotting studies will help confirm diagnosis.
Dermatitis herpetiformis	• Usually presents as tiny vesicles and erosions. • Most often clustered on elbows, knees, shoulders, sacrum, and buttocks. • Blisters not trauma-induced. • Pruritus is intense. • May be associated with gluten sensitivity.
Erythema multiforme major	• Typical target lesions may be present. • Only occasionally bullous, and bullae are not trauma-induced. • Oral mucous membrane erosions common. • Palms and soles usually involved. • History of herpes simplex virus infection or drug ingestion may be present.

Look-alikes *(continued)*

Disorder	Differentiating Features
Epidermolysis bullosa acquisita	• Acquired autoimmune blistering disease, not genetic. • Direct fluorescence and immunoblotting studies will help confirm diagnosis.
Linear IgA dermatosis	• Acquired autoimmune blistering disorder, not genetic • "Cluster of jewels" pattern (annular grouping of bullae) often noted • Blisters not trauma-induced • Mucosal involvement not as extensive as EB

How to Make the Diagnosis

- Skin biopsy is required to confirm the diagnosis.
- Biopsy material is sent for routine histopathology, immunomapping, and, occasionally, electron microscopy.
- Molecular analysis is available for most major subtypes of EB.
- Prenatal diagnosis is possible.

Treatment

- Treatment is palliative and supportive.
- Avoidance of trauma, treatment of infections, pain control, and nutritional counseling are all vital.
- Bullae may be drained with sterile needle and syringe for pain control.
- Antibiotic ointment and protective dressings can be applied to areas of open or blistered skin to promote healing and prevent secondary infection.
- Patient/family education, psychologic support, and referral to support group organizations are important.

Treating Associated Conditions

- Multidisciplinary treatment teams are important to decrease morbidities associated with EB.
- Care teams may include representation from primary care/pediatrics, dermatology, nursing, plastic surgery, ophthalmology, gastroenterology, general surgery, hematology, dentistry, and nutrition.
- Growth failure is treated with aggressive nutritional rehabilitation; may require gastrostomy tube placement for infants with severe forms of EB.
- Esophageal involvement with dysphagia may require dietary modifications or dilatation procedures.
- Mitten-hand deformities require physical therapy and surgical intervention (degloving procedures).

Prognosis

- Prognosis depends on the subtype of EB.
- Children with most forms of EBS, non-Herlitz JEB, and DDEB tend to have a fairly good prognosis.
- Epidermolysis bullosa simplex, Dowling-Meara , may be severe during infancy and occasionally fatal.
- Herlitz JEB and JEB with pyloric atresia have a poor prognosis.
- Patients with RDEB have a chronic course marked by complications and diminished quality of life. Squamous cell carcinoma, if it occurs, is usually rapidly progressive and invasive, leading to death in most of these patients.

When to Worry or Refer

- Patients with possible EB should be referred to an experienced dermatologist for confirmation of the diagnosis and coordination of multidisciplinary care.
- Because of the increased risk of cutaneous squamous cell carcinoma, any suspicious lesion in patients with RDEB should be biopsied.

Resources for Families

- Dystrophic Epidermolysis Bullosa Research Association (debra) of America: Provides information, support, and resources for patients who have epidermolysis bullosa and their families.
  www.debra.org
- debra UK: Located in the United Kingdom, this organization provides information for patients who have epidermolysis bullosa and their families.
  www.debra.org.uk
- Epidermolysis Bullosa Medical Research Foundation: Dedicated to supporting research in EB. Provides information for patients and families.
  www.ebkids.org

Linear IgA Dermatosis

Introduction/Etiology/Epidemiology

- Also known as chronic bullous disease of childhood
- A rare, acquired immunobullous disorder
- Most often occurs in children younger than 5 years
- Occasionally preceded by an upper respiratory illness
- Some reports of occurrence following vaccinations, although causality is not proven

Signs and Symptoms

- Vesiculobullous lesions occur on the extremities, face, and trunk.
- Bullae may form a ring around margins of an older crusted lesion, forming the "cluster of jewels" configuration (Figure 80.1).
- Pruritus tends to be mild, but pain may be significant.
- Mucous membranes may be involved.
  - Oral erosions most common type of mucous membrane involvement.
  - Eye involvement occurs less commonly.

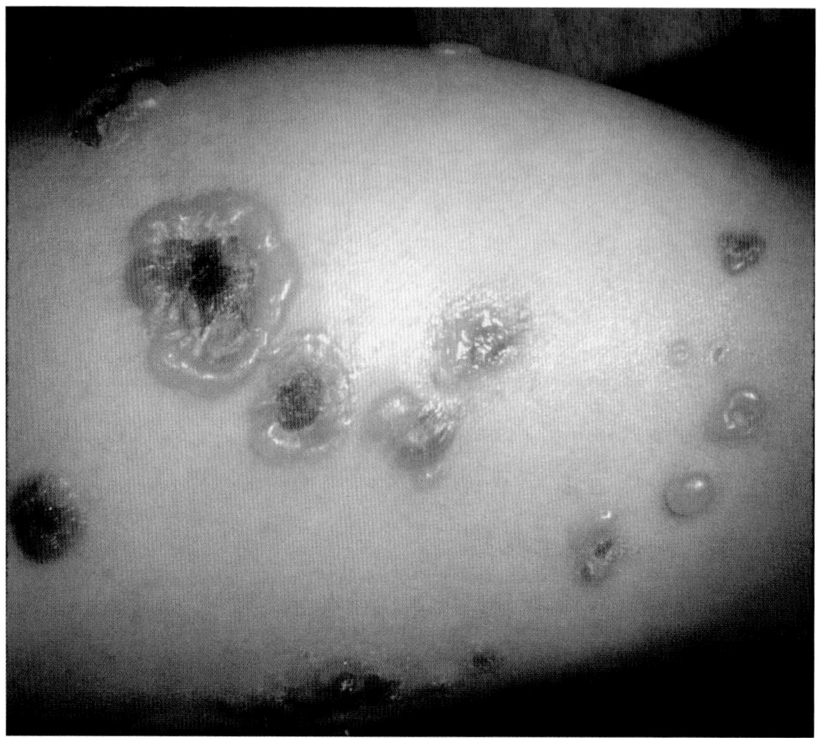

Figure 80.1. Linear IgA dermatosis lesions showing bullae surrounding a crust—the "cluster of jewels" configuration.

Look-alikes

Disorder	Differentiating Features
Bullous impetigo	• Does not usually present as a recurrent or chronic condition. • Involvement more focal. • Mucous membranes not involved. • Blisters rupture easily, leaving superficial erosions with peripheral collarettes of scale.
Herpes simplex virus infection	• Most often clustered vesicles and erosions on an erythematous base • Usually more focal
Bullous pemphigoid	• Urticarial plaques present in addition to tense blisters. • Pruritus common with early lesions. • Direct fluorescence and immunoblotting studies will help confirm diagnosis.

Look-alikes *(continued)*

Disorder	Differentiating Features
Dermatitis herpetiformis	• Usually presents as tiny vesicles and erosions. • Most often clustered on elbows, knees, shoulders, sacrum, and buttocks. • Pruritus is intense. • May be associated with gluten sensitivity.
Stevens-Johnson syndrome	• Typical target lesions may be present. • Only occasionally bullous. • Oral mucous membrane erosions common. • Palms and soles usually involved. • History of *Mycoplasma* or herpes simplex virus infection or drug ingestion may be present.
Epidermolysis bullosa	• Inherited (not acquired) mechanobullous disease. • Usually begins in neonatal period or during early infancy. • Blisters induced by trauma. • Certain subtypes may reveal nail dystrophy, milia, extensive scarring, mitten deformities of the hand. • Immunomapping of skin biopsy specimens confirms diagnosis.
Bullous lupus erythematosus	• Other features of systemic lupus erythematosus (SLE) usually present. • Concentrated in sun-exposed areas. • Antinuclear antibody (and other serologic studies) will confirm diagnosis of SLE. • Direct immunofluorescence and immunoblotting studies help confirm the diagnosis.
Epidermolysis bullosa acquisita	• Blisters induced by trauma. • Scarring common. • Direct fluorescence and immunoblotting studies will help confirm diagnosis.
Bullous insect bites	• Typically occur in the summer months. • Pruritus present. • Linear groupings of lesions may be present. • Central punctum may be visualized. • Other, more typical urticarial papules may be present.

How to Make the Diagnosis

- The diagnosis is suggested clinically and confirmed by skin biopsy.
- Histopathologic analysis reveals a subepidermal blister.
- Direct immunofluorescence examination shows a linear band of IgA along the dermal-epidermal junction.

Treatment

- After confirming normal glucose-6-phosphate dehydrogenase levels, dapsone is used initially at a dose of 0.5 to 1 mg/kg per day.
- Patients on dapsone require monitoring for decreased hemoglobin and leukopenia, as well as hepatotoxicity (rare).
- Systemic steroids may be useful during acute stage of therapy (often in conjunction with dapsone) but should not be used chronically.
- For dapsone-resistant disease, other treatment options include sulfapyridine, erythromycin, azathioprine, colchicine, mycophenolate mofetil, and intravenous Ig.

Treating Associated Conditions

- If conjunctival involvement is present, regular ophthalmologic evaluations are indicated.

Prognosis

- Most children with linear IgA dermatosis experience spontaneous remission within 5 years of onset, but treatment of the disorder can be challenging.

When to Worry or Refer

- Dermatology referral should be made early for diagnostic confirmation and initiation of therapy.

Resources for Families

- DermNet NZ: Provides information about the disease. **http://dermnetnz.org/immune/linear-iga.html**

Genodermatoses

CHAPTER

81

Ichthyosis

Introduction/Etiology/Epidemiology

- Ichthyosis refers to a large group of heterogeneous skin disorders having the common clinical feature of thick fishlike scale.
- The most common form is ichthyosis vulgaris, with an incidence of 1:250.
- The forms most likely to be encountered will be discussed here.

Signs and Symptoms

- Ichthyosis vulgaris: incidence 1:250 autosomal-dominant inheritance
  - Usually not present at birth.
  - Fine brown-gray scale most prominent on distal extremities (Figure 81.1); flexural areas are spared.
  - Striking accentuation of palmar and plantar skin creases.
  - Often accompanies atopic dermatitis.
  - Diagnosis: clinical.
  - May be associated with mutation in profilaggrin gene (*FLG*).
- X-linked recessive ichthyosis: incidence 1:2,000 to 1: 6,000
  - The molecular defect is absence of cholesterol sulfate sulfohydrolase (steroid sulfatase).
  - Female carriers have deficient placental steroid sulfatase and associated perinatal problems, including delayed onset of labor and failure to progress.
  - Often presents at birth with diffuse erythema and exfoliation.
  - "Dirty" brown fine scale that involves the flexures, preauricular areas, lateral neck, and flanks; palms and soles are spared (Figure 81.2).
  - 50% of patients and 30% of carriers have corneal opacities.
  - Patients with X-linked recessive ichthyosis have an increased incidence of cryptorchidism and may have increased risk of testicular cancer.
  - Diagnosis: clinical, enzyme assay, fluorescent in situ hybridization.

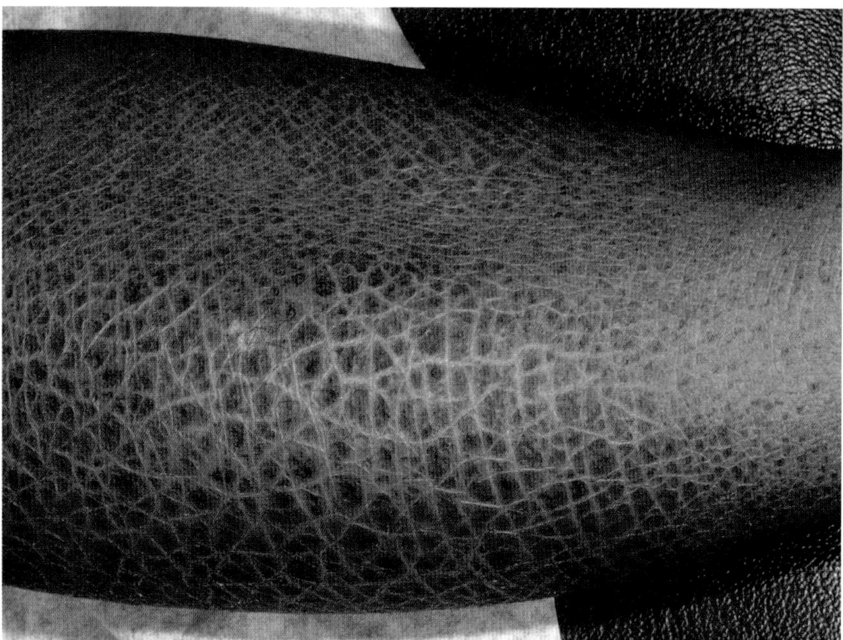

Figure 81.1. In ichthyosis vulgaris, fine scales with a "pasted on" appearance are observed on the distal extremities.

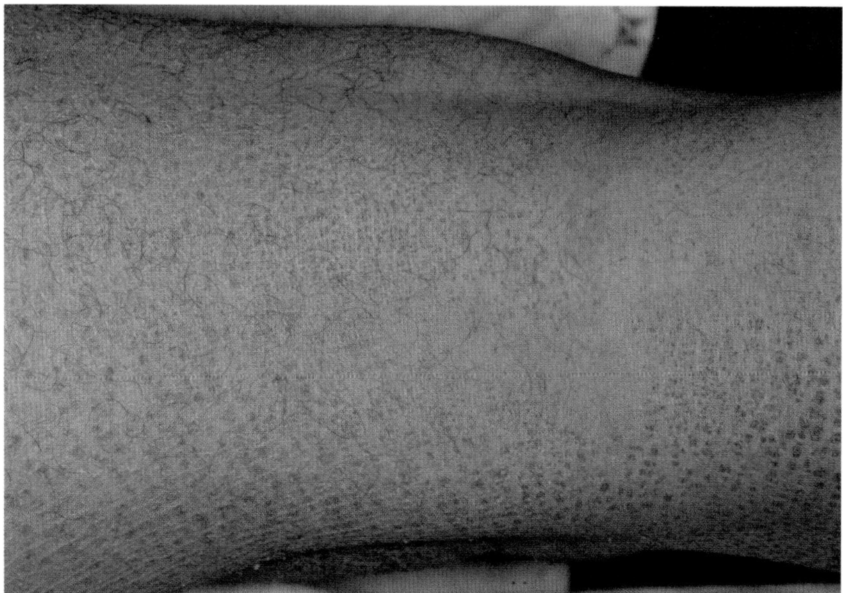

Figure 81.2. X-linked recessive ichthyosis.

- Lamellar ichthyosis: incidence 1:300,000 autosomal-recessive inheritance
  - One of the more severe ichthyoses.
  - Usually present at birth.
    - Often, the neonate is covered with a collodion membrane (Figure 81.3) and exhibits ectropion and eclabium.
    - Neonates may have increased transepidermal water loss and resulting hypernatremic dehydration.
  - Characterized by thick, platelike scale over the entire body (Figure 81.4), ectropion, eclabium, entrapment of hair, entrapment of sweat ducts (leading to hyperthermia from reduced sweating), and abnormal nails.
  - Once the lamellar scales have matured and dried, water retention (ie, sweat retention) becomes more problematic.
  - Diagnosis: clinical, histopathology, electron microscopy, molecular genetic testing.
  - Often related to mutation in transglutaminase 1.

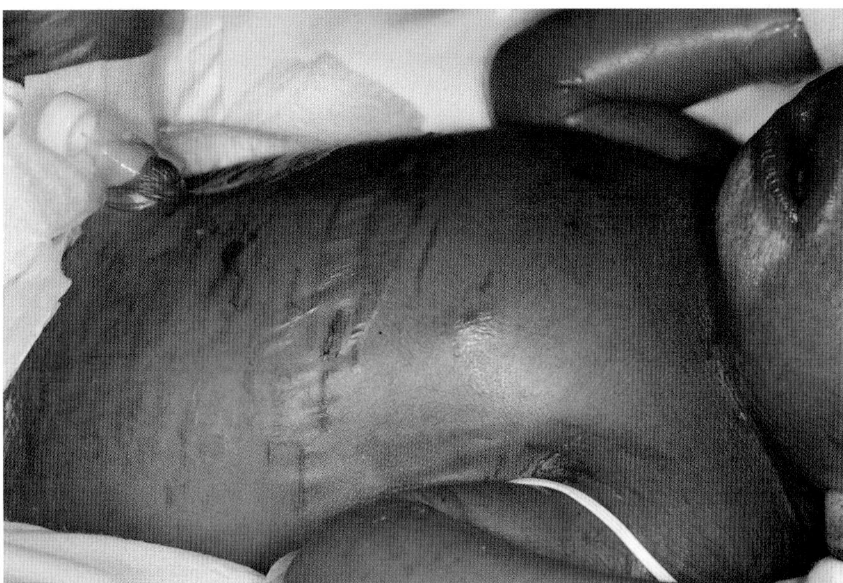

Figure 81.3. Collodion baby: this neonate is covered with a thick membrane and there is mild eclabium.

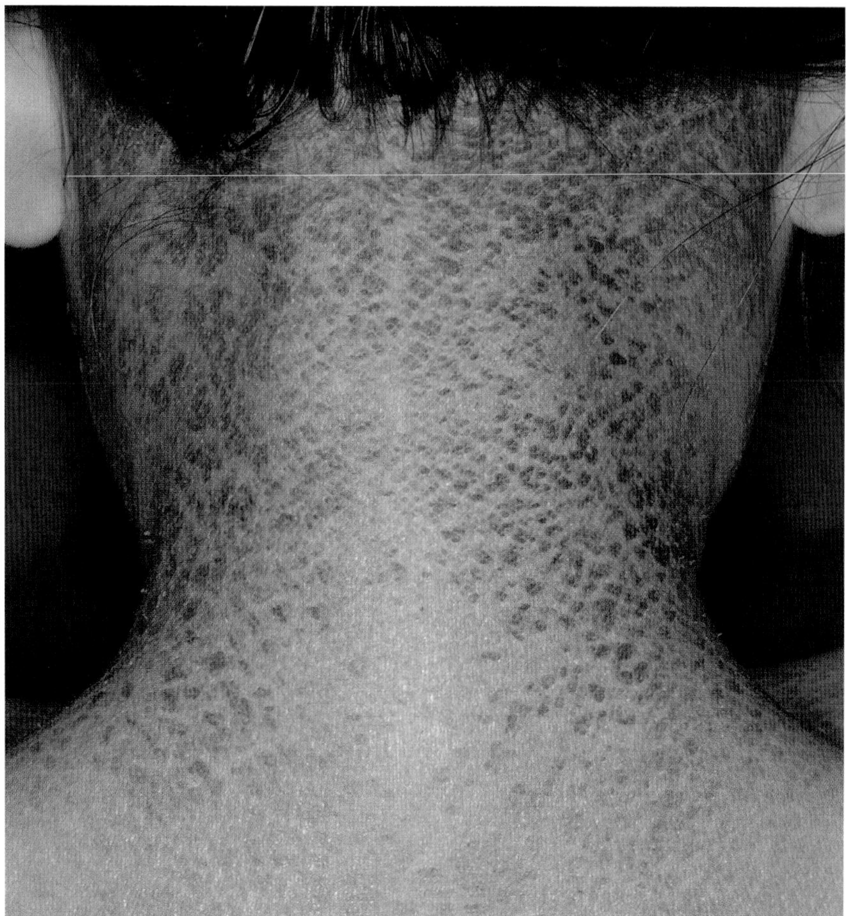

Figure 81.4. Lamellar ichthyosis is characterized by thick, platelike scales.

- Congenital ichthyosiform erythroderma (CIE): incidence 1:100,000 to 1:200,000 autosomal-recessive inheritance
  - Clinically similar to lamellar ichthyosis in onset (birth with collodion membrane), chronicity, and proclivity to encase scalp, eyelids (causing ectropion), and lips (causing eclabium).
  - Unique features of CIE are the presence of erythroderma and fine whitish scale on trunk (Figure 81.5).
  - Distal extremities, as in lamellar ichthyosis, exhibit thick, dark, large, platelike scales.
  - Some patients may improve after puberty.

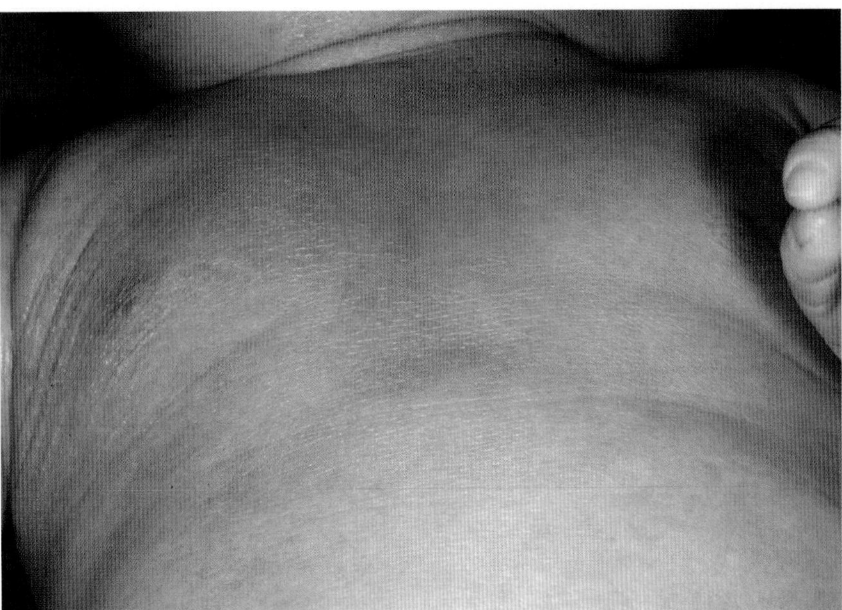

Figure 81.5. Patients who have nonbullous congenital ichthyosiform erythroderma exhibit diffuse erythema and fine scaling.

- Diagnosis: clinical, histopathology, electron microscopy, molecular genetic testing.
- May be related to mutations in transglutaminase 1, *ALOXE3,* or *ALOX12B.*

- Epidermolytic hyperkeratosis (formerly bullous congenital ichthyosiform erythroderma): incidence 1:300,000 autosomal-dominant inheritance
  - Presents as a severe blistering disease in the newborn. Sheets of epidermis are shed, leaving a widespread glistening redness of the skin (ie, erythroderma).
  - Patches of thick, dark scales develop within the first few weeks of life, especially around flexures.
    - Scales become dark, thickened, and quill-like (Figure 81.6).
    - Blistering diminishes by age 1 year, but skin remains fragile and may blister with trauma in older children.
  - Diagnosis: clinical, histopathology, molecular genetic testing.
  - Caused by mutations in keratin 1 (*KRT1*) or keratin 10 (*KRT10*) genes.

Look-alikes

The features described previously assist in differential diagnosis.

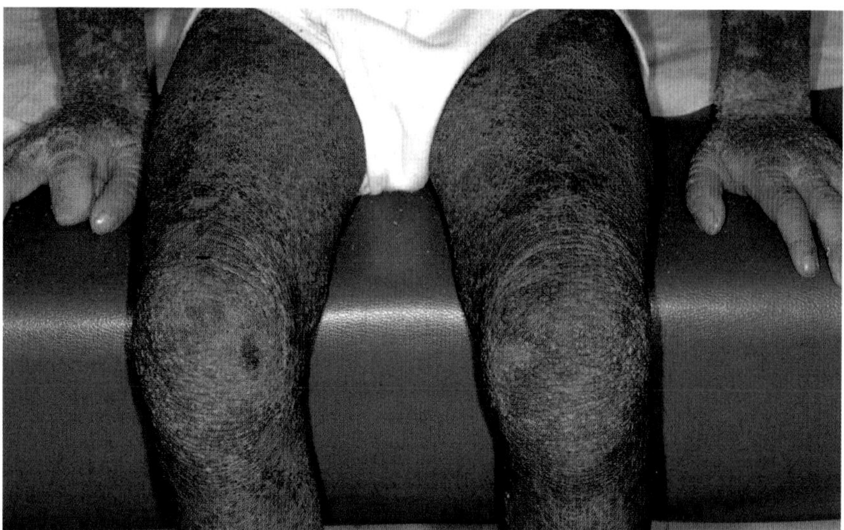

Figure 81.6. Epidermolytic hyperkeratosis. The skin takes on a cobblestone appearance on the extremities.

How to Make the Diagnosis

- Diagnosis is based on clinical features and testing for individual disorders (as discussed previously).
- Mutation analysis is available for diagnostic confirmation and prenatal testing.

Treatment

- Newborns: careful attention to the fluid and electrolyte balance, temperature, protein intake, and infection risk.
- Older children: The specific type of ichthyosis will dictate therapy. Children with types other than ichthyosis vulgaris are best managed in consultation with a pediatric dermatologist. Elements of treatment include
  - Application of an emollient
  - Application of a keratolytic (used with caution if the skin surface is compromised due to concerns about systemic absorption)
  - Preservation of range of motion when thick scale surrounds joints
  - Use of systemic retinoids for severe cases

Treating Associated Conditions

- Ichthyosis may be the cutaneous manifestation of a variety of other disorders. Consider this possibility if the patient exhibits abnormalities of the central nervous, cardiovascular, or skeletal systems or if the patient has hepatomegaly or experiences metabolic disturbances.

Prognosis

- Prognosis depends on the type of ichthyosis. The prognosis is excellent for ichthyosis vulgaris; those with more severe forms will experience lifelong difficulties with dry skin and thick scale.

When to Worry or Refer

- Severe platelike scale, ectropion, metabolic disturbance, and other anomalies

Resources for Families

- Foundation for Ichthyosis & Related Skin Types: Provides information and support for patients and families, as well as links to health care professionals. **www.firstskinfoundation.org**

CHAPTER
82

Incontinentia Pigmenti

Introduction/Etiology/Epidemiology

- X-linked dominant disorder that is usually lethal in male embryos (although rare cases may result from mosaicism or XXY genotype)
- Due to a mutation in the nuclear factor-kB essential modulator (*NEMO*) gene

Signs and Symptoms

- Four stages are recognized.
  - Stage 1
    - Often presents at birth with vesicles on erythematous bases distributed in a linear arrangement on limbs or in a whorled pattern on the trunk (conforming to Blaschko lines) (Figure 82.1).
    - Vesicles occur in crops for weeks to months.
  - Stage 2
    - Begins at about 1 month of age and consists of warty, red-brown papules with scale (Figure 82.2)
    - Typically resolves by 4 to 6 months of age
  - Stage 3
    - Linear and swirled hyperpigmentation (along Blaschko lines) (Figure 82.3)
    - May persist for years
  - Stage 4
    - Hypopigmented atrophic streaks (Figure 82.4)
    - Follicular atrophoderma
    - Observed in some patients
- Important to recognize that not all stages may present clinically and there may be overlap between stages.
- Other clinical features include alopecia, dystrophic nails, pegged teeth (common), ocular abnormalities (vascular abnormalities that may threaten vision, optic atrophy, microphthalmos, cataracts, myopia; strabismus may be seen as a late complication as a result of prolonged sensory deprivation), and central nervous system anomalies (seizures, developmental delay).

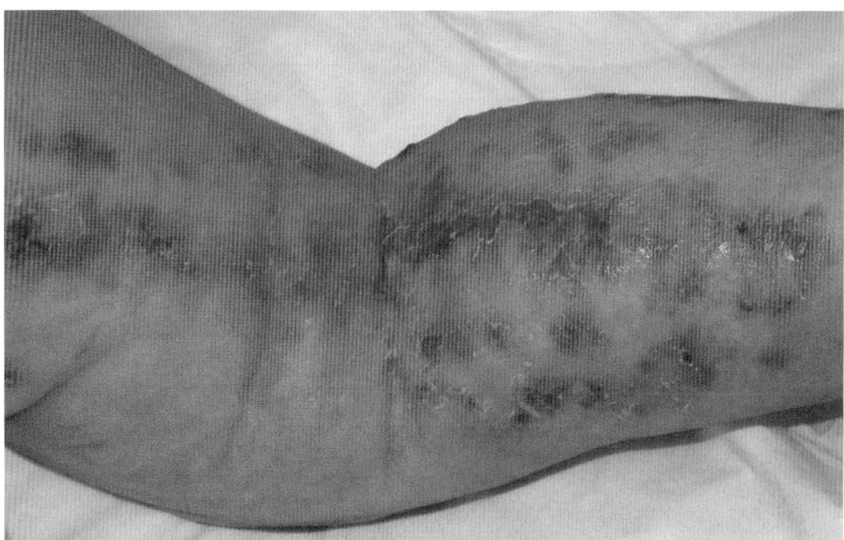

Figure 82.1. In the first stage of incontinentia pigmenti, vesicles and crusting appear in a linear arrangement on the limbs or in a whorled distribution on the trunk.

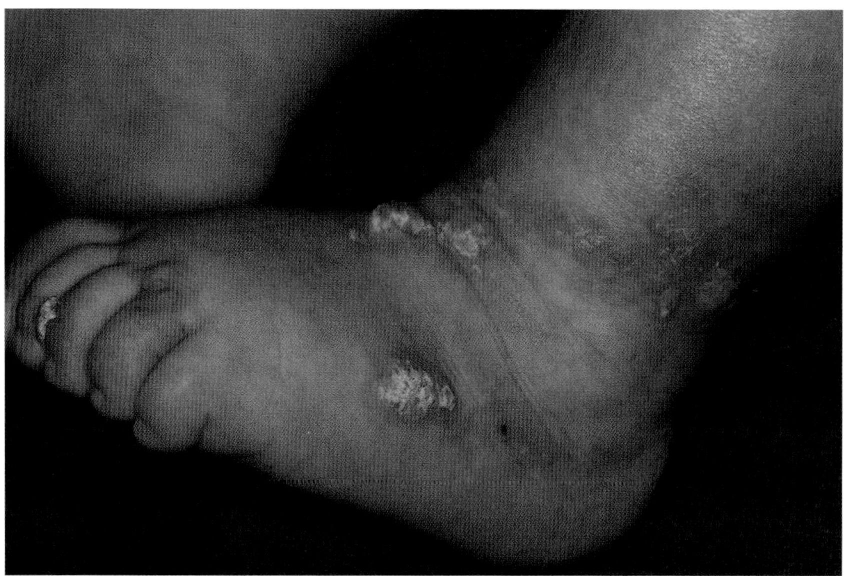

Figure 82.2. Warty papules in this infant, who has the second stage of incontinentia pigmenti.

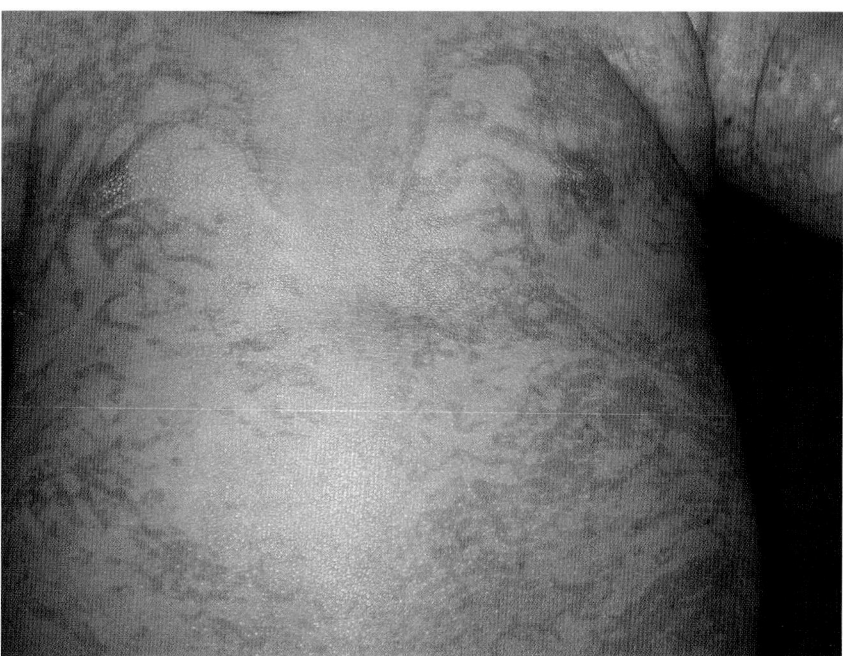

Figure 82.3. Whorled and linear hyperpigmentation, arranged along the lines of Blaschko, are observed in the third stage of incontinentia pigmenti.

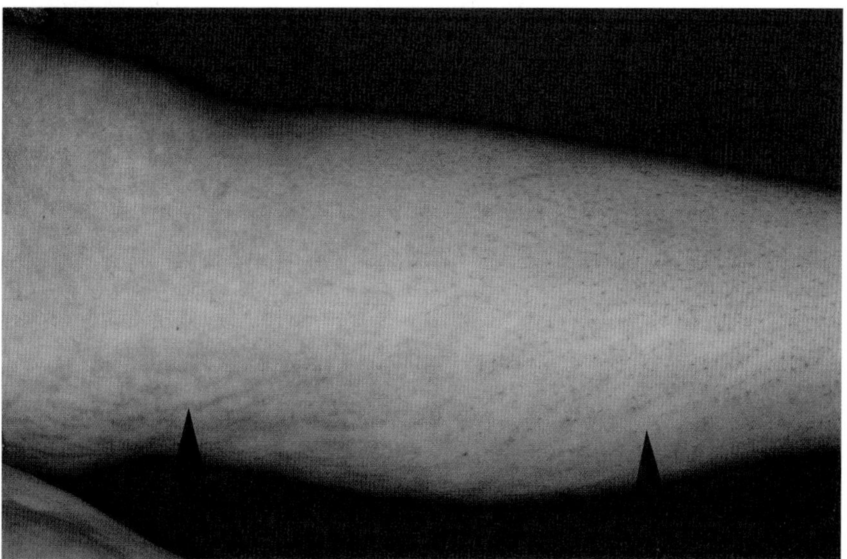

Figure 82.4. Hypopigmented atrophic streaks (arrows) are observed in the fourth stage of incontinentia pigmenti.

Look-alikes

The differential diagnosis of vesicles appearing in the neonatal period is presented here (in descending order of frequency of occurrence). In none of these disorders are vesicles distributed in a linear or whorled pattern as they are in incontinentia pigmenti.

Disorder	Differentiating Features
Erythema toxicum	• Individual vesicles or pustules on erythematous bases
Miliaria crystallina	• Fragile vesicles without surrounding erythema
Bullous impetigo	• Flaccid bullae or ruptured bullae forming round or oval crusted erosions; vesicles occasionally are present. • Gram stain or bacterial culture will reveal *Staphylococcus aureus.*
Scabies	• Occurs rarely during the first month of life • Generalized eruption; may have vesicles but usually will be accompanied by erythematous papules or nodules and burrows • Palm and sole involvement common
Neonatal herpes simplex virus infection	• Typically, clustered vesicles on an erythematous base (although solitary vesicles occasionally occur). • Vesicles concentrated on head, particularly at sites of trauma (eg, that caused by a scalp electrode). • Infants may have signs of sepsis (in disseminated disease) or seizures or coma (in central nervous system disease).
Infantile acropustulosis	• Usually begins in first months of life (not in first days) • Recurrent vesicles or pustules that are limited to the hands and feet, including palms, soles, wrists, and ankles
Eosinophilic pustular folliculitis	• Papules and pustules typically located on scalp • Marked pruritus present • Exhibits chronic, intermittent course

How to Make the Diagnosis

- Diagnosis is made clinically based on the appearance and distribution (ie, linear and whorled) of lesions and confirmed with skin biopsy.
- Exclude other diagnoses of importance (eg, herpes simplex virus infection, impetigo).
- Skin biopsy can be used to confirm the diagnosis (during stage 1) when necessary.
- Mutation analysis is available for diagnostic confirmation.

Treatment

- Infants in the vesicular stage should be treated with a topical antibiotic ointment applied to open areas to prevent secondary bacterial infection.
- Warty stage lesions may improve temporarily with application of keratolytic agents containing urea or salicylic acid.
  - Beware of the increased percutaneous absorption of these agents, which might lead to systemic toxicity.
  - Application of an emollient to the warty lesions may suffice, as they eventually resolve spontaneously.
- Pediatric ophthalmologic consultation should be obtained as soon after birth as possible, with close follow-up during the first 3 years.
- Male patients should have a karyotype performed, and genetics consultation should be considered.
- Early dental evaluation is recommended with appropriate follow-up.
- Additional evaluation should be based on observation of other features, such as seizures, developmental delay, or skeletal anomalies.

Treating Associated Conditions

- Neurodevelopmental, ocular, skeletal, and dental problems should be addressed as they develop.

Prognosis

- Prognosis is generally excellent but is influenced by involvement of other areas, particularly the central nervous system.

When to Worry or Refer

- Refer all patients for dental and ophthalmologic evaluation.
- Refer to neurology, genetics, or orthopedic surgery if clinically indicated.

Resources for Families

- Incontinentia Pigmenti International Foundation: Provides information about incontinentia pigmenti and links to support groups.
  www.ipif.org
- National Institute of Neurological Disorders and Stroke: Provides information about incontinentia pigmenti and links to relevant organizations.
  www.ninds.nih.gov/disorders/incontinentia_pigmenti/incontinentia_pigmenti.htm

CHAPTER 83

Neurofibromatosis (NF)

Introduction/Etiology/Epidemiology

- Neurofibromatosis (NF) is a cluster of syndromes sharing common features.
  - Neurofibromatosis type 1 is transmitted as an autosomal-dominant trait (50%) or occurs as a spontaneous mutation (50%). The gene responsible is located on chromosome 17 and encodes the protein neurofibromin.
  - Inheritance of NF2 is autosomal dominant, with 50% spontaneous new mutations. The gene responsible for NF2 is located on the long arm of chromosome 22 and encodes the protein merlin.

Signs and Symptoms

- Neurofibromatosis 1
  - 2 or more of the following clinical features are necessary for the diagnosis of NF1:
    - Café au lait macules (Figure 83.1).
      - 6 or more measuring more than 0.5 cm in infants and children or more than 1.5 cm in postpubertal individuals. (Nearly 90% of children who have ≥6 café au lait macules ultimately will be diagnosed as having NF1.)
      - Nearly all patients who have NF1 meet this criterion.

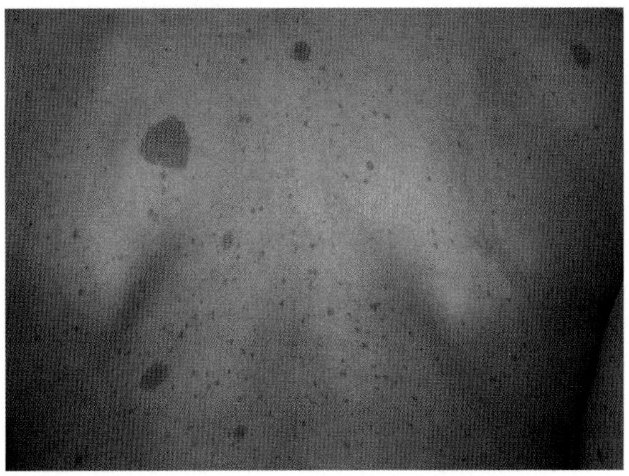

Figure 83.1. Multiple café au lait macules in a patient who has neurofibromatosis type 1.

- 2 or more neurofibromas of any type (Figure 83.2) or 1 or more plexiform neurofibroma (Figure 83.3).
- Axillary or inguinal freckling (Figure 83.4); occurs in 90% of patients.
- Optic glioma.
- 2 or more Lisch nodules (iris hamartomas); these are rarely seen prior to 3 years of age (Figure 83.5).
- Characteristic osseous lesion (eg, dysplasia of the sphenoid bone or dysplasia or thinning of long bone cortex).
- First-degree relative with a diagnosis of NF1.

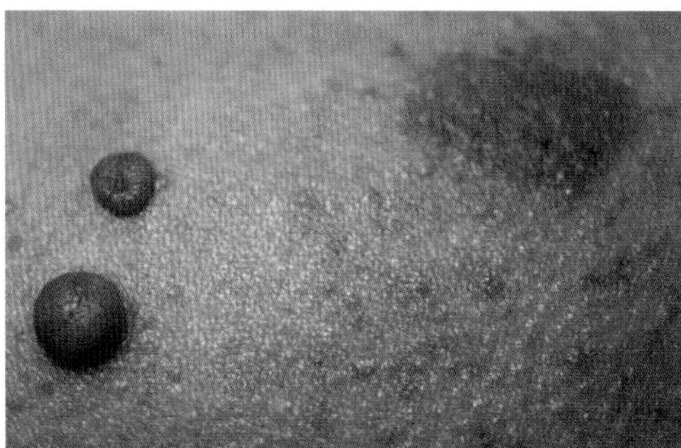

Figure 83.2. Neurofibromas and a café au lait macule in a patient who has neurofibromatosis type 1.

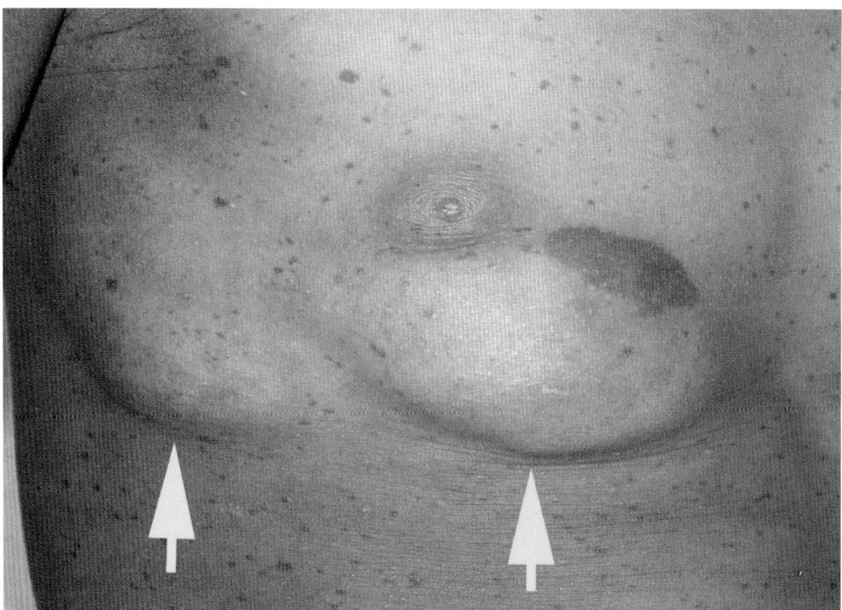

Figure 83.3. Plexiform neurofibromas (large, subcutaneous masses, arrows) in a patient who has neurofibromatosis type 1.

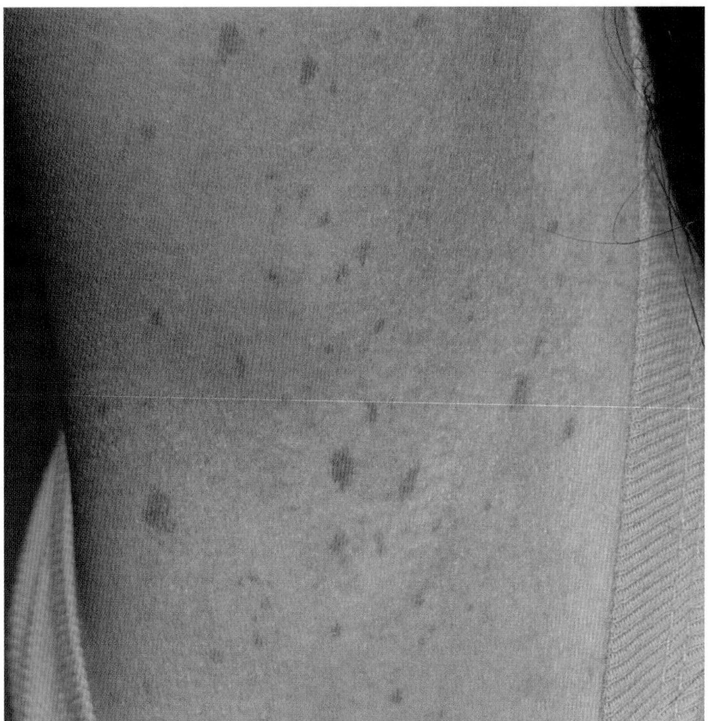

Figure 83.4. Axillary freckling in a patient who has neurofibromatosis type 1.

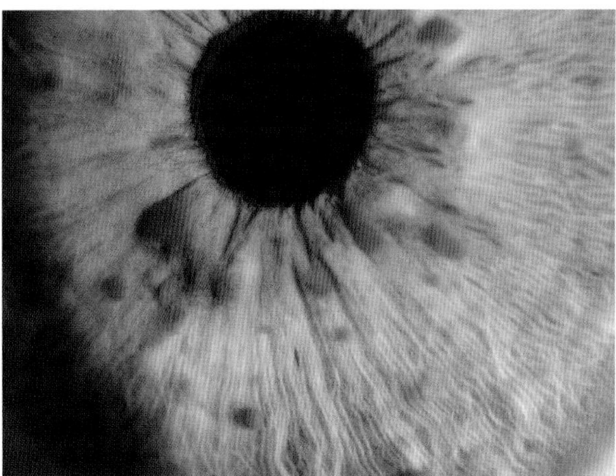

Figure 83.5. Lisch nodules, iris hamartomas, are observed in patients who have neurofibromatosis type 1.

- Other common features observed in patients who have NF1 include
  - Macrocephaly (independent of tumors or severity).
  - Short stature.
  - Precocious puberty.
  - Scoliosis.
  - Hypertension (may be due to renal artery stenosis or pheochromocytoma).
  - Learning disabilities observed in as many as 40% of children; attention-deficit/hyperactivity disorder (ADHD) and autism spectrum disorder also may occur.
  - Intellectual disability seen in approximately 5% of patients.
  - Seizure disorders occur in as many as 7% of individuals.

- Neurofibromatosis 2 (bilateral acoustic neuroma syndrome)
  - Diagnosis requires the presence of one of the following:
    - Bilateral vestibular schwannomas
    - Affected first-degree relative with NF2 AND
      - Unilateral vestibular schwannoma OR
      - Any 2 of meningioma, schwannoma, glioma, neurofibroma, or posterior subcapsular lenticular opacities
    - Unilateral vestibular schwannoma AND any 2 of meningioma, schwannoma, glioma, neurofibroma, or posterior subcapsular lenticular opacities
    - Multiple meningiomas AND
      - Unilateral vestibular schwannoma OR
      - Any 2 of schwannoma, glioma, neurofibroma, or cataract
  - Other features include
    - Fewer cutaneous neurofibromas than in patients who have NF1
    - Small numbers of large pale café au lait macules

Look-alikes

The constellation of features observed in patients who have NF1 generally suggests the diagnosis and excludes other disorders. Some diseases characterized by multiple café au lait macules are presented as follows.

Disorder	Differentiating Features
McCune-Albright syndrome	• Large segmental café au lait macule(s) • Bony abnormalities (eg, polyostotic fibrous dysplasia) • Endocrine abnormalities
Silver-Russell syndrome	• Triangular face • Short stature • Skeletal asymmetry • Abnormal pubertal development
Bloom syndrome	• Short stature • Facial telangiectasias and erythema • Narrow face, prominent nose and ears
Watson syndrome	• Mental retardation, pulmonary stenosis, axillary freckling
Multiple café au lait macules without NF	• Multiple café au lait macules without other features of NF1 (Some of these patients may have Legius syndrome, characterized by multiple café au lait macules and, in some cases, intertriginous freckling, lipomas, macrocephaly, learning disabilities, ADHD, and developmental delay.)

How to Make the Diagnosis

- The diagnosis of NF1 or NF2 is usually made clinically, satisfying the criteria listed previously. Molecular genetic testing is available for NF1 and NF2 and may be used to confirm a clinical diagnosis or evaluate a patient in whom diagnostic uncertainty exists. It may also be used in counseling affected individuals who are planning a pregnancy or in prenatal diagnosis once pregnant.

Treatment

- There is no specific therapy for NF1. Management is directed primarily at identifying and treating complications. Those providing health care for patients who have NF1 should consult the American Academy of Pediatrics policy statement, "Health Supervision for Children With Neurofibromatosis" (*Pediatrics.* 2008;121[3]:633–642). Elements of surveillance include
  - Genetic evaluation.
  - At all health maintenance visits monitor growth, head circumference, and blood pressure; perform a complete examination concentrating on cutaneous, ophthalmologic, neurologic, and skeletal systems; and assess development and behavior, vision, and hearing.
  - Head magnetic resonance imaging (MRI): The role of this procedure (eg, to determine if an optic glioma is present) in asymptomatic individuals is controversial.
- There is no specific therapy for NF2. Management should include
  - Genetic evaluation
  - Surveillance for vestibular schwannomas by MRI, audiometry, or auditory brain stem–evoked response

Treating Associated Conditions

- Neurofibromatosis 1: Learning disabilities, optic gliomas, plexiform neurofibromas, and other complications should be addressed if they develop.
- Neurofibromatosis 2: Vestibular schwannomas or hearing loss should be addressed if present.

Prognosis

- The prognosis for NF is variable, depending on the severity of involvement and development of malignancy.
- The spectrum of severity ranges from individuals with minimal effect on quality of life to those with profound effect or who require multiple procedures and coordinated multispecialty care.

When to Worry or Refer

- Neurofibromatosis 1: development of pain in or sudden growth of a plexiform neurofibroma; sudden changes in visual acuity; development of headache, hypertension, scoliosis, or abnormalities of long bones.
- Neurofibromatosis 2: development of hearing loss, tinnitus, difficulties with balance, headache, or other signs of increased intracranial pressure.
- Subspecialties that may be involved in the care of patients with NF include genetics, neurology, ophthalmology, surgery (orthopedic, general, plastic), dermatology, otolaryngology, and oncology.

Resources for Families

- Children's Tumor Foundation: Education and links to support and physicians for patients who have neurofibromatosis and their families.
  www.ctf.org
- Neurofibromatosis Network: Provides support and information for patients and families.
  www.nfnetwork.org
- Neurofibromatosis Clinical Trials Consortium: Information about ongoing clinical trials and links to 13 NF clinical centers.
  www.uab.edu/nfconsortium

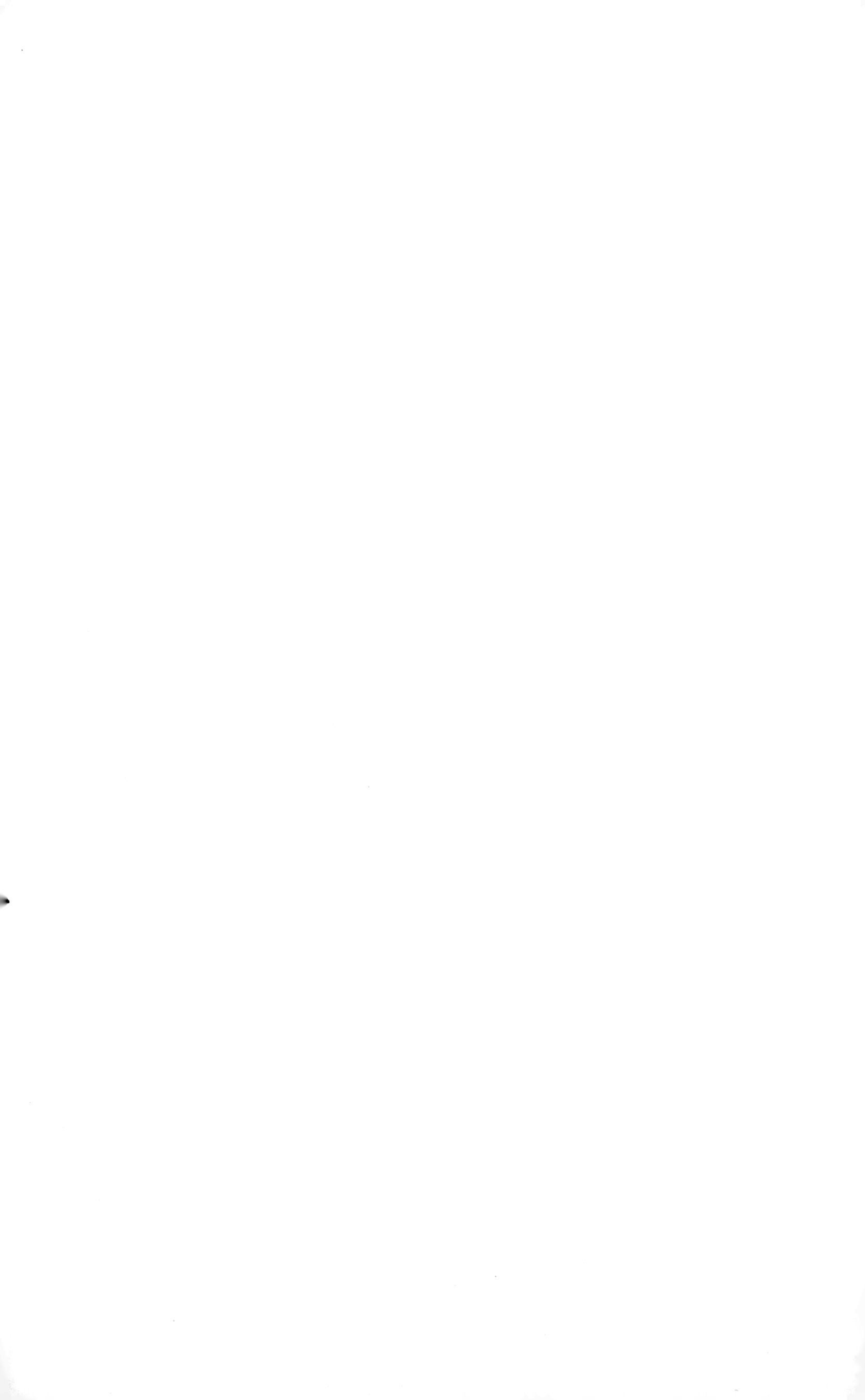

CHAPTER

84

Tuberous Sclerosis Complex (TSC)

Introduction/Etiology/Epidemiology

- Tuberous sclerosis complex (TSC) is a neurocutaneous syndrome with highly variable features.
- Tuberous sclerosis complex is caused by mutations in 2 genes: *TSC1* on chromosome 9 (encoding hamartin) and *TSC2* on chromosome 16 (encoding tuberin).
- The disorder is transmitted as an autosomal-dominant trait with high penetrance but markedly variable expressivity; two-thirds of cases represent new mutations.

Signs and Symptoms

Tuberous sclerosis complex involves abnormalities of the following systems:

- Skin
  - Hypomelanotic macules (ie, ash leaf macules): present at birth or soon thereafter; occur in 87% to 100% of patients (Figure 84.1)
  - Facial angiofibromas (ie, adenoma sebaceum)
    - Erythematous papules located in the nasolabial folds, nose, cheeks, or chin (Figure 84.2)
    - Appear between 2 and 6 years of age; occur in 47% to 90% of patients
  - Shagreen patches: plaques with a peau d'orange texture usually observed in the lumbosacral region (Figure 84.3); occur in 20% to 80% of patients
  - Fibrous facial plaques: connective tissue nevi that may be present at birth
  - Ungual fibromas: usually appear after puberty; observed in 17% to 80% of patients (Figure 84.4)
- Brain: subependymal nodules (90%), seizures (80%), cortical tubers (70%), mental retardation/developmental delay (50%), autism spectrum disorder (16%–61%)
- Kidney: angiomyolipomas (70%), cysts

- Heart: rhabdomyomas (47%–67%), arrhythmias
- Eye: astrocytic hamartoma of the retina, optic disc, or both (up to 50% of patients)
- Lungs: lymphangioleiomyomatosis (LAM) (30% of women)

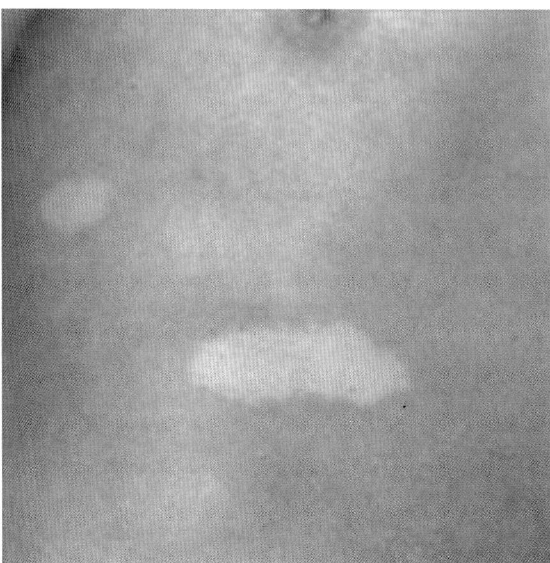

Figure 84.1. Ash leaf macules on the chest of a child who has tuberous sclerosis complex.

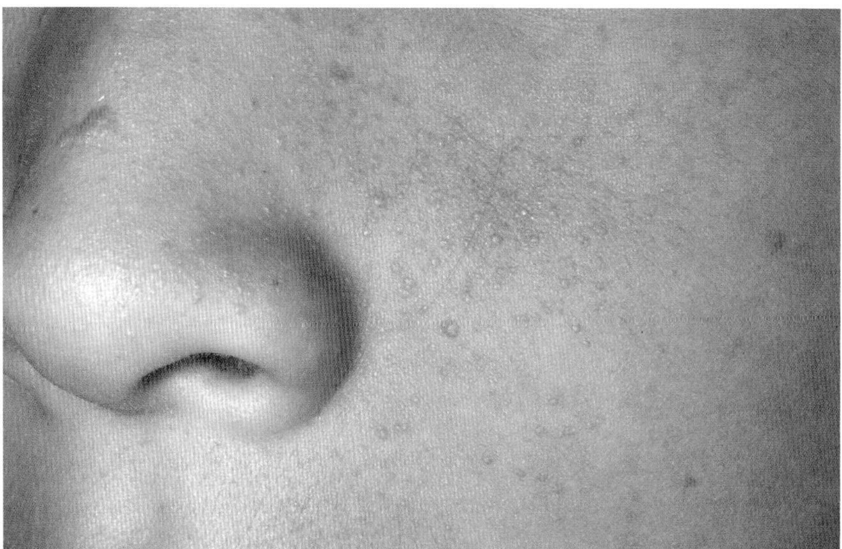

Figure 84.2. Facial angiofibromas are pink papules that may mimic the lesions of acne.

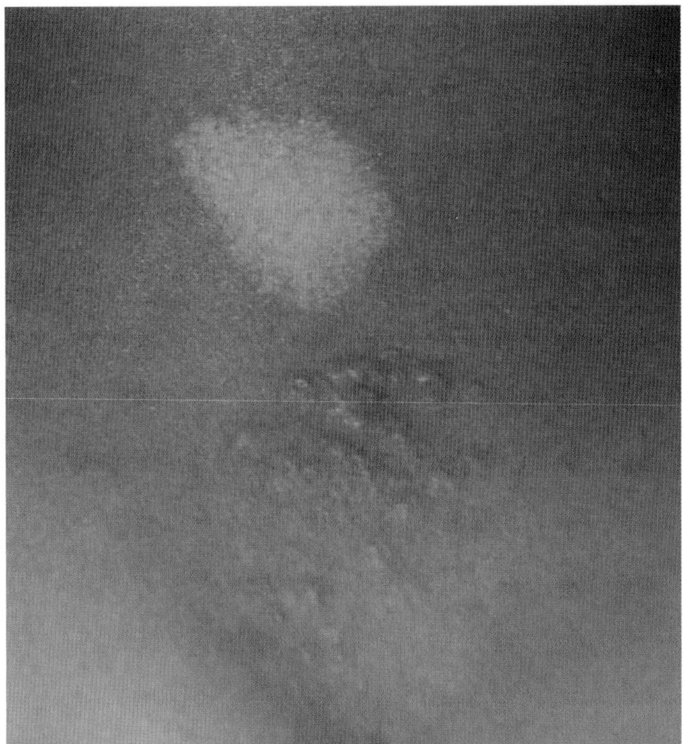

Figure 84.3. Shagreen patches have an orange-peel or cobblestone texture and often are located over the lumbosacral spine. This patient also has a hypomelanotic patch.

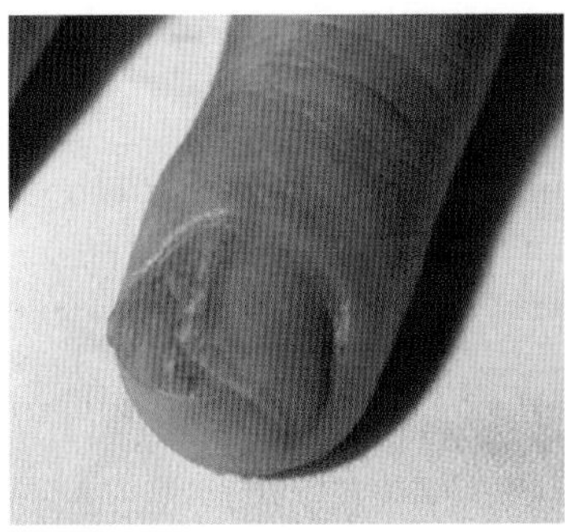

Figure 84.4. Ungual fibromas usually appear after puberty in patients who have tuberous sclerosis complex.

Look-alikes

The constellation of clinical findings suggests the diagnosis of TSC and excludes other disorders. The differential diagnosis of ash leaf macules and angiofibromas is presented here; however, in each of the conditions listed, other features of TSC would be absent.

Disorder	Differentiating Features
Ash Leaf Macules	
Vitiligo	• Acquired disorder. • Affected areas exhibit complete pigment loss (ie, depigmentation), not hypopigmentation. • Predilection for elbows, knees, ankles, hips, fingers, and periorificial regions.
Pityriasis alba	• Acquired disorder • Poorly defined areas of macular hypopigmentation often with associated scale • Atopic history common
Tinea versicolor	• Acquired disorder. • Seen mainly in postpubertal individuals. • Well-defined hypopigmented macules and patches located on the trunk, upper arms, or neck. • Lesions often have associated fine scale and may be pruritic.
Pigmentary mosaicism–nevus depigmentosus type	• Present at birth but may not become noticeable for months to years • Hypopigmentation with a shaggy border • Usually occurs unilaterally and respects the midline • Typically larger than an ash leaf macule • Geographic or segmental distribution common
Pigmentary mosaicism–hypomelanosis of Ito type	• Present at birth but may not become noticeable for months to years • Hypopigmentation that follows the lines of Blaschko (lines representing patterns of embryonic cell migration from the neural crest); presents as streaky lines on the extremities and whorls on the trunk
Piebaldism	• Congenital absence of pigmentation localized to one area. • Associated poliosis (depigmentation of hair) may be present when involving face/scalp. • Rare associations with other abnormalities (eg, Waardenburg syndrome).
Nevus anemicus	• Congenital area of pallor (may resemble hypopigmentation) resulting from diminished vascular flow to the affected region. • Diascopy (compressing the lesion with a glass slide) will cause blanching of surrounding normal skin, causing border of the lesion to disappear.

Angiofibromas	
Acne	• Often appears later than angiofibromas • Comedones (ie, blackheads and whiteheads) and pustules usually present • Involvement of forehead, chest, shoulders, and back common • Early acne usually limited to "T-zone" (forehead, middle face/chin, nose)
Molluscum contagiosum	• Usually translucent papules that may have a central umbilication • Usually not symmetrically distributed and may be present at other (non-facial) sites
Periorificial dermatitis	• Typically exhibits small pustules and acneiform papules. • Erythema and scaling may be present, especially in nasolabial folds. • Concentrated in perioral, perinasal, and periorbital regions.
Keratosis pilaris	• Small, rough-feeling (sandpaper), skin-colored or erythematous papules. • Keratin plug emerging from follicular orifice may be observed or palpated. • Often located at other sites (eg, upper arms, thighs, buttocks).

How to Make the Diagnosis

- Definite TSC requires the presence of 2 major features or 1 major and 2 or more minor features.
- Possible TSC requires the presence of 1 major feature or 2 or more minor features.
- Mutation analysis is available for diagnostic confirmation and prenatal diagnosis.

Major Features

- 3 or more hypomelanotic macules (at least 5 mm in diameter)
- Facial angiofibromas (≥3) or forehead plaques
- Nontraumatic ungual fibroma (≥2)
- Shagreen patch (connective tissue nevus)
- Multiple retinal hamartomas
- Cortical dysplasias (includes tubers and cerebral white matter radial migration lines)
- Subependymal nodule

- Subependymal giant cell astrocytoma
- Cardiac rhabdomyoma
- Lymphangioleiomyomatosis
- Angiomyolipoma (≥2)

Minor Features

- "Confetti" hypopigmented macules
- Dental enamel pits (≥3)
- Intraoral fibromas (≥2)
- Retinal achromic patch
- Multiple renal cysts
- Nonrenal hamartoma

Treatment

- Prompt diagnosis, treatment of the seizure disorder, surveillance for additional features and complications, and genetic counseling form the fundamental approach to management.
- Multidisciplinary care is vital; subspecialties which may be involved in TSC patient care include genetics, neurology, ophthalmology, dermatology, nephrology, cardiology, oncology, pulmonology, orthopedic surgery, and dentistry.
- Essential studies if considering the diagnosis include brain magnetic resonance imaging (MRI), neurodevelopmental testing, ophthalmologic evaluation, electrocardiography, echocardiography, and abdominal MRI (preferred over renal ultrasonography). For additional information, consult Krueger and Northrup (*Pediatr Neurol.* 2013;49[4]:255–265).
- Several clinical trials are underway investigating the use of topical or systemic inhibitors of mammalian target of rapamycin (mTOR) for various manifestations of TSC.
  - Everolimus has been approved for use in the treatment of subependymal giant cell astrocytoma associated with TSC.
  - mTOR inhibitors are used to treat growing renal angiomyolipoma and severe lung disease caused by LAM.
  - Topical mTOR inhibitors (especially sirolimus [rapamycin]) are being used to treat facial angiofibromas.

Treating Associated Conditions

- Complete evaluation, as noted previously, should identify most of the associated problems; these should be managed appropriately.
- Brain MRI should be repeated every 1 to 3 years through adolescence.
- Abdominal MRI (preferred over renal ultrasonography) should be performed every 1 to 3 years.
- Chest computed tomography should be performed if pulmonary symptoms are present (particularly in adult women to assess for pulmonary LAM).

Prognosis

Prognosis depends on

- The extent of neurologic involvement and the development of central nervous system complications. (Central nervous system tumors are the leading cause of morbidity and mortality.)
- Complications in other organ systems
  - Renal: second leading cause of early death in patients who have TSC
  - Cardiovascular: rhabdomyomas (often regress spontaneously), cardiac arrhythmias
  - Pulmonary: pulmonary lymphangiomyomatosis (usually affects adult women)

When to Worry or Refer

- Presence of brain, cardiac, renal, or pulmonary tumors.
- Consider referral for neurodevelopmental testing.

Resources for Families

- National Institute of Neurological Disorders and Stroke: Provides information about tuberous sclerosis and links to organizations providing support.
  www.ninds.nih.gov/disorders/tuberous_sclerosis/tuberous_sclerosis.htm
- Tuberous Sclerosis Alliance: Provides support and information (in English and Spanish) for affected patients and their families. The organization also maintains a list of TSC clinics in the United States.
  www.tsalliance.org
- Tuberous Sclerosis Association: A site in the United Kingdom that provides information for patients and medical providers.
  www.tuberous-sclerosis.org
- National Institutes of Health: Clinical trials site has information on clinical studies for TSC.
  www.nih.gov/health/clinicaltrials/CTgovSearchTips.htm

Hair Disorders

CHAPTER 85

Alopecia Areata

Introduction/Etiology/Epidemiology

- Alopecia areata is a common cause of non-scarring hair loss (alopecia) in children and adults.
- Prevalence is estimated at approximately 0.2% of the population, and lifetime risk is believed to be between 1% and 2%.
- Genetic and environmental factors may be important; approximately 1 in 5 patients has an affected family member. Recent studies have identified nucleotide polymorphisms that appear to be associated with alopecia areata.
- Believed to be an organ-specific autoimmune disease; melanocyte peptides are the suspected antigen.
- Patients may be more frequently affected by atopic diseases such as asthma, allergic rhinitis, and atopic dermatitis.
- May be associated with other autoimmune/systemic disorders, including thyroid disease, vitiligo, diabetes, systemic lupus erythematosus, and inflammatory bowel disease; risk of potential associations remains unclear and controversial.
- Also rarely reported in association with HIV and other immunodeficiency diseases.

Signs and Symptoms

- Most patients have a history of asymptomatic sudden hair loss, which is often rapidly progressive.
- The affected scalp usually has round to oval, smooth, well-circumscribed patches of complete hair loss (Figure 85.1).
- Alopecia may range from a small solitary patch to many patches of variable size (Figure 85.2).

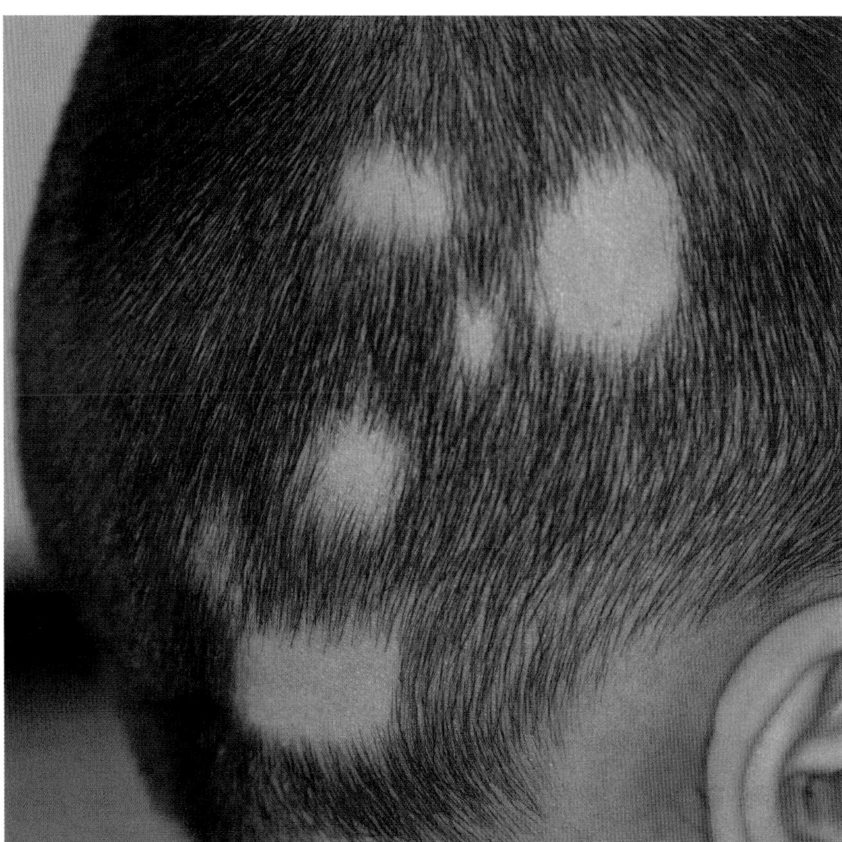

Figure 85.1. Smooth, well-defined patches of complete hair loss in a child with alopecia areata.

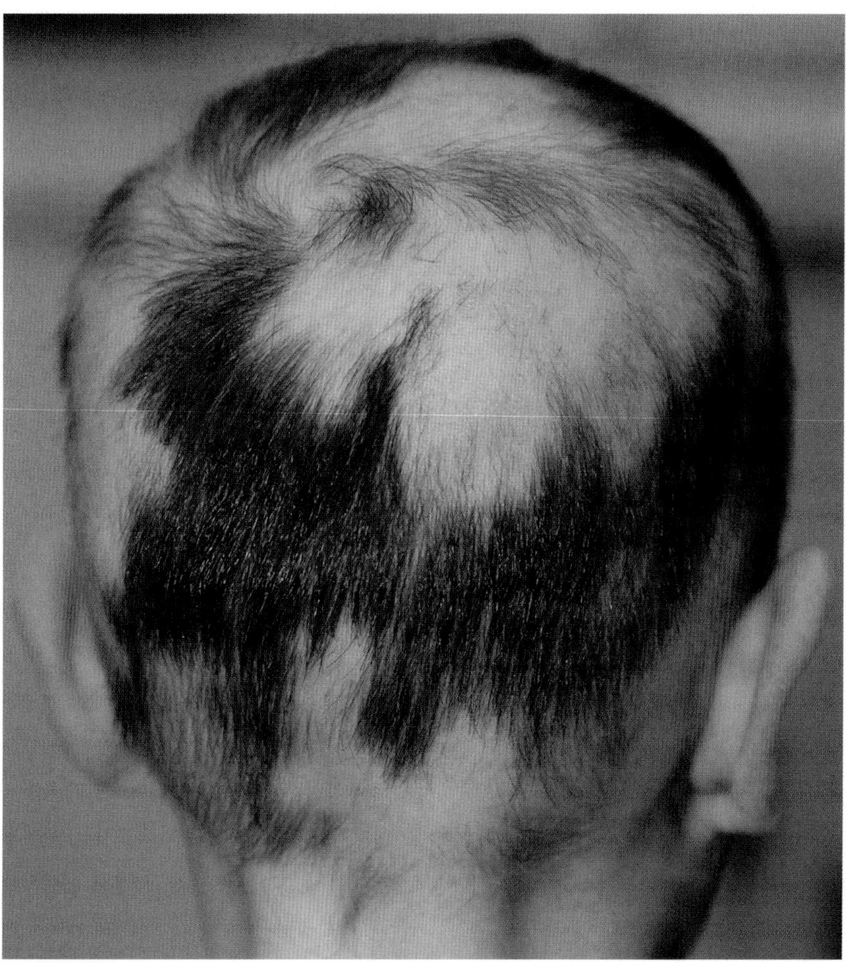

Figure 85.2. Extensive patchy hair loss in a child with alopecia areata.

- Less commonly, a patient may present with an *ophiasis* distribution in which there is circumferential hair loss extending around the temporal and occipital hairlines; this form has a poorer prognosis.
- Occasionally, the condition can progress to complete loss of all scalp hair (*alopecia totalis*) (Figure 85.3) or complete alopecia of all hair-bearing surfaces, including lashes, brows (Figure 85.4), and body hair (*alopecia universalis*).
- Rarely, alopecia areata may present with diffuse hair thinning that may resemble telogen effluvium.
- Usually, there are no associated scalp findings of scale or inflammation, although histologically, there is evidence of a perifollicular lymphocytic infiltration.
- In some patients, finding of exclamation point hairs (short hairs that taper proximally and are thicker distally) can further support the diagnosis.
- Dermoscopy (magnified light examination) reveals tapered hairs and yellow perifollicular dots; this modality may be used by dermatologists if the diagnosis is in question.
- Nail changes (not specific for alopecia areata) include
  - Multiple small pits (often linear) (Figure 85.5)
  - Trachyonychia (thin nails with a diffuse sandpaper-like texture)
  - Separation of the nail plate from the nail bed (onycholysis)

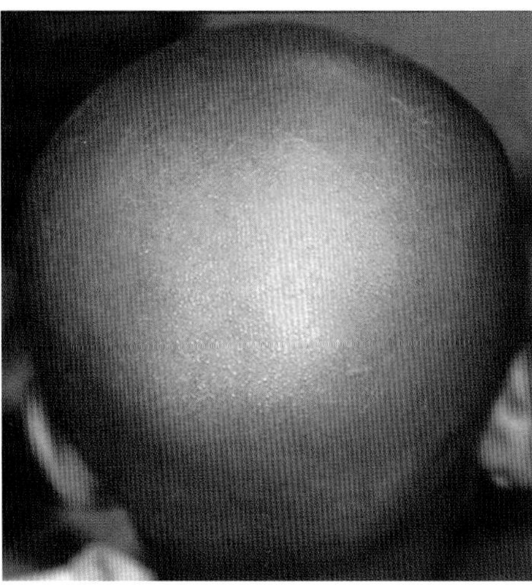

Figure 85.3. Nearly complete hair loss in a child with severe alopecia areata (alopecia totalis).

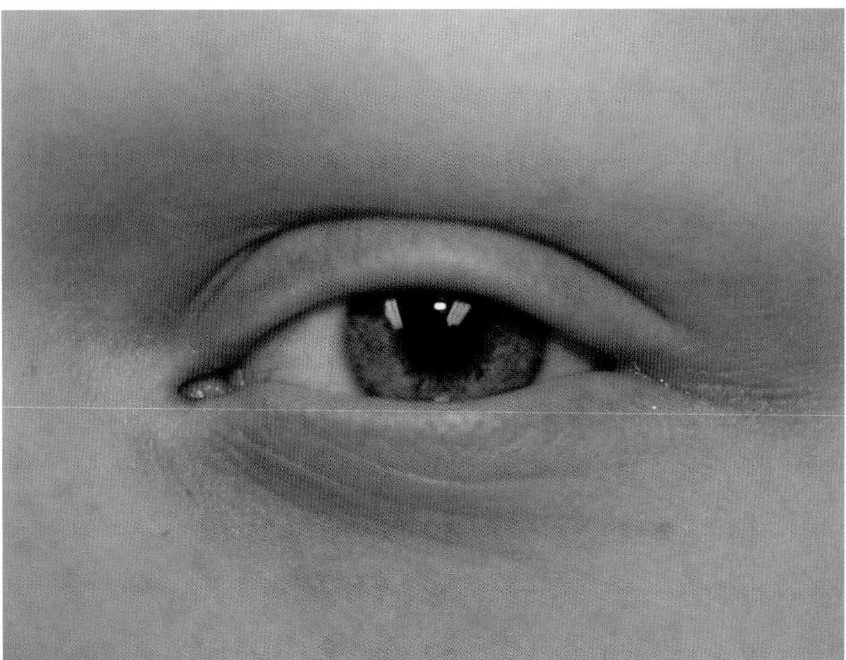

Figure 85.4. Complete loss of eyelashes and eyebrows in this child with alopecia universalis.

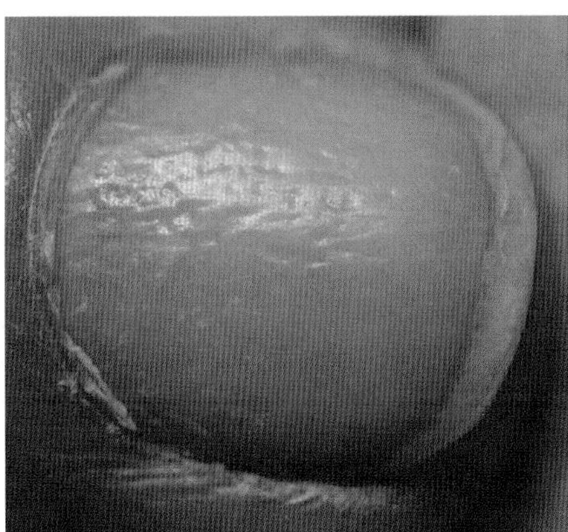

Figure 85.5. Multiple small nail pits may be observed in patients who have alopecia areata.

Look-alikes

Nail changes would not be present in any of the conditions listed herein.

Disorder	Differentiating Features
Tinea capitis	• Scaling or inflammation of the scalp usually present. • Black dot hairs may be observed. • Regional lymphadenopathy (cervical, suboccipital) may be present. • Fungal culture or potassium hydroxide preparation result is positive.
Traction alopecia	• Symmetric bilateral involvement typical • Thinning or complete hair loss, especially around hairline or in areas where hair is parted • Most common in African American girls; hair styling usually suggestive with tight braids or heavy hair adornments
Trichotillomania	• Irregularly shaped areas of incomplete alopecia. • Hairs of differing lengths in affected regions. • Broken-off hairs are present. • Secondary findings (excoriations, crusting) or features of nail-biting may be present.
Loose anagen syndrome	• Typical onset in preschool years. • No complete hair loss; rather, diffusely thin and lusterless hair. • Hair grows slowly; history of no (or few) haircuts common. • Hair mount of easily extracted hairs confirms diagnosis (reveals ruffled cuticle and dystrophic anagen bulb).
Telogen effluvium	• Usually diffuse thinning without areas of complete hair loss • Typically associated with preceding physical/emotional trauma or illness, which is believed to trigger conversion from anagen to telogen phase of hair growth • Self-limited; gradual improvement within months
Androgenetic alopecia	• Not typically seen in younger children • Classic distribution: symmetric over vertex and frontal hairline • May occur in adolescent males or, less commonly, females • May be associated with signs of hyperandrogenism

How to Make the Diagnosis

- Diagnosis is usually a clinical one, based on the typical findings.
- In some patients, there may be associated loss of eyebrows or eyelashes and characteristic nail changes.
- Skin biopsy rarely necessary to confirm the diagnosis; findings include perifollicular lymphocytic infiltration.

Treatment

- The most commonly used first-line therapy for alopecia areata is topical or intralesional corticosteroids.
  - Used primarily in mild to moderate patchy disease; often not practical in patients with extensive hair loss.
  - Patients receiving high-potency topical steroids or injected steroids should be monitored for cutaneous atrophy; hypothalamic-pituitary-adrenal axis suppression possible with chronic long-term corticosteroid therapy (mainly with ultra-potent topical preparations or repeated intralesional therapy).
  - Intralesional steroid injections usually not tolerated well in younger children and, hence, used infrequently before 10 to 12 years of age.
- Other topical treatments for patchy/localized alopecia areata include
  - Minoxidil
  - Calcineurin inhibitors (tacrolimus or pimecrolimus)
  - Anthralin ("short contact" therapy)
  - Immunotherapy (contact sensitization with squaric acid or other agents)
  - Excimer laser therapy
- For alopecia totalis, some clinicians use more aggressive systemic immunosuppressive modalities, but careful analysis of the risk versus benefit ratio must be considered. Systemic corticosteroids may be considered for select patients, and usually only as a bridge to halt severe progression of hair loss, while topical therapies are also started; potential side effects make this a rarely utilized modality in young children.
- Intermittent recurrence of disease activity is common in patients with alopecia areata.
- Hair loss can be devastating for the patient as well as family members; in patients or family members struggling with the effect of chronic or extensive hair loss, referral to a psychologist may be helpful.
- Education about other resources, including the National Alopecia Areata Foundation, may be very beneficial (see Resources for Families).
- Hair prosthesis should be considered for children with severe loss who express interest in this modality.

Treating Associated Conditions

- Because alopecia areata can occur more commonly in the setting of other autoimmune disorders, a comprehensive family history and review of systems should be obtained for other autoimmune disorders, including thyroid disease, type 1 diabetes, and inflammatory bowel disease.
- Laboratory workup should be based on findings from the history and physical examination.
- Alopecia areata has been reported in the setting of autoimmune polyglandular syndromes.

Prognosis

- Because response to therapy is unpredictable, prognosis is difficult to predict and extremely variable.
- Many children with an isolated episode of localized patchy hair loss will have spontaneous hair regrowth without therapy.
- Children with rapid and extensive hair loss, especially when progressing to complete loss, usually respond poorly to therapy.
- Prepubertal onset and family history of alopecia areata portend a poorer prognosis.

When to Worry or Refer

- Referral to a pediatric dermatologist should be considered in children with more extensive or chronic hair loss or when the diagnosis of alopecia areata is uncertain.
- Referral may also be beneficial if the primary care physician is not experienced in treating the disorder.
- If the patient has a second autoimmune disorder or a first-degree relative who has 2 autoimmune disorders, consultation with a pediatric endocrinologist is warranted.

Resources for Families

- American Academy of Pediatrics: HealthyChildren.org.
  www.HealthyChildren.org/hairloss
- National Alopecia Areata Foundation: Provides information, support, and resources for patients and families.
  www.naaf.org
- Locks of Love: Public nonprofit organization that provides hairpieces to financially disadvantaged children in the United States and Canada.
  www.locksoflove.org

Loose Anagen Syndrome

Introduction/Etiology/Epidemiology

- In loose anagen syndrome, the actively growing anagen hairs (see human hair growth phases in Chapter 87, Telogen Effluvium) are poorly anchored and more easily removed from the scalp than normal.
- Characteristically seen in children, typically blonde girls between 2 and 5 years of age, although it may occur in males and in patients with darker hair.
- Possibly an autosomal-dominant disorder, although many cases appear to be sporadic.

Signs and Symptoms

- Classic presentation is a child presenting with fine, limp hair that does not grow well (Figures 86.1 and 86.2).
- Parent may report that the child does not need haircuts because the hair grows so slowly.
- Hair loss may be patchy or diffuse, and the hair is often irregular in length.
- Hairs are easily removed from the scalp with gentle traction, although shedding is cyclic, so inability to extract hair does not rule out the diagnosis.
- Usually no associated nail or skin alterations or systemic manifestations.

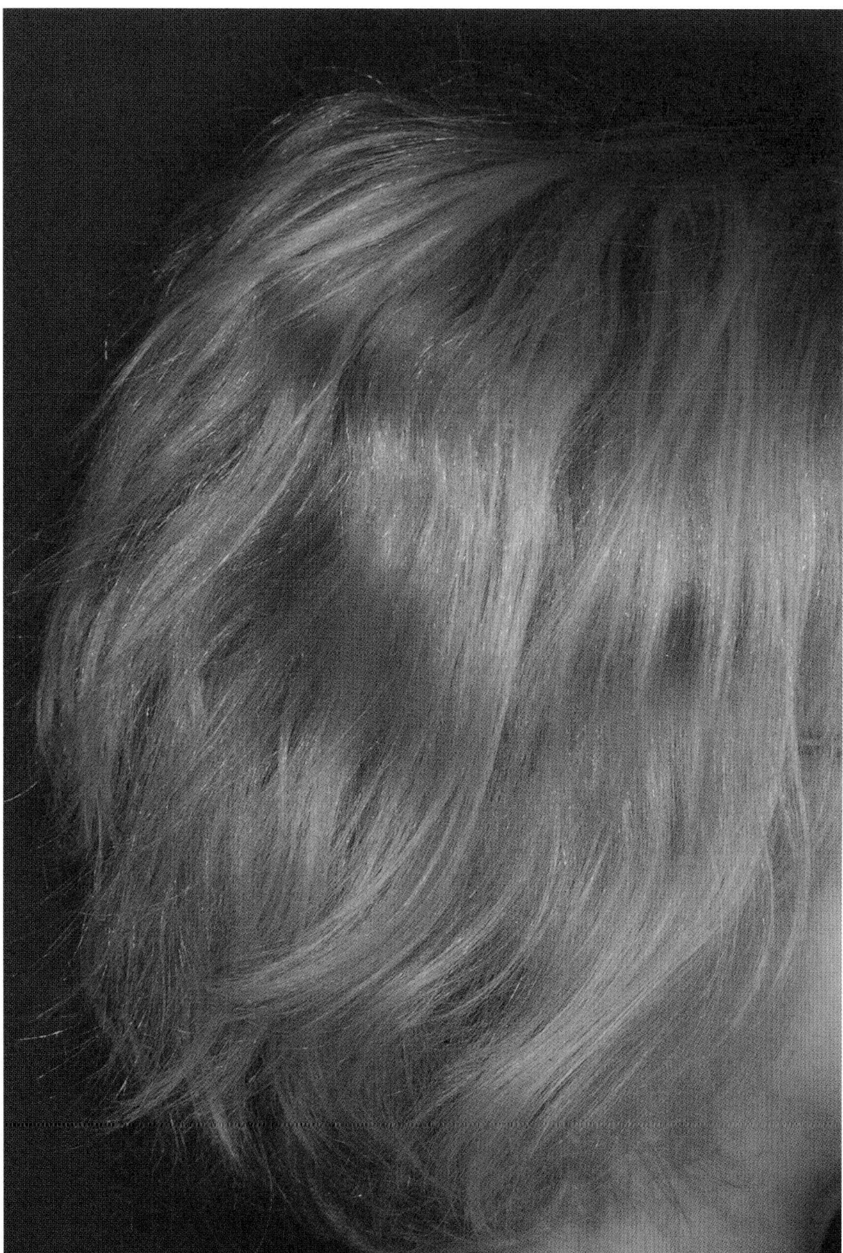

Figure 86.1. Typical appearance of a patient with loose anagen syndrome: short, fine, blonde hair that does not grow well.

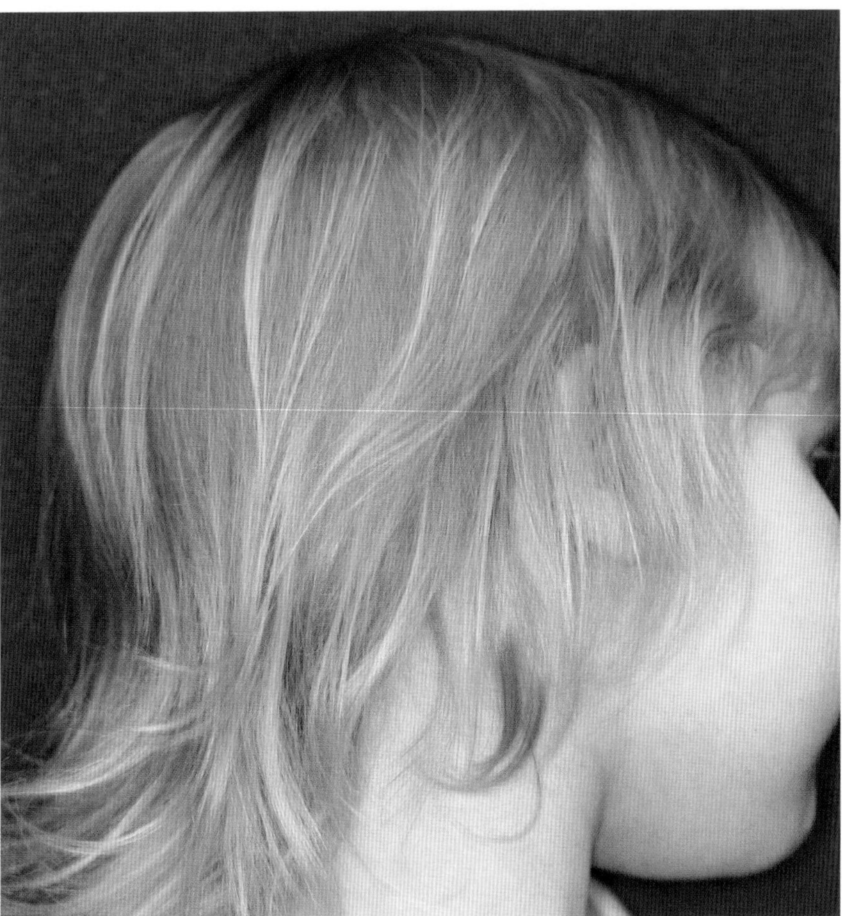

Figure 86.2. Fine, short, lightly pigmented hair that does not grow well in a young girl with loose anagen syndrome.

Look-alikes

Disorder	Differentiating Features
Telogen effluvium	• Acquired condition; affected children usually have history of previously normal hair texture and rate of growth. • History of inciting trigger (eg, febrile illness, surgery, anesthesia) common. • Hairs of normal length. • Hair pull reveals multiple telogen hairs rather than dystrophic anagen hairs. • Improves spontaneously over 3 to 6 months.
Alopecia areata	• Usually causes patches of complete alopecia; may have loss of eyebrows or eyelashes • May have associated nail pitting • May see exclamation point hairs
Trichotillomania	• Acquired condition; usually localized, not diffuse. • Areas of hair loss often have angulated borders. • Hairs of differing lengths in affected areas. • Broken-off hairs are present. • Easily extracted anagen hairs not present.
Ectodermal dysplasia	• Distinct facial features (dark circles under eyes, frontal bossing, full lips) • May have associated nail/skin/dental abnormalities • Congenital condition; usually does not improve with age • Large group of inherited disorders that may have additional systemic manifestations
Hair shaft abnormalities (eg, trichorrhexis nodosa, monilethrix)	• Structural abnormalities of the hair shaft often result in hair fragility and breakage, leading to sparse, short hair that appears dry or lusterless. • Microscopic examination of hairs often diagnostic, but consultation with a pediatric dermatologist advised if this diagnosis is being considered.

How to Make the Diagnosis

- The diagnosis is usually suggested clinically.
- Diagnostic confirmation can be made by performing a gentle hair pull and examining the extracted anagen hairs microscopically. The distinctive microscopic findings include a ruffled cuticle and distorted anagen hair bulb (Figure 86.3).

Treatment

- There is no treatment available for loose anagen syndrome.
- Gentle hairstyling should be encouraged to minimize further hair loss.

Prognosis

- The prognosis is good; the condition usually improves over time.
- Although the condition has been reported in the setting of Noonan syndrome, most patients do not have systemic associations.

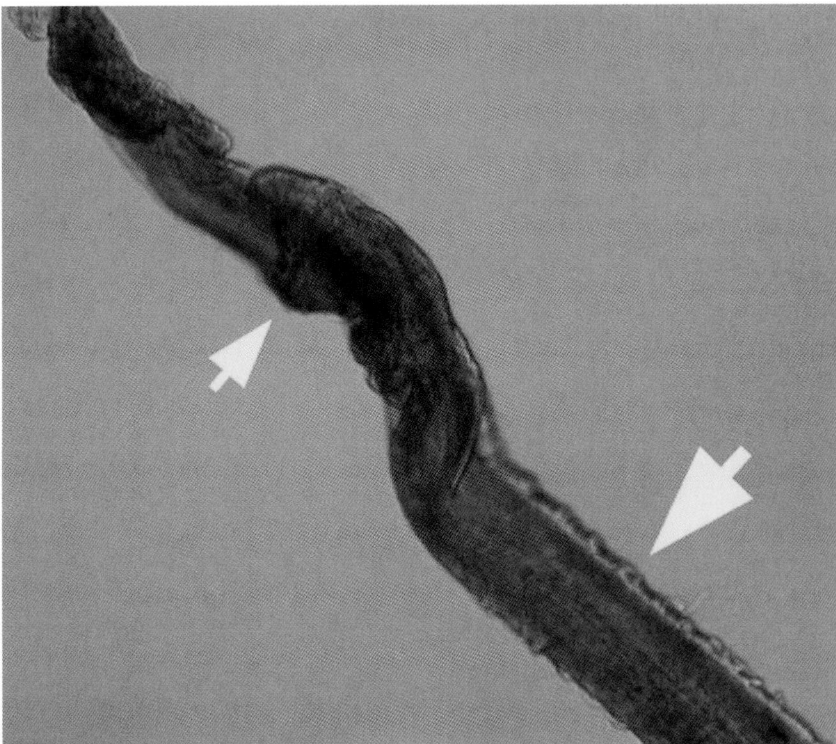

Figure 86.3. Typical microscopic appearance of a dysplastic anagen hair in a patient who has loose anagen syndrome. Note the "ruffled sock" appearance of the cuticle (large arrow) and the distorted bulb (small arrow).

When to Worry or Refer

- If associated nail, dental, or cutaneous alterations are present, referral to evaluate for possible ectodermal dysplasia or other genodermatoses should be considered.
- Consider referral when the diagnosis is in question, if other abnormalities of the hair shaft are detected on microscopic examination, or in children with potential systemic abnormalities.

CHAPTER 87

Telogen Effluvium

Introduction/Etiology/Epidemiology

- One of the most common forms of non-scarring alopecia in children.
- Human hair follicle has 3 distinct phases.
  - Anagen phase: approximately 80% to 90% of hairs in this growing phase; can last from 2 to 6 years (average 3 years)
  - Catagen phase: brief, approximately 3-week period of involution
  - Telogen phase: resting phase typically lasting 3 months; approximately 10% of hairs at any time; an average of 50 to 100 telogen hairs shed daily and simultaneously replaced
- It is unclear what stimuli trigger anagen hairs to enter the catagen phase under normal circumstances, although there are several known events that may interrupt the normal hair cycle and cause large numbers of hairs to prematurely enter the catagen, then telogen phase in concert (resulting in greater than normal hair loss).
  - Most common forms of telogen effluvium include physiological hair loss of newborns and postpartum women (in which case childbirth is believed to be the trigger).
  - There are also several physical injuries and illnesses that may cause large numbers of anagen hairs to prematurely enter the telogen phase, including
    - High fever
    - Surgery
    - General anesthesia
    - Serious infections
    - Thyroid disease (hypothyroidism or hyperthyroidism)
    - Iron deficiency
    - Malnutrition related to underlying medical problems (eg, celiac disease, anorexia nervosa) or crash diets insufficient in calories or protein
    - Essential fatty acid, zinc, or biotin deficiency
    - Medications (eg, angiotensin-converting enzyme inhibitors, anticonvulsants [eg, valproic acid, carbamazepine], β-blockers, cimetidine, lithium, oral contraceptives)

- Usually, the onset of hair loss occurs 6 weeks to 4 months after the preceding trigger event/condition.

Signs and Symptoms

- Patients usually present with a history of increased shedding of the hair or hair falling out at the root (often noticed after washing or brushing hair).
- Process is generally diffuse and very subtle, even undetectable, to the clinician.
- Condition usually is much more apparent to the affected patient or family members and may be more noticeable when comparing the child's appearance with photographs taken prior to the onset.
- Patients lack other symptoms, and the scalp generally appears normal with no evidence of scale or inflammation.
- There usually are no completely bald areas but rather diffuse thinning of the scalp hair (Figures 87.1 and 87.2).
- It may occasionally be associated with Beau lines on the nails (horizontal bands or grooves in same area of several or all nails).

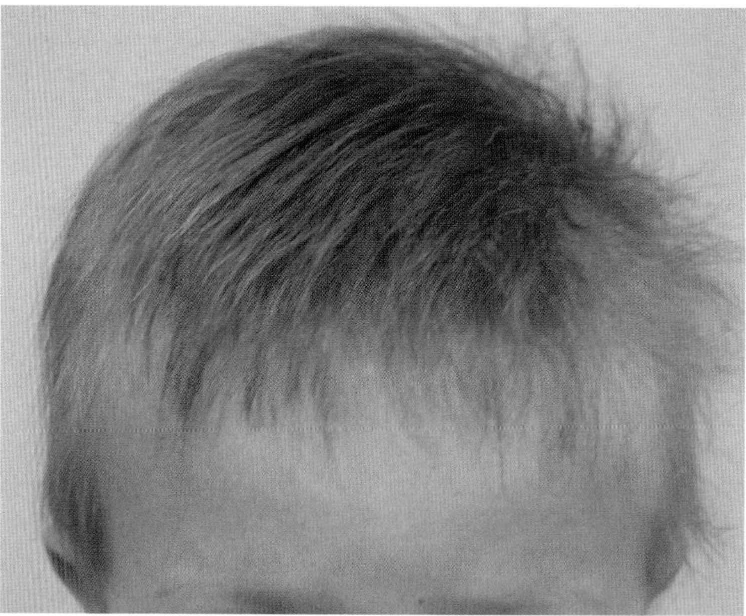

Figure 87.1. Diffuse thinning of scalp hair typical of telogen effluvium. This child experienced complete regrowth of the scalp hair within several months.

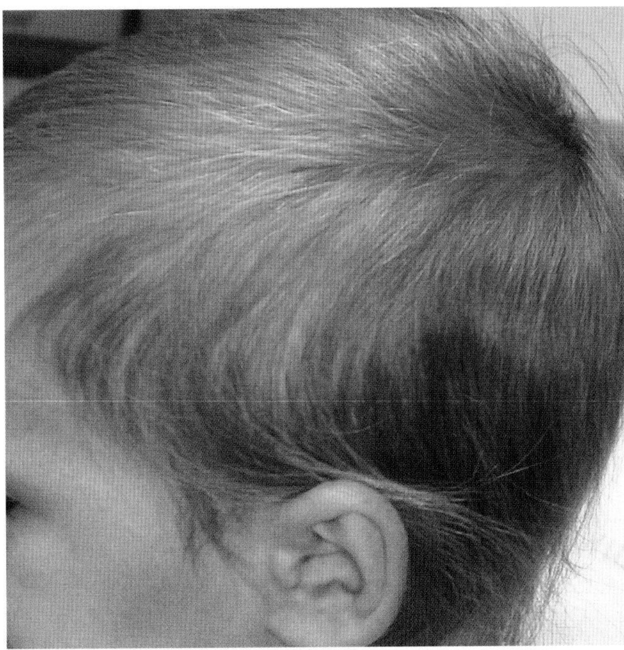

Figure 87.2. Diffuse thinning of the scalp hair in this child with telogen effluvium.

Look-alikes

Disorder	Differentiating Features
Tinea capitis	• Usually causes localized hair loss. • Scaling or inflammation of the scalp usually present. • Black dot hairs may be observed. • Regional lymphadenopathy (cervical, suboccipital) may be present. • Fungal culture or potassium hydroxide preparation is positive.
Traction alopecia	• Usually causes localized hair loss with symmetric bilateral involvement • Thinning or complete hair loss, especially around hairline or in areas where hair is parted • Most common in African American girls; hair styling usually suggestive with tight braids or heavy hair adornments
Trichotillomania	• Usually causes localized hair loss. • Irregularly shaped areas of incomplete alopecia. • Hairs of differing lengths in affected areas. • Broken-off hairs are present.
Alopecia areata	• Usually causes localized hair loss (occasionally may be widespread) • Round or oval areas of complete alopecia • May have associated nail pitting
Loose anagen syndrome	• Typically long history of diffusely thin and lusterless hair. • Hair grows slowly; history of no (or few) haircuts common. • Hair mount of easily extracted hairs confirms the diagnosis (reveals ruffled cuticle and dystrophic anagen bulb).

How to Make the Diagnosis

- The diagnosis of telogen effluvium is most commonly made based on a clinical history of hair shedding beginning 2 to 4 months after a significant physical illness, injury, or other stressful event.
- Examination usually reveals an absence of scalp changes, and hair loss is usually diffuse and subtle.
- Hair pull examination can be done by firmly placing a lock of hair between the thumb and forefinger and applying steady traction. If more than 6 hairs are removed, this is suggestive of active hair shedding.
- Microscopic examination of extracted hairs can confirm the pulled hairs are in the telogen phase. Typical appearance of telogen hair reveals nonpigmented root with club shape.
- If clinical examination is suggestive of telogen effluvium but there is no supportive history, other hair loss disorders should be considered.
  - Careful diet history and growth evaluation should be obtained to rule out underlying nutritional deficiencies or history of crash dieting.
  - A medication history also should be elicited.
  - Laboratory investigation for iron deficiency anemia or thyroid disease should be considered.
- Cessation of hair loss within 3 to 4 months followed by gradual regrowth is consistent with the diagnosis.

Treatment

- The clinician's main responsibility is to provide reassurance to the patient or parents about the expectation of complete regrowth of hair, usually within 6 months.
- Treatment should be directed toward any underlying medical conditions, such as correction of iron deficiency anemia or thyroid disease, or management of any identified nutritional deficiencies.

Prognosis

- The prognosis for telogen effluvium is excellent.
- Complete hair regrowth usually occurs within 6 months.

When to Worry or Refer

- If an underlying trigger cannot be elicited via comprehensive history, physical examination, or laboratory studies, the clinician should consider referral to a dermatologist.
- If progressive hair loss persists for more than 6 months, dermatology referral is recommended.

Resources for Families

- American Hair Loss Association: Provides information about various causes of hair loss.
  www.americanhairloss.org

CHAPTER 88

Traction Alopecia

Introduction/Etiology/Epidemiology

- Traction alopecia is a common cause of hair loss that is most commonly seen in African American children, particularly girls.
- The condition is due to styling with tight braids, cornrows, or ponytails, especially when using heavy hair adornments that increase tension further on the already-stressed hair.
- African American hair has inherently lower strength, which may predispose to hair loss under conditions of increased tension or weight on the hair.

Signs and Symptoms

- Usually characterized by thinning of the hair, particularly around the frontal and parietotemporal hairlines.
  - Alopecia or thinning of the hair may extend circumferentially around the hairline, depending on how the hair is styled.
  - Hair loss also may be observed between the tight braids where the hair has been parted (Figures 88.1 and 88.2).
  - Fine vellus hairs may be observed in affected areas.
- There usually are no associated scalp changes, although occasionally, perifollicular inflammation can be observed, including erythema or papules and pustules (most often representing sterile folliculitis related to application of greasy pomades).

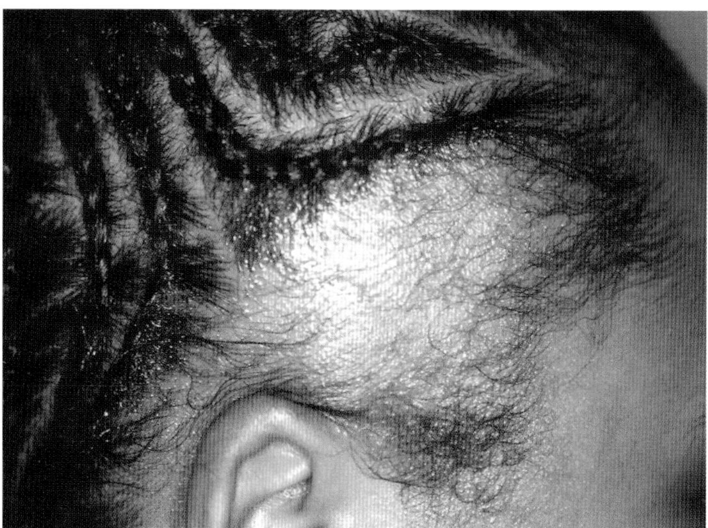

Figure 88.1. Marked thinning of the temporal scalp due to traction alopecia. Note the hairstyle with many small, tight braids typically seen in children with this disorder.

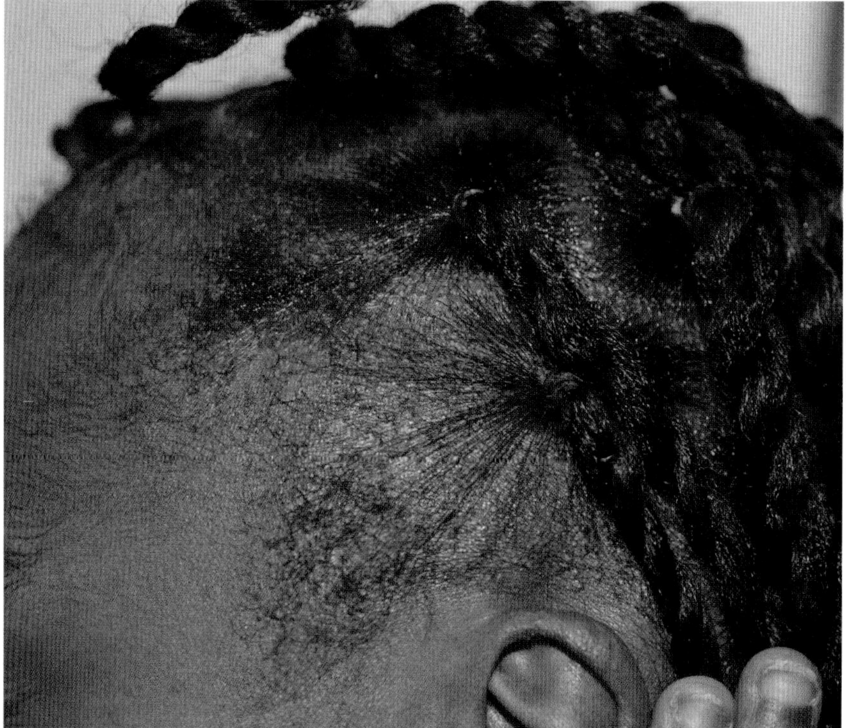

Figure 88.2. Partial alopecia involving the hairline in this child with traction alopecia. Note the tightly pulling braids and multiple hair adornments.

Look-alikes

Presented here are causes of localized hair loss. Hair loss is usually not symmetric in any of these conditions.

Disorder	Differentiating Features
Tinea capitis	• Scaling or inflammation of scalp usually present. • Black dot hairs may be observed. • Regional lymphadenopathy (cervical, suboccipital) may be present. • Fungal culture or potassium hydroxide preparation is positive.
Trichotillomania	• Irregularly shaped areas of incomplete alopecia. • Hairs of differing lengths in affected areas. • Broken-off hairs are present.
Alopecia areata	• Round or oval areas of complete alopecia. • Lesions may be scattered throughout scalp, rather than limited to frontal or parietotemporal hairlines or areas between braids. • Nail pits may be present.

How to Make the Diagnosis

- The diagnosis usually is made clinically based on the pattern of hair loss.
- When suspecting traction alopecia, a careful history should be obtained on hairstyling practices, including braids, ponytails, hair adornments, and chemical processing or heat-related procedures.

Treatment

- The mainstay of treatment is aimed at changing the hairstyling practices to ones that avoid any undue tension, trauma, or weight on the involved hair.
- Loose hairstyles without braids or hair adornments should be encouraged.
- Gentle treatment of the hair with avoidance of chemical processing or heat-related procedures also should be emphasized.

Treating Associated Conditions

- Sterile folliculitis is treated best by withdrawing the application of greasy pomades to the scalp.
- If follicular pustules are present, bacterial and fungal cultures should be performed to rule out bacterial infection and tinea capitis, respectively.

Prognosis

- If the condition is recognized promptly and the appropriate changes made in hairstyling, the prognosis is excellent, with complete regrowth of hair expected.
- In patients with more chronic traction alopecia (years), permanent hair loss may result.

When to Worry or Refer

- Consider referral to a dermatologist if the diagnosis is in doubt or for those patients with chronic symptoms because permanent hair loss may result.

Trichotillomania

Introduction/Etiology/Epidemiology

- Trichotillomania (hair-pulling disorder), the loss of hair due to hair pulling, plucking, or twisting, is a common cause of hair loss in children.
- Classified in the past as an impulse control disorder and, more recently, in *Diagnostic and Statistical Manual of Mental Disorders, 5th Edition,* as an obsessive-compulsive disorder.
- Seen more frequently in children and adolescents than adults and more common in females.
- Exact frequency is unknown, but some reports indicate prevalence of up to 1 in 200 persons by 18 years of age.
- May involve pulling or twisting of the hairs of the scalp (most commonly affected site), eyelashes, eyebrows, or other hair-bearing areas.
- Most patients/parents deny pulling or twisting (some may not even be cognizant of the behavior), which can make accurate diagnosis a challenge.
- An often-chronic condition that may vary greatly in severity, from a short-lived habit with localized hair loss to a more severe condition with associated psychologic or psychiatric morbidity.
- Affected patients often have an associated sense of tension prior to the act of hair pulling or twisting, which is typically followed by a sense of relief or gratification.

Signs and Symptoms

- Localized well-circumscribed areas of hair loss, often with angular or irregular borders (Figures 89.1 and 89.2).
- Careful examination reveals hairs of variable length within the affected region (unlike the complete hair loss of alopecia areata) (Figure 89.3).

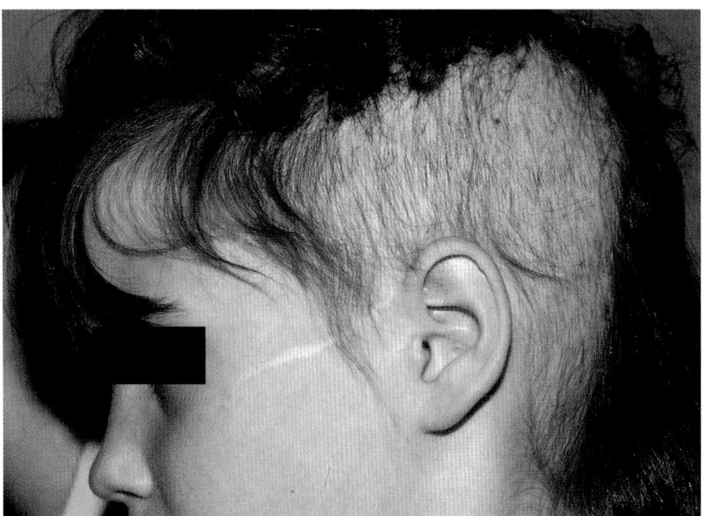

Figure 89.1. Trichotillomania. There is a well-defined patch of relative alopecia within which hairs are of differing lengths. The hair in the affected area has a bristlelike feel.

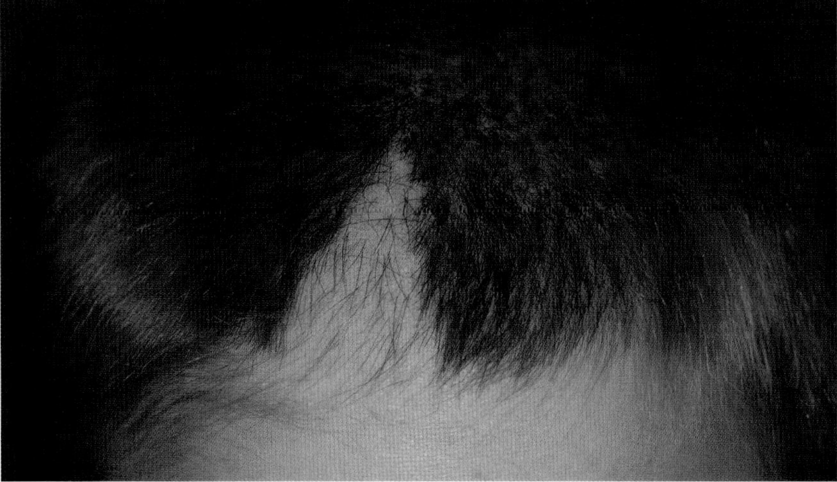

Figure 89.2. Trichotillomania. Irregular patch of alopecia with broken-off hairs in this school-aged boy with a history of obsessive-compulsive behavior and anxiety.

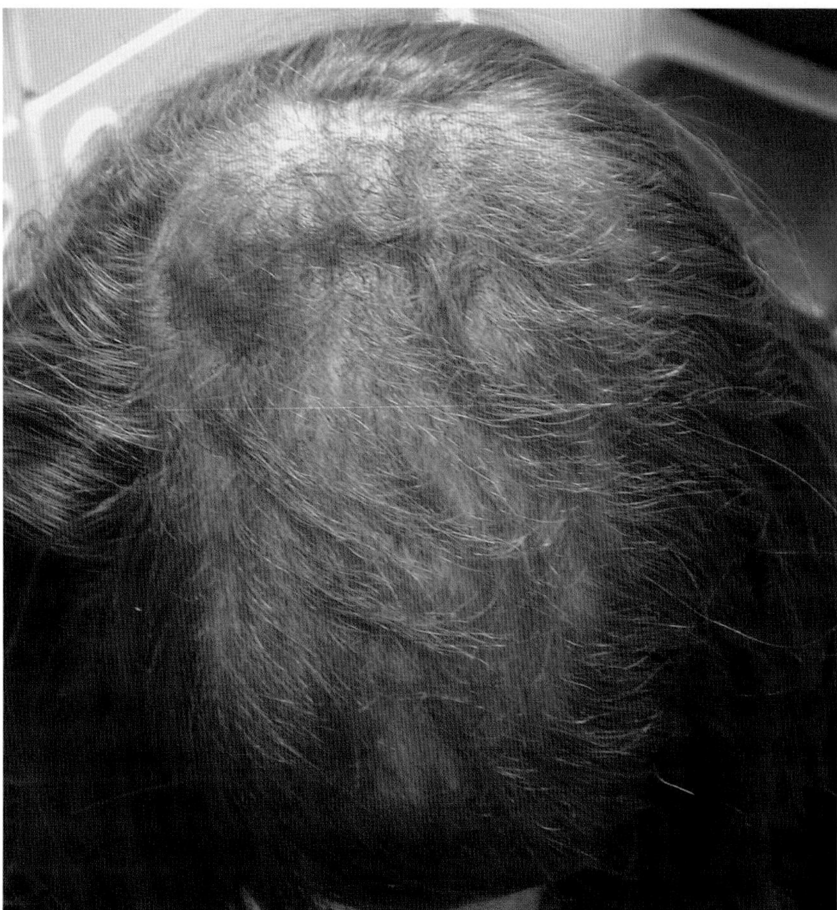

Figure 89.3. Trichotillomania involving the vertex scalp. Note the well-demarcated area of affected scalp and variation in hair length within the affected areas.

- Frontal, temporal, and parietal scalp usually affected; eyelashes and eyebrows involved less often (Figures 89.4 and 89.5).
- Affected area often has a rough, bristlelike texture due to hair stubble (see Figure 89.1).
- Usually no associated scalp abnormalities, although some erosions may be present.
- Classically occurs on the contralateral side of the dominant hand.
- Associated findings may include nail biting (onychophagia), skin or nose picking, and lip biting.

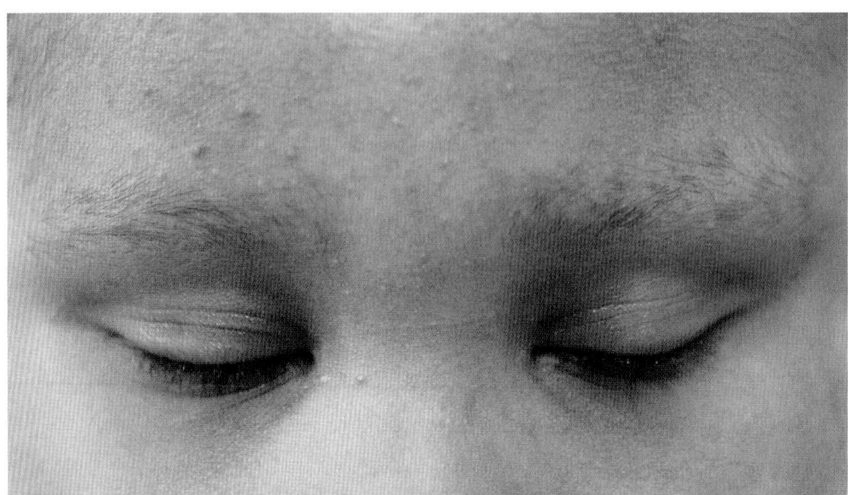

Figure 89.4. Patchy, irregular loss of eyebrows and eyelashes in this patient with trichotillomania.

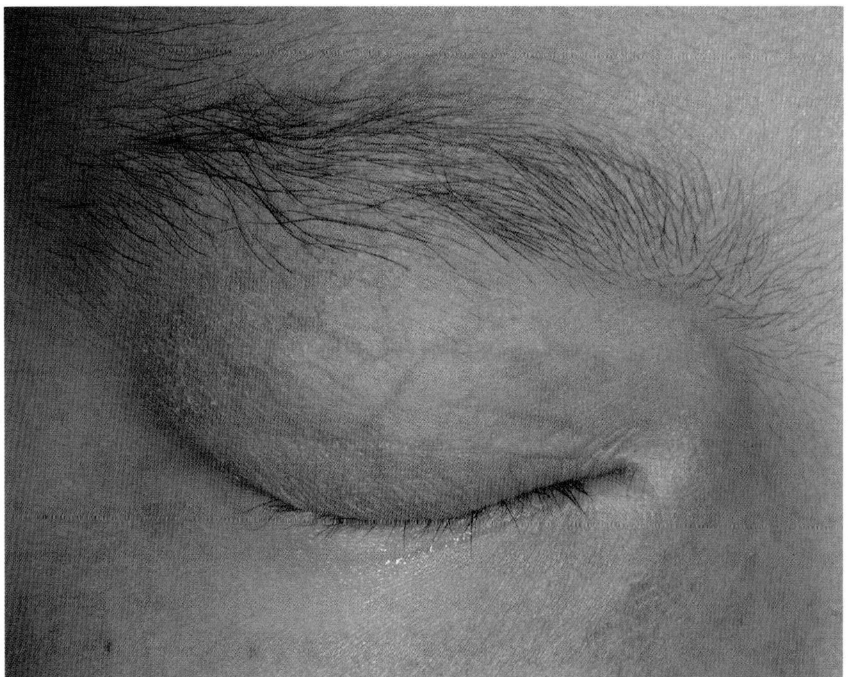

Figure 89.5. Trichotillomania localized to the eyelashes. Note the lashes of differing lengths within the affected upper eyelid margin.

Look-alikes

Disorder	Differentiating Features
Tinea capitis	• Black dot hairs may be observed. • Regional lymphadenopathy (cervical, suboccipital) may be present. • Fungal culture or potassium hydroxide preparation is positive.
Alopecia areata	• Round or oval areas (angular borders not observed) of complete hair loss. • Exclamation point hairs may be observed. • Nail pitting may be present. • Hairs have similar length during regrowth phase. • Broken-off hairs are absent.
Traction alopecia	• Symmetric bilateral involvement present. • Thinning or complete hair loss, especially around hairline or in areas where hair is parted. • Broken-off hairs are typically absent.

How to Make the Diagnosis

- The diagnosis can be very challenging because many patients and parents deny the behavior of hair pulling or twisting.
- In younger children, parents may observe and report the behavior of hair pulling or twisting, while in older children and adolescents, the behavior is usually carried out in private and family members are not aware of the habit.
- The diagnosis is made clinically based on the characteristic pattern of irregular and bizarre patterns of hair loss, presence of broken-off hairs, and exclusion of other potential causes (eg, tinea capitis).
- Although generally not necessary, skin biopsy may be helpful in making the diagnosis. Histologic findings include follicular plugging, melanin casts, trichomalacia, hemorrhage, and an increase in catagen hair follicles.
- Special care and sensitivity must be used when the potential diagnosis of trichotillomania is discussed with the patient and family members.

Treatment

- There are no specific therapies for trichotillomania.
- Close collaboration with a child psychologist or psychiatrist is often necessary to reverse the behavior.
  - In some patients, behavior modification strategies alone can be helpful.
  - In others, a combination of behavior modification and pharmacologic therapy, such as selective serotonin reuptake inhibitors, may be necessary, but evidence for effectiveness of medication intervention is limited.

Treating Associated Conditions

- Psychiatric comorbidities (eg, obsessive-compulsive disorder, depression, anxiety disorder) should be addressed by a pediatric psychologist or psychiatrist; such comorbidities are unlikely in younger patients.
- Trichophagia and trichobezoar should be considered in patients presenting with symptoms suggestive of gastric obstruction.

Prognosis

- Patients with trichotillomania are a heterogeneous group, so the prognosis varies from excellent in those individuals with an isolated habit to poor in individuals who have associated psychiatric morbidity.
- In general, younger children appear to have a more favorable outcome than those with a later onset of disease.

When to Worry or Refer

- Referral to a pediatric dermatologist may be helpful when the diagnosis is uncertain.
- Once the diagnosis is suspected, patients may benefit from referral to a behavioral pediatrician, child psychologist, or psychiatrist experienced in the disorder.

Resources for Families

- Trichotillomania Learning Center: Provides information, resources, and links for patients and families.
  www.trich.org
- Trichotillomania Support Online: Web site in the United Kingdom that provides information and support for patients who have trichotillomania.
  www.trichotillomania.co.uk

Skin Disorders in Neonates/Infants

CHAPTER 90

Aplasia Cutis Congenita

Introduction/Etiology/Epidemiology

- Aplasia cutis congenita (ACC) is a congenital defect of the skin that results in localized absence of the epidermis, dermis, and, occasionally, subcutaneous tissue.
- The cause is unknown and most cases are sporadic, although autosomal-dominant inheritance has been suggested in some reports. A link with maternal antithyroid medication (especially methimazole) use during pregnancy has been suggested.
- Aplasia cutis congenita is a feature of Adams-Oliver (with transverse limb defects and vascular and cardiac abnormalities) and oculocerebrocutaneous (Delleman) syndromes and may occur in those who have trisomy 13.

Signs and Symptoms

- Usually presents as a solitary, round, oval, or stellate-shaped, 1- to 2-cm ulcer (Figure 90.1) or scar (Figure 90.2) located on the scalp near the origin of the hair whorl (although other body sites occasionally are affected). A minority of patients have multiple lesions (typically 2 or 3).
- In some patients, the defect is covered by a thin membrane and surrounded by long dark hairs (the hair collar sign; Figure 90.3). This membranous form of ACC is postulated to represent a mild form of cranial neural tube closure defect.
- Large lesions (>4 cm) may be associated with underlying skull defects that may predispose to sagittal sinus hemorrhage or thrombosis, local infection, or meningitis.

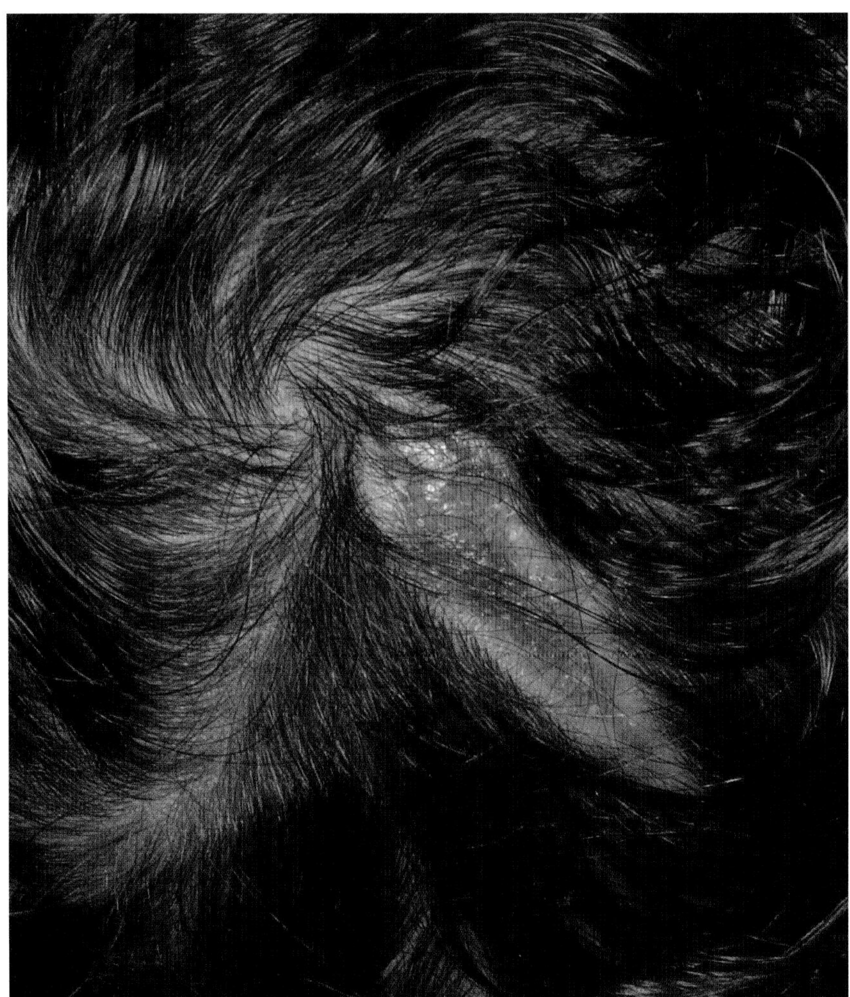

Figure 90.1. Stellate ulcer with overlying crust characteristic of aplasia cutis congenita.

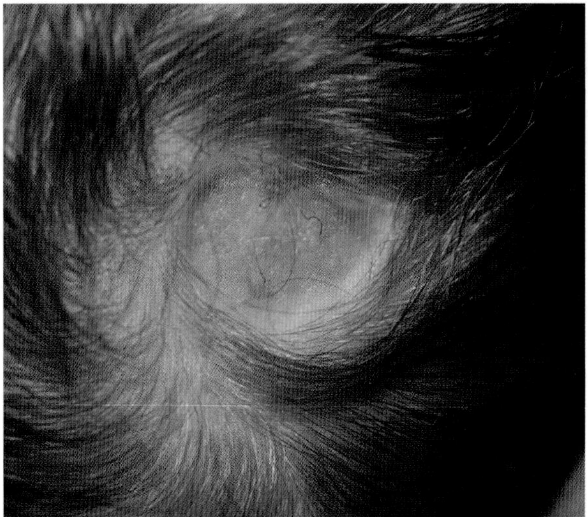

Figure 90.2. Aplasia cutis congenita presenting as an atrophic scar.

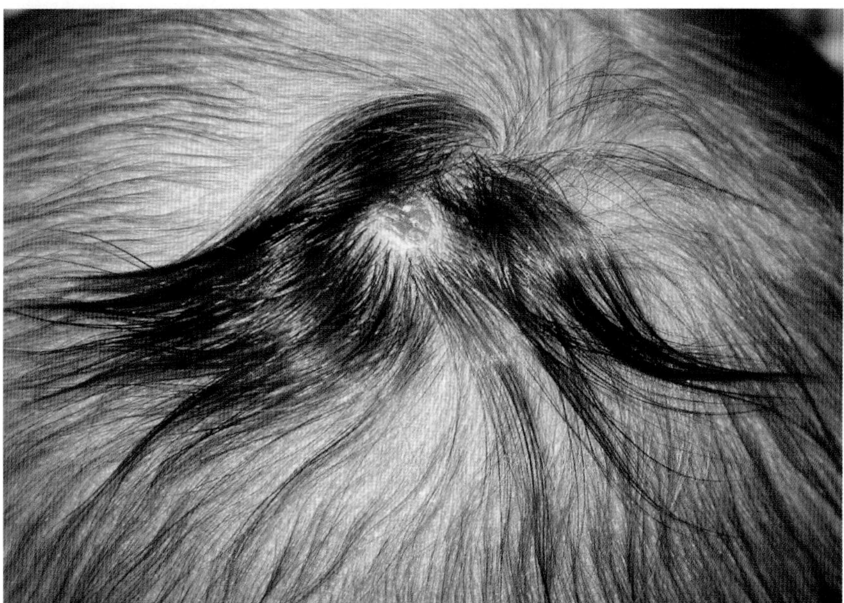

Figure 90.3. Aplasia cutis congenita in which a thin membrane is surrounded by long dark hairs (the hair collar sign).

Look-alikes

Disorder	Differentiating Features
When Presenting as an Ulcer	
Herpes simplex virus infection	• Usually presents as clustered vesicles on an erythematous base (not a solitary large ulcer) • Lesions usually not present at birth
Trauma from forceps	• May cause a scalp erosion (more superficial than an ulcer), and shape and location likely to be different than seen in ACC
Trauma from scalp electrode	• Usually produces an erosion (more superficial than an ulcer) and is typically smaller than ACC
Epidermolysis bullosa	• Typically more superficial than ACC, with denudation and eroded patches • Usually presents with multiple sites of involvement • Oral mucosal involvement occasionally present
When Presenting as a Scar	
Nevus sebaceous	• Usually presents as a verrucous (warty) plaque; however, some lesions are quite flat in neonates and may mimic a scar. • Often yellow-orange to tan in color. • If left untreated, texture becomes more elevated and verrucous in the peri-pubertal and postpubertal years.

How to Make the Diagnosis

- The diagnosis is usually made clinically based on the appearance of the lesion(s).

Treatment

- For small ulcers, local wound care to prevent secondary bacterial infection is sufficient. Lesions presenting as scars require no treatment.
- Large lesions require plastic surgery consultation and imaging.

Prognosis

- Excellent for small lesions; atrophic scars will persist and ulcers will heal with atrophic scars. Large lesions may be associated with underlying skull defects that may predispose to sagittal sinus hemorrhage or thrombosis, local infection, or meningitis. For such patients, plastic surgical consultation is recommended.

When to Worry or Refer

- Obtain plastic surgery consultation for patients with large lesions or deeper involvement.

Resources for Families

- US National Library of Medicine Genetics Home Reference: Nonsyndromic aplasia cutis congenita.
  http://ghr.nlm.nih.gov/condition/nonsyndromic-aplasia-cutis-congenita

Diaper Dermatitis

Introduction/Etiology/Epidemiology

- One of the most common skin disorders of infancy

Signs and Symptoms

Table 91.1. Common Forms of Diaper Dermatitis

Condition	Cause	Clinical Features	Treatment
Irritant dermatitis (Figure 91.1)	• Moisture, friction, enzymes in stool	• Erythematous patches that involve the lower abdomen, buttocks, and thighs • Convex surfaces involved; inguinal folds often spared	• Frequent diaper changes • Topical barrier cream or ointment at all diaper changes • Topical low-potency corticosteroid twice daily as adjunctive therapy
Candidiasis (Figure 91.2)	• Infection with *Candida* species (primary or complicating existing irritant dermatitis)	• Erythematous patches that involve the convexities and inguinal creases • Satellite papules and pustules • Scaling at the margins of involved areas	• Topical antifungal preparation (eg, nystatin, clotrimazole)
Seborrheic dermatitis (Figure 91.3)	• Cause unknown • Associated with sebaceous gland function • May represent an inflammatory response to yeasts of the genus *Malassezia* (*Pityrosporum*)	• Begins at 3–4 weeks of age and resolves by the end of the first year of life. • Salmon-pink patches with greasy scale that involve the convexities and inguinal creases. • Involvement of the scalp, face, retroauricular creases, umbilicus, or chest may be present.	• Skin: topical low-potency corticosteroid or antifungal preparation (eg, nystatin, clotrimazole) • Scalp: oil massage and brushing or antiseborrheic shampoo (eg, one containing pyrithione zinc or selenium sulfide)

Table 91.1. Common Forms of Diaper Dermatitis *(continued)*

Condition	Cause	Clinical Features	Treatment
Bullous impetigo (Figure 91.4)	• Infection with *Staphylococcus aureus* that elaborates epidermolytic toxin	• Flaccid blisters filled with clear or purulent fluid. • Blisters rupture rapidly, leaving round or oval crusted erosions with a rim of scale.	• Oral antistaphylococcal antibiotic (The agent selected depends on local antibiotic resistance patterns.)
Folliculitis (Figure 91.5)	• Infection of hair follicles with *S aureus*	• Pustules with surrounding erythema that are centered around hair follicles	• Many lesions: oral antistaphylococcal antibiotic (the agent selected depends on local antibiotic resistance patterns). • Few lesions: topical antibiotic (eg, mupirocin, clindamycin, retapamulin). • Bleach baths may be useful for patients with persistent/recurrent infections.
Intertrigo (Figure 91.6)	• Rubbing of apposed skin surfaces complicated by heat and moisture	• Erythema and superficial erosions located in the inguinal creases • May become secondarily infected with *Candida* species or *Streptococcus pyogenes*, less commonly *S aureus*	• Absorbent powder (to reduce moisture and friction) • Antifungal preparation (if candidal infection) or antibiotic (if bacterial infection)
Jacquet erosive diaper dermatitis (Figure 91.7)	• Multiple factors, including moisture, friction, enzymes in stool • Considered a variant of irritant dermatitis	• Well-defined shallow ulcers or ulcerated nodules	• Topical low-potency corticosteroid twice daily and barrier preparation at all diaper changes

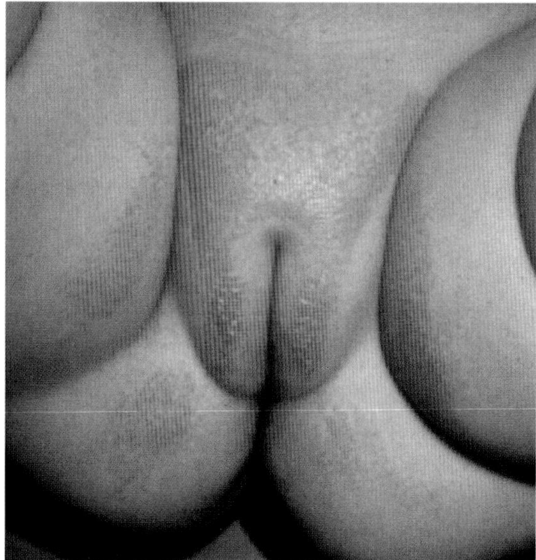

Figure 91.1. Irritant diaper dermatitis. Erythematous patches sparing the skinfolds.

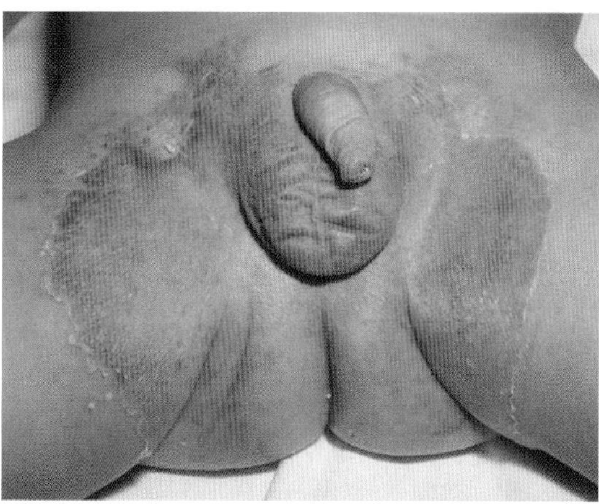

Figure 91.2. Erythematous patches that involve the creases and convexities are characteristic of candidal diaper dermatitis. Satellite lesions and scaling are present.

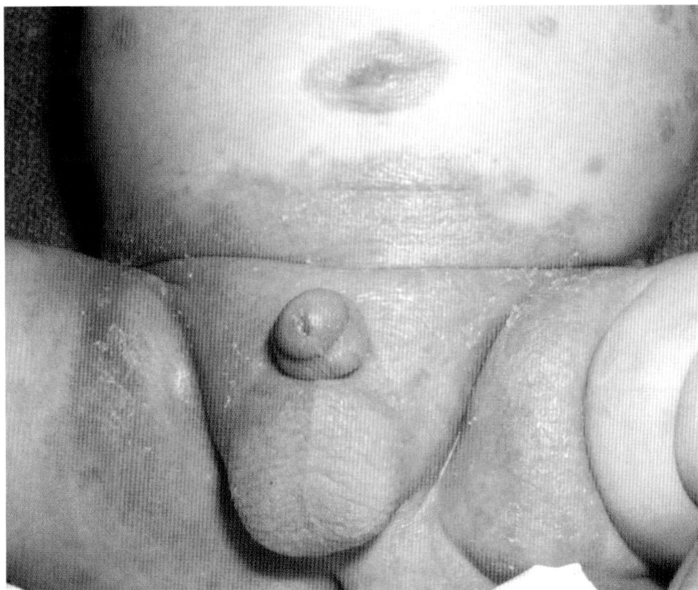

Figure 91.3. Salmon-pink patches with greasy scale involve the creases and convexities in seborrheic dermatitis.

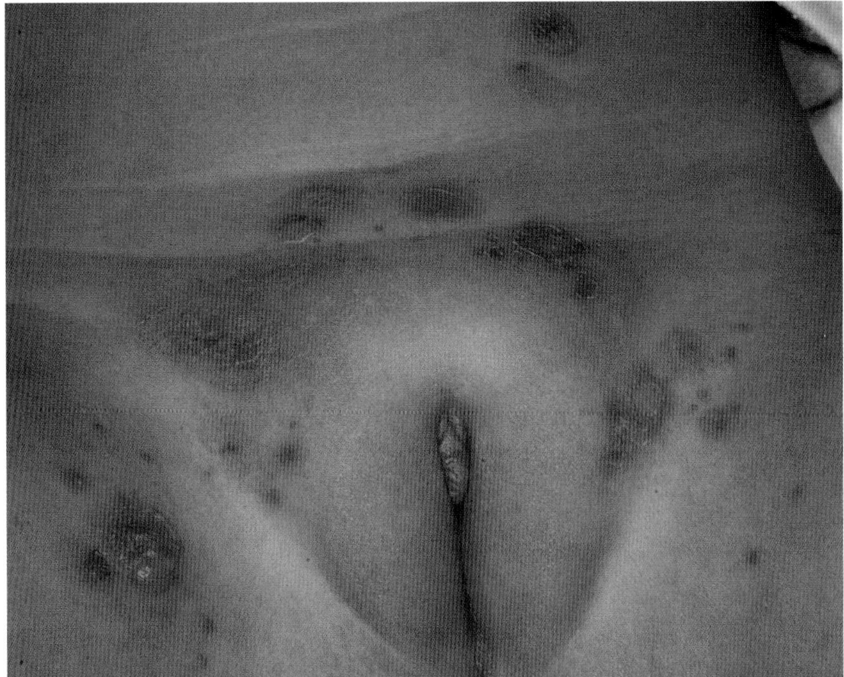

Figure 91.4. Flaccid bullae that rupture easily leaving round, crusted erosions occur in bullous impetigo.

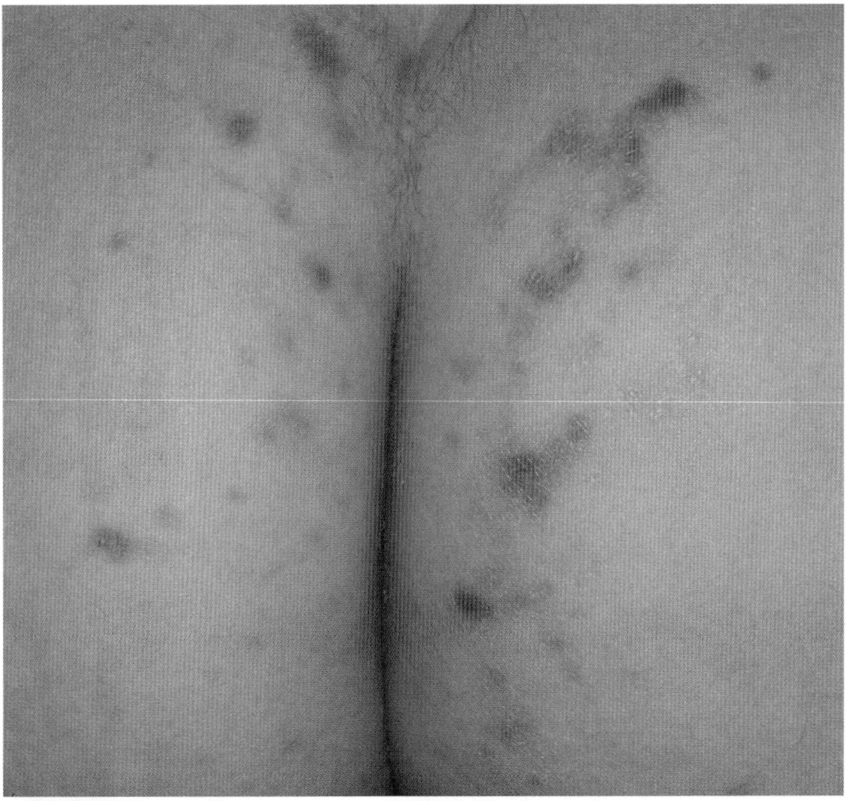

Figure 91.5. Folliculitis often involves the buttocks. There are erythematous papules centered around hair follicles. Frequently, patients also have pustules.

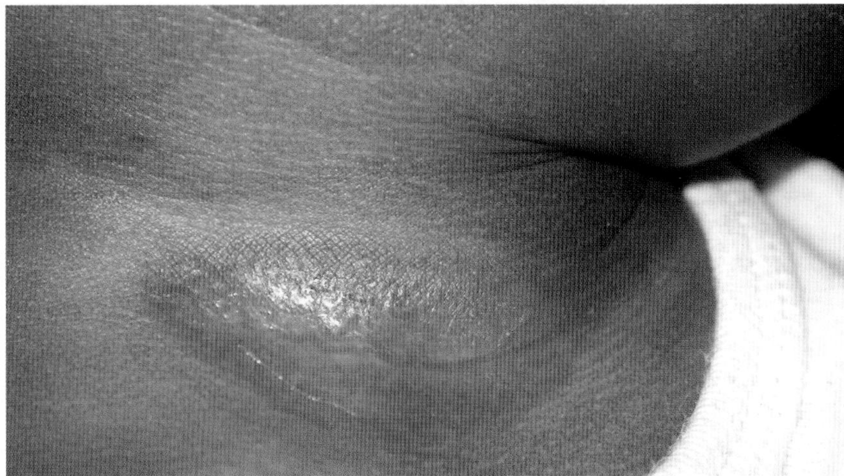

Figure 91.6. Intertrigo, shown here involving the neck, produces superficial erosions in areas where moist skin surfaces are in apposition.

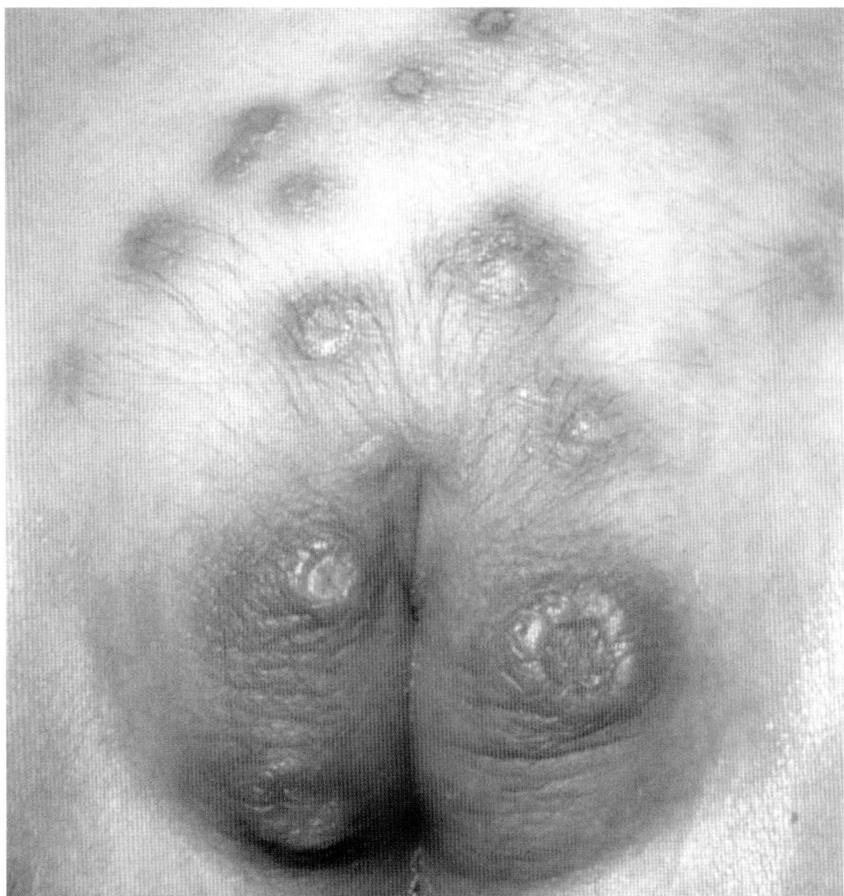

Figure 91.7. Jacquet erosive diaper dermatitis. Well-defined shallow ulcers and ulcerated nodules.

Table 91.2. Uncommon Forms of Diaper Dermatitis

Condition	Cause	Clinical Features	Treatment
Psoriasis (Figure 91.8)	• Unknown	• Erythematous scaling papules or plaques (scaling of the scalp and umbilicus may be present). • Lesions in the diaper area often lack scale characteristic of lesions located elsewhere. • May be difficult to distinguish from seborrheic dermatitis.	• Topical emollient and topical low-potency corticosteroid
Acrodermatitis enteropathica (Figure 91.9)	• Autosomal-recessive disorder. • Defective transport protein causes impaired zinc absorption.	• Often begins when infants are weaned from human to cow milk formula. • Scaling erythematous eruption located around the mouth and in the diaper area. • Infants may have sparse hair, diarrhea, or failure to gain weight.	• Oral zinc supplementation • Topical low-potency corticosteroid
Langerhans cell histiocytosis (Figure 91.10)	• Rare disorder; Langerhans cells (antigen-processing cells in the skin) accumulate in skin or other organs.	• Lesion types: vesicles or pustules (often with a hemorrhagic crust); erythematous, orange, or yellow-brown papules or nodules; petechiae; erosions (in the diaper area). • Areas affected: scalp, palms and soles, skinfolds, diaper area. • Other features: Affected infants may have hepatosplenomegaly, lymphadenopathy.	• Refer to pediatric dermatologist or pediatric oncologist for evaluation.
Congenital syphilis (Figure 91.11)	• Intrauterine infection with *Treponema pallidum*	• Symptoms: rash, bloody diarrhea, rhinorrhea, irritability, pain with movement (Parrot pseudoparalysis) • Skin lesions: condyloma lata (ie, flat-topped papules and plaques located in the diaper area or at the angles of the mouth), scaling copper-colored papules and plaques on the trunk and extremities, or vesicles and bullae	• Consult with a pediatric infectious disease specialist on evaluation and therapy.

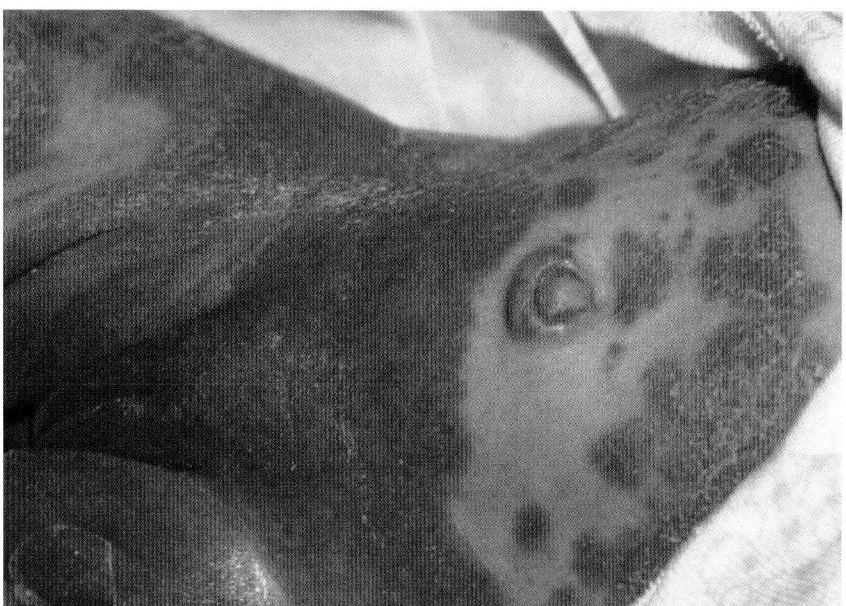

Figure 91.8. Psoriasis in the diaper area produces erythematous patches or plaques. Unlike lesions elsewhere, scale may be absent.

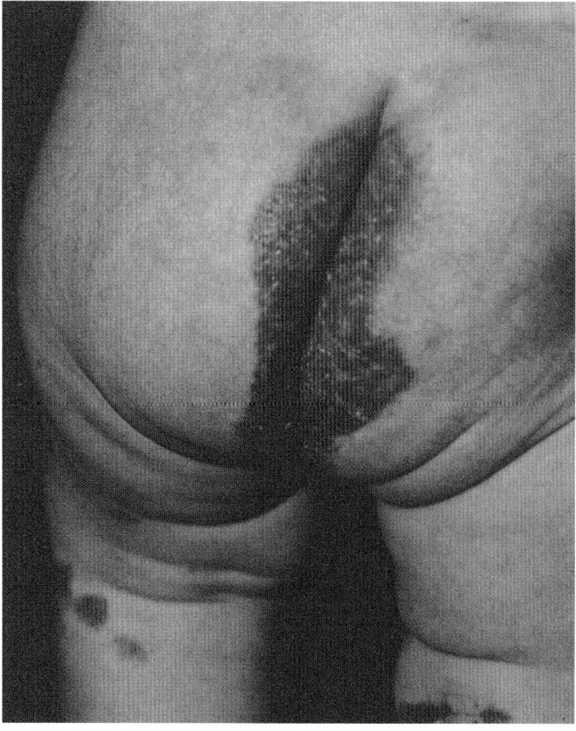

Figure 91.9. Acrodermatitis enteropathica causes erythematous patches in the diaper area and around the mouth.

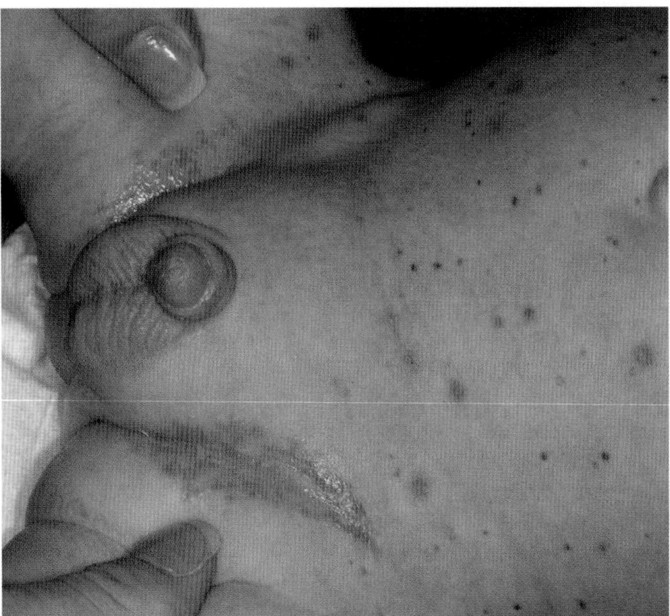

Figure 91.10. Erythematous papules of Langerhans cell histiocytosis.

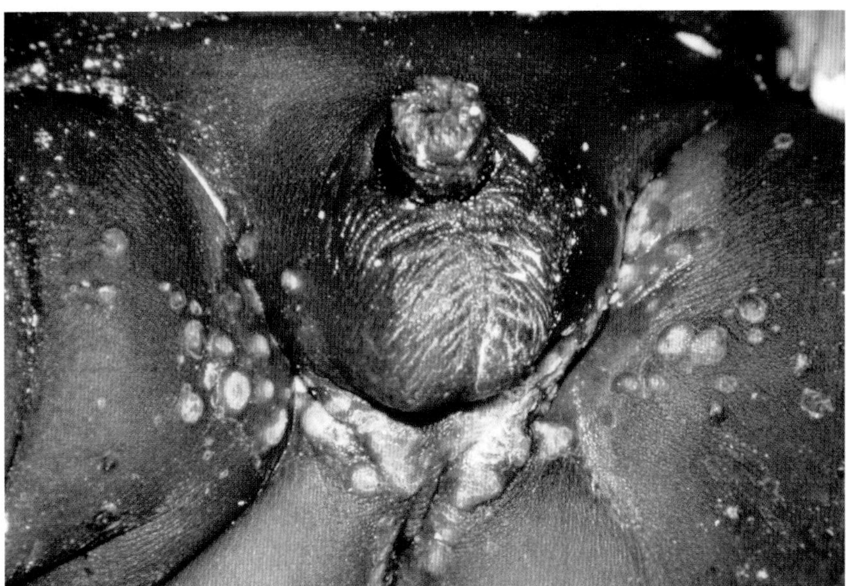

Figure 91.11. Condylomata lata, flat-topped papules and plaques, occur in the diaper area in congenital syphilis.

When to Worry or Refer

- Infants should be referred if appropriate therapy fails (to consider alternate diagnoses and possibly perform skin biopsy).
- Infants suspected of having Langerhans cell histiocytosis should be referred for evaluation to a pediatric dermatologist or pediatric oncologist.
- Consultation with a pediatric infectious disease specialist is warranted for infants suspected of having congenital syphilis.

Resources for Families

- American Academy of Pediatrics: HealthyChildren.org.
  www.healthychildren.org/English/health-issues/conditions/infections/pages/Thrush-and-Other-Candida-Infections.aspx
- MedlinePlus: Information for patients and families (in English and Spanish) sponsored by the National Library of Medicine and National Institutes of Health.
  www.nlm.nih.gov/medlineplus/yeastinfections.html

CHAPTER 92

Eosinophilic Pustular Folliculitis

Introduction/Etiology/Epidemiology

- Rare disorder of unknown cause that usually begins during the first days or weeks after birth

Signs and Symptoms

- Pruritic papules and pustules occur on the scalp (Figure 92.1) and occasionally the face, neck, and trunk.
- Crops of new lesions appear as others resolve, leading to a chronic relapsing course.

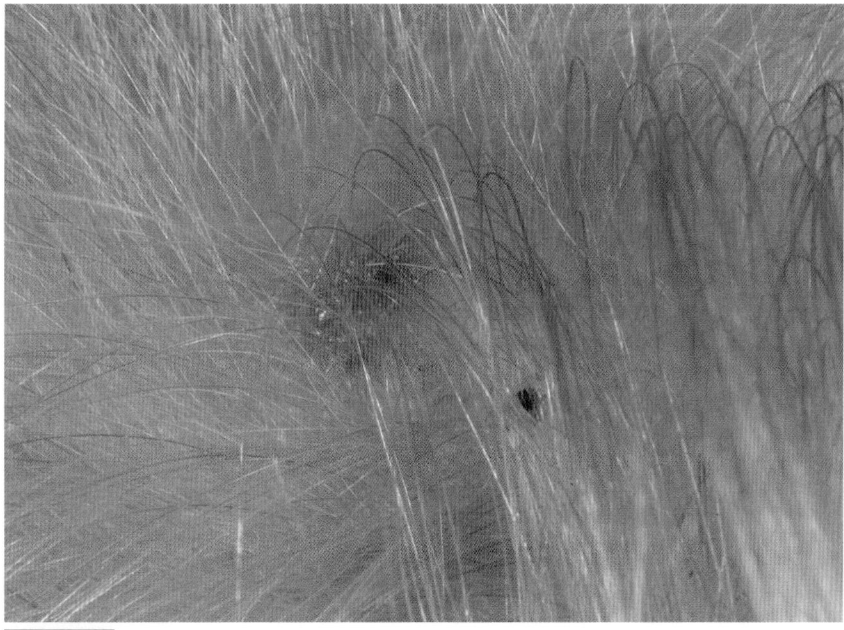

Figure 92.1. Ruptured pustules on the scalp in an infant who has eosinophilic pustular folliculitis.

Look-alikes

- Eosinophilic pustular folliculitis may be confused with infantile acropustulosis, erythema toxicum, and transient neonatal pustular melanosis, although its localization to the scalp helps to differentiate it from these disorders.
- See Look-alikes in Chapter 93, Erythema Toxicum, to assist in differentiating eosinophilic pustular folliculitis from other disorders characterized by vesiculopustules.

How to Make the Diagnosis

- The diagnosis may be suspected clinically and can be supported by finding a predominance of eosinophils on Wright stain of pustule fluid or skin biopsy.

Treatment

- There is no specific treatment.
- A sedating oral antihistamine or topical corticosteroid may provide relief if pruritus is severe.

Prognosis

- Usually resolves spontaneously in several months to 5 years

When to Worry or Refer

- Referral generally is required to confirm the diagnosis.
- In some infants, eosinophilic pustular folliculitis may be a presenting feature of hyperimmunoglobulinemia E syndrome, which is characterized by immunodeficiency with very high IgE levels, atopic dermatitis, bony abnormalities, and recurrent cutaneous and sinopulmonary infections.

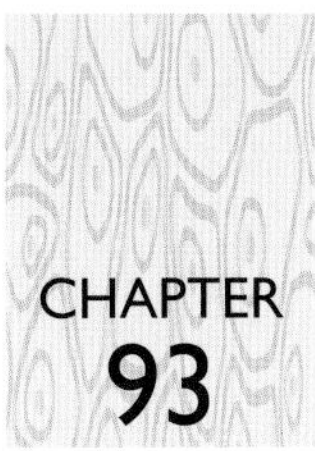

CHAPTER
93

Erythema Toxicum

Introduction/Etiology/Epidemiology

- Occurs in approximately 50% of newborns; rarely observed in premature neonates.
- Cause is unknown.

Signs and Symptoms

- Usually begins at 24 to 48 hours after birth; rarely, lesions may be present at birth or appear as late as 10 days of life.
- Appears as discrete, blotchy erythematous macules or patches, each with a central papule, vesicle, or pustule (Figures 93.1 and 93.2).

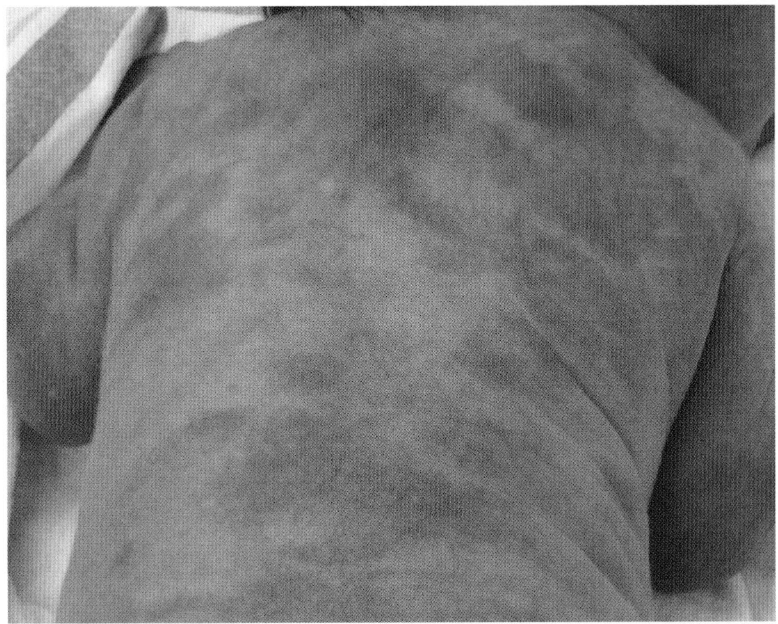

Figure 93.1. Erythematous macules, each with a central papule, are typical of erythema toxicum.

- Occasionally, there may be clusters of papules, vesicles, or pustules that form an erythematous plaque.
- Palms and soles are spared.
- New lesions appear for several days; the process lasts a week or less.

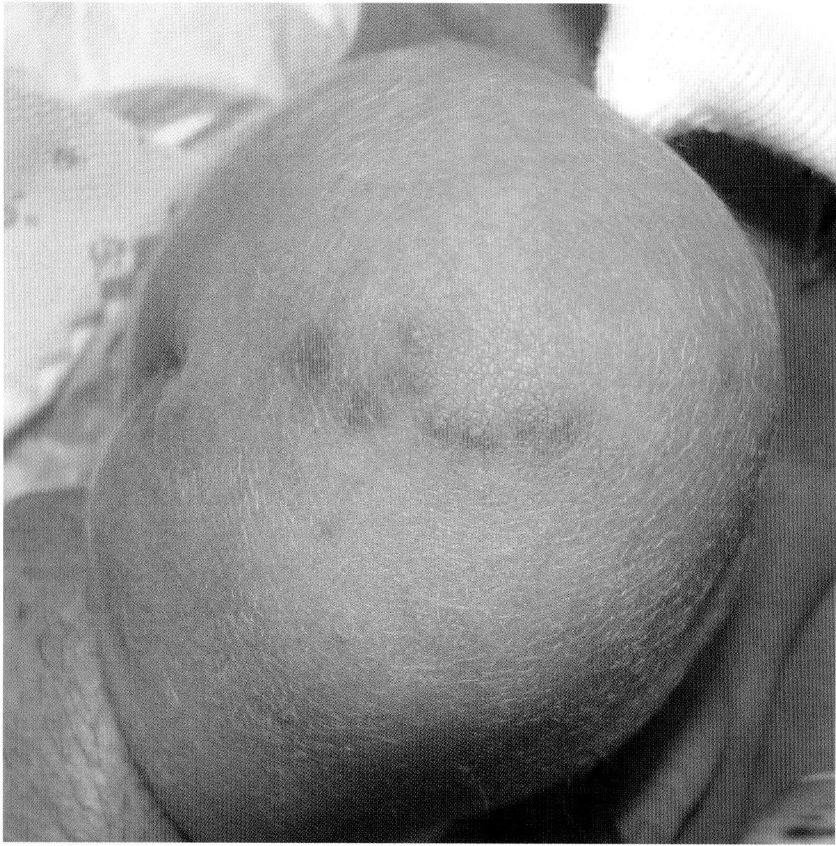

Figure 93.2. Erythematous papules of erythema toxicum located on the knee.

Look-alikes (in descending order of frequency of occurrence)

Disorder	Differentiating Features
Transient neonatal pustular melanosis	• Most often seen in African American newborns; rare in other racial groups. • Pustules (without erythema) or ruptured pustules that appear as small freckle-like hyperpigmented macules surrounded by a rim of scale. • Pustular fluid contains neutrophils.
Miliaria crystallina	• Fragile vesicles without surrounding erythema
Neonatal acne (also termed neonatal cephalic pustulosis)	• Papules and pustules typically limited to face (Some neonates may have lesions on scalp and upper chest.)
Staphylococcal folliculitis	• White to slightly yellow pustules with surrounding rim of erythema. • Hair may be noted protruding centrally. • Gram stain or bacterial culture will reveal *Staphylococcus aureus.*
Bullous impetigo	• Flaccid bullae or ruptured bullae forming round or oval crusted erosions; vesicles occasionally present. • Gram stain or culture will reveal *S aureus.*
Scabies	• Occurs rarely during the first month of life. • Generalized eruption; may have vesicles but usually will be accompanied by erythematous papules or nodules and burrows. • Palmoplantar involvement common. • Mineral oil preparation of scrapings of papules will reveal mites, eggs, or fecal material.
Neonatal herpes simplex virus infection	• Typically clustered vesicles on an erythematous base (although solitary vesicles occasionally occur). • Lesions concentrated on the head, particularly at sites of trauma (eg, that caused by a scalp electrode). • Neonates may have signs of sepsis (in disseminated disease) or seizures or coma (in central nervous system disease). • Tzanck smear, direct fluorescence examination, viral culture, or polymerase chain reaction (cerebrospinal fluid) will confirm diagnosis.
Congenital candidiasis	• Widespread rash composed of tiny erythematous papules, pustules, and scaling. • Potassium hydroxide preparation of scale or a pustule roof will reveal pseudohyphae or spores. • Palmoplantar involvement common. • Nail changes (yellow discoloration, ridging) may be present.
Infantile acropustulosis	• Usually begins in first months of life (not in first days). • Vesicles or pustules limited to hands and feet, including palms, soles, wrists, and ankles. • Episodes last 5–10 days and reappear every 2–4 weeks.

Look-alikes (in descending order of frequency of occurrence) *(continued)*

Disorder	Differentiating Features
Incontinentia pigmenti	• Vesicles on erythematous base appear at birth or within the first 2 weeks. • Arranged in linear fashion on extremities or in a swirled pattern on trunk (along lines of Blaschko).
Eosinophilic pustular folliculitis	• Papules and pustules typically located on scalp • Exhibits chronic, intermittent course

How to Make the Diagnosis

- The diagnosis is made clinically. If uncertainty exists, performance of a Wright stain of vesicular fluid will reveal a predominance of eosinophils.
- Performance of a Tzanck smear, viral culture, direct fluorescence examination, polymerase chain reaction, Gram stain, or bacterial culture will assist in excluding infectious causes.
- Skin biopsy rarely is required to exclude incontinentia pigmenti.

Treatment

- No treatment is required.

Prognosis

- Resolves spontaneously; does not recur.

When to Worry or Refer

- Obtain consultation if presentation is atypical (eg, suggesting an alternate diagnosis like herpes simplex virus infection, incontinentia pigmenti).

Resources for Families

- MedlinePlus: Information for patients and families (in English and Spanish) sponsored by the National Library of Medicine and National Institutes of Health.
  www.nlm.nih.gov/medlineplus/ency/article/001458.htm

CHAPTER 94

Infantile Acropustulosis

Introduction/Etiology/Epidemiology

- Uncommon disorder of unknown cause, although it is possible that, in some cases, it represents a cyclical immune hyperreactivity to past scabies infestation

Signs and Symptoms

- May be present at birth but most often begins during the first months of life.
- Extremely pruritic, tense vesiculopustules appear on the hands and feet (Figure 94.1), including the palms and soles and sides of the digits.
- In occasional patients, a few lesions may be present on the trunk, proximal extremities, or scalp.
- Individual lesions last 5 to 10 days and then spontaneously resolve; the process recurs every 2 to 4 weeks.

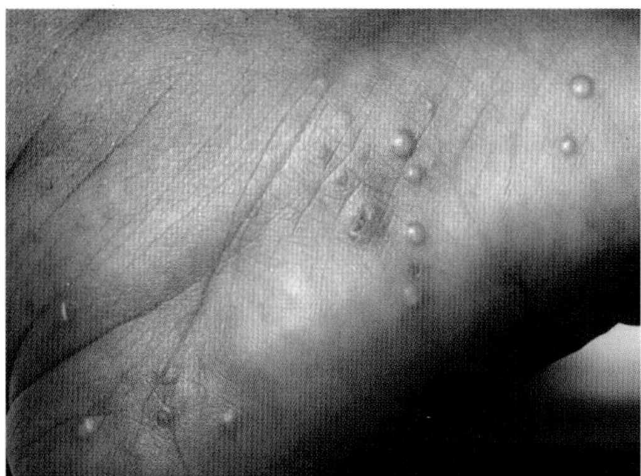

Figure 94.1. Tense vesiculopustules on the foot in infantile acropustulosis.

Look-alikes

- Most often, infantile acropustulosis is confused with scabies; however,
  - In infants, scabies produces a generalized eruption that is not limited to the hands and feet and is unlikely to recur multiple times.
  - A mineral oil preparation of scrapings of papules in scabies will reveal mites, eggs, or fecal material.
- Infantile acropustulosis also may be confused with dyshidrotic eczema, but this condition occurs rarely in infancy. (This condition is characterized by recurring deep-seated vesicles concentrated on the lateral aspects of the digits.)
- See Look-alikes in Chapter 93, Erythema Toxicum, to assist in differentiating infantile acropustulosis from other disorders characterized by vesiculopustules.

How to Make the Diagnosis

- The diagnosis usually is made clinically based on the history of recurrences and the location and appearance of lesions.
- If uncertainty exists, a Wright stain of vesicular fluid will reveal a predominance of neutrophils and eosinophils.
- Gram stain reveals no organisms and a mineral oil preparation reveals no evidence of scabies.

Treatment

- If symptoms are mild, no therapy is required.
- If pruritus is severe, consider
  - Potent topical corticosteroid applied to lesions twice daily during flares
  - Oral sedating antihistamine to provide relief from pruritus
- Dapsone may be used in severe cases (use with caution due to potential for hemolytic anemia and methemoglobinemia), although it is rarely necessary.

Prognosis

- Usually resolves within 1 to 2 years

When to Worry or Refer

- Consider referral if diagnosis is uncertain or if severe pruritus does not respond to standard therapy.

Intertrigo

Introduction/Etiology/Epidemiology

- Rubbing of moist skin surfaces results in superficial erosions.
- Often becomes secondarily infected with *Candida* species; also may be secondarily infected with *Streptococcus pyogenes* or, less commonly, *Staphylococcus aureus.*

Signs and Symptoms

- Erythema and superficial erosions located in the skinfolds (eg, anterior neck fold, axillae, inguinal creases) (Figure 95.1).
- If secondary candidal infection is present, the area often is bright red and satellite lesions are present.
- Secondary *S pyogenes* (or, occasionally, *S aureus*) infection is suggested by persistent lesions that are superficially eroded, painful, and malodorous.

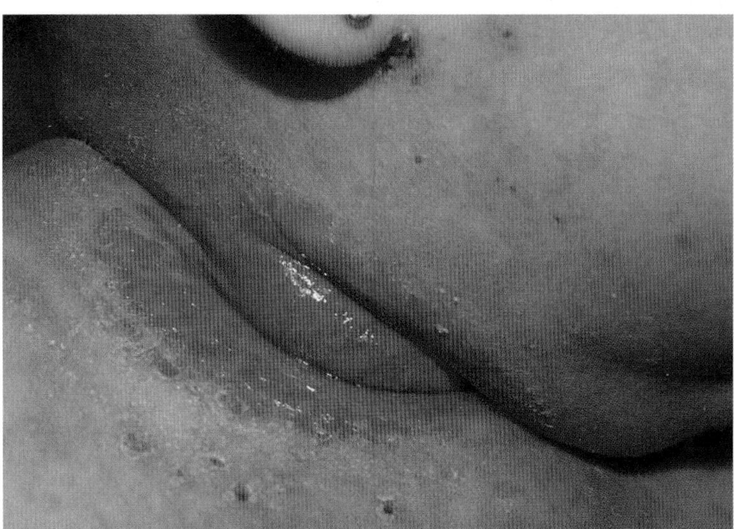

Figure 95.1. Intertrigo is characterized by erythematous superficial erosions located in the skinfolds. This infant had secondary infection with *Streptococcus pyogenes.*

Look-alikes

Disorder	Differentiating Features
Seborrheic dermatitis	• Begins at 3–4 weeks and resolves by end of first year • Salmon-pink patches with greasy scale • Usually involves several sites (eg, retroauricular folds, anterior neck fold, axillae, diaper area) symmetrically (not a single site, as in intertrigo)
Candidal diaper dermatitis	• Bright red, erythematous patch that involves inguinal creases, as well as convexities of the proximal thighs and lower abdomen. • Satellite lesions and scale may be present. • Potassium hydroxide preparation will reveal pseudohyphae and spores.
Tinea cruris	• Erythematous patch involving proximal medial thigh and inguinal fold. • Border somewhat elevated and has associated scale. • Potassium hydroxide preparation will reveal branching hyphae.
Erythrasma	• Erythematous to brown patch • Coral red fluorescence on Wood lamp examination

How to Make the Diagnosis

- The diagnosis is made clinically.

Treatment

- Apply an absorbent powder (to reduce moisture) or a greasy emollient (to reduce friction).
- For more severe cases, apply a low-potency topical corticosteroid.
- Treat with an antifungal preparation (if candidal infection) or oral antibiotic (if streptococcal or staphylococcal infection) suspected.

Prognosis

- Excellent

When to Worry or Refer

- Patients should be referred if the diagnosis is uncertain or fails to respond to therapy.

Resources for Families

- MedlinePlus: Information for patients and families (in English and Spanish) sponsored by the National Library of Medicine and National Institutes of Health. **www.nlm.nih.gov/medlineplus/ency/article/003223.htm**

Miliaria

Introduction/Etiology/Epidemiology

- Obstruction of eccrine ducts. Three forms are recognized.
  - Miliaria rubra (prickly heat or heat rash): caused by deep intraepidermal obstruction of eccrine ducts accompanied by an inflammatory response
  - Miliaria crystallina: caused by superficial obstruction that results in trapping of sweat
  - Miliaria pustulosa: often considered a variant of miliaria rubra but with a more intense inflammatory response
- Occurs in infants who are in warm environments, febrile, or dressed overly warmly.

Signs and Symptoms

- Miliaria rubra: erythematous papules located on the forehead, upper trunk, or flexural areas (eg, neck folds) or under clothing, bandages, or monitor leads (Figure 96.1)
- Miliaria crystallina: fragile, non-inflamed, small vesicles filled with clear fluid (Figure 96.2)
- Miliaria pustulosa: pustules with surrounding erythema that are located in the areas described for miliaria rubra (see Figure 96.1)

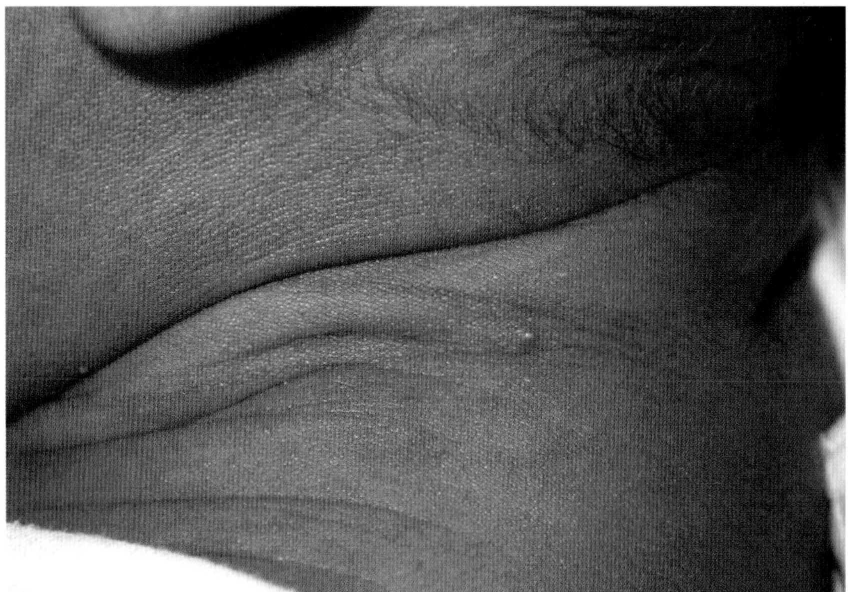

Figure 96.1. Erythematous papules (miliaria rubra) and pustules (miliaria pustulosa) located in the skinfolds of the neck.

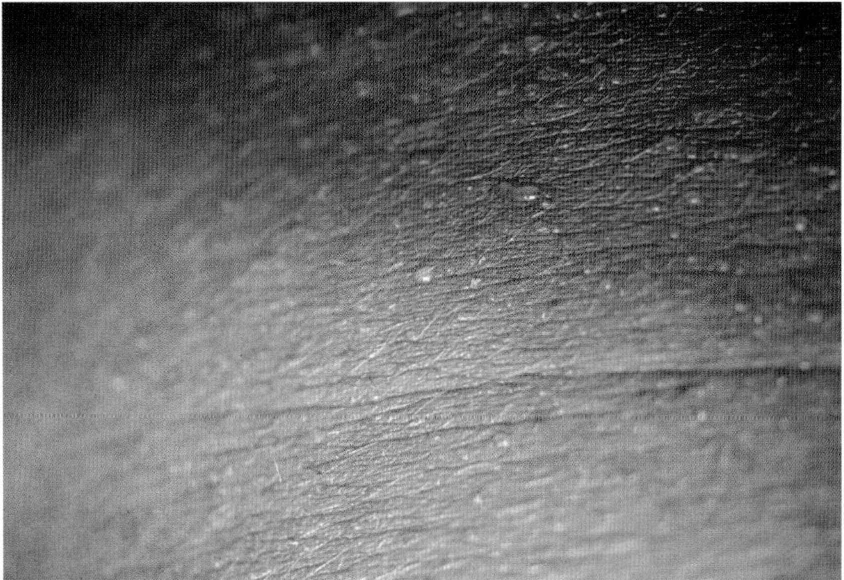

Figure 96.2. Miliaria crystallina is characterized by fragile superficial vesicles without surrounding erythema.

Look-alikes

- Miliaria crystallina occasionally may be mistaken for herpes simplex virus infection; however, the lesions of miliaria crystallina have no associated erythema.
- Miliaria pustulosa and rubra may mimic staphylococcal folliculitis; however, a Gram stain of pustular contents would reveal no organisms and a bacterial culture would be sterile.
- See Look-alikes in Chapter 93, Erythema Toxicum, to assist in differentiating miliaria from other disorders characterized by vesiculopustules.

How to Make the Diagnosis

- The diagnosis is made clinically.

Treatment

- The best management is prevention. Avoid environmental overheating, overdressing infants, and applying thick emollients (that may obstruct eccrine ducts).
- For infants with established miliaria, provide an air-conditioned environment, if possible. Cool baths or sponge baths may be helpful.

Prognosis

- Resolves spontaneously

When to Worry or Refer

- Referral is warranted only if diagnostic uncertainty exists.

Resources for Families

- American Academy of Pediatrics: HealthyChildren.org. **www.healthychildren.org/English/ages-stages/baby/bathing-skin-care/Pages/Your-Newborns-Skin-Birthmarks-and-Rashes.aspx**

Nevus Sebaceous (of Jadassohn)

Introduction/Etiology/Epidemiology

- Hamartoma of sebaceous and apocrine glands and epidermal elements present in 0.3% of newborns.
- Usually appears as an isolated finding; rarely associated with neurologic, ocular, or skeletal abnormalities (ie, epidermal nevus or Schimmelpenning syndrome).

Signs and Symptoms

- Usually presents at birth as a solitary, well-circumscribed, round or oval plaque.
- Typically located on the scalp, where it is associated with alopecia (Figure 97.1), or face, where it may be linear (Figure 97.2).
- Lesions are yellow, yellow-brown, orange, or pink and have a velvety or verrucous texture.
- At puberty, androgenic stimulation causes lesions to become more elevated and develop a rough surface.

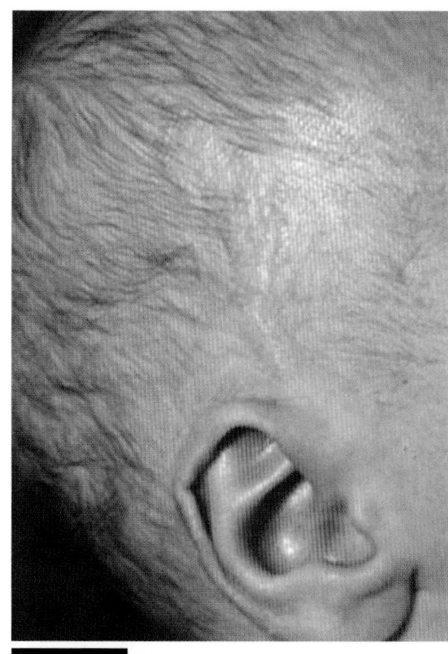

Figure 97.1. Nevus sebaceous. Yellow-tan hairless plaque located on the scalp.

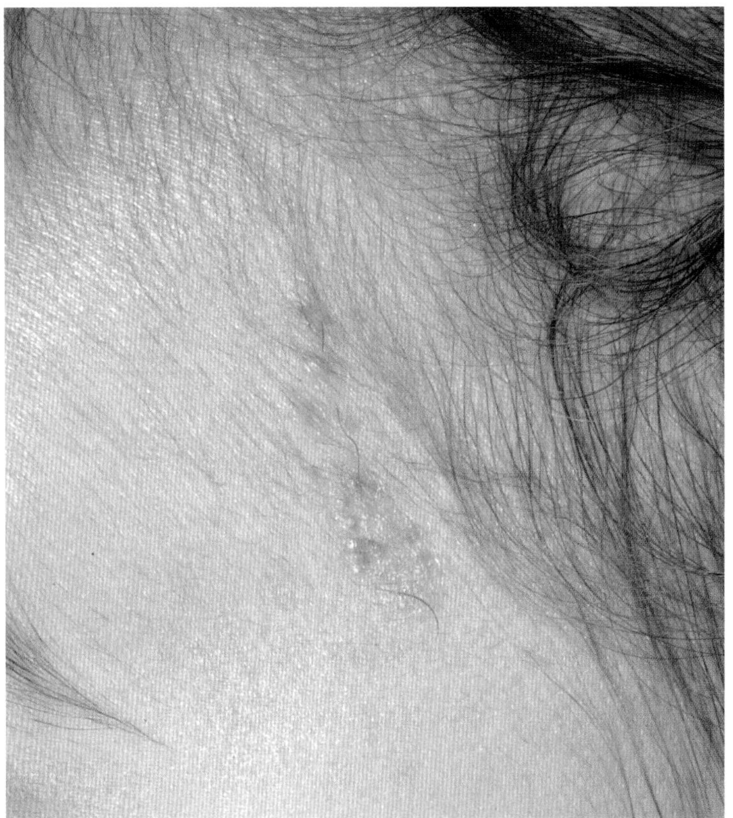

Figure 97.2. A linear nevus sebaceous located on the face.

Look-alikes

Disorder	Differentiating Features
Aplasia cutis congenita	• Presents at birth as an ulcer or scar • Rarely has a yellow color; does not change at puberty
Epidermal nevus	• May be difficult to differentiate from nevus sebaceous • Often has rougher surface and more brown in color
Juvenile xanthogranuloma	• One or more yellow-orange papules or dome-shaped non-verrucous plaques • Usually acquired (not present at birth)

How to Make the Diagnosis

- The diagnosis may be suspected clinically and can be confirmed by skin biopsy.

Treatment

- No treatment is required during infancy or childhood.
- Because there is a small risk of developing an adnexal tumor or basal cell carcinoma within the nevus after puberty, some advise elective excision at this time. Another option is to excise only those nevi that develop suspicious changes (eg, a nodule within the nevus) or those that are cosmetically significant.

Prognosis

- Most sebaceous nevi exhibit a benign course, although there is a small chance of malignant transformation, as discussed previously.

When to Worry or Refer

- Changes in a nevus sebaceus (eg, development of a nodule) should prompt referral to a dermatologist.
- If concern exists about the epidermal nevus syndrome (eg, the nevus sebaceus is extensive or linear and associated with developmental delay, seizures, or ophthalmologic abnormalities [eg, coloboma of the eyelid]), consultations with a pediatric dermatologist, neurologist, medical geneticist, or pediatric ophthalmologist should be sought, as indicated.

CHAPTER 98

Transient Neonatal Pustular Melanosis

Introduction/Etiology/Epidemiology

- Occurs in 5% of African American neonates; rare in other racial groups
- Cause unknown

Signs and Symptoms

- Present at birth.
- May present as pustules without surrounding erythema (Figure 98.1) or ruptured pustules that appear as small (several millimeters) hyperpigmented macules, often with a rim of surrounding scale (Figures 98.2 and 98.3).
- Lesions may occur at any location, but the forehead, chin, neck, and trunk most often are affected; the palms and soles occasionally are involved.
- Pustules resolve in several days; hyperpigmented macules resolve in 3 to 4 months.

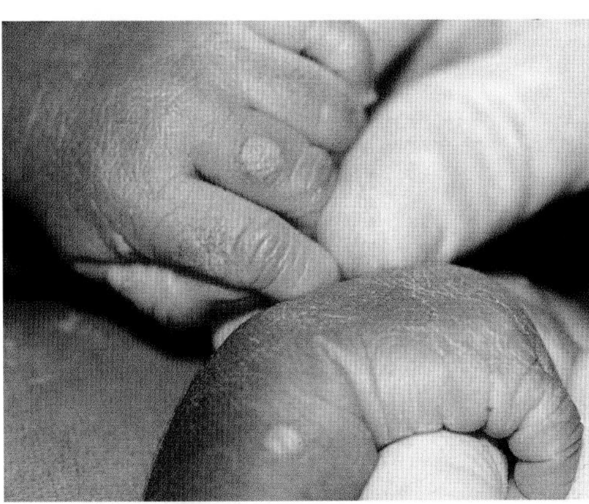

Figure 98.1. Pustules without surrounding erythema may be observed in neonates who have transient neonatal pustular melanosis.

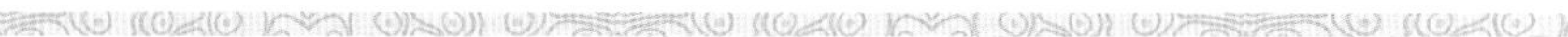

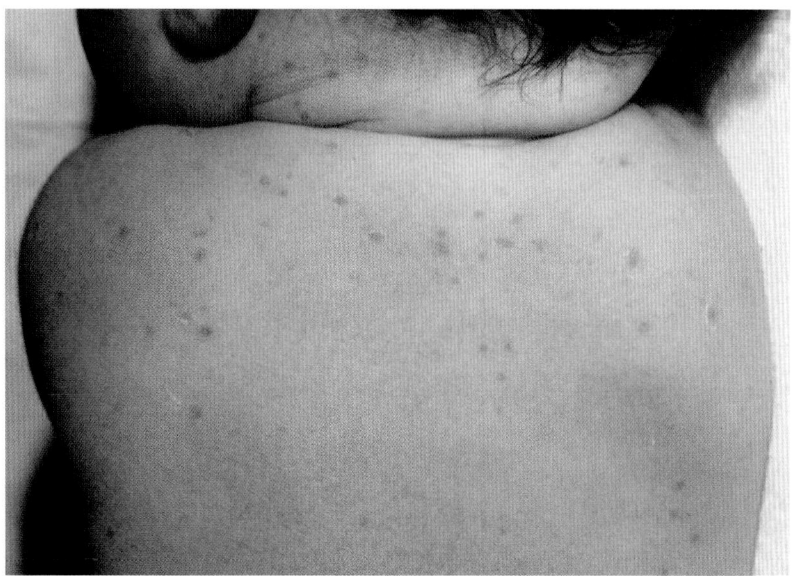

Figure 98.2. Hyperpigmented macules, some with a rim of scale, are seen in transient neonatal pustular melanosis.

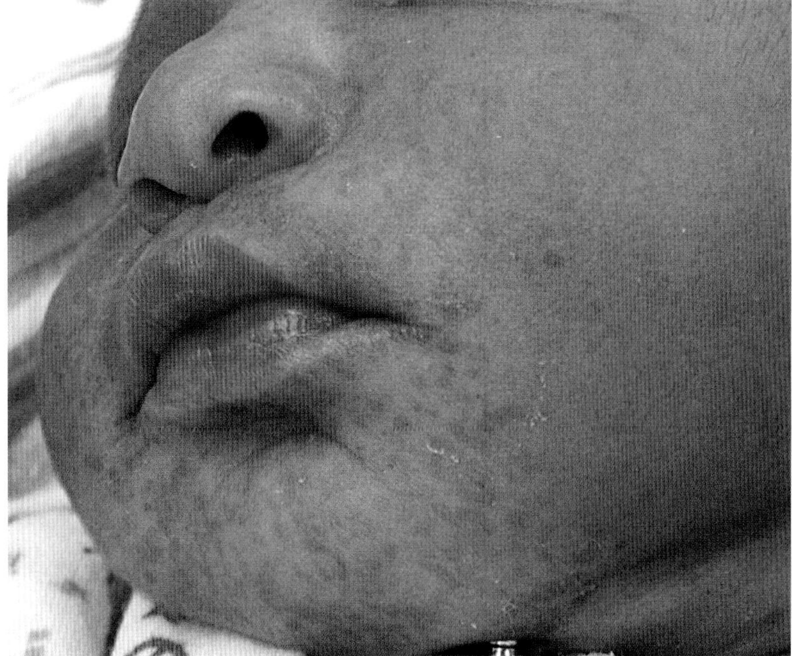

Figure 98.3. Transient neonatal pustular melanosis. Hyperpigmented macules on the chin. Note the collarettes of scale present in some areas.

Look-alikes

- The differential diagnosis includes miliaria, staphylococcal folliculitis, and congenital candidiasis (although these disorders produce lesions that exhibit erythema); infantile acropustulosis (lesions typically are pruritic and limited to the hands and feet); and congenital herpes simplex virus infection (lesions often are clustered and lack hyperpigmentation).
- See Look-alikes in Chapter 93, Erythema Toxicum, to assist in differentiating transient neonatal pustular melanosis from other disorders characterized by vesiculopustules.

How to Make the Diagnosis

- The diagnosis is made clinically. If uncertainty exists, performance of a Wright stain of vesicular fluid will reveal a predominance of neutrophils. Gram stain reveals no organisms.
- Performance of a Gram stain and bacterial culture of pustule fluid will exclude staphylococcal folliculitis, the condition with which transient neonatal pustular melanosis is most often confused. A potassium hydroxide preparation will exclude congenital candidiasis.

Treatment

- No treatment is required.

Prognosis

- Resolves spontaneously; does not recur.
- Hyperpigmented macules may take 3 to 6 months to resolve.

When to Worry or Refer

- In view of the age of onset and typical clinical appearance, referral rarely is necessary.

Resources for Families

- American Academy of Pediatrics: HealthyChildren.org. **www.HealthyChildren.org/Birthmarks**
- WebMD: Information for families is contained in the Health A-Z topics. **www.webmd.com/children/tc/newborn-rashes-and-skin-conditions-topic-overview**

Acute Drug/Toxic Reactions

CHAPTER 99

Drug Hypersensitivity Syndrome

Introduction/Etiology/Epidemiology

- A severe cutaneous drug eruption in combination with systemic manifestations.
- Also known as drug reaction with eosinophilia and systemic symptoms (DRESS) and drug-induced hypersensitivity syndrome.
- Classic triad consists of fever, skin rash, and internal organ (usually liver) involvement.
- Occurs 1 to 8 weeks (most common: 2–4 weeks) after starting the drug.
- Most often occurs following initial exposure to the medication.
- Potentially life-threatening.
- Most common causative drugs include anticonvulsant agents (mainly the aromatic agents, including phenytoin, carbamazepine, and phenobarbital; also lamotrigine), sulfonamides (mainly trimethoprim-sulfamethoxazole; rarely, furosemide), dapsone, minocycline, and allopurinol; nonsteroidal anti-inflammatory drugs also occasionally implicated.
- Etiology involves impaired detoxification of drug metabolites and may involve coinfection with human herpesvirus 6.
- May be a familial predisposition.

Signs and Symptoms

- Fever and malaise early.
- Rash begins as exanthematous eruption, becoming more edematous and erythematous and with confluence of lesions (Figure 99.1).
- Eruption may become vesicular, bullous, or purpuric; may simulate/progress to Stevens-Johnson syndrome/toxic epidermal necrolysis.
- Mucous membranes may be involved.
- Characteristic facial edema develops, especially periorbital (Figure 99.2).

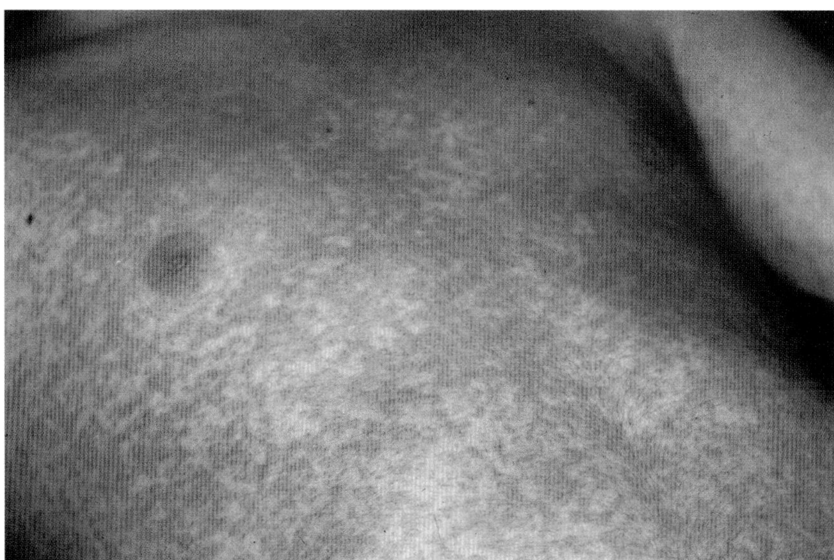

Figure 99.1. Drug hypersensitivity syndrome. This patient developed an eruption of erythematous macules and papules during his second week of carbamazepine therapy. Fever and hepatitis were also present.

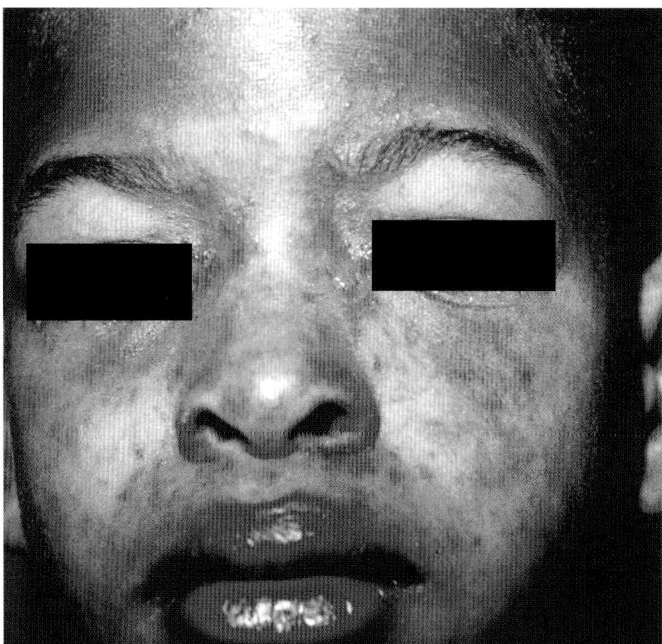

Figure 99.2. Drug hypersensitivity syndrome. Therapy with phenytoin resulted in a widespread skin eruption in this child, including facial involvement with prominent periorbital edema. He also had lip swelling, fever, lymphadenopathy, and hepatitis.

- Cervical lymphadenopathy common.
- Liver is the most common extracutaneous site of involvement; may progress to fulminant hepatitis.
- Other involvement may include nephritis, pneumonitis, thyroiditis, and myocarditis; thyroid involvement may be delayed, with hypothyroidism noted up to 2 to 3 months following the acute reaction.

Look-alikes

Disorder	Differentiating Features
Simple exanthematous drug eruption	• Lacks facial edema, lymphadenopathy, hepatitis, atypical lymphocytosis • Fever less common
Viral exanthem	• Less severe skin eruption • Usually lacks facial edema, hepatitis • Fever more commonly low grade, transient • History of drug ingestion lacking
Cutaneous lymphoma	• Lacks facial edema, hepatitis • Fever uncommon • History of drug ingestion lacking • Histopathologic features confirmatory

How to Make the Diagnosis

- The diagnosis is suggested by fever and a severe rash in the presence of facial edema, lymphadenopathy, and a history of ingestion of an implicated drug.
- Supportive laboratory findings include atypical lymphocytosis and eosinophilia, as well as elevation of liver transaminases; thyroid testing should be performed at baseline and, if normal, repeated in 2 to 3 months.
- Skin biopsy, when performed, reveals dense lymphocytic infiltrate with eosinophils in the dermis.
- Patch testing may be useful diagnostically, especially with carbamazepine and phenytoin, but exact sensitivity and specificity of this type of testing is unclear.
- Lymphocyte toxicity assays may be useful in confirming the triggering medication but not readily available.

Treatment

- Offending agent should be immediately discontinued once the diagnosis has been recognized.
- Systemic corticosteroids have been used for severe or progressive disease, with a gradual (3–4 week) taper, although their use is controversial.
- Antihistamines and topical corticosteroids may be useful for pruritus, and oral antipyretics may be useful in decreasing erythroderma and symptoms. Antipyretics should be used with caution in patients with liver involvement, especially when coadministered with systemic corticosteroids.
- Severely progressive disease has been treated with intravenous immunoglobulin and, rarely, liver transplantation.

Treating Associated Conditions

- Hypothyroidism should be treated appropriately, if present.

Prognosis

- The long-term outcome depends on the degree of extracutaneous involvement.
- Rapid recognition and prompt discontinuation of the causative agent may be associated with a better prognosis, although some patients will continue to progress.
- If the reaction is secondary to an aromatic anticonvulsant (eg, phenytoin, carbamazepine, phenobarbital, primidone), it is vital that substitution of another anticonvulsant from this group be avoided, given the high risk of cross-reactivity.

When to Worry or Refer

- Consider drug hypersensitivity syndrome or dermatology consultation in the patient presenting with a severe skin eruption accompanied by fever and lymphadenopathy.
- If hepatitis is noted, consultation with gastroenterology or hepatology should be requested.

Erythema Multiforme (EM)

Introduction/Etiology/Epidemiology

- Erythema multiforme (EM; previously called erythema multiforme minor) is a reactive inflammatory disorder of limited duration that may become recurrent.
- Causes include infection and medications.
- Recurrent EM in children is due largely to recurrent herpes simplex virus (HSV) infection.

Signs and Symptoms

- Begins as erythematous, blanching, round or oval papules or plaques.
- Lesions then develop a target appearance, with central dusky to violaceous color (Figure 100.1) (sometimes with a central vesicle, bulla [Figure 100.2], or crust) surrounded by concentric white (sometimes) and red rings, the latter 2 representing vasoconstriction or vasodilation, respectively.
- A single mucosal surface (usually lips) may be involved.
- The disease lasts 7 to 10 days before resolving spontaneously.

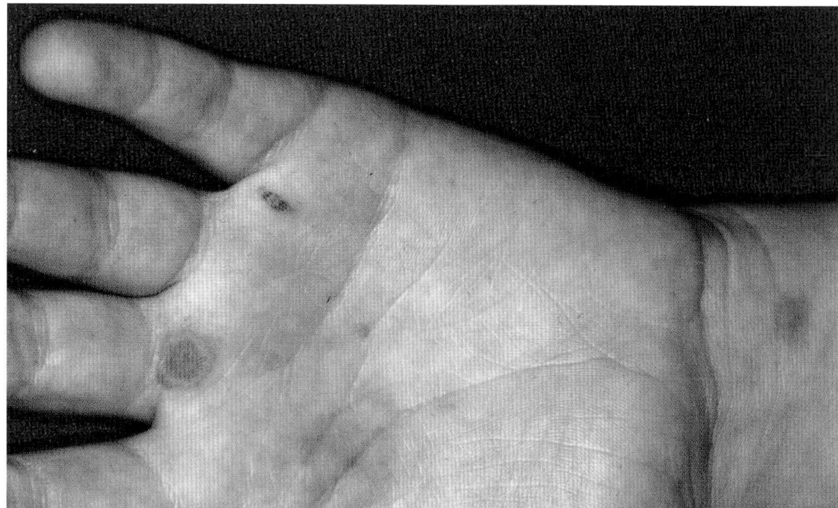

Figure 100.1. Erythema multiforme. Target lesions are erythematous papules or plaques that develop a central violaceous discoloration.

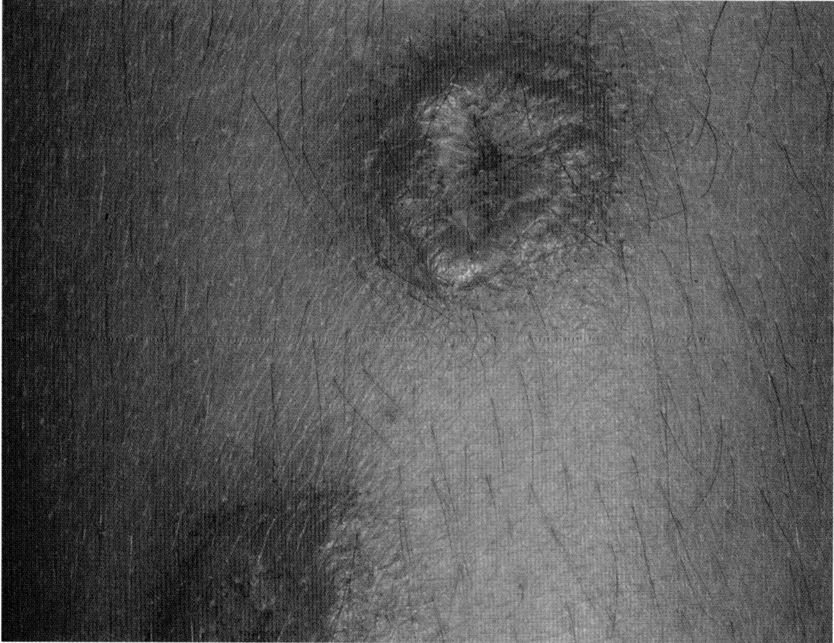

Figure 100.2. Erythema multiforme. Target lesions may develop central bullae or vesicles.

Look-alikes

Disorder	Differentiating Features
Urticaria	• Erythematous blanching wheals that resolve or change in 24 hours or sooner. • Occasionally, lesions may become centrally dusky, but no vesicle or crust formation. • Although lesions may become annular, true target lesions do not occur. • In "urticaria multiforme," annular, polycyclic, and occasionally dusky urticarial papules and plaques occur and may be mistaken for EM.
Stevens-Johnson syndrome toxic epidermal necrolysis (TEN)	• Prodromal symptoms (eg, fever, sore throat, malaise) precede appearance of rash by as much as 14 days. • Patients are systemically ill. • Target lesions may be few in number or atypical in their appearance (especially in TEN). • Erythematous macules or patches that develop bullae and erosions. • Extensive mucosal involvement with 2 or more sites affected. • Stevens-Johnson syndrome often associated with *Mycoplasma pneumoniae* infection. • TEN often associated with reaction to systemic drug.
Serum sickness or serum sickness–like eruption	• Large, often purple, urticarial-appearing plaques present. • Target lesions and blistering absent. • Fever, arthralgia, or arthritis constant features. • Periarticular swelling often present. • Ambulatory children may refuse to walk during episode.

How to Make the Diagnosis

- The diagnosis of EM is made clinically and may be confirmed by skin biopsy.
- Presence of target lesions concentrated on the palms, soles, arms, and legs.
- Target lesions exhibit peeling, blistering, or crusting in the center of some lesions.
- Involvement of no more than one mucosal surface.

Treatment

- Consider antiviral prophylaxis for presumed HSV infection if EM is recurrent.
- If pruritus is significant, an antihistamine may be prescribed.
- Corticosteroid therapy is not indicated.

Prognosis

- Erythema multiforme resolves spontaneously, leaving only occasional postinflammatory hyperpigmentation.
- Recurrent EM may indicate HSV infection and reactivation. In such cases, antiviral prophylaxis may be required to prevent EM recurrences.

Resources for Families

- MedlinePlus: Information for patients and families (in English and Spanish) sponsored by the National Library of Medicine and National Institutes of Health.
  https://www.nlm.nih.gov/medlineplus/ency/article/000851.htm
- WebMD: Information for families is contained in Skin Problems and Treatments Health Center.
  www.webmd.com/skin-problems-and-treatments/erythema-multiforme

CHAPTER 101

Exanthematous and Urticarial Drug Reactions

Introduction/Etiology/Epidemiology

- Drug reactions or eruptions may present in a variety of morphologic forms.
- May include exanthematous (morbilliform), urticarial, pustular, and blistering presentations.
- Exanthematous form is the most common type of cutaneous drug eruption.
- Urticarial form is the second most common type of cutaneous drug eruption.
- Exanthematous eruptions may present anytime within first 2 weeks of starting the medication; urticarial eruptions tend to present more rapidly (ie, immediate reactions).
- These reactions are frequently responsible for premature discontinuation of treatment.
- Increased risk in patients on multiple medications and those with concomitant viral infection; classic example is the exanthematous eruption that occurs after ingestion of penicillin-class antibiotics in patients with acute Epstein-Barr virus infection.
- Most common cause of a drug eruption is an antimicrobial agent.
- Penicillin-cephalosporin cross-reactivity is generally overemphasized in the literature and classic teachings. Penicillin-allergic patients are at a very mildly (1%–3%) increased risk of reaction to first-generation cephalosporins (ie, cefadroxil, cefazolin, cephalexin, cephalothin, and cephaloridine) and to the second-generation cefamandole; there appears to be no increased risk associated with the use of other cephalosporins in these patients.

Signs and Symptoms

- Exanthematous eruption
  - Generalized erythematous macules and papules (Figure 101.1).
  - May appear morbilliform (measles-like) or scarlatiniform (scarlet fever–like).
  - Often begins on the head and upper trunk, with cephalocaudad extension.
  - Lesions may become confluent and are often pruritic.
  - Rarely progresses to erythroderma or exfoliation.
  - Etiologies include antibiotics (especially ß-lactams, sulfonamides), barbiturates, anticonvulsants, angiotensin-converting enzyme (ACE) inhibitors, gold, and nonsteroidal anti-inflammatory agents.

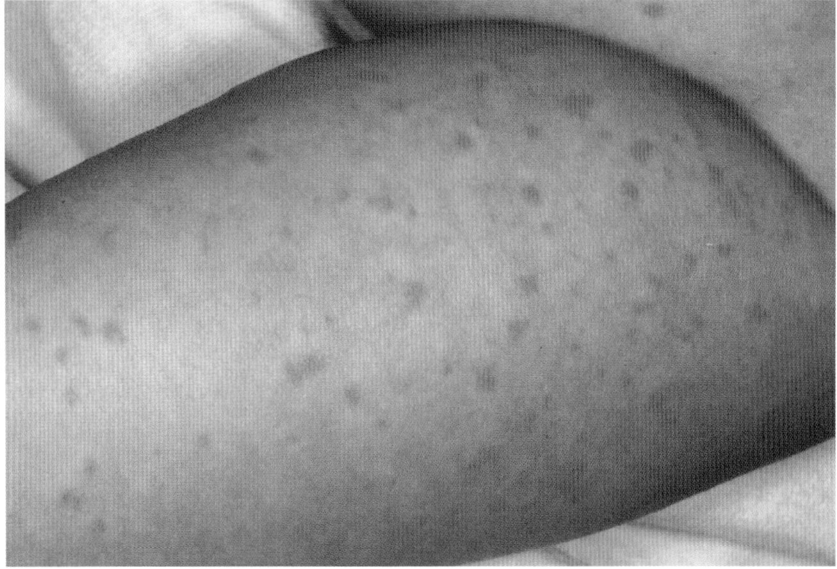

Figure 101.1. Exanthematous drug eruption. These erythematous macules and papules occurred during therapy with amoxicillin.

- Urticarial eruption
  - Pruritic, edematous wheals of various sizes (Figure 101.2).
  - May appear annular, arcuate, or polycyclic.
  - Individual lesions last no longer than 24 hours, but new lesions may continue to develop.
  - When deeper subcutaneous or dermal tissues are involved (eg, lips, eyes, mucous membranes), it is termed *angioedema.*
  - Etiologies include antibiotics (especially sulfonamides, ß-lactams), anticonvulsants, ACE inhibitors, azole antifungal agents, narcotic analgesics, salicylates, and radiocontrast dye.

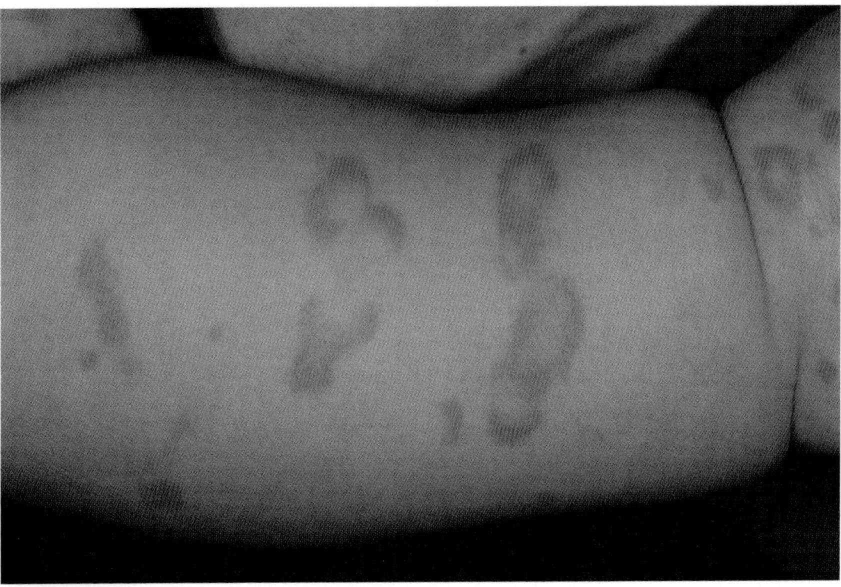

Figure 101.2. Urticarial drug eruption. These urticarial papules and plaques occurred 2 days following initiation of oral sulfonamide therapy.

Look-alikes

Disorder	Differentiating Features
Exanthematous Drug Eruption	
Viral exanthem	• Associated infectious symptomatology. • Lack of preceding drug ingestion. • At times, the 2 may be indistinguishable.
Scarlet fever	• Accentuation of eruption in skinfolds • Circumoral pallor • Pharyngitis and strawberry tongue • Rapid testing or culture result positive for *Streptococcus pyogenes*
Miliaria rubra (prickly heat)	• Tends to predominate in occluded areas (eg, skinfolds) • Lack of preceding drug ingestion • Often a history of overheating, swaddling, overapplication of greasy topical products (eg, petrolatum) • Resolves rapidly with cooling and avoidance of occlusion
Drug hypersensitivity syndrome	• Marked facial edema, with periorbital accentuation • Cervical lymphadenopathy common • Fever often present • Atypical lymphocytosis, eosinophilia, and hepatitis on laboratory monitoring • Classically develops 2 to 4 weeks following drug ingestion
Graft-versus-host disease (GVHD)	• Susceptible patient (eg, following stem cell transplantation) • Palms, soles, posterior auricular scalp involved • Associated diarrhea, bilirubin elevation • Characteristic changes of GVHD noted on skin biopsy samples
Urticarial Drug Eruption	
Erythema multiforme	• True target lesions with 3 zones (central duskiness, surrounded by pallor, and then peripheral erythema) • Palm and sole involvement common • Usually lack of preceding drug ingestion • Occasional single mucous membrane involvement • Commonly associated with recurrent herpes simplex virus infection in children
Serum sickness–like eruption	• Purple appearance of urticarial lesions ("purple urticaria") • Fever common • Periarticular swelling and pain with ambulation • Occasional proteinuria
Kawasaki disease	• High fever common (for ≥5 days, to meet diagnostic criteria) • Conjunctival injection (nonpurulent), oral mucosal hyperemia, lip fissuring, strawberry tongue present • Cervical lymphadenopathy common • May have accentuation of rash with desquamation in perineum • Risk of coronary artery aneurysms

How to Make the Diagnosis

- The diagnosis is entertained based on the cutaneous findings and presenting history.
- Development of a timeline of drug ingestion and development of the eruption may be useful in patients receiving multiple medications; often, however, the exact culprit may be difficult to confirm.
- Ruling out other potential explanations may be necessary with laboratory testing or medical imaging.
- Skin biopsy occasionally helpful.

Treatment

- Withdrawal of the causative agent usually results in spontaneous resolution.
- Therapy is generally symptomatic and may include oral antihistamines and topical antipruritic preparations. The latter include topical corticosteroids, camphor and menthol preparations, calamine, and witch hazel; topical diphenhydramine is available but should be avoided, as it may result in contact sensitization (with allergic contact dermatitis).
- "Treating through" the cutaneous eruption may be considered for patients with an exanthematous drug eruption in whom the treatment is extremely important and when there is no satisfactory substitute; requires close clinical follow-up.
- Systemic corticosteroids rarely indicated for exanthematous or urticarial drug eruptions.

Treating Associated Conditions

- In patients for whom an infectious exanthem cannot be excluded, appropriate examination, testing (when indicated), and parental education should be offered.

Prognosis

- Uncomplicated exanthematous and urticarial drug eruptions resolve completely and without permanent sequelae.

When to Worry or Refer

- Consider dermatology referral when
    - Atypical cutaneous features are present.
    - The skin eruption is unusually severe or associated with extracutaneous findings.
    - The diagnosis is in question.

Resources for Families

- MedlinePlus: Information for patients and families (in English and Spanish) sponsored by the National Library of Medicine and National Institutes of Health.
  https://www.nlm.nih.gov/medlineplus/ency/article/000819.htm

Fixed Drug Eruption

Introduction/Etiology/Epidemiology

- Common drug eruption in children and adults.
- Characterized by recurrence of the eruption at same location on the body after repeat ingestion of etiologic medication.
- May involve skin or mucosal sites.
- May occur as a single lesion (Figure 102.1) or in a generalized form (Figure 102.2).
- Common causes include sulfonamides, nonsteroidal anti-inflammatory agents, acetaminophen, tetracycline, and pseudoephedrine; also reported in association with fluconazole, dextromethorphan, sildenafil, metronidazole, and phenylephrine.
- Latent period of 1 to 2 weeks after first exposure, 12 to 24 hours following subsequent exposures.
- "Fixed food eruption" has been described with similar clinical features in association with ingestion of licorice, asparagus, cashew nut, peanut, lentils, quinine (in tonic water), and tartrazine (in artificially colored cheese crisps).

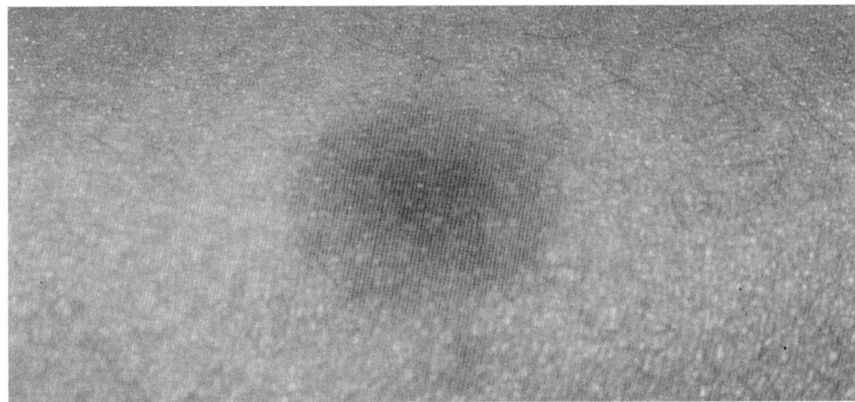

Figure 102.1. Fixed drug eruption. This single lesion occurred in response to sulfonamide ingestion.

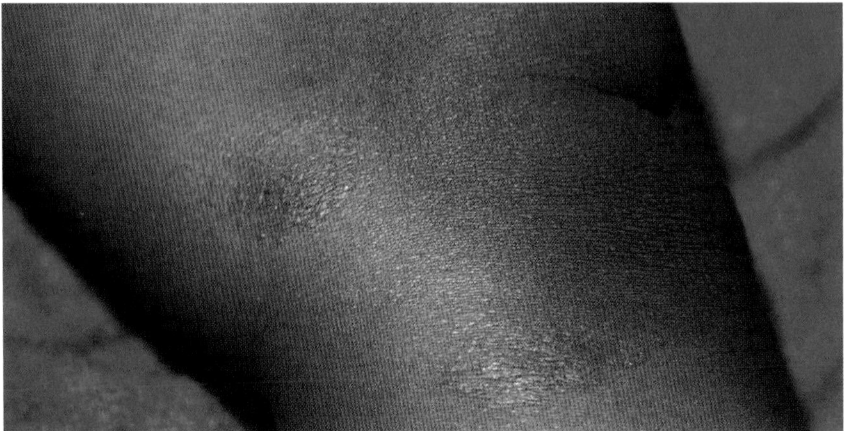

Figure 102.2. Fixed drug eruption. This child had multiple lesions, felt to be due to acetaminophen or pseudoephedrine.

Signs and Symptoms

- Sharply demarcated, red to violaceous plaques.
- Occasionally, a central blister or erosion is present.
- Acute inflammation resolves over several days, leaving hyperpigmentation, which may persist for months to years.
- Sites of predilection include lips, face, extremities, and genitalia.
- On readministration of the drug (or food), lesions recur in same location or locations.

Look-alikes

Disorder	Differentiating Features
Arthropod bite	• Usually pruritic • Resolves without recurrence in same location • History of preceding drug ingestion lacking
Erythema multiforme	• Multiple lesions typical (less common with fixed drug eruption) • Symmetric palm and sole lesions common • May not always be able to distinguish
Urticaria	• Rapid resolution of lesions over hours • Persistent hyperpigmentation rare • Mixture of annular, solid, and arcuate patterns
Herpes simplex virus infection	• May be considered in the differential diagnosis of genital fixed drug eruption • Painful • Blisters, erosions, or crusting consistently present • History of sexual activity or concerns for sexual abuse present • History of preceding drug ingestion lacking

How to Make the Diagnosis

- Fixed drug eruption should be suspected clinically based on examination findings and drug ingestion history.
- History of recurrence with drug ingestion is supportive.
- Histologic findings (if skin biopsy performed) are confirmatory.

Treatment

- No treatment is necessary.
- Acute inflammation subsides over days, pigmentation over months to years.
- Drug can occasionally be readministered without exacerbation, although recurrence is likely.

Prognosis

- Fixed drug eruptions resolve completely, although the pigmentation may take months to years to fade.
- Fixed drug eruption is not indicative of a risk for more serious reactions to the offending agent.

When to Worry or Refer

- Consider referral when the diagnosis is in question.

Serum Sickness–Like Reaction

Introduction/Etiology/Epidemiology

- Characterized by fever, rash, and arthralgias.
- More common in children.
- Usually occurs 1 to 3 weeks after starting implicated medication, occasionally earlier.
- Distinguished from "true" serum sickness by absence of immune complexes, hypocomplementemia, vasculitis, and kidney disease.
- Potential causes include cefaclor (classic descriptions), other cephalosporins, penicillin, amoxicillin, tetracyclines, sulfonamides, clarithromycin, bupropion, and ß-blockers; occasional reports in association with efalizumab, rituximab, infliximab, transfusions, and influenza vaccine.
- Occasionally, presents without history of preceding drug ingestion.

Signs and Symptoms

- Eruption may be morbilliform or, more commonly, urticarial (Figure 103.1).
- Classic feature is "purple urticaria," with violaceous hue in skin lesions (Figures 103.2 and 103.3).
- Periarticular swelling and pain with ambulation are common.
- Toddlers often refuse to bear weight on legs.
- Fever is often present, and lymphadenopathy is common.

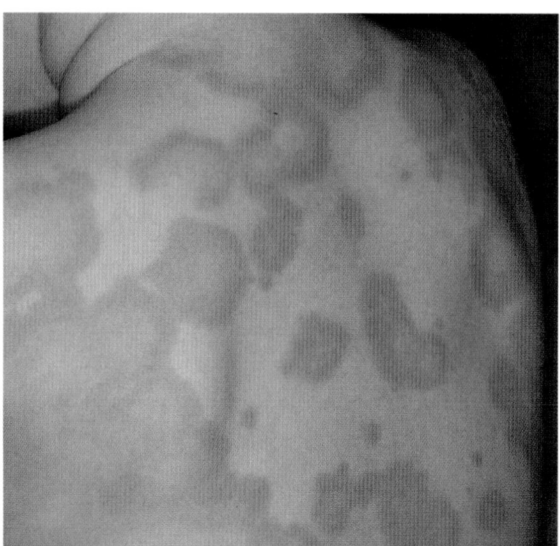

Figure 103.1. Serum sickness–like reaction. Urticarial papules and plaques are seen in this patient, who also had marked periarticular swelling.

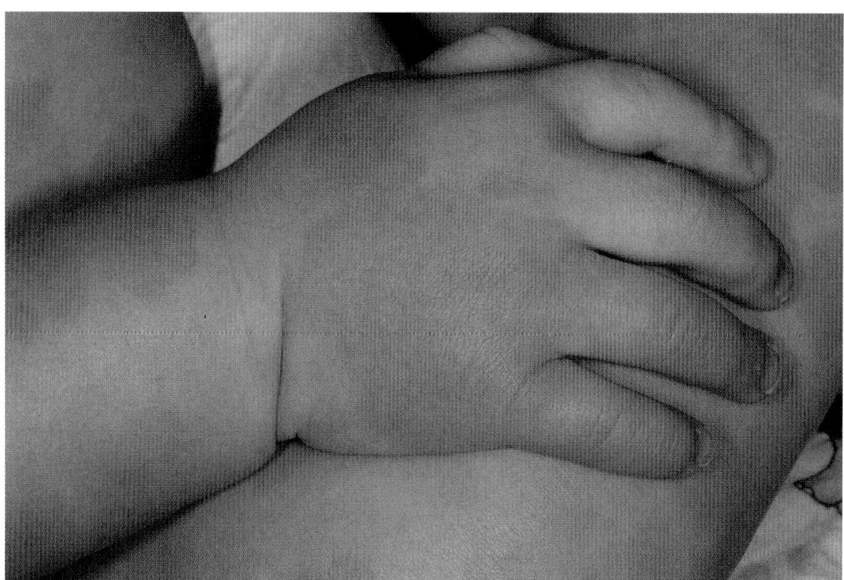

Figure 103.2. Serum sickness–like reaction. Hand swelling and urticarial plaques with a purple hue are seen in the same patient as in Figure 103.1.

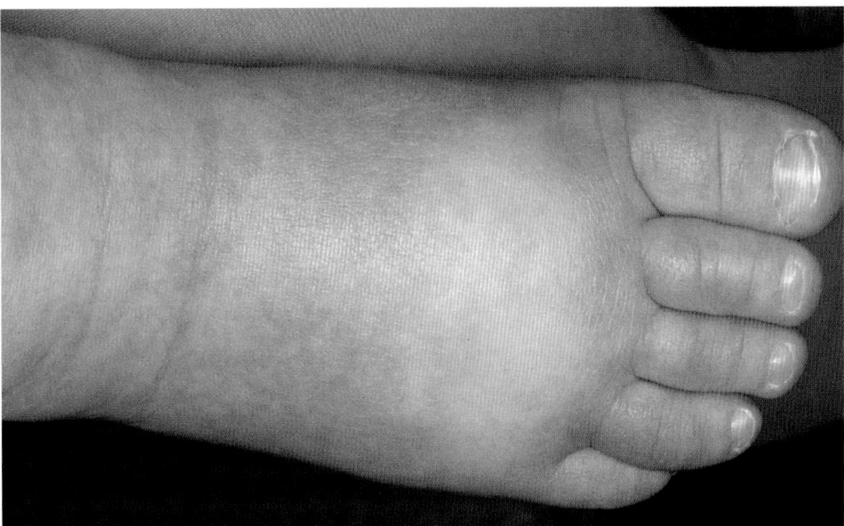

Figure 103.3. Serum sickness–like reaction. Periarticular and foot swelling, along with markedly purple, urticarial plaques, are seen in this toddler, who was receiving amoxicillin-clavulanate therapy for otitis media.

Look-alikes

Disorder	Differentiating Features
Urticaria	• More transient, with individual lesions resolving within 24 hours • Usually lacks violaceous appearance • Pruritus more common • Fever less common
Erythema multiforme	• Classic target lesions, with 3 zones of color: central duskiness (often with a vesicle or crust), surrounded by a pale ring and a peripheral red or purple ring • Palm and sole involvement common • Fever often absent • Lack of preceding drug ingestion history • May be recurrent, often in association with herpes simplex virus infection
Kawasaki disease	• Conjunctival injection, oral mucosal hyperemia, lip fissuring usually present • May have accentuation of rash with desquamation in perineum • Cervical lymphadenopathy common • Lack of preceding drug ingestion history

How to Make the Diagnosis

- The diagnosis of serum sickness–like eruption should be considered in the febrile child presenting with purple urticaria and periarticular swelling following medication (especially antibiotic) ingestion.

Treatment

- The offending medication should be discontinued.
- Oral antihistamines and antipyretics may provide symptom relief.
- Nonsteroidal anti-inflammatory agents will offer relief of joint pain and may accelerate the resolution of swelling.
- In patients with severe symptoms, systemic corticosteroids may be helpful and should be tapered over 3 to 4 weeks to prevent a rebound in symptoms.
- Cross-reaction of the specific cephalosporin or penicillin with other ß-lactams is unusual; avoidance of all ß-lactam antibiotics is probably unnecessary but is recommended by some experts.

Prognosis

- Most patients with serum sickness–like eruption recover fully with no long-term sequelae.

When to Worry or Refer

- Consider dermatology referral when the diagnosis is in question or when symptoms are severe and therapy is being considered.

Stevens-Johnson Syndrome (SJS)

Introduction/Etiology/Epidemiology

- Stevens-Johnson syndrome (SJS) (previously called erythema multiforme [EM] major) is a more serious condition that may not be related to EM. Many believe that SJS and toxic epidermal necrolysis (TEN) are variants of the same disease, differing in the extent of body surface involvement.
- Stevens-Johnson syndrome is a systemic illness of acute onset, often triggered by infection (eg, with *Mycoplasma pneumoniae*, Epstein-Barr virus, cytomegalovirus) or medications (eg, sulfonamides, antiepileptic drugs, acetaminophen, nonsteroidal anti-inflammatory drugs).
- Early in the course of the disease, SJS may have a presentation similar to that of EM (eg, targetoid lesions on extremities).
- The incidence of SJS is about 1 in 500,000 per year.
- Recurrence of SJS may occur in up to 18% of patients and may be delayed for up to 7 years.

Signs and Symptoms

- Often begins with prodromal symptoms of fever, headache, cough, sore throat, arthralgias, or malaise that precede the onset of the rash by up to 14 days.
- Patients develop target lesions or areas of erythema that form blisters that rupture, leaving erosions (Figures 104.1 and 104.2). The skin may appear dull and dusky before the blistering phase begins.
- Extensive mucosal surface erosions (involving ≥2 sites) are common; these may involve the eye (eyelids, conjunctiva, cornea), mouth (Figure 104.3), esophagus, or respiratory tract.
- Complications include interstitial pneumonitis, nephritis, and blindness. The severity of ocular sequelae is related to the severity of eye involvement early in the disease course.
- Dehydration from poor oral intake may be seen in patients with moderate to several oral mucosal involvement.

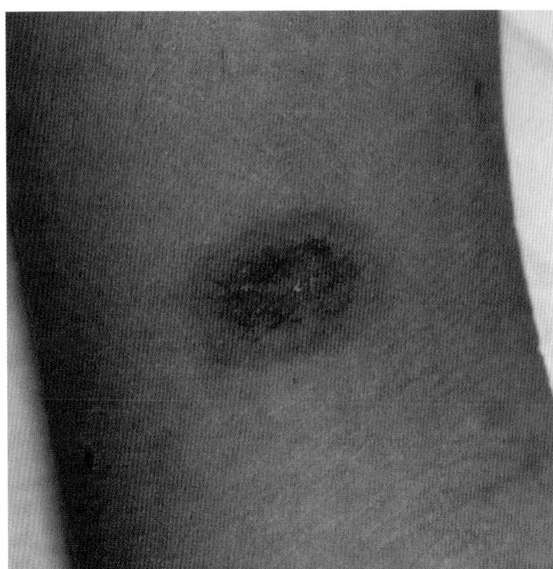

Figure 104.1. Target lesion in a patient who has Stevens-Johnson syndrome.

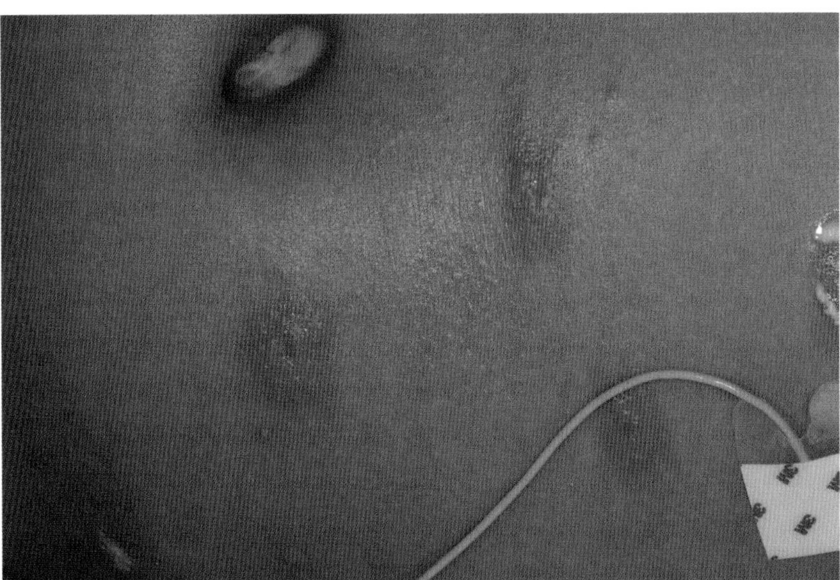

Figure 104.2. Erythematous erosions in a patient who has Stevens-Johnson syndrome.

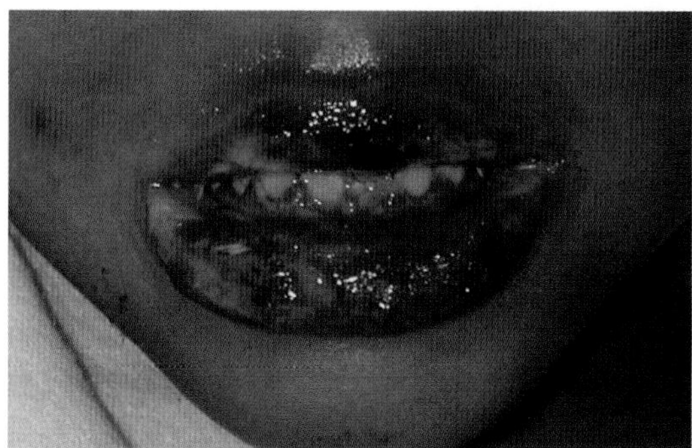

Figure 104.3. Extensive ulceration of the lips and oral mucosa are observed in Stevens-Johnson syndrome.

Look-alikes

Disorder	Differentiating Features
Urticaria	• Erythematous blanching wheals that resolve or change in 24 hours or sooner. • Occasionally, lesions may become centrally dusky, but no vesicle or crust formation. • Although lesions may become annular, true target lesions do not occur. • Mucosal erosions do not occur.
Kawasaki disease	• Eruption typically morbilliform, without vesicles or crusting. • Patients have nonpurulent conjunctival injection, not purulent conjunctivitis as observed in SJS. • Patients may have erythema and cracking of lips but not mucosal ulcers.
Serum sickness or serum sickness–like eruption	• Large, often purple, urticarial-appearing plaques present. • Target lesions, blistering, mucosal erosions absent. • Fever, arthralgia, or arthritis are constant features. • Periarticular swelling often present. • Ambulatory children may refuse to walk during episode.
Staphylococcal scalded skin syndrome	• Radial ("sunburst") erosions and crusting around mouth. • Sunburn-like erythema concentrated in skinfolds. • Superficial erosions develop but intact blisters uncommon (in contrast to SJS); Nikolsky sign present. • Oral erosions and ulcers absent. • Target lesions absent.
Toxic epidermal necrolysis (TEN)	• Target lesions may be present, but also dusky erythematous patches that rapidly form bullae and erosions. • Widespread detachment of the epidermis usually present. • More extensive skin involvement in TEN (>30% of body surface area [BSA]); in SJS, <10% of BSA is involved, while in SJS-TEN, 10% to 30% is involved. • More often drug-related.

How to Make the Diagnosis

- Presence of prodromal symptoms.
- Target lesions, blisters, or erosions.
- Involvement of 2 or more mucosal surfaces.
- Patients are systemically ill and may acutely decompensate.

Treatment

- Treatment is largely supportive.
- Identify and rapidly remove or treat the suspected precipitant.
- The role of systemic steroids remains controversial.
- Patients who have severe SJS may benefit from
  - Hospitalization (in a burn or other intensive care unit if there are extensive erosions) with careful attention to fluids, nutrition, eye care (including consultation with ophthalmology), and possibility of secondary bacterial infection
  - Intravenous Ig administration
- Avoid repeat exposure to offending medications, when identified.

Treating Associated Conditions

- Infectious causes (eg, *M pneumoniae* pneumonia) should be identified and treated if possible.

Prognosis

- SJS usually lasts 1 to 2 weeks, but complicated cases may resolve more slowly. Severe ocular sequelae may result.
- Most pediatric patients with SJS heal fully without permanent sequelae.
- The Score of Toxic Epidermal Necrolysis (SCORTEN) severity-of-illness scale has been used to predict mortality of SJS and TEN in adults and has also been shown to be useful in predicting morbidity in children when calculated within the first day of hospital admission.

When to Worry or Refer

- Ocular involvement in SJS should prompt ophthalmologic consultation.
- Widespread cutaneous blistering may require hospitalization in a burn or other intensive care setting.

Resources for Families

- Stevens Johnson Syndrome Foundation: Provides information, phone support, and referrals.
  www.sjsupport.org

Toxic Epidermal Necrolysis (TEN)

Introduction/Etiology/Epidemiology

- Toxic epidermal necrolysis (TEN) is a severe, potentially life-threatening multisystem illness characterized by generalized tender erythema, widespread bulla formation, and loss of the epidermis.
- Most cases of TEN are caused by drugs. The most common offending agents are antibiotics, antiepileptics, sulfonamides, and nonsteroidal anti-inflammatory agents.
- The incidence is estimated to be 0.5 to 1.2 cases per million per year.

Signs and Symptoms

- Conjunctival injection, ocular foreign body sensation and itching, fever, skin tenderness, and constitutional symptoms (eg, malaise, myalgias, arthralgias, nausea, vomiting, diarrhea) often precede the eruption by several days.
- The onset is abrupt with generalized tender erythema, progressing rapidly to dusky gray color with sloughing and development of large bullae (Figure 105.1).
- Sloughing skin removes the entire epidermis, including the pigmented layer, so the base is devoid of pigment (Figure 105.2).
- Glistening red and white patches resemble the base of a second-degree burn.
- Nikolsky sign is present (gentle lateral pressure on an area of dusky erythema or the edge of a bulla leads to separation of the skin).
- Mucosal surfaces are tender, eroded, and crusted.
  - Oral mucosa is painful and ulcerated.
  - Conjunctivae erode and ulcerate.
  - Urethral involvement is common, occasionally leading to dysuria, urethral stricture.
  - Respiratory mucosa may be involved.

- Other organ systems involved include
  - Renal (acute interstitial nephritis)
  - Gastrointestinal (mucosal sloughing and bleeding)
  - Pulmonary (tracheal and bronchial mucosal erosion, pneumonitis)

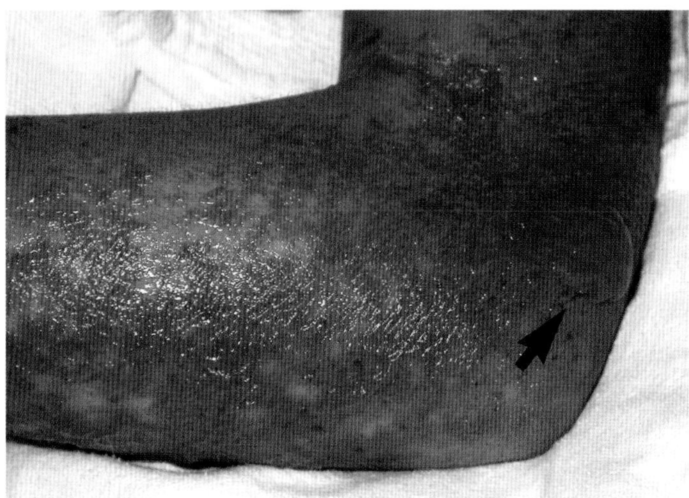

Figure 105.1. In toxic epidermal necrolysis, flaccid bullae appear (arrow) and rapidly rupture.

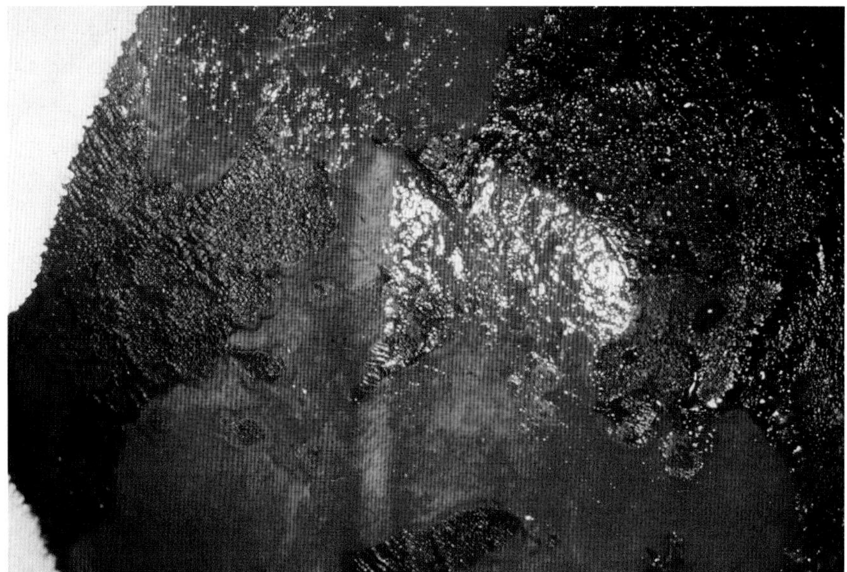

Figure 105.2. Toxic epidermal necrolysis is characterized by shedding of large areas of necrotic epidermis.

Look-alikes

Disorder	Differentiating Features
Stevens-Johnson syndrome (SJS)	• May have blister formation, but less severe than in TEN (<10% of body surface area [BSA] is involved, whereas in TEN, >30% of BSA is affected); 10% to 30% BSA is considered SJS-TEN overlap. • More often related to infection (eg, *Mycoplasma pneumoniae*) than drugs in children.
Staphylococcal scalded skin syndrome	• Often begins with rhinorrhea and periorificial crusting. • Blisters form and rupture, leading to superficial exfoliation, but the pigmented epithelium is retained below the blister. • Constitutional symptoms milder and disease less severe. • Oral and conjunctival mucosae spared.
Kawasaki disease	• Eruption typically morbilliform, without presence of vesicles, bullae, or crusting. • Patients have nonpurulent conjunctival injection but not the purulent conjunctivitis or erosions as seen in TEN. • Patients may have erythema and cracking of lips but not mucosal erosions. • Rash accentuated in flexural locations (especially the groin).
Toxic shock syndrome	• Patients exhibit diffuse erythema and may have superficial desquamation, but bullae and erosions absent. • Rash accentuated in flexural locations. • Nikolsky sign absent. • Hypotension required for definitive diagnosis.
Acute generalized exanthematous pustulosis	• Large areas of erythema with numerous superimposed small pustules • Bullae and erosions absent

How to Make the Diagnosis

- The diagnosis is suspected clinically based on
  - Acute onset of a severe illness with rapid progression of generalized erythema to blistering and loss of the epidermis associated with mucosal and systemic features
  - Presence of Nikolsky sign
  - Loss of the pigmented epithelium with the blister roof
- Skin biopsy or frozen section, as needed.

Treatment

- Admission to an intensive care or burn unit is imperative.
- Supportive care includes maintenance of fluid and electrolyte status, infection control, emollients over the denuded areas, and parenteral nutrition.
- Topical antibacterial ointments or creams are often useful, but beware the use of topical sulfa-based agents in patients whose TEN was triggered by sulfonamides.
- Remove the offending drug.
- Intravenous Ig should be considered; shown in some studies to be beneficial.
- Systemic steroids are generally contraindicated due to increased mortality risk in patient population.

Treating Associated Conditions

- Monitor for and address renal, gastrointestinal, and pulmonary complications.
- Ophthalmologic consultation is indicated; aggressive lubrication is always recommended, and amniotic membrane transplantation to the ocular surface is occasionally considered for aggressive ocular disease.
- Severe urethral involvement may cause urinary retention, requiring indwelling catheter placement.

Prognosis

- Mortality in drug-induced TEN is approximately 20%.
- Mortality in idiopathic TEN approaches 50%.
- Neutropenia, severe hypoproteinemia, and extensive surface area involvement are poor prognostic factors.
- Long-term complications affect the eyes (eg, dry eye syndrome, aberrant lashes, impaired tear production, corneal scarring, blindness), skin (eg, dyspigmentation), and nails (eg, deformities).

When to Worry or Refer

- All patients with TEN should be referred to an experienced burn center or intensive care unit.

Resources for Families

- WebMD: Information for families is contained in Children's Health. **http://children.webmd.com/toxic-epidermal-necrolysis**

Urticaria

Introduction/Etiology/Epidemiology

- Acute urticaria (lasting <6 weeks) is a common condition of childhood; chronic urticaria (lasting ≥6 weeks) is uncommon.
- Erythema results from vasodilation, and wheals are produced by fluid leaking from blood vessels into the surrounding dermis.
- Histamine is the primary mediator in response to a variety of antigens (eg, infectious agents, drugs, foods, insect venom).
- Physical urticaria may be triggered by heat, cold, pressure, vibration, sunlight, water, or exercise.

Signs and Symptoms

- Lesions appear abruptly as pruritic, pink to red raised wheals of variable size and shape (eg, arcs, rings, plaques) (Figures 106.1 and 106.2).
- Lesions are transient, usually resolving in 0.5 to 3 hours, reappearing in other locations.
- Lesions may become large and annular in appearance (ie, central clearing occurs); referred to by some as urticaria multiforme.
- By definition, a lesion of urticaria must change or resolve within 24 hours of its appearance.

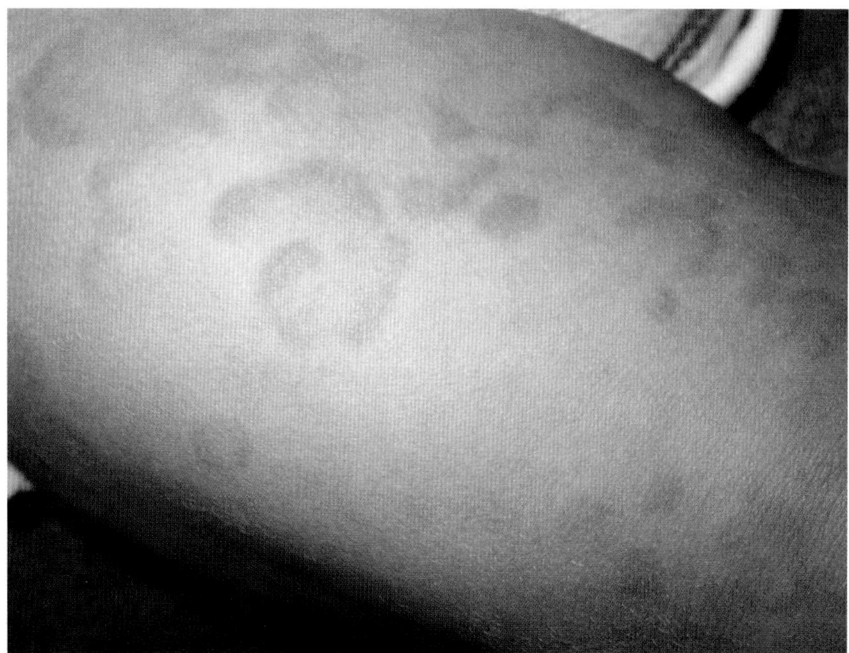

Figure 106.1. Urticaria. Erythematous wheals with multiple shapes, including papules and incomplete rings.

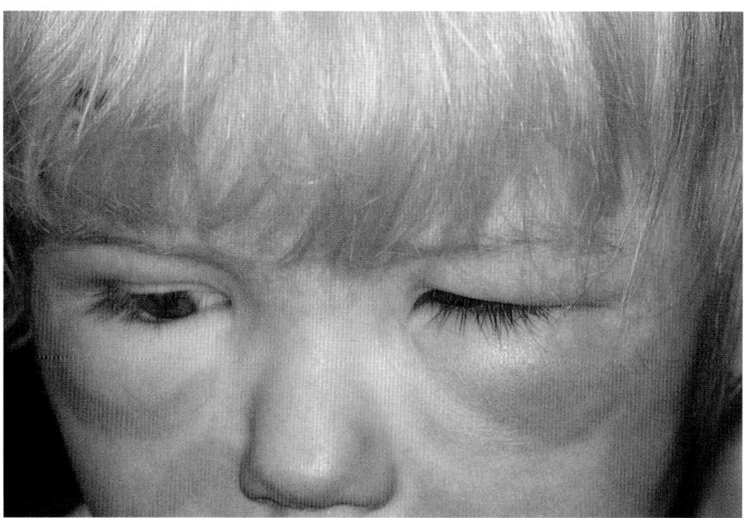

Figure 106.2. This child who has urticaria also exhibits angioedema, an indistinct swelling around the eyes.

Look-alikes

Disorder	Differentiating Features
Erythema multiforme (EM)	• Lesions of urticaria resolve or change shape in a few hours, whereas those of EM remain fixed in location for the duration of the illness (ie, 7–14 days). • Lesions of EM centrally dark and dusky and often develop a central blister or crust. • Unlike the lesions of urticaria, those of EM often located on extremities and face with relative sparing of trunk.
Henoch-Schönlein purpura (HSP)	• Vasculitis, so lesions will remain fixed and become purpuric over time. • Generally confined to lower body and legs. • Abdominal pain, arthralgias, arthritis, or hematuria may accompany the cutaneous findings of HSP.
Serum sickness or serum sickness–like eruption	• Giant, often purple, urticarial plaques common. • Fever, arthralgias, and arthritis constant features. • Periarticular swelling often present. • Ambulatory children may refuse to walk during episode.
Papular urticaria	• Random pattern of urticarial-appearing papules, often with central puncta, that remain fixed in location for weeks and tend to recur in similar distribution pattern • Vesiculation or trauma due to scratching common
Urticarial vasculitis	• Often associated with burning or pain • Individual lesions last longer than 24 hours or may have a purpuric or hyperpigmented appearance • May be associated with autoimmune disease, hepatitis, hypocomplementemia, or arthritis

How to Make the Diagnosis

- The main discriminating features are erythematous wheals that resolve or change shape within 24 hours.
- Abrupt onset, following exposure to specific triggers of histamine release.
- Identification of the trigger agent is usually difficult. Examples include infectious agents (eg, *Streptococcus pyogenes*, Epstein-Barr virus, adenovirus, parasites), drugs (eg, penicillin, opiates, nonsteroidal anti-inflammatory agents, insulin, blood products), foods (eg, nuts, eggs, shellfish, strawberries), systemic diseases (eg, collagen vascular disease, inflammatory bowel disease, thyroiditis), and insect stings.
- If uncertainty about the diagnosis of urticaria exists, administration of subcutaneous epinephrine will cause lesions to resolve.

Treatment

- Oral antihistamines are effective in symptomatic management of urticaria. First-generation agents, such as diphenhydramine hydrochloride (5 mg/kg per day in 4 divided doses) or hydroxyzine hydrochloride (2–4 mg/kg per day in 3–4 divided doses), are most commonly used.
- If sedation occurs or first-generation agents are ineffective, a second-generation (eg, cetirizine, loratadine) or third-generation (eg, desloratadine, fexofenadine, levocetirizine) antihistamine may be prescribed, reserving the first-generation agent for bedtime.
- Although controversial, the addition of an H_2-receptor antagonist (eg, cimetidine, ranitidine) may be effective when H_1 agents alone are ineffective.
- Systemic corticosteroids represent second-line therapy for severe disease; steroids generally are not advisable given the risk of rebound flare on discontinuation and side effect profile when used for prolonged periods.
- Treatment should be maintained for 5 to 7 days after urticaria has resolved to prevent relapse; longer duration of antihistamine therapy may be necessary in chronic urticaria.
- If the offending trigger can be identified, avoidance or treatment is recommended.

Treating Associated Conditions

- Subcutaneous extension of lesions (ie, angioedema) may occur.
  - Patients exhibit indistinct swelling of the eyelids, lips, extremities, or genitalia. Occasionally, there is involvement of the oral cavity or airway.
  - Management of uncomplicated angioedema associated with urticaria is as described in the preceding sections. Intramuscular epinephrine should be considered if there is evidence of respiratory compromise.
- Anaphylaxis
  - Anaphylaxis is a medical emergency that occurs when massive histamine release causes airway edema, laryngospasm, profound hypotension, and cardiovascular collapse.
  - Airway compromise is responsible for most deaths.
  - Epinephrine must be administered emergently, along with antihistamines and, often, a corticosteroid.
- Heredity angioedema (caused by C1 esterase inhibitor deficiency) presents with swelling of the face, throat, or extremities or abdominal pain (without associated urticaria). Diagnosis is confirmed by measuring the C1 esterase inhibitor level.

Prognosis

- Acute urticaria often resolves within 1 to 2 weeks.
- Chronic urticaria may last for years, but it resolves spontaneously within 5 years in 30% to 55% of patients.

When to Worry or Refer

- Recurrent episodes of urticaria, chronic urticaria, or a single episode of anaphylaxis merit referral for allergy evaluation.

Resources for Families

- American Academy of Pediatrics: HealthyChildren.org.
  www.HealthyChildren.org/hives
  https://www.healthychildren.org/English/tips-tools/symptom-checker/Pages/symptomviewer.aspx?symptom=Hives
- American Academy of Dermatology: Hives.
  https://www.aad.org/public/diseases/itchy-skin/hives
- MedlinePlus: Information for patients and families (in English and Spanish) sponsored by the National Library of Medicine and National Institutes of Health.
  https://www.nlm.nih.gov/medlineplus/ency/article/000845.htm
- WebMD: Information for families is contained in the Health A-Z topics.
  www.webmd.com/skin-problems-and-treatments/guide/hives-urticaria-angioedema

Cutaneous Manifestations of Rheumatologic Diseases

Juvenile Dermatomyositis (JDM)

Introduction/Etiology/Epidemiology

- Rare inflammatory vasculopathy primarily involving the skin and muscle with potential for multisystem compromise.
- A subset of patients has no evidence of muscle disease; termed *dermatomyositis sine myositis.*
- Bimodal age peaks: childhood (5–10 years) and adulthood (45–55 years).
- Incidence of approximately 2 to 7 cases per million children per year.
- Approximately equal gender ratio in prepubertal patients; increased ratio of female to male patients in adults (approximately 10:1).
- In approximately 10% to 20% of patients, overlap of juvenile dermatomyositis (JDM) with other connective tissue disease exists.
- Although dermatomyositis in adult patients may be a marker for occult malignancy, this association is not seen in children.
- Etiology/pathogenesis of JDM is poorly understood; believed to be autoimmune in nature, and patients may have familial/genetic predisposition.

Signs and Symptoms

Cutaneous

- Juvenile dermatomyositis has pathognomonic skin changes that may vary greatly in severity; characteristic inflammatory and telangiectatic skin findings are seen in around 3 out of 4 affected children.
- Pink to violet–colored discoloration of eyelids (heliotrope) and cheeks in malar distribution with associated edema of affected skin (Figures 107.1 and 107.2).
- Erythema and telangiectasias may be present on the extensor extremities, neck, and hairline.
- Photosensitivity is common, with relative sparing of sun-protected sites.

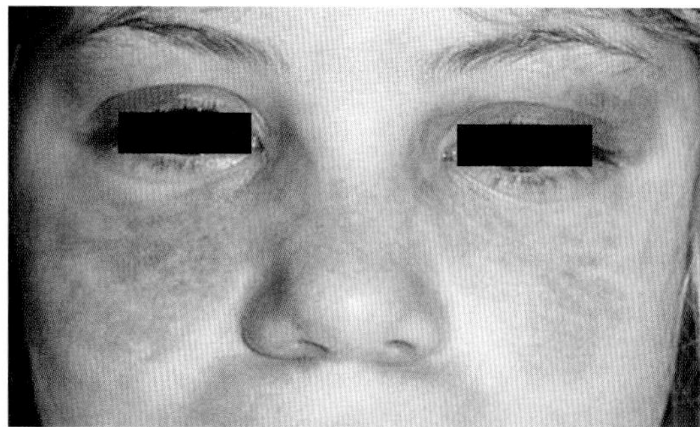

Figure 107.1. Heliotrope rash and telangiectatic erythema of the cheeks in a school-aged girl with juvenile dermatomyositis.

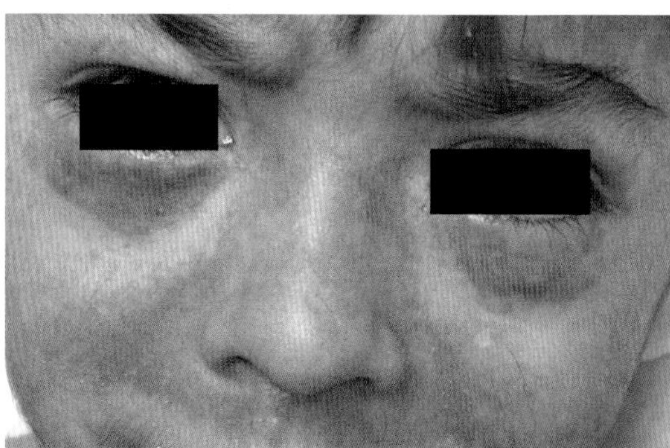

Figure 107.2. More pronounced erythematous to violaceous patches on the face of this child with darker skin who has juvenile dermatomyositis.

- Gottron sign or papules: pink to red telangiectatic macules (Gottron sign) or flat-topped lichenoid papules (Gottron papules), most often located over the proximal interphalangeal and metacarpophalangeal joints; less often involve the distal interphalangeal joints (Figure 107.3).
  - May be scaly
  - Occasionally appear symmetrically over the extensor extremities (elbows, knees) and may resemble lesions of psoriasis
- Dilated capillaries (telangiectasias) of the proximal nail folds (may need ophthalmoscope or dermatoscope to visualize) (Figure 107.4). May also see areas of capillary dropout within these areas of capillary dilation. These periungual changes appear to correlate with skin disease activity.
- Calcinosis cutis occurs in up to one-quarter of affected children. Variably sized calcium deposits can present as firm papules or nodules, usually located over the joints of the elbows or knees (Figure 107.5).
  - More common in childhood than in adult patients.
  - Usually a later finding; rarely seen at time of initial presentation.
  - Occasionally become secondarily infected.
  - Can become disabling if extensive.

- Severity of calcinosis seems to correlate with severity of inflammation and overall disease severity.
- Seen less frequently with aggressive and early therapy.

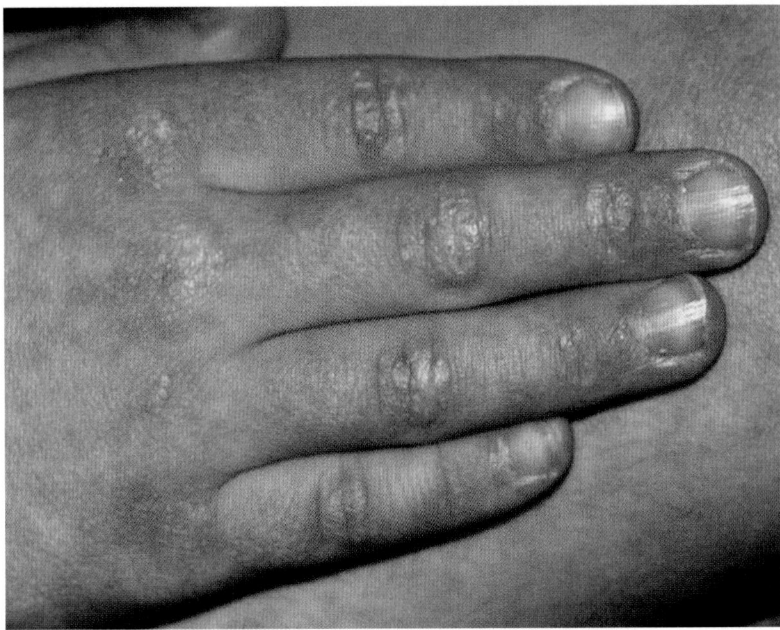

Figure 107.3. Typical Gottron papules (erythematous to violaceous, flat-topped papules) overlying the knuckles in this patient with juvenile dermatomyositis.

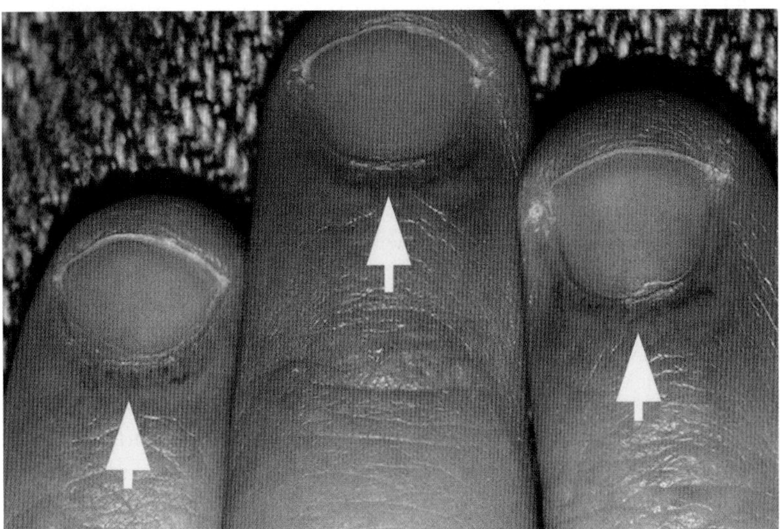

Figure 107.4. Dilated capillaries of the nail folds (arrows) in a patient who has juvenile dermatomyositis.

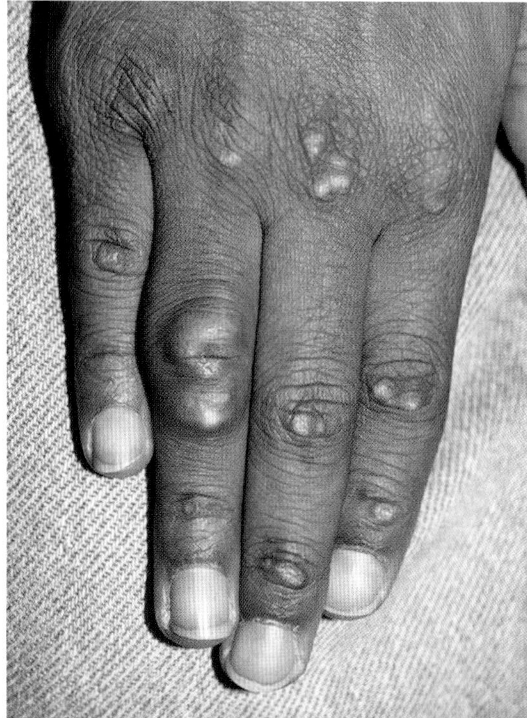

Figure 107.5. Calcinosis cutis of the fourth finger as well as Gottron papules on the knuckles of this patient with a long history of juvenile dermatomyositis.

- Widespread edema of the skin may be seen in more severe cases.
- Poikilodermatous changes (ie, atrophy, telangiectasias, and hypopigmentation and hyperpigmentation within same region of skin) may be seen in chronic disease; often, there is a distinct violaceous discoloration of the skin.
- Localized or widespread ulcerations may occur; extensive ulcerations believed to be associated with poor prognosis.
- Inflammation of the scalp with associated scarring or non-scarring alopecia seen occasionally in children with JDM; more often seen in affected adults.
- Lipodystrophy may be seen occasionally in association with panniculitis and may be generalized or partial.
- Acanthosis nigricans (velvety hyperpigmentation of the neck, axillae) is occasionally seen in patients with JDM, especially those with lipodystrophy.

Systemic

- Symmetric proximal muscle weakness may accompany or follow skin changes.
  - Usually involves the anterior neck flexors, the hip and shoulder girdle, and core musculature
  - May present with difficulty climbing stairs, raising arms to brush hair, or rising from lying to sitting and sitting to standing positions
  - May or may not have associated muscle pain or tenderness to palpation
- May involve other striated muscle and result in symptoms of dysphagia, dysphonia, choking, or nasal speech.
- In severe disease, can progress to involve respiratory muscles and lead to restrictive lung disease.
- Arteritis can occasionally lead to myocarditis, pericarditis, mucosal ulcerations of the gastrointestinal tract, or microscopic hematuria.
- Fatigue and loss of energy are reported in most patients on presentation.
- A nondestructive arthritis may occur in up to half of affected children.

Look-alikes

Disorder	Differentiating Features
Psoriasis	• Psoriatic lesions of knees and elbows may resemble those of JDM but usually contain thicker, micaceous (silvery-white) scale. • May have associated nail changes (pitting, onycholysis). • No dilated capillaries of nail folds. • No calcinosis cutis. • Facial involvement less common (but more common in pediatric psoriasis compared with adults). • Histology distinctive. • Usually improves (rather than being exacerbated) with sun exposure.
Allergic contact dermatitis	• May have more marked edema of eyelids and affected skin • More acute onset than JDM • Severe pruritus usually present
Systemic lupus erythematosus	• Usually less eyelid involvement. • Distinct systemic manifestations. • Photosensitivity a prominent feature, often with butterfly facial erythema. • Erythema of the dorsal fingers usually spares the areas over joints. • Serologic studies may help distinguish the 2 disorders.

Look-alikes *(continued)*

Disorder	Differentiating Features
Scleroderma/CREST syndrome (**c**alcinosis, **R**aynaud phenomenon, **e**sophageal involvement, **s**clerodactyly, **t**elangiectasia)	• May have similar telangiectatic changes around the nails as in JDM • May have symptoms of dysphagia in both conditions • May also have calcinosis cutis in CREST syndrome • Sclerodactyly (thickening/tightness of the fingers and toes) or generalized induration not typically seen in JDM • Distinctive histologic changes on skin biopsy
Atopic dermatitis	• Often with earlier onset (infancy or toddler years) • Usually associated with more severe pruritus • Predilection for neck and flexural extremities (extensor surfaces in infants)
Cutaneous T-cell lymphoma	• Rare in children • Poikilodermatous form seen mainly in adults • Characteristic histologic features
Postinfectious myopathy/myositis	• No associated skin changes • Usually self-limited, lasting days to weeks
Collagen vascular disease–associated myositis/myopathy	• May or may not have associated dermatologic alterations. • Systemic lupus erythematosus–associated myositis generally does not have significant elevation of muscle enzymes. • May have other systemic alterations not typically seen in JDM.

How to Make the Diagnosis

- There is no single diagnostic test for JDM.
- The diagnosis is suggested clinically by the combined findings of pathognomonic skin changes and associated symmetric proximal muscle weakness.
- Supportive diagnostic evidence includes
  - Elevated skeletal muscle enzymes
    - Creatine phosphokinase
    - Aldolase
    - Aspartate aminotransferase and lactate dehydrogenase (may also be elevated because they are released from damaged muscle tissue)
    - Alanine aminotransferase
  - Characteristic histologic changes on skin biopsy (epidermal atrophy, interface dermatitis, mucin deposition).
  - Characteristic histology from muscle biopsy (usually deltoid or quadriceps). This procedure has been largely replaced by magnetic resonance imaging (MRI), which reveals increased signal intensity on fat-suppressed T2-weighted images; MRI may also be helpful in following the clinical course of muscle involvement.

- Characteristic electromyography findings.
- Some myositis-specific antibodies may be present and may help in predicting prognosis.

Treatment

- Most patients are managed by pediatric rheumatologists; pediatric dermatologists are often involved at diagnosis, when patients present with cutaneous signs/symptoms.
- While muscle disease is usually quite responsive to therapy, cutaneous disease may be very resistant to multiple treatment modalities.
- Mainstays of treatment include
  - Photoprotection.
    - Daily use of broad-spectrum sunscreen with sun protection factor 30 or higher
    - Use of protective clothing
    - Avoidance of prolonged sun exposure
  - Topical steroids or topical calcineurin inhibitors (eg, pimecrolimus, tacrolimus) may be helpful for any associated pruritus but rarely modify the course of cutaneous disease.
  - Systemic corticosteroids (oral or pulsed intravenous [IV]); high-dose pulsed IV steroids are increasingly used by specialists who treat JDM.
  - Immunosuppressive therapy/steroid-sparing agents.
    - Methotrexate
    - Hydroxychloroquine (low dose), often used for inflammatory skin disease (although effectiveness is controversial)
    - Intravenous immunoglobulin
    - Cyclosporine
    - Azathioprine
    - Pulsed cyclophosphamide
    - Rituximab
    - Tumor necrosis factor α–antagonists including infliximab and etanercept (although some patients appear to worsen on these therapies)
  - Autologous stem cell transplantation (in some severe cases).
  - Physical therapy.

Treating Associated Conditions

- Arthritis, gastrointestinal tract vasculopathy with ulceration or hemorrhage, malabsorption, and interstitial lung disease may occur and require specific evaluation as indicated.
- Calcinosis is very difficult to treat; reported therapies include increasing systemic immunosuppression, bisphosphonates, sodium thiosulfate, surgery.

Prognosis

- The prognosis is variable but seems quite favorable for most children treated aggressively with corticosteroids. Many will become disease-free after 2 to 4 years and remain so off of therapy.
- Control of skin disease and muscle disease does not correlate well; muscle disease is usually quite responsive to corticosteroid therapy, while dermatologic manifestations often are recalcitrant and persistent despite good control of muscle disease.

When to Worry or Refer

- All patients with skin or muscle symptoms suggestive of JDM should be referred to a pediatric rheumatologist and dermatologist to confirm the clinical diagnosis and for ongoing management.
- Prompt and accurate diagnosis as well as aggressive systemic management is critical in the presence of muscle or systemic manifestations.

Resources for Families

- Cure JM Foundation: Provides information and support for patients who have juvenile dermatomyositis.
  www.curejm.com

Morphea

Introduction/Etiology/Epidemiology

- Also referred to as localized scleroderma, morphea is an uncommon autoimmune inflammatory sclerosing disorder of the skin and subcutaneous tissue.
- While the term *scleroderma* and the characteristic hardening (sclerosis) of the skin can be confused with systemic sclerosis, rarely does morphea progress to systemic disease. For this reason, the term *morphea* is preferred over localized scleroderma.
- Incidence estimated to be 0.4 to 1 per 100,000 individuals, and the condition is 2 to 3 times more common in females than males; recent studies suggest morphea is more prevalent in white females.
- Mean age of onset in children is 5 to 8 years; however, morphea has been described in infants, and there are even case reports of congenital morphea.
- While most have disease limited to the skin and subcutaneous tissue, a subset of patients may have associated extracutaneous findings.
- Divided into several subtypes; clinical features vary depending on the subtype of morphea.
- Disease severity ranges from a solitary area of induration (hardening of skin) to severe, disfiguring disease affecting skin, subcutaneous tissue, and even underlying muscle and bone.
- Occasionally observed in the setting of other connective tissue disorders, including juvenile idiopathic arthritis, systemic lupus erythematosus, systemic sclerosis, Sjögren syndrome, juvenile dermatomyositis, polymyositis, and eosinophilic fasciitis.

Signs and Symptoms

Skin Findings

- Begins insidiously as a gradual hardening of the skin.
- May begin with an inflammatory stage that presents with erythema or a violaceous discoloration of the skin (Figure 108.1); at times, this can resemble a port-wine stain (capillary malformation).
- With time, the redness fades and the affected area of skin becomes indurated and often ivory-colored and shiny in appearance.
- In contrast, some lesions become hyperpigmented with time (see Figure 108.1). These changes usually evolve gradually over several months.

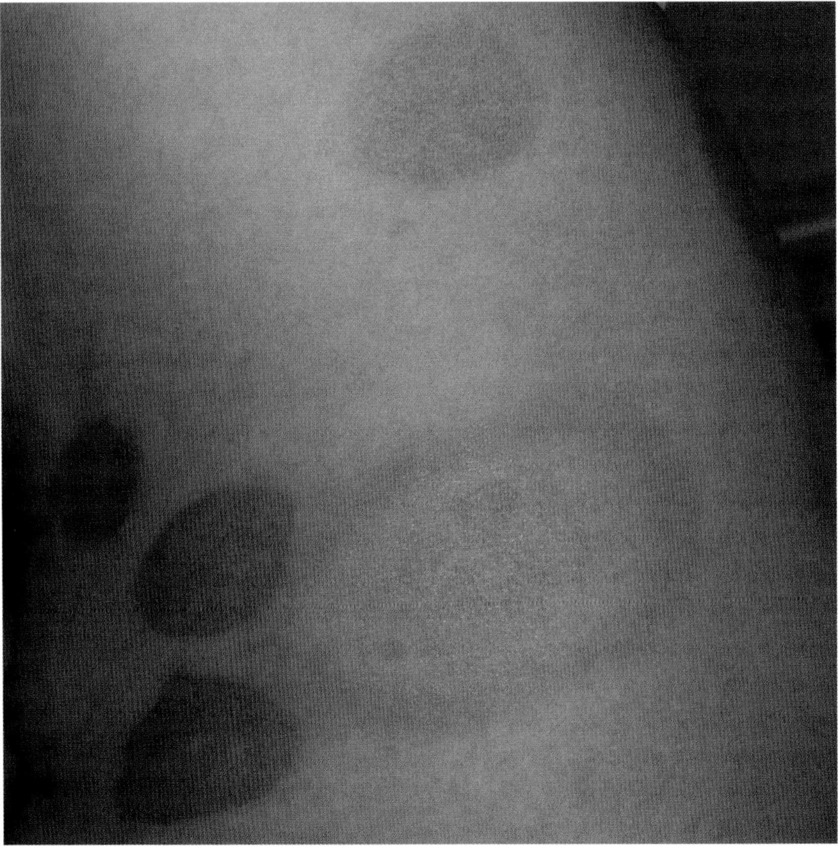

Figure 108.1. Circumscribed (plaque) morphea. There is a new lesion in the center of the photograph. It is an erythematous patch with a more intensely erythematous to violaceous border. Resolving lesions are seen as hyperpigmented patches.

- Overall clinical appearance varies depending on the subtype. There is no universally agreed-on classification of morphea, but a recently proposed classification system divides morphea into 5 subtypes.
  - Linear scleroderma
  - Circumscribed (plaque) morphea
  - Generalized morphea
  - Pansclerotic morphea
  - Mixed subtype
- Linear scleroderma is the most common type of morphea in children and most often affects the face and extremities.
  - Hardening of the skin or subcutaneous tissue (as well as the associated hypopigmentation or hyperpigmentation) spreads in a linear distribution, most commonly over an extremity (Figure 108.2) or on the face (Figure 108.3).
  - Early findings of erythema and violaceous discoloration are more subtle in linear versus circumscribed (plaque) morphea; the early erythema can occasionally be confused with a port-wine stain.
  - When involving the forehead and scalp, referred to as *en coup de sabre* (cut of a saber) (Figures 108.4 and 108.5). Tends to have a unilateral distribution in most children; the skin gradually becomes more atrophic and develops a depressed, groove-like appearance.
  - More extensive hemifacial involvement may occur; it is termed *progressive facial hemiatrophy* (or Parry-Romberg syndrome).
  - Scalp involvement may be associated with alopecia (see Figure 108.4); can also spread inferiorly to involve the periorbital region, nose, and mouth; may become quite disfiguring due to marked atrophy.
  - Morphea may be associated with significant atrophy of the skin and subcutaneous tissue; when involving a limb, this can result in circumferential and linear undergrowth of the affected extremity.
  - When extending over a joint, morphea may result in contractures and impaired mobility or range of motion, which can be permanent.
- Circumscribed (plaque) morphea is the second most common subtype of morphea in children.
  - May present with one or more plaques of affected skin, most often located on the trunk. Affected skin usually begins with an oval or round circumscribed area of induration.
  - Often begins with erythematous or violaceous discoloration (see Figure 108.1), which gradually evolves to the characteristic ivory color with increasing induration; as the process progresses, the erythema or violet hue fades.
  - Circumscribed morphea can be further categorized as superficial or deep, depending on the depth of skin and soft tissue involvement.

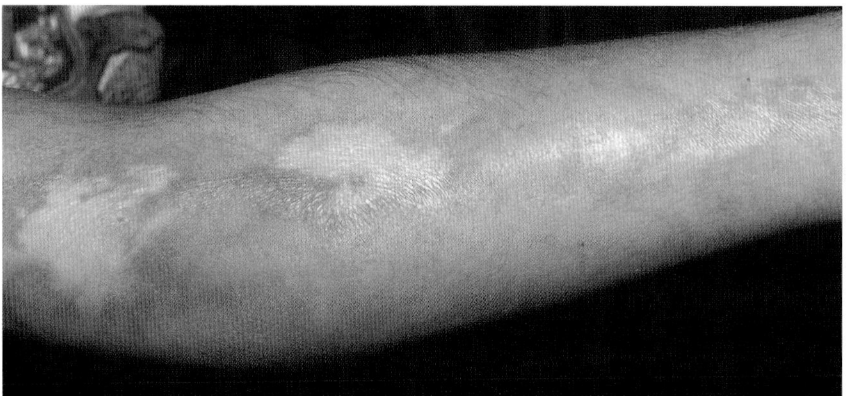

Figure 108.2. Linear morphea involving the arm. The lesions are ivory-colored and indurated. Hyperpigmentation is developing.

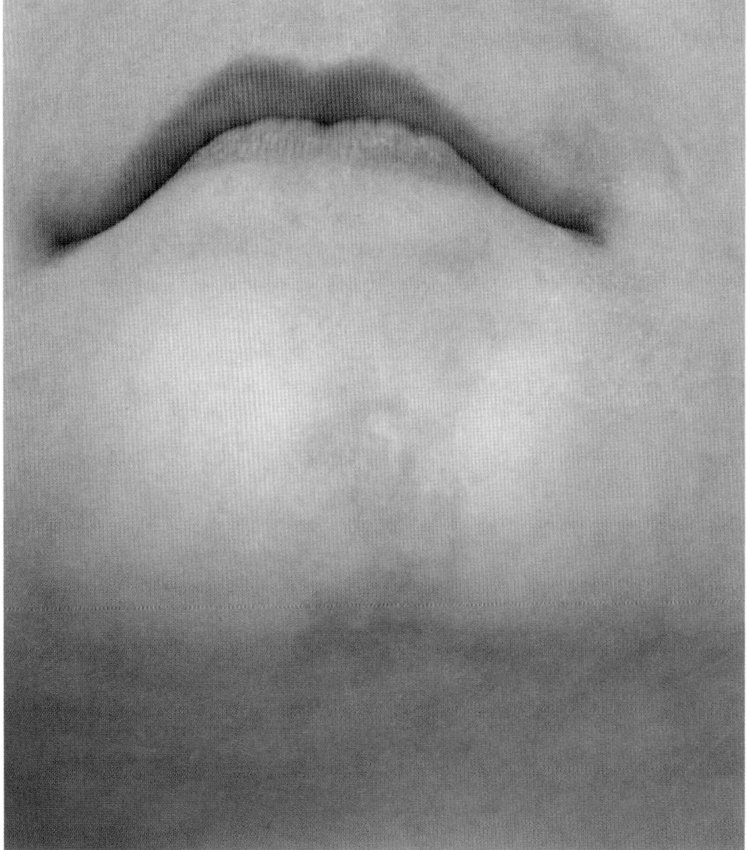

Figure 108.3. Linear morphea involving the face. Note the atrophy affecting the chin to the left of midline.

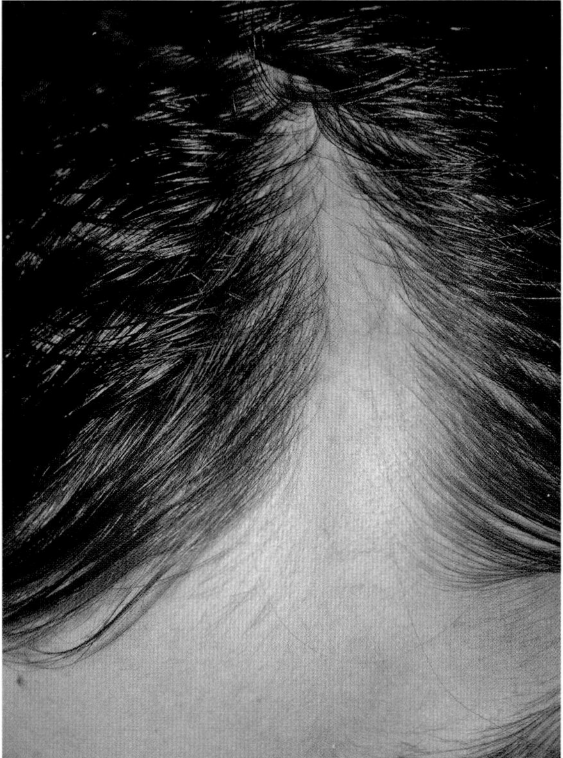

Figure 108.4. *En coup de sabre* form of linear morphea. There is a linear area of atrophy and alopecia involving the frontal scalp.

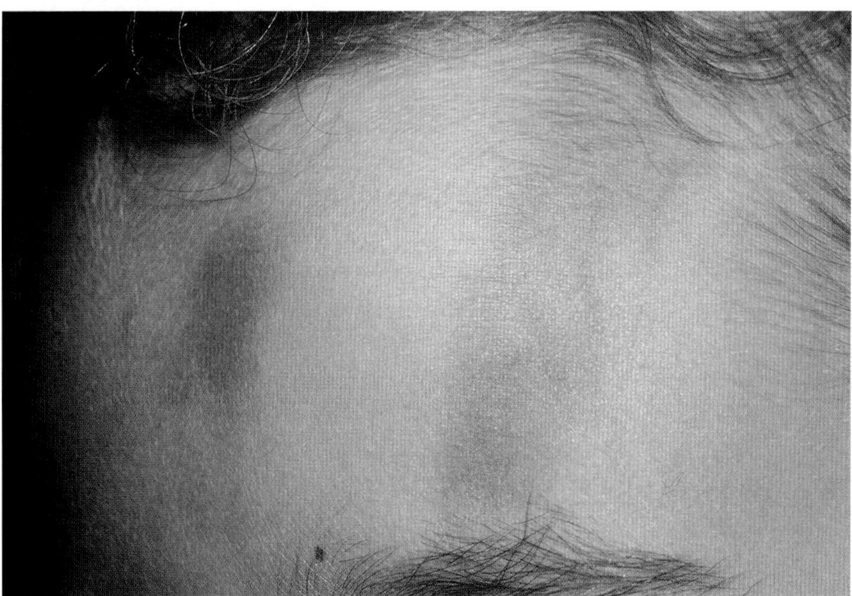

Figure 108.5. In this child with the *en coup de sabre* form of linear morphea, resolving lesions have become hyperpigmented.

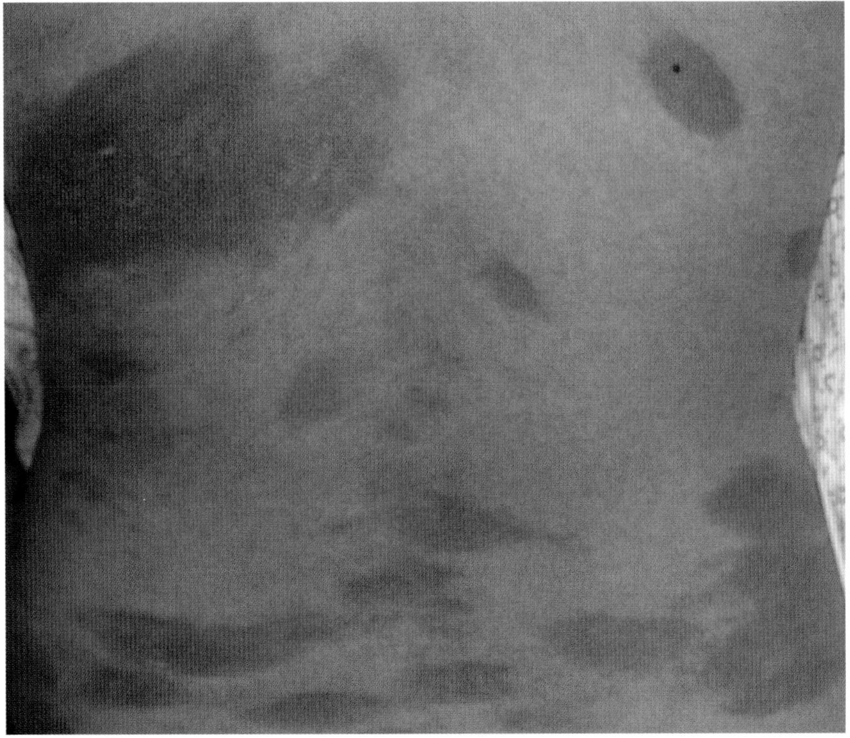

Figure 108.6. Generalized morphea. Multiple lesions involving the trunk have become hyperpigmented and many are atrophic.

- Generalized morphea is defined by some experts as multiple plaques of morphea covering at least 30% of the body.
  - Recent classification defines generalized morphea as 4 or more individual plaques measuring more than 3 cm (which may become confluent), involving at least 2 of 7 anatomic sites (head/neck, right or left arm, right or left leg, anterior trunk, posterior trunk) (Figure 108.6).
- Pansclerotic morphea is a rare subtype involving the skin, subcutaneous tissue, muscle, and bone, often on an extremity.
  - Usually results in circumferential involvement with significant cosmetic and functional compromise; skin may show pitting edema or diffuse painful areas with a puckered or peau d'orange texture.
- Mixed subtype
  - Some patients do not fall clearly into any of the subtypes of morphea and have features of more than one subtype, most commonly a combination of linear and circumscribed (plaque) morphea.

Other Clinical Signs

In recent years, it has become increasingly apparent that a subset of patients with morphea may have associated extracutaneous symptoms. A multicenter study of 750 patients with juvenile localized scleroderma (morphea) revealed that nearly one-quarter had extracutaneous features. A more recent study concluded that the risk of extracutaneous symptoms was greater in patients with disease onset prior to 10 years of age.

- Articular findings are most common and include arthralgias and arthritis. Articular abnormalities are more common in linear scleroderma and may affect the involved or uninvolved (by morphea) joints or extremities.
- Neurologic abnormalities have been reported, primarily with linear morphea of the upper face. Central nervous system abnormalities include headaches, seizures, peripheral neuropathy, and behavioral or learning abnormalities. Headaches appear to be most common and may meet criteria for migraines. Magnetic resonance imaging abnormalities, including white matter abnormalities, intracerebral atrophy, and calcifications, have been reported in some patients.
- Ocular abnormalities may include episcleritis, uveitis, keratitis, xerophthalmia, glaucoma, and papilledema. Ophthalmologic evaluation is recommended for patients with linear morphea in the en coup de sabre distribution.
- Vascular involvement (most commonly Raynaud phenomenon), gastroesophageal reflux or dysphagia, and abnormalities of the cardiac, pulmonary, and renal systems are infrequently associated with morphea.
- Likelihood of patients with morphea developing systemic sclerosis is exceedingly low (<1% risk).
- Psychologic implications may result from this chronic disease and its potential cosmetic and functional sequelae.

Look-alikes

Disorder	Differentiating Features
Capillary malformation (port-wine stain)	• May resemble early inflammatory stage of morphea. • Usually present at birth, unlike most morphea. • Usually stable during first several years of life. • Flat and smooth, not firm or indurated on palpation. • Some capillary malformations are associated with overgrowth (but not typically atrophy) of underlying tissues.
Lichen striatus	• May resemble early lesions of linear morphea • Lichenoid papules that coalesce in a linear/band-like pattern • No firmness or induration of the affected skin • Self-limited condition that often resolves spontaneously over 1–2 years • May leave persistent hypopigmentation but no atrophy of affected skin
Lichen sclerosis et atrophicus (LSA)	• May also show sclerotic white plaques with atrophy • Most often involves the female and male genitalia • More likely to be associated with severe pruritus than morphea • Extragenital LSA more likely to be associated with skin dryness than morphea • Sclerotic white scar-like lesions usually smaller than morphea; may have guttate ("teardrop") pattern • More likely to see telangiectasias or follicular plugging in LSA than with morphea • Hemorrhagic blisters occasionally present
Atrophoderma of Pasini and Pierini	• Considered by some clinicians to be a superficial variant of morphea. • Hyperpigmented (brown to gray to blue) patches seen most commonly on the back. • Lesions lack induration. • Face, hands, and feet usually spared. • Lesion borders are sharply defined; described as having "cliff-drop" borders that range from 1–8 mm in depth. • Duration of many years to decades with benign course.
Linear atrophoderma of Moulin	• Atrophic plaques that are linear and may follow the lines of Blaschko. • Inflammation, induration, and pigmentary changes are all absent.
Acrodermatitis chronica atrophicans	• Cutaneous manifestation of chronic Lyme disease. • Violaceous plaques of the distal extensor extremities that may become indurated, hyperpigmented, and atrophic. • Primarily seen in Europe, linked to *Borrelia* infection (connection between *Borrelia* infection and morphea remains controversial). • May have associated arthritis and neuropathy. • Primarily in adult women, occurring several months to years after initial infection. • Lyme antibody titers may be positive.

Look-alikes *(continued)*

Disorder	Differentiating Features
Systemic sclerosis (scleroderma)	• Generalized disorder that may affect many organs in addition to the skin: lungs, kidneys, heart, gastrointestinal track, joints. • Much less common in children than adults. • Nail fold capillary changes in nearly all patients similar to those seen in juvenile dermatomyositis. • Frequently associated with Raynaud phenomenon (often first sign of systemic sclerosis). • Often associated with characteristic facial features: pinched nose, pursed lips, small oral aperture. • Sclerodactyly (shiny tapered fingertips with limited range of motion) seen in most patients. • Other common features include arthralgias, decreased joint mobility, weight loss, fatigue, gastrointestinal symptoms, shortness of breath with exertion. • Telangiectasias, calcification, and ulceration of the skin may occur (rarely seen in morphea). • Skin involvement is diffuse, not linear or well circumscribed.
Chronic graft-versus-host disease, sclerodermatous type	• History of preceding at-risk procedure (ie, bone marrow or stem cell transplantation) and immunosuppressed host. • Widespread sclerodermatous plaques may be seen, similar to systemic sclerosis or generalized morphea. • May be associated with cutaneous ulceration, nail dystrophy, scarring alopecia, and joint contractures. • Erosions of the oral mucous membranes often present. • Systemic manifestations may include gastrointestinal, hepatic, pulmonary, cardiac, hematologic aberrations. • Skin biopsy usually shows interface dermatitis in addition to dermal sclerosis.
Eosinophilic fasciitis	• Generalized infiltration/induration of skin of the trunk and extremities; classically spares hands, feet, and face (although hands and feet occasionally involved). • Abrupt onset of painful skin swelling. • Cobblestoned or puckered appearance of the skin may be present. • Usually responds well to systemic steroids. • Usually not well circumscribed or linear in distribution. • Associated with striking peripheral eosinophilia (but may rapidly correct on administration of systemic steroids), elevated erythrocyte sedimentation rate, and hypergammaglobulinemia.

Look-alikes *(continued)*

Disorder	Differentiating Features
Nephrogenic systemic fibrosis (nephrogenic fibrosing dermopathy)	• Usually seen in patients with renal insufficiency and exposure to gadolinium-based contrast media • Often associated with a hypercoagulable state • Poorly defined, indurated plaques usually distributed symmetrically on the extremities • Frequently associated with joint contractures, pain, and decreased mobility • May develop fibrosis of heart, lungs, and skeletal muscle
Progeria	• Premature aging syndrome. • Diagnosis should be considered in young infants who present with widespread sclerodermatous plaques. • Other characteristic features include thin and beaked nose, midfacial duskiness and hypoplasia, micrognathia, slow growth. • Prominent skin vasculature, especially over the scalp. • Small face with birdlike appearance. • Caused by mutation in *LMNA* gene.

How to Make the Diagnosis

- In most children, morphea is diagnosed based on clinical features. Skin biopsy can be helpful to confirm a clinical diagnosis, though, when uncertain.
- Blood analyses may be used to screen for associated systemic autoimmune or rheumatologic disease but are not helpful in diagnosing morphea.
- Patients with more extensive skin disease or associated extracutaneous symptoms may benefit from comprehensive physical and laboratory evaluation by a pediatric rheumatologist.

Treatment

- Patients with morphea are usually treated by a pediatric dermatologist or pediatric rheumatologist.
- Clinical follow-up is challenging, and there is no consistently used tool to measure improvement or deterioration in disease; photographic comparisons, ultrasound, and thermography have all been used with variable consistency and utility; the Localized Scleroderma Cutaneous Assessment Tool (LoSCAT) and modified LoSCAT have been found useful in evaluating patient disease progression and for use in clinical trials.

- Treatment modality depends primarily on the severity of the patient's morphea and may vary from close clinical observation to multidisciplinary management with the use of topical and systemic agents.
  - Patients with mild, localized morphea are most frequently managed with topical corticosteroids, calcipotriene (vitamin D analogue), or topical immunomodulators (tacrolimus or pimecrolimus).
  - Patients with more extensive disease and associated psychosocial or functional impairment are usually treated with systemic immunosuppressive therapies, most commonly oral or intravenous pulsed corticosteroids or methotrexate. Mycophenolate mofetil has been used to treat severe or methotrexate-resistant morphea with success, as have oral calcitriol and rituximab.
  - Phototherapy (particularly psoralen plus UV-A light or UV-A1) has been used with success in the treatment of morphea, especially in adults. There is less experience with light therapy in the treatment of childhood morphea.

Treating Associated Symptoms

- Careful history and physical examination should be performed in all patients with morphea to screen for associated clinical symptoms or physical findings. While morphea is confined to the skin and subcutaneous tissues in most patients, there is an important subset of patients who may have associated systemic symptoms.
- Extracutaneous involvement may be articular, neurologic (primarily in patients with en coup de sabre distribution), vascular, ocular, and gastrointestinal in nature. Patients should be treated as necessary by a pediatric rheumatologist, pediatric dermatologist, or other appropriate subspecialist depending on the nature and extent of involvement.
- Physical and occupational therapy referrals should be initiated, as indicated.

Prognosis

- Most patients with morphea have active disease for 3 to 5 years, followed by a period of spontaneous remission. However, there can be considerable variability depending on the disease subtype and its extent. In some cases, there may be significant psychosocial and functional impairment.
- A minority of affected children may continue to have morphea during adulthood, and another subset may experience relapse of active disease even after a several-year period of remission.

- Patients with limited plaque morphea usually do well with spontaneous remission after several years of disease activity. However, lesions of morphea can leave permanent pigmentary changes and atrophy of the affected skin, even after the active disease subsides.
- Severe linear morphea can result in limited range of motion and atrophy of affected extremities, resulting in discrepancies in length and circumference between affected and unaffected limbs.

When to Worry or Refer

- Children suspected of having cutaneous manifestations of morphea should be referred to a dermatologist or pediatric dermatologist for confirmation of the diagnosis and potential treatment.
- Patients with facial involvement, widespread skin lesions, aggressive progression of disease, or linear scleroderma overlying joints may merit management with systemic medications or phototherapy.
- Patients with extensive or aggressive cutaneous disease may benefit from referral to a pediatric rheumatologist for evaluation of potential extracutaneous involvement and potential systemic therapy.
- Patients with severe morphea are often comanaged by pediatric dermatology and rheumatology specialists.

Resources for Families

- Mayo Clinic: Diseases and conditions. **www.mayoclinic.org/diseases-conditions/morphea/basics/definition/con-20028397**

CHAPTER 109

Systemic Lupus Erythematosus (SLE)

Introduction/Etiology/Epidemiology

- A multisystem autoimmune disorder with protean skin manifestations resulting from immune complex deposition and end-organ damage.
- More common in females than males; approximately 80% of children and adults with systemic lupus erythematosus (SLE) are female; however, in prepubescent children, the male to female ratio may be more equal.
- Presents most often in postpubertal females (20% of cases are diagnosed in the first 2 decades of life), especially African Americans, Asians, Hispanics, and Native Americans.
- Median age of onset in childhood SLE is 11 to 12 years of age.
- Exact cause remains poorly understood; believed to be related to genetic and environmental factors; hormonal factors may also play a role.
- Extracutaneous targets most commonly include joints, hematologic system, lungs, heart, kidneys, and central nervous system.
- Around 80% of patients with SLE will have skin involvement at some point in their course and often as the presenting feature.
- Advances in early diagnosis and treatment have improved survival and quality of life for affected individuals; nevertheless, SLE can lead to significant morbidity and even mortality.

Signs and Symptoms

- Malar erythema often seen; redness occurs in a butterfly distribution over the cheeks, sparing the nasolabial folds, and often appears after sun exposure.
  - Edema often present along with facial erythema.
  - Occasionally, rash has a papular component.
  - Malar skin eruption usually transient and non-scarring.

- Erythematous patches and papules over the dorsal fingers may occur and usually spare the areas overlying joints (in contrast with juvenile dermatomyositis).
- Discoid lupus erythematosus (DLE) lesions are a cutaneous manifestation seen in approximately 10% of children with SLE; they are seen more commonly in adult SLE.
  - Lesions usually are located on face or scalp and are usually round or coin-shaped, annular (central clearing present), hyperpigmented, and, often, scaly (Figures 109.1 and 109.2).
  - Central atrophy may be present.
  - Lesions vary in size, usually 1 to 3 cm.
  - Often, lesions resolve with chronic pigmentary change (hypopigmentation or hyperpigmentation) and scarring (Figure 109.3).
  - Approximately 25% to 30% of children with DLE will eventually progress to SLE.
- Nonscarring alopecia (hair loss) is commonly seen in SLE but is nonspecific; it most often presents as thinning of the hair in the temporal scalp regions.
- Nasal/oral/palatal ulcerations (Figure 109.4), nail fold telangiectasias, petechial or purpuric lesions, livedo reticularis, erythema nodosum, photosensitivity, and small ice pick–like scars of the fingertips are other cutaneous features of SLE.

Other Clinical Findings

- Fever, malaise, weight loss, and arthralgias or arthritis are common in children with SLE.
- Additional signs and symptoms include fatigue, abdominal pain, muscle weakness, lymphadenopathy, hepatosplenomegaly, anorexia, weight loss, night sweats, and Raynaud phenomenon (blanching of fingertips with cold exposure followed by cyanosis and a reactive hyperemia on rewarming).
- Pulmonary (most often pleuritis) and cardiac (including pericarditis, myocarditis, valvular disease, and coronary artery vasculitis) manifestations may also occur in children with SLE.

Lupus Variants

Discoid Lupus Erythematosus

- Discoid lesions may be seen in the setting of SLE or in patients with skin disease only.

- Discoid lupus erythematosus is also known as chronic cutaneous lupus erythematosus.
- Skin lesions present as annular, scaly plaques with pigmentary change and atrophy (see Figures 109.1 and 109.2). Early discoid lesions may occasionally be confused with tinea corporis (ringworm).
- Scarring may occur.
- Lesions of DLE are often exacerbated by sun exposure.

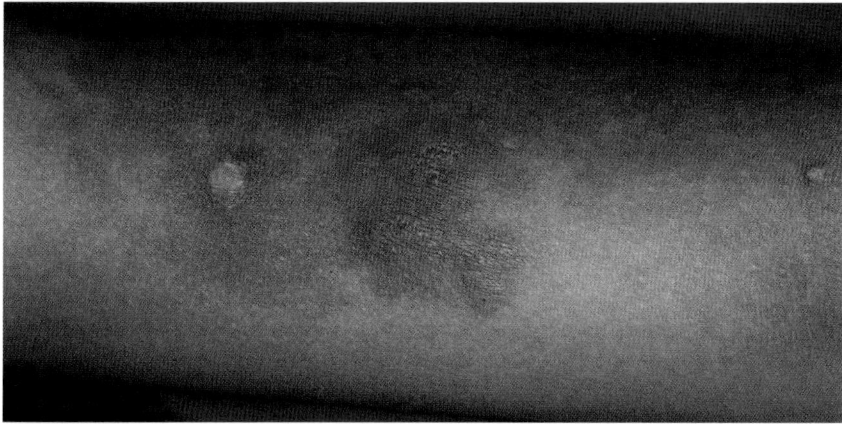

Figure 109.1. Lesions of active discoid lupus erythematosus on the arm in addition to areas of postinflammatory hyperpigmentation and scarring in sites of previous lesions.

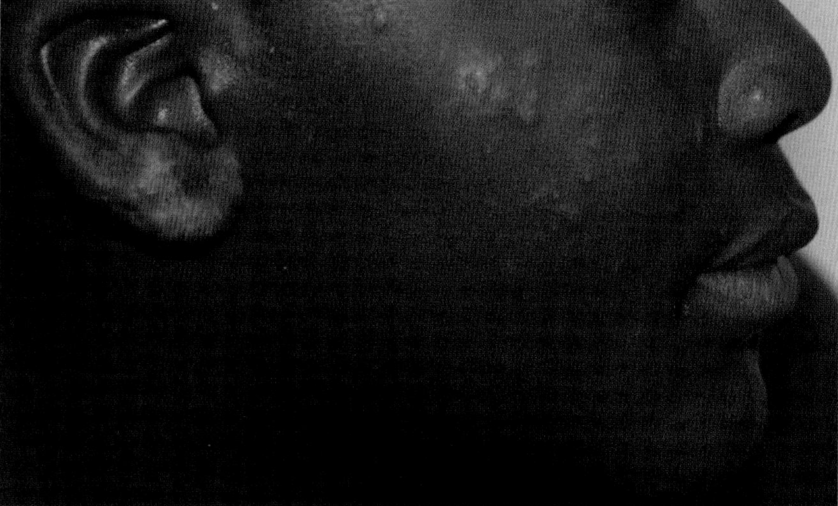

Figure 109.2. Multiple erythematous papules and plaques on the face of a boy with chronic cutaneous (discoid) lupus erythematosus. Note the cutaneous atrophy of several lesions, particularly on the earlobe, a characteristic location for lupus lesions.

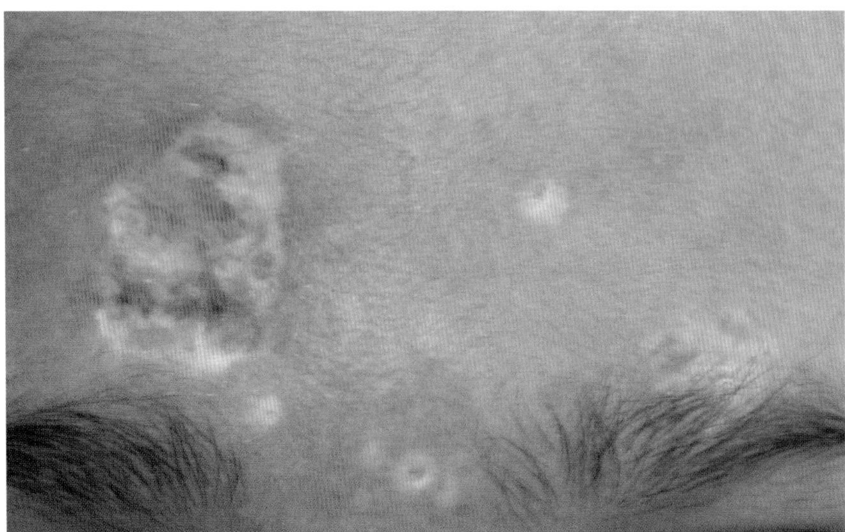

Figure 109.3. Atrophic scarring plaques on the face of a teenaged girl with systemic lupus erythematosus.

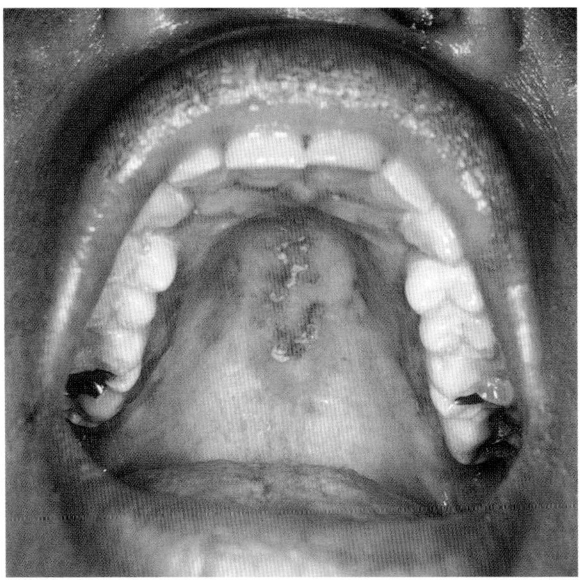

Figure 109.4. Palatal ulcerations in this young adult woman with systemic lupus erythematosus.

Subacute Cutaneous Lupus Erythematosus

- Subacute cutaneous lupus erythematosus (SCLE) is a subtype of lupus characterized by significant photosensitivity; it only occasionally occurs in children.
- Lesions usually appear in a sun-exposed distribution, and in most, the condition is milder in severity than SLE.
- Lesions are often annular or psoriasis-like in configuration (Figure 109.5).
- Postinflammatory pigmentary changes common, but scarring does not occur.
- Most patients have positive anti–SS-A (anti-Ro) antibody, which is associated with photosensitivity; pregnant women with anti–SS-A antibody (whether or not they have overt SLE or SCLE) are at risk of having a neonate with neonatal lupus erythematosus (NLE); anti–SS-B (anti-La) antibody is also associated with SCLE.
- Approximately 15% of patients with SCLE develop significant systemic disease with time; in general, though, patients with SCLE may have a better prognosis than those who have SLE.

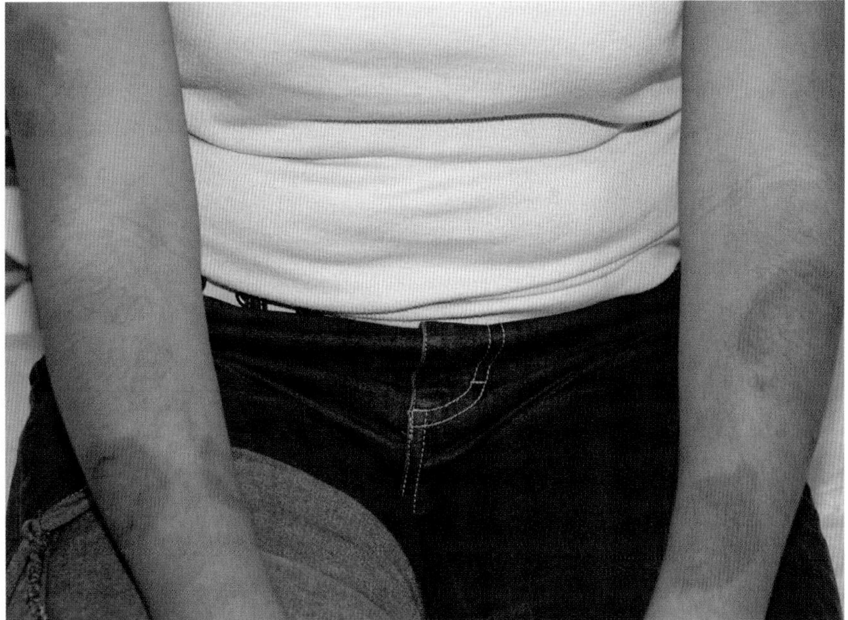

Figure 109.5. Large edematous, erythematous, arcuate, and annular plaques on the arms of this teenaged female with subacute cutaneous lupus erythematosus.

Neonatal Lupus Erythematosus

- A distinct type of lupus seen in newborns and young infants that results from transplacentally acquired autoantibodies, most often anti–SS-A (anti-Ro) antibody or anti–SS-B (anti-La) antibody, potentially in association with congenital heart block.
- Antibodies to U1 ribonucleoprotein (RNP) may also be associated with NLE and are usually not associated with congenital heart block.
- Most common target organs in NLE are the skin and heart.
- Approximately half of patients with NLE have cutaneous manifestations.
- Neonatal lupus erythematosus is the most common cause of congenital heart block; unfortunately, it often results in third-degree heart block requiring pacemaker placement.
- Cutaneous features usually present between 2 and 8 weeks of life; often, parents report exacerbation or appearance following sun exposure.
- Skin lesions usually develop between birth and 8 weeks of age and are distributed most commonly on the face and head; they are usually annular in configuration and erythematous or telangiectatic; they are often mildly scaly and may resemble lesions of tinea corporis (Figure 109.6), seborrheic dermatitis, or atopic dermatitis. Mild atrophy may be present.
- While some infants with NLE have lesions in a photodistribution (in areas of sun exposure), others may have more generalized eruptions involving skin never exposed to the sun (Figure 109.7).
- There may be a distinct periorbital accentuation, termed the "raccoon eyes" appearance.
- Lesions of NLE are self-limited and usually resolve by 6 months of age without scarring.
- Approximately 10% of infants may develop hepatic or hematologic alterations (usually self-limited).
- Less than half of mothers have a known diagnosis of autoimmune disease; mothers are most likely to have (or eventually develop) SCLE, SLE, or Sjögren syndrome.
- Infants with cutaneous findings suggestive of NLE should be evaluated for cardiac, hematologic, or hepatic abnormalities; serologic studies usually confirm the diagnosis and should be performed on infant and mother.
- Skin biopsy is rarely indicated.
- Asymptomatic mothers of infants with NLE should have a comprehensive rheumatologic evaluation and be followed closely for connective tissue disease.
- There is an increased risk of having another infant with NLE in subsequent pregnancies.

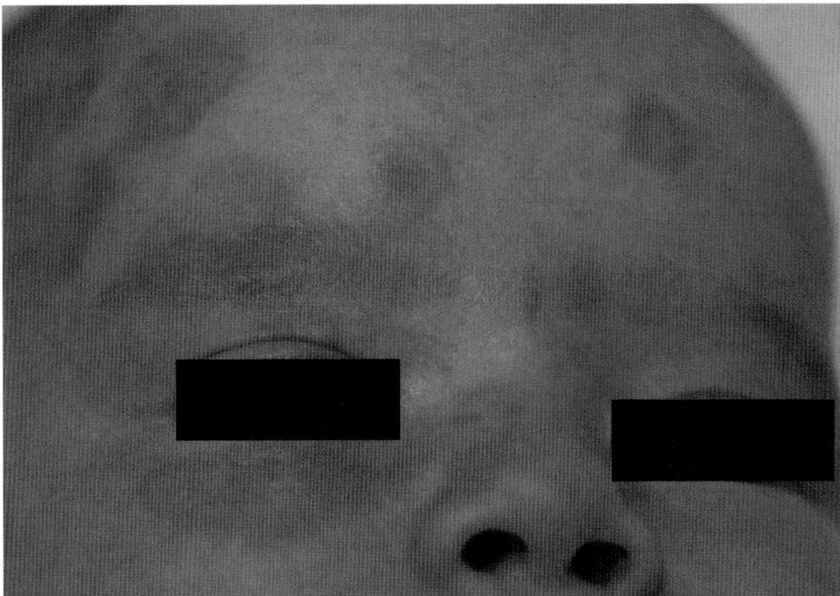

Figure 109.6. Multiple annular plaques with dusky atrophic centers on the face and scalp of this 1-month-old with neonatal lupus erythematosus (NLE). His mother had no previous history of connective tissue disease but was later diagnosed with systemic lupus erythematosus. Her subsequent pregnancy resulted in a second child with cutaneous NLE.

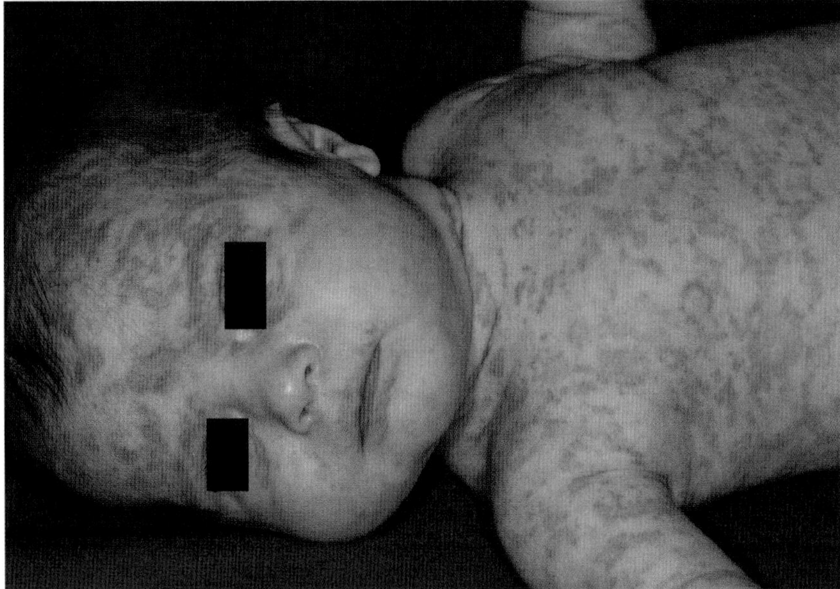

Figure 109.7. Young infant with widespread erythematous, slightly atrophic patches and plaques secondary to neonatal lupus erythematosus. Note the prominent involvement of the periorbital region, forehead, and scalp.

Look-alikes

Disorder	Differentiating Features
Systemic Lupus Erythematosus	
Juvenile idiopathic arthritis, systemic subtype	• Evanescent hive-like lesions. • Usually no malar erythema. • High-spiking fevers common, often correlate with the presence of skin eruption. • Skin findings may exhibit Koebner phenomenon.
Juvenile dermatomyositis	• Proximal muscle weakness in most patients; less common in SLE. • Arthritis usually absent. • Distribution of cutaneous lesions over extensor surfaces of arms and legs. • Heliotrope rash (periorbital distribution). • May have malar rash, which often does not spare nasolabial folds. • Skin changes often show lilac-colored hue. • Calcinosis cutis in some patients. • Gottron sign (erythema) or papules (lichenoid papules) present over knuckles, elbows, knees. • Periungual erythema and nail fold telangiectasias.
Drug hypersensitivity syndrome (sulfa, minocycline, aromatic anticonvulsants, lamotrigine)	• Usually classic triad of fever, rash, and lymphadenopathy • History of drug ingestion, usually preceding syndrome by 3–8 weeks • Increased eosinophils and atypical lymphocytes on complete blood cell count • Histologic findings distinct from those of lupus • Sudden onset of diffuse cutaneous eruption; distinct facial/periorbital edema often present • Eventual exfoliation; some patients with generalized exfoliative erythroderma • Frequent liver involvement; occasionally a fulminant hepatitis
Rosacea	• No systemic abnormalities. • Often more prominent in the nasolabial folds and over medial cheeks. • Inflammatory papules and pustules may be present. • Facial telangiectasias common. • May involve the eyes (ocular rosacea). • Chronic waxing and waning course. • Exacerbated by sunlight, heat, alcohol, hot beverages, spicy foods.
Polymorphous light eruption	• Lacks systemic associations • Typically presents in late spring with initial sun exposure of the season • Edema and erythema of the face, ears, arms, and dorsal hands

Look-alikes *(continued)*

Disorder	Differentiating Features
Subacute Cutaneous Lupus Erythematosus	
Psoriasis	• Most often occurs on knees, elbows, scalp, umbilicus, gluteal crease. • Lesions are plaques, typically thicker than SCLE lesions, and have silvery to white (micaceous) adherent scale. • May have associated nail findings. • Typically improves (rather than worsens) in sunlight. • Negative serologic studies for lupus erythematosus.
Tinea corporis	• Plaques usually have more scaling and may have central clearing. • Inflammatory papules/pustules may be present. • No accentuation in sun-exposed sites. • Positive potassium hydroxide preparation or fungal culture. • Negative serologic studies for lupus erythematosus.
Granuloma annulare	• Annular lesions lack scale and are not exacerbated by sunlight. • Most often distributed on dorsal feet, ankles, wrists, and legs. • No systemic abnormalities in most patients. • Negative serologic studies for lupus erythematosus. • Resolves spontaneously over 2–4 years.
Neonatal Lupus Erythematosus	
Seborrheic dermatitis	• May also have scalp dermatitis, usually with greasy yellow scaling. • Erythema and maceration may occur in the neck, inguinal and axillary folds, and umbilicus (and, less often, the popliteal and antecubital fossae). • Onset in early infancy. • Usually self-limited with spontaneous clearing by 6–12 months of age. • No association with congenital heart block.
Tinea corporis/faciei	• Positive potassium hydroxide preparation or fungal culture. • Negative serologic studies for lupus erythematosus. • May have more scale or inflammatory papules/pustules. • No accentuation in sun-exposed areas. • No periorbital accentuation. • History of known exposure may be present.
Psoriasis	• Facial involvement less common • Often shows significant diaper and umbilical involvement in infant • No accentuation in sun-exposed sites • Typically improves (rather than worsening) with sun exposure • Negative serologic studies for lupus erythematosus
Atopic dermatitis	• Pruritus very common. • Associated excoriations or crusting may be present. • Lichenification (thickening of skin in chronically rubbed sites) often present. • Lesions not typically annular. • Atopic diathesis often present. • Negative serologic studies for lupus erythematosus.

How to Make the Diagnosis

- A thorough history, review of systems, and physical examination are critical in the accurate diagnosis of lupus. Helpful physical findings in SLE include
  - Malar erythema
  - Nasal or oral ulcerations
  - Diffuse non-scarring alopecia
  - Raynaud phenomenon
  - Periungual telangiectasia
  - Vasculitis (red/purple macules and papules on hands or small ulcerations of the fingertips)
  - Lymphadenopathy
  - Erythema of the palms
- When a diagnosis of SLE is suspected, the following laboratory evaluation should be considered:
  - Antinuclear antibody profile (including anti-dsDNA, anti-Sm, anti–SS-A [anti-Ro], anti–SS-B [anti-La], anti-RNP antibodies)
  - Antiphospholipid antibody and lupus anticoagulant panels
  - Complete blood cell count with differential and platelet count
  - Chemistries to include liver and renal function
  - Complement levels (C3, C4, total hemolytic complement)
  - Erythrocyte sedimentation rate (less commonly, C-reactive protein)
  - Urinalysis with microscopic examination and first-morning spot protein to creatinine ratio
- Serologic studies may aid in confirming the diagnosis of lupus and may also help with categorization of subtype and prognosis.
  - Antinuclear antibody almost always positive in SLE but is also positive in 5% to 10% of the general population.
    - Five distinct staining patterns
      - Speckled: least specific (may be seen with Scl-70, Smith, RNP, SS-A and SS-B antibodies)
      - Homogeneous: associated with anti-nucleoprotein antibodies
      - Shaggy/peripheral: associated with anti-dsDNA antibodies
      - Centromere: associated with CREST syndrome (**c**alcinosis, **R**aynaud phenomenon, **e**sophageal dysmotility, **s**clerodactyly, and **t**elangiectasias; also known as limited cutaneous systemic sclerosis)
      - Nucleolar pattern: often seen in diffuse or limited cutaneous systemic sclerosis (scleroderma)

- If high clinical suspicion of lupus, check for anti-native dsDNA antibodies; these are highly specific for SLE and present in about half of patients; often associated with renal disease.
- Antibodies against small nuclear (sn) RNPs
  - Anti-Smith: specific for SLE; present in 20% SLE patients; associated with higher risk for renal disease
  - Anti-RNP: may be seen in SLE, scleroderma, or mixed connective tissue disease
  - Anti–SS-A (anti-Ro): seen in about 30% of SLE patients and approximately half of patients with Sjögren syndrome, as well as in patients with SCLE and NLE; strong association with photosensitivity
  - Anti–SS-B (anti-La): positive in about 10% patients with SLE; often seen in association with anti–SS-A (anti-Ro) antibody; also seen in SCLE and NLE
- Antiphospholipid antibody: Occurs in 30% to 50% of adult lupus patients and can also occur in patients with antiphospholipid antibody syndrome; associated with higher incidence of thrombotic events; skin findings may include livedo reticularis or cutaneous ulcerations.
- In general, patients with SLE should meet 4 of the following 11 criteria (American College of Rheumatology 1997 revised criteria for classification of SLE):
  1. Malar rash
  2. Discoid rash
  3. Photosensitivity
  4. Oral ulcerations
     a. Oral or nasopharyngeal ulcers, usually painless
  5. Arthritis
     a. Two or more joints
     b. Nonerosive arthritis
  6. Serositis (pleuritis or pericarditis)
  7. Renal disease (persistent proteinuria or cellular casts)
  8. Neurologic manifestations (seizures, psychosis)
  9. Hematologic disorder (≥1 of the below findings on >1 occasion)
     a. Hemolytic anemia
     b. Leukopenia (<4,000/mm^3)
     c. Lymphopenia (<1,500/mm^3)
     d. Thrombocytopenia (<100,000/mm^3)

10. Immunologic disorder (≥1 of the following)
    a. Anti-DNA antibody to native DNA in abnormal titer
    b. Anti-Sm antibody
    c. Positive finding of antiphospholipid antibodies based on an abnormal serum level of IgG or IgM anticardiolipin antibodies, a positive test result for lupus anticoagulant using a standard method, or a false-positive serologic test for syphilis known to be positive for at least 6 months and confirmed by *Treponema pallidum* immobilization or fluorescent treponemal antibody absorption test
11. Antinuclear antibody (in absence of drugs known to cause drug-induced lupus)

Treatment

- Patients who have SLE should be followed closely by a pediatric rheumatologist, and a multidisciplinary approach should be employed for those who have significant systemic disease.
- Cutaneous manifestations may be managed in conjunction with a pediatric or adult dermatologist.
- Treatment of cutaneous disease may include (depends on severity and response to treatment)
    - Photoprotection
        - Avoidance of excessive sun exposure, especially between 10:00 am and 4:00 pm.
        - Protective clothing.
        - Daily broad-spectrum sunscreen use with high sun protection factor (>30); products containing titanium dioxide or zinc oxide are optimal.
    - Topical corticosteroids
    - Topical calcineurin inhibitors (tacrolimus, pimecrolimus)
    - Intralesional corticosteroids
    - Systemic agents for more severe skin disease
        - Hydroxychloroquine (alone or in combination with quinacrine)
        - Oral retinoids
        - Dapsone
        - Methotrexate
        - Clofazimine
        - Thalidomide
        - Azathioprine

- Treatment of systemic disease usually requires one or a combination of the following systemic medications:
  - Prednisone.
  - Azathioprine.
  - Mycophenolate mofetil.
  - Cyclophosphamide.
  - Rituximab.
  - Belimumab, an anti–B-lymphocyte stimulator antibody, was recently approved for treatment of SLE in adults; there is minimal experience in treatment of childhood SLE.
- In addition, nonsteroidal anti-inflammatory agents can be used for musculoskeletal symptoms and serositis but should not be used in patients with nephritis.

Treating Associated Conditions

- Patients with SLE are likely to need concurrent care from multiple specialists depending on the degree of end-organ involvement.
- Those with significant renal disease often benefit from collaborative care with a nephrologist.
- Those with neuropsychiatric disease may require specialty care directed at central nervous system complications.
- Due to the chronic and potentially disabling nature of lupus, the disorder can be associated with significant psychologic morbidity, and care from an appropriate specialist may be very beneficial.

Prognosis

- The prognosis for patients with SLE is quite variable and depends on the organ systems involved.
- Patients who have diffuse proliferative glomerulonephritis and associated hypertension often have a poorer prognosis.
- Infection is a major cause of death and is usually related to use of systemic corticosteroids or other immunosuppressive agents.
- Patients with DLE generally have a good prognosis.
- Children with NLE have a good overall prognosis; those with congenital heart block often require pacemaker placement.

When to Worry or Refer

- Children suspected of having cutaneous or systemic manifestations of lupus should be referred to a rheumatologist or dermatologist for confirmation of diagnosis and management.
- If a patient with SLE acutely develops cytopenias and fever, the diagnosis of *macrophage activation syndrome* should be considered and is often accompanied by hyperferritinemia and hypertriglyceridemia; these patients should immediately be evaluated by a pediatric rheumatologist.
- Infants suspected of having NLE should undergo immediate cardiac evaluation, including electrocardiography, to assess for congenital heart block; mothers of these infants should be referred for rheumatologic evaluation.

Resources for Families

- Lupus Foundation of America: Provides information, support, and links for patients and families.
  www.lupus.org
- S.L.E. Lupus Foundation: Provides information and support for patients and families.
  www.lupusny.org
- The Lupus Initiative: Provides information and support for patients, families, and medical professional. Sponsored by the American College of Rheumatology.
  www.thelupusinitiative.org

Nutritional Dermatoses

Acrodermatitis Enteropathica (AE)

Introduction/Etiology/Epidemiology

- Acrodermatitis enteropathica (AE) is an autosomal-recessive disorder that results in a characteristic acral and periorificial eruption, diarrhea, and alopecia.
  - Acrodermatitis enteropathica is caused by mutations in the SLC39A4 gene that encodes an intestinal transporter required for zinc absorption from the small intestine.
- Acquired zinc deficiency (eg, due to excessive losses [eg, chronic diarrhea], dietary restriction, administration of total parenteral nutrition with inadequate zinc supplementation) results in symptoms and signs analogous to those of AE. An unusual form of acquired zinc deficiency may occur in breastfed infants whose mothers produce zinc-deficient milk.

Signs and Symptoms

- In formula-fed neonates and infants, the symptoms of AE typically appear days to weeks following birth when zinc stores become depleted. In breastfed infants, AE becomes manifest shortly after weaning. This delay in onset is thought to be the result of enhanced bioavailability of zinc in human milk.
- Rash is often the first sign of disease.
  - The rash of AE is acral (ie, on the extremities) and periorificial (ie, around the mouth, nose, eyes, and anus) (Figures 110.1–110.3). The digits may be involved with periungual erythema and swelling.
  - Lesions are erythematous patches with well-defined borders. Scaling, erosions, crusting, vesicles, and bullae may occur.
- The most common associated symptoms are alopecia and diarrhea. Others include anorexia, behavioral changes (eg, irritability, apathy), failure to thrive, ocular symptoms (eg, blepharitis, conjunctivitis), and recurring bacterial or fungal infections.

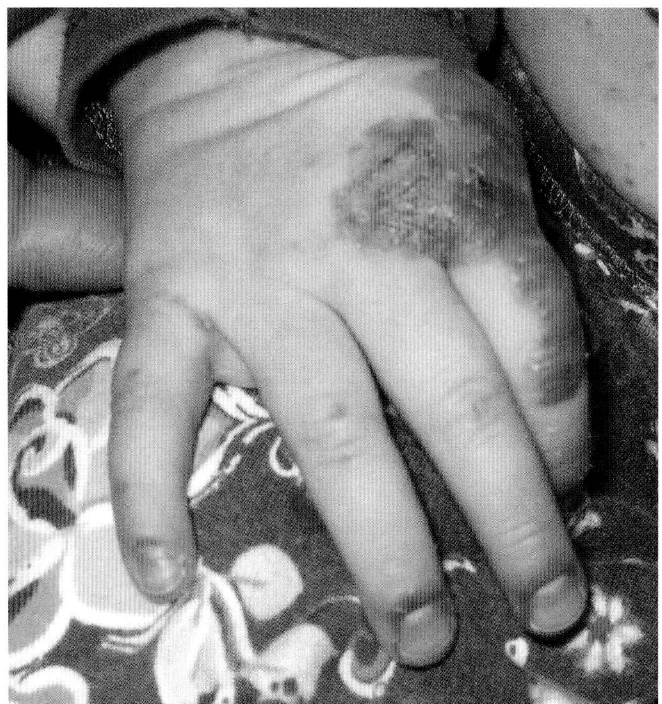

Figure 110.1. Acrodermatitis enteropathica. Erythema, scaling, and crusting on the hand.

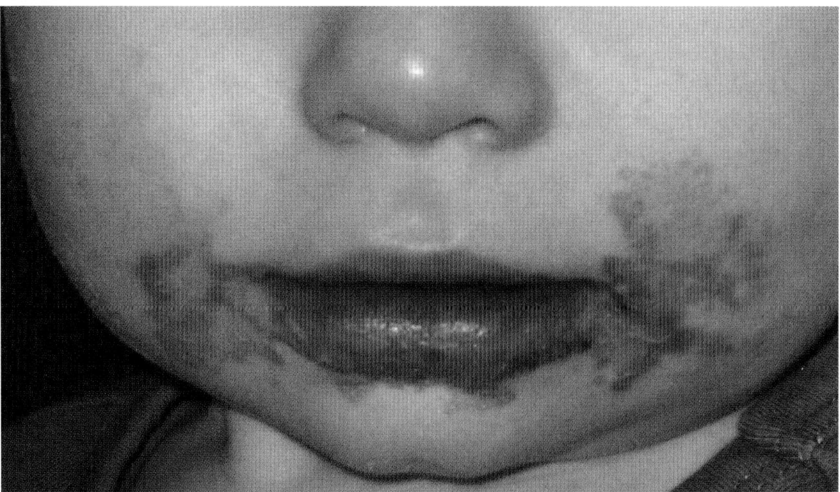

Figure 110.2. Acrodermatitis enteropathica. Erythema and crusting around the mouth of the patient shown in Figure 110.1.

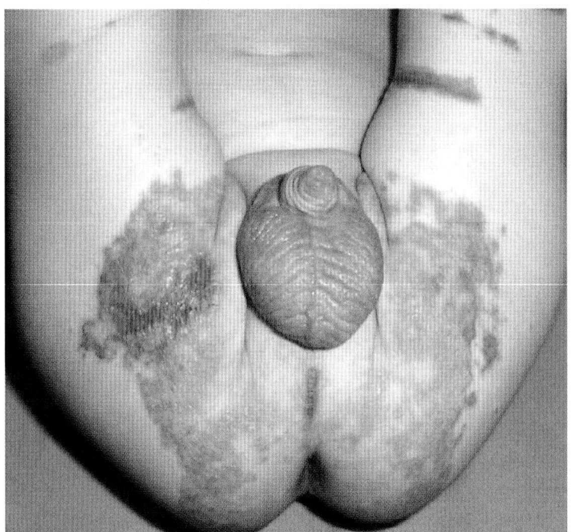

Figure 110.3. Erythema and crusting in the diaper area of an infant who has acrodermatitis enteropathica.

Look-alikes

Kwashiorkor, essential fatty acid deficiency (including the rash seen in cystic fibrosis), vitamin B_{12} deficiency, isoleucine deficiency, certain organic acid disorders, and biotin deficiency may produce an eruption similar to that of AE. The acral and periorificial distribution of the rash of AE may help to distinguish it from other disorders.

Disorder	Differentiating Features
Atopic dermatitis	• Diaper area usually spared. • Trunk often affected in infants (uncommon in AE). • Facial involvement (eg, cheeks) occurs frequently, but perioral and periorbital involvement uncommon. • Pruritus usually present.
Crusted impetigo	• Distribution usually not as extensive as AE. • Lesions appear as erosions with a yellow crust; erythematous patches are typically absent.
Irritant diaper dermatitis	• Rash limited to the diaper area
Psoriasis	• Diaper area involvement may mimic that of AE, but typical psoriatic lesions (ie, erythematous papules and plaques with thick scale) may be present elsewhere. • Erosive changes absent.
Seborrheic dermatitis	• Scalp involvement common (ie, cradle cap). • Skin lesions often have "greasy" scale. • Perioral and periorbital involvement uncommon. • Erosive changes absent.

How to Make the Diagnosis

- The presence of AE is suggested by the acral and periorificial distribution of the erosive rash and the presence of lesions with well-defined borders.
- A serum zinc level 50 mcg/dL or lower supports the clinical diagnosis; care should be exercised to collect blood in correct tubes, given potential zinc contamination of some materials.
- Low serum alkaline phosphatase is often present.
- Rapid response of the rash and other symptoms to zinc supplementation supports the diagnosis.

Treatment

- Oral zinc supplementation (usually lifelong in AE): Supplementation should begin at a dose of 1 to 3 mg/kg daily of elemental zinc. A suspension can be prepared by a compounding pharmacy. The daily dose may be divided twice or 3 times a day and is best administered 1 to 2 hours before a feeding or meal.
  - Zinc sulfate (23% elemental zinc): 5 to 15 mg/kg daily
  - Zinc gluconate (14% elemental zinc): 7 to 21 mg/kg daily
- Irritability, anorexia, diarrhea, and the rash improve within days (Figure 110.4).
- Monitor zinc level periodically (every 3–6 months) and adjust dose accordingly.

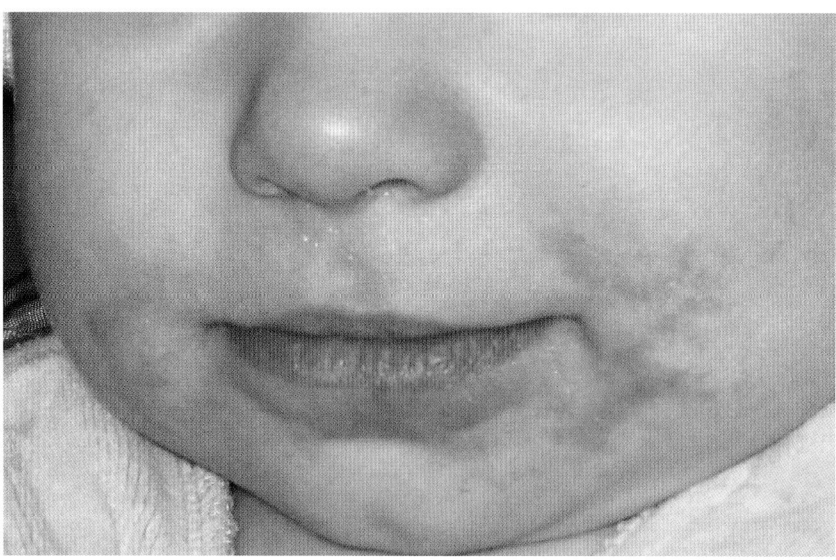

Figure 110.4. The patient shown in Figure 110.2 ten days after beginning zinc supplementation. The perioral eruption has improved greatly.

- Adverse effects include
  - Zinc may cause nausea or vomiting (may be lessened by using the gluconate form).
  - Because zinc may interfere with the absorption of copper, some recommend periodic measurement of the serum copper concentration.

Prognosis

- Excellent, although lifetime zinc supplementation generally is required for neonates or infants who have AE

When to Worry or Refer

- Consider consultation or referral if the patient fails to respond to zinc therapy. If the patient has an acquired form of zinc deficiency, identification and treatment of the underlying cause are necessary.

Resources for Families

- National Organization for Rare Disorders: Acrodermatitis enteropathica. **http://rarediseases.org/rare-diseases/acrodermatitis-enteropathica**
- National Center for Advancing Translational Sciences Genetic and Rare Diseases Information Center: Acrodermatitis enteropathica. **http://rarediseases.info.nih.gov/gard/5723/acrodermatitis-enteropathica/resources/1**

Kwashiorkor

Introduction/Etiology/Epidemiology

- Kwashiorkor is a disorder characterized by insufficient protein intake in the setting of adequate caloric intake. The typical skin findings include a "flaky paint" rash and alopecia.
- It usually is considered a disease of children residing in areas of famine. However, the disease has been reported in developed countries when children are fed protein-deficient diets or have malabsorption or failure to thrive due to neglect. Some examples include
  - Infants fed rice milk by parents in an attempt to manage food allergies
  - Infants fed protein-deficient diets to treat underlying diseases (eg, nonketotic hyperglycemia, glutaric aciduria type 1)
  - Infants who have diseases characterized by malabsorption (eg, Crohn disease, cystic fibrosis)
  - Infants fed diluted formula by caregivers in an attempt to make the formula last longer or intentionally limit calories
  - Infants fed inappropriately by their caregivers because of mental illness or unusual feeding practices or beliefs

Signs and Symptoms

- Systemic symptoms include fatigue, lethargy, and irritability. As protein deprivation continues, individuals exhibit growth failure, generalized edema, and a protuberant abdomen (due to hepatomegaly [from fatty infiltration] or ascites).
- The diffuse rash of kwashiorkor is composed of well-defined erythematous patches with overlying scale. The scale edges are elevated, an appearance similar to that of peeling paint chips (Figures 111.1–111.3). This finding has led to the term "flaky paint dermatosis."
- Other cutaneous abnormalities include loss of skin pigment and thinning and diminished pigmentation of the hair.

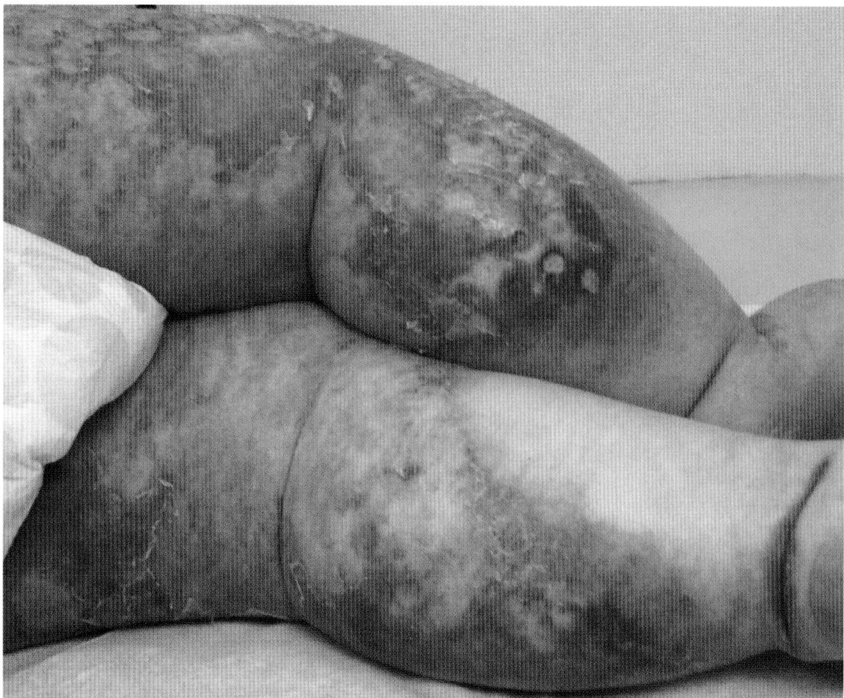

Figure 111.1. Toddler who had kwashiorkor and zinc deficiency. There are well-defined erythematous patches.

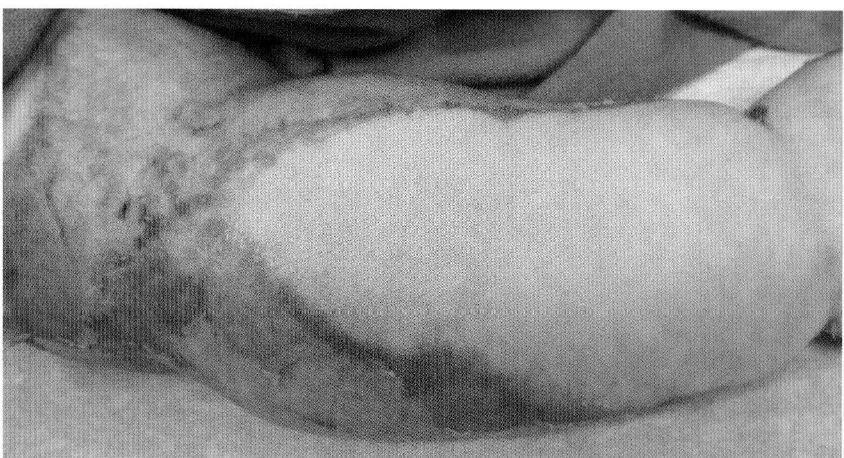

Figure 111.2. Sharply marginated patches with "flaky paint" scale are present in the patient shown in Figure 111.1.

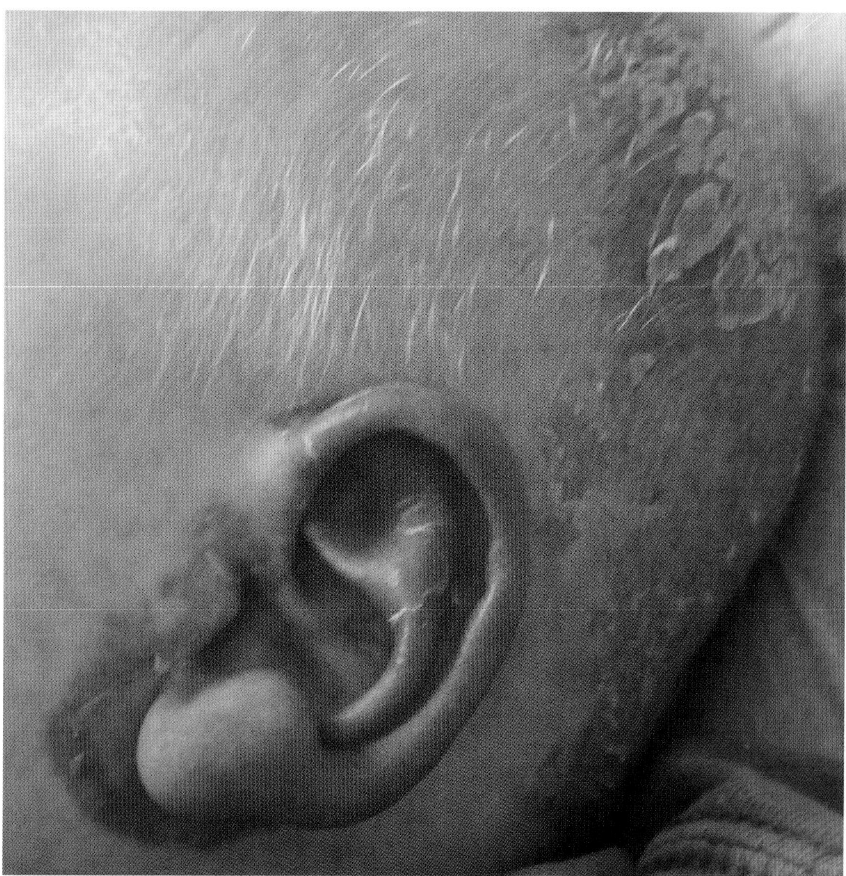

Figure 111.3. Scalp involvement in kwashiorkor with a prominent flaky paint appearance.

Look-alikes

The presence of edema, hypoproteinemia, and hypoalbuminemia helps to differentiate kwashiorkor from other disorders that may produce a similar eruption, including those characterized by nutritional deficiency (eg, of essential fatty acids, vitamin B_{12}, isoleucine, zinc, biotin).

Disorder	Differentiating Features
Acrodermatitis enteropathica (AE)	• It may be difficult to distinguish AE from kwashiorkor clinically, and the 2 entities may coexist. • Periorificial and acral involvement common (unlike kwashiorkor). • Edema, hypoproteinemia, hypoalbuminemia absent. • Serum zinc concentration reduced.
Atopic dermatitis	• Edema, hypoproteinemia, hypoalbuminemia absent • "Flaky paint" appearance of scale absent • Characteristic distribution by age
Crusted impetigo	• Distribution usually not as extensive as in kwashiorkor • Edema, hypoproteinemia, hypoalbuminemia absent • "Flaky paint" appearance of scale absent
Psoriasis	• Edema, hypoproteinemia, hypoalbuminemia absent. • Typical psoriatic lesions (ie, papules and plaques with thick adherent scale) usually present (scale does not have the "flaky paint" appearance), although diaper involvement may reveal minimal scaling. • Preference for scalp, umbilicus, diaper region in infants.
Seborrheic dermatitis	• Edema, hypoproteinemia, hypoalbuminemia absent • "Flaky paint" appearance of scale absent (scale often characterized as "greasy") • Preference for scalp, umbilicus, diaper region in infants

How to Make the Diagnosis

- The diagnosis is suspected clinically based on the appearance of the rash and presence of edema.
- The presence of hypoproteinemia and hypoalbuminemia supports the diagnosis.

Treatment

- Institution of a diet or parenteral nutrition containing appropriate amounts of protein is paramount. Depending on the underlying cause of protein deficiency, this may require consultation with colleagues in nutrition, gastroenterology, or other disciplines.
- Investigation for coexisting nutritional deficiencies (eg, AE) may be appropriate.

Prognosis

- Treatment early in the course of the disease is associated with excellent prognosis.
- In severe cases, death may occur, caused by electrolyte disturbances or immunodeficiency resulting in infection.

When to Worry or Refer

- If kwashiorkor is suspected, prompt laboratory evaluation and initiation of nutritional restitution is vital.
- If abuse or neglect is suspected, a referral to child protective services should be made.

Resources for Families

- MedlinePlus: Information for patients and families (in English and Spanish) sponsored by the National Library of Medicine and National Institutes of Health.
  www.nlm.nih.gov/medlineplus/ency/article/001604.htm

Other Disorders

Erythema Nodosum

Introduction/Etiology/Epidemiology

- Erythema nodosum (EN) is a reactive inflammatory disorder of the subcutaneous fat (ie, panniculitis) that has a limited duration and resolves spontaneously.
- Potential triggers include infections (*Streptococcus pyogenes* is most common trigger in children; others include *Mycoplasma pneumoniae, Yersinia enterocolitica,* tuberculosis, and cutaneous fungal infections), medications (estrogen in oral contraceptives, sulfonamides), and inflammatory disorders such as inflammatory bowel disease or sarcoidosis.
- Erythema nodosum is the most common panniculitis in all age groups. It is rare in those younger than 2 years. Incidence increases with age with peaks in teens and young adults. Among children with EN, there is a slight female predominance.

Signs and Symptoms

- Red, tender, raised 1- to 3-cm nodules and plaques often start on the shins (Figure 112.1).
- In children, lesions may also develop on thighs, arms, face, trunk, and, very rarely, palms or soles.
- Lesions do not ulcerate or leave scars.
- May turn purple/violaceous before resolution.
- About 10% of children with EN may have arthralgias.
- Lasts up to 6 weeks and may intermittently recur for a few months.
- Recurrences after resolution are unusual.

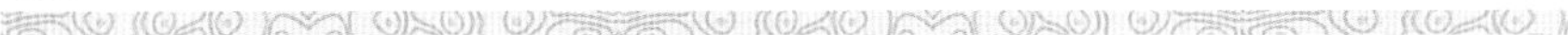

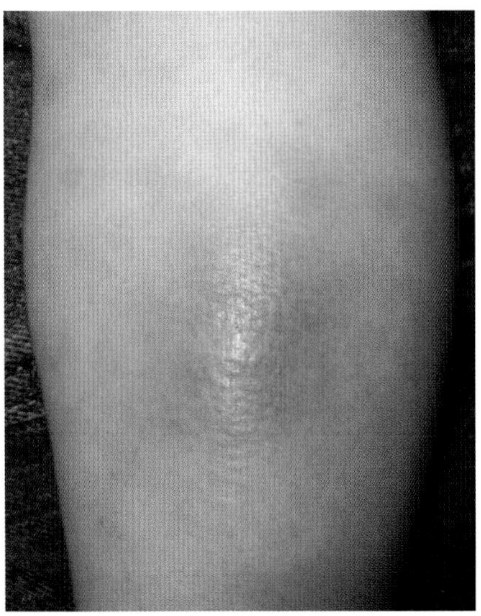

Figure 112.1. A tender red nodule on the shin characteristic of erythema nodosum.

Look-alikes

Disorder	Differentiating Features
Eccrine hidradenitis	• Confined to palms and soles • Mainly occurs in summer; teens and preteens • No history of antecedent infection
Bruises, ecchymoses	• Often a history of trauma • Rare recrudescence • Typically undergo color evolution from purple to green and yellow
Cellulitis	• Usually unifocal • Associated fever often present • Less nodular, usually more of a patch or thin plaque
Arthropod bites	• Rarely tender; usually very pruritic • Often see small puncta at bite site
Vasculitis	• Palpable purpura with no blanching. • Often progressive. • Lesions range from small petechiae to larger ecchymotic or purpuric papules or nodules.

How to Make the Diagnosis

- Diagnosis of EN can usually be made clinically but may be confirmed by skin biopsy if uncertainty exists.
- If the patient is healthy and a cause is not immediately apparent, consider screening tests, including measurement of antistreptolysin-O or anti-deoxyribonuclease B titers, complete blood cell count, chest radiography, and testing for tuberculosis (purified protein derivative or interferon gamma receptor assay).

Treatment

- Treat or remove underlying cause, if identified.
- If pain is significant, advise rest, leg elevation, and a nonsteroidal anti-inflammatory drug.
- Persistent cases may require a brief oral corticosteroid course; other reported therapies include colchicine, salicylates, and potassium iodide.

Prognosis

- Excellent. Erythema nodosum usually resolves spontaneously in 2 to 6 weeks, with rare long-term recurrence risk.

When to Worry or Refer

- Atypical, prolonged, or severe course.
- Concern exists for a systemic illness precipitating EN (eg, inflammatory bowel disease).

Resources for Families

- MedlinePlus: Information for patients and families (in English and Spanish) sponsored by the National Library of Medicine and National Institutes of Health.
  https://www.nlm.nih.gov/medlineplus/ency/article/000881.htm
- WebMD: Information for families is contained in the Health A-Z topics.
  www.webmd.com/skin-problems-and-treatments/erythema-nodosum

Henoch-Schönlein Purpura

Introduction/Etiology/Epidemiology

- Henoch-Schönlein purpura (HSP) is a systemic small vessel vasculitis with IgA immune complexes. It is the most common vasculitis of childhood.
- Etiology of HSP is unknown, but frequent occurrence after acute infections (especially upper respiratory tract infection or streptococcal pharyngitis) suggests infectious triggers. Immunizations and medications have been implicated, although less often.
- Most commonly seen between 2 and 11 years of age, with a mean age of 6 years; slight male predominance.
- Incidence is estimated to be 10 to 30 cases per 100,000 per year younger than 17 years.

Signs and Symptoms

- Classic tetrad of nonthrombocytopenic palpable purpura, arthralgias, abdominal pain, and renal involvement.
- Skin
  - Rash begins as urticarial macules and plaques on legs and buttocks, progressing to palpable purpura (Figures 113.1 and 113.2); petechiae may be present.
  - Forearms, elbows, trunk, and face (ears) may be involved in younger children, along with hand and foot edema. The rash often involves pressure points or dependent areas.
  - Occasional oral and nasal mucosal involvement.
  - Lesions develop in crops, with newer urticarial lesions intermixed with older palpable purpura.
  - Occasionally, patients may develop blisters, ulcers, or necrosis.

- Renal involvement occurs in 20% to 50% of patients.
  - Spectrum of disease ranges from microscopic hematuria or minimal proteinuria to nephritic or nephrotic syndrome (5%); 2% to 5% of patients progress to end-stage renal failure.
  - May not appear until weeks after the onset of disease but usually within 3 months of onset; therefore, serial urine evaluations (typically every 1–2 weeks) recommended for several months (most suggest for 3–6 months) following the diagnosis.
- Gastrointestinal involvement occurs in 50% to 70% of children.
  - Colicky abdominal pain, vomiting, and gross or occult bleeding are most common.
  - Intussusception in 2% to 4%, usually involving the small bowel; more common in boys.
- Musculoskeletal
  - Arthralgias occur in 60% to 80% of children with HSP; rarely true arthritis.
  - Ankles and knees most commonly affected.
- Other
  - Rarely, central nervous system (eg, headache, seizures, behavioral changes) or lung involvement (ie, infiltrates or diffuse alveolar hemorrhage) may occur.
  - Infrequent scrotal involvement with purpura (Figure 113.3) or pain that may mimic testicular torsion.

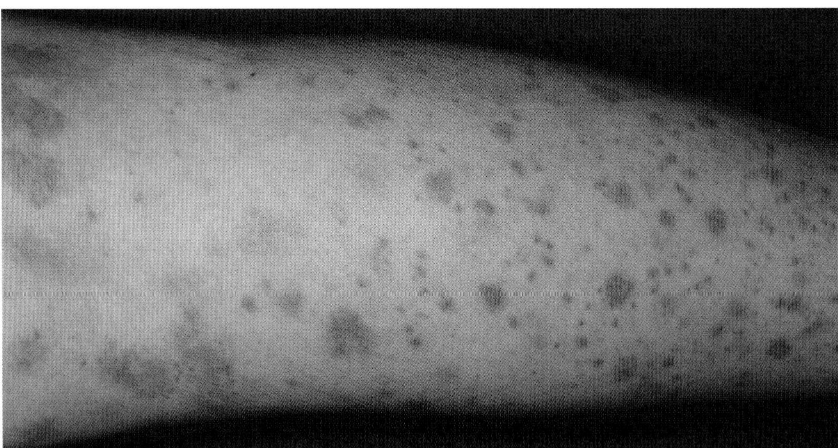

Figure 113.1. A mixture of urticarial, violaceous, and purpuric plaques is typical of Henoch-Schönlein purpura.

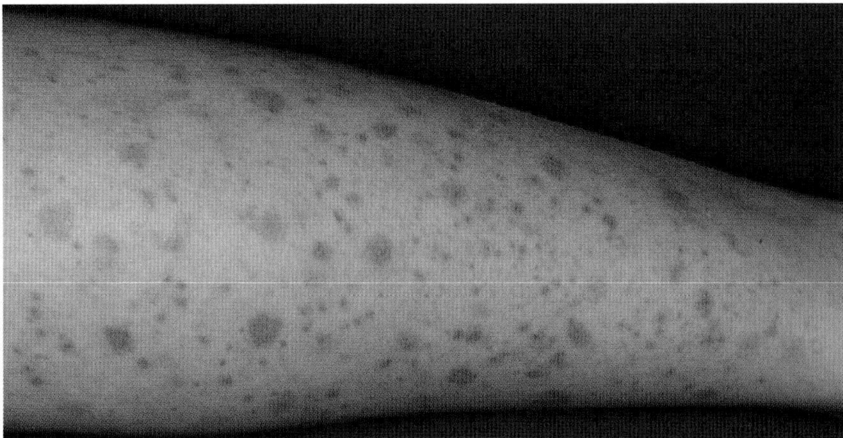

Figure 113.2. Pink and purpuric macules and papules on the leg of a patient with Henoch-Schönlein purpura.

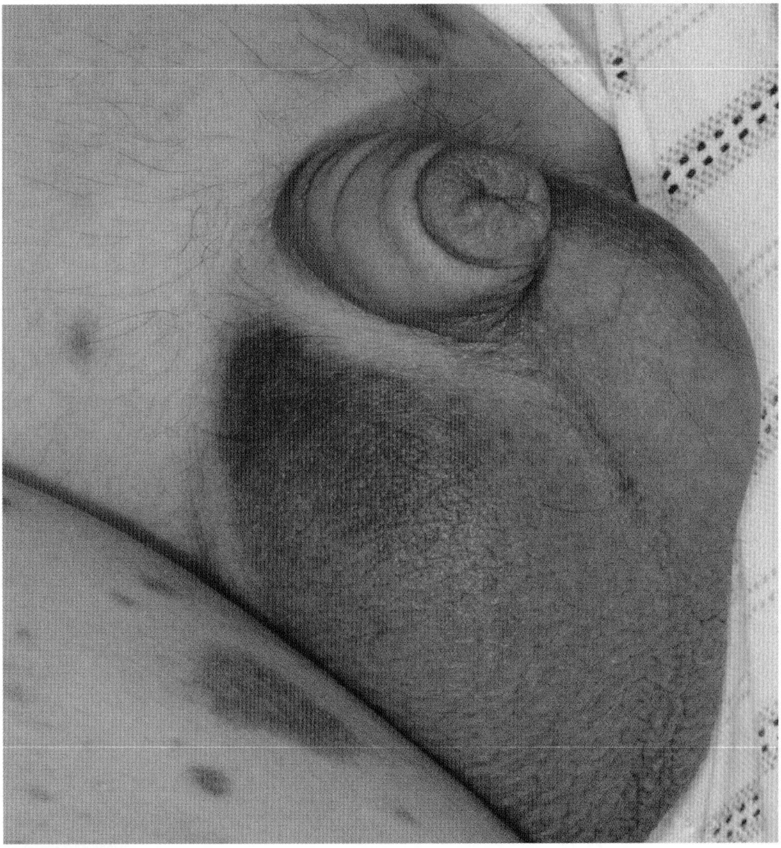

Figure 113.3. Purpura involving the scrotum in a patient with Henoch-Schönlein purpura and scrotal pain.

Look-alikes

Disorder	Differentiating Features
Acute hemorrhagic edema of infancy	• Younger children (4 months–3 years) • Cockade (medallion-like) purpura • Facial, hand, and foot edema • No systemic features • IgA deposition usually absent on histology of skin biopsy • Benign self-limited course
Septic vasculitis	• Febrile and often toxic-appearing; shock may be present. • Progressive course. • Often a more widespread distribution. • Multisystem disease.
Hypersensitivity vasculitis	• Often induced by medication • Lesions often more widespread • Often presents with petechiae and small purpuric papules
Ecchymoses, benign	• Usually no renal, gastrointestinal, or joint concerns • Skin lesions typically fewer in number • Usually limited to areas overlying bony prominences (eg, anterior tibial surfaces)
Ecchymoses associated with child abuse	• Usually no renal, gastrointestinal, or joint associations. • Skin lesions typically fewer in number. • Historical context important. • Other features of abuse may be present (eg, retinal hemorrhage, bony fractures).
Urticaria	• May mimic early HSP • Purpura absent • Lesions usually widespread and transient (resolving within 24 hours)

How to Make the Diagnosis

- The clinical presentation is usually highly suggestive, especially when the classic tetrad (lower body purpura, arthralgias, abdominal pain, renal involvement) is present.
- No laboratory tests are specific to HSP, making it largely a clinical diagnosis.
- Skin biopsy (when necessary) is usually confirmatory on histology and immunofluorescence study (demonstrating leukocytoclastic vasculitis with IgA1 deposits and neutrophil infiltration of small blood vessel walls).
- Renal biopsy, if needed, reveals proliferative glomerulonephritis with IgA1 deposition.

Treatment

- Most patients require only supportive care.
- If severe joint or abdominal pain or with severe skin involvement, consider oral corticosteroid therapy.
- Must assess renal function and urinalysis long-term, given possible delayed presentation of renal disease in HSP.
- Treatment of renal involvement depends on severity. In patients with significant nephritis or nephrosis, consultation with a pediatric nephrologist is warranted.
- Some evidence that treatment with systemic corticosteroids may reduce intussusception risk or renal disease progression. Steroid use does not prevent recurrence.

Prognosis

- Excellent in most. Typically resolves in 4 to 6 weeks.
- Recurrences in one-third of patients, usually within 3 to 4 months.
- Severity of nephritis predicts outcome.

When to Worry or Refer

- Renal insufficiency or rapidly progressive kidney disease, nephritic/nephrotic syndrome
- Concern for intussusception
- Acute scrotal pain or swelling (when concern exists for testicular torsion)
- Central nervous system involvement (eg, change in mental status or behavior, seizures)
- Hemoptysis

Resources for Families

- MedlinePlus: Information for patients and families (in English and Spanish) sponsored by the National Library of Medicine and National Institutes of Health.
  https://www.nlm.nih.gov/medlineplus/ency/article/000425.htm
- WebMD: Information for families is contained in the Health A-Z topics.
  www.webmd.com/skin-problems-and-treatments/henoch-schonlein-purpura-causes-symptoms-treatment

Kawasaki Disease

Introduction/Etiology/Epidemiology

- Also known as acute febrile mucocutaneous lymph node syndrome.
- Acute multisystem vasculitis of children, usually younger than 5 years; involves small- and medium-sized muscular arteries.
- Most common cause of acquired heart disease in children in developed nations.
- Etiology remains unknown; research suggests a provocative infectious agent that enters through the upper respiratory tract and a possible genetic predisposition (many candidate genes identified).
- A marked seasonality has been observed, with studies suggesting the possible role of tropospheric wind currents in spreading the causative agent.
- No diagnostic test exists.
- Coronary artery aneurysms may develop in up to 25% of untreated patients (2%–4% with appropriate therapy).

Signs and Symptoms

- Diagnosis is based on fulfillment of diagnostic criteria, which consist of fever for at least 5 days and 4 of the following 5 clinical features:
  - Bilateral bulbar conjunctival injection (nonexudative), classically with perilimbic sparing (Figure 114.1)
  - Oral mucosa changes, including erythematous, fissured lips (Figure 114.2); strawberry tongue (Figure 114.3); pharyngeal erythema
  - Nonsuppurative cervical lymphadenopathy (at least 1.5 cm and often unilateral)
  - Edema and erythema of the hands and feet (early) (Figure 114.4); periungual desquamation in subacute phase
  - Polymorphous rash

- Fevers are usually high (≥39°C).
- Irritability is common and may reflect cerebral vasculitis or aseptic meningitis.
- Rash may be exanthematous (macular, papular), urticarial, scarlet fever–like, or erythema multiforme–like in character; pustular presentations have also been observed.
- Accentuation of skin eruption frequently noted in perineal and genital regions (Figure 114.5); may be desquamative; is considered an important clue to the diagnosis.
- BCG vaccination site erythema and induration may be noted.
- Vesicles, bullae, and purpura are usually not seen; peripheral gangrene may rarely occur (Figure 114.6).
- A psoriasis-like skin eruption may be present, especially during the convalescent phase.
- In addition to coronary aneurysms, other cardiac complications may include myocarditis, valvulitis, pericardial effusion, and myocardial infarction.
- Incomplete or atypical Kawasaki disease may occur, especially in infants, in which patients do not fulfill classic diagnostic criteria; in a child with unexplained fever and some diagnostic features, this diagnosis should be considered.

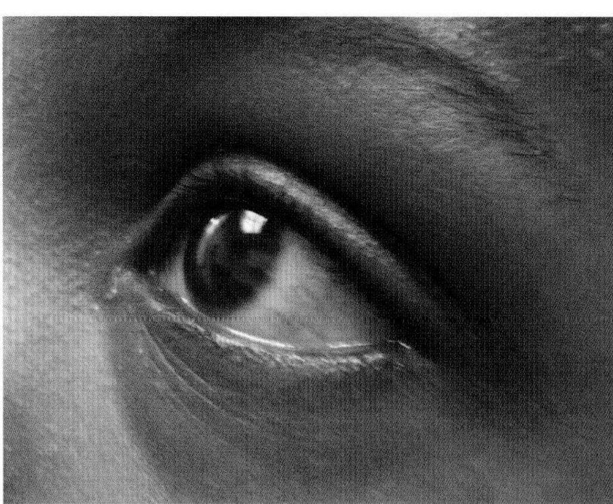

Figure 114.1. In Kawasaki disease, nonexudative conjunctival injection is present, often with perilimbic sparing.

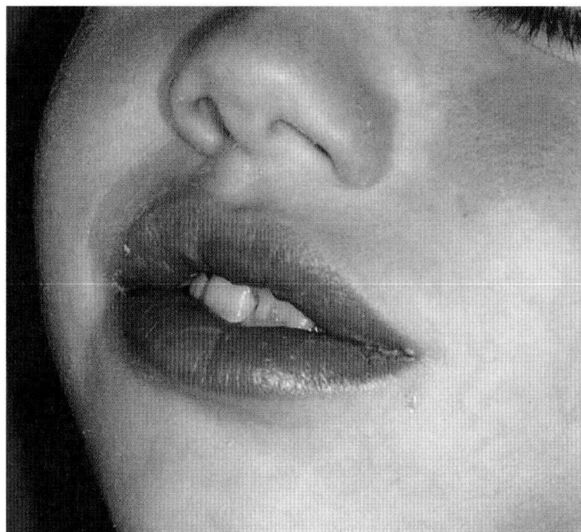

Figure 114.2. Kawasaki disease. Hyperemia, edema, and fissuring of the lips.

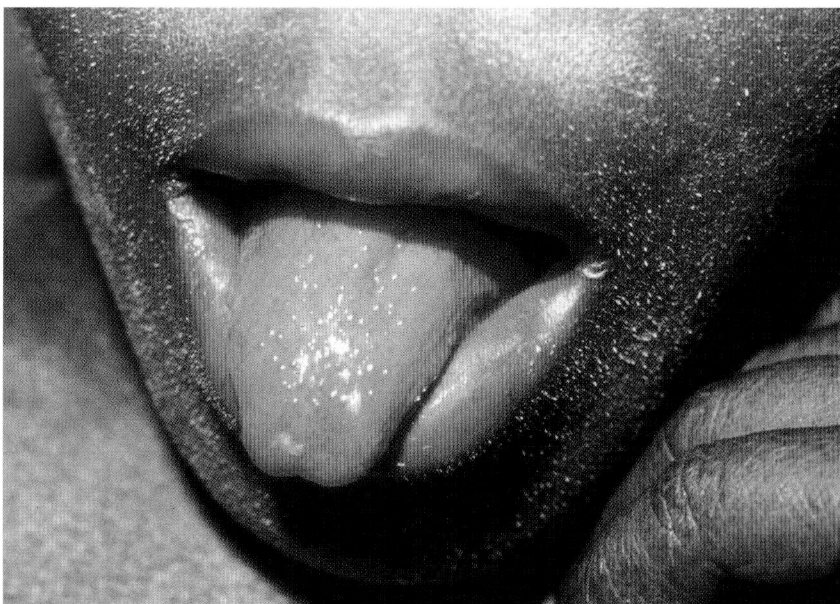

Figure 114.3. Kawasaki disease. Strawberry tongue was present in this boy with severe coronary aneurysms.

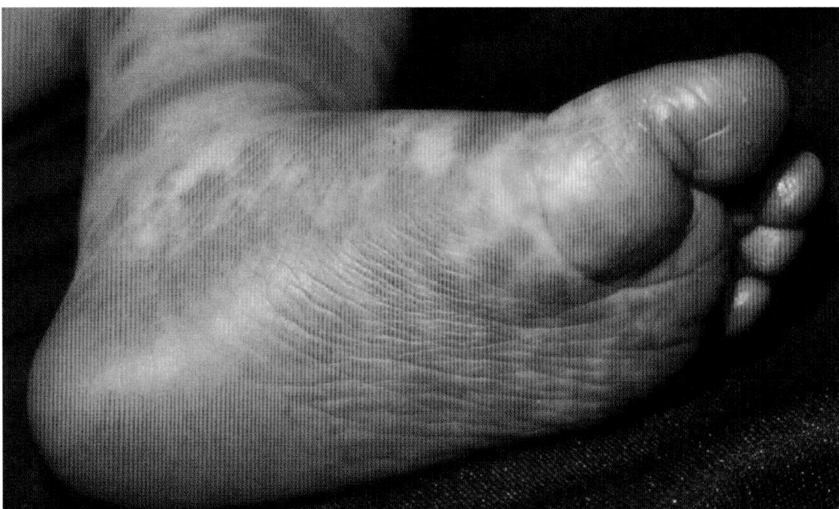

Figure 114.4. Kawasaki disease. Erythematous patches and plaques with foot swelling.

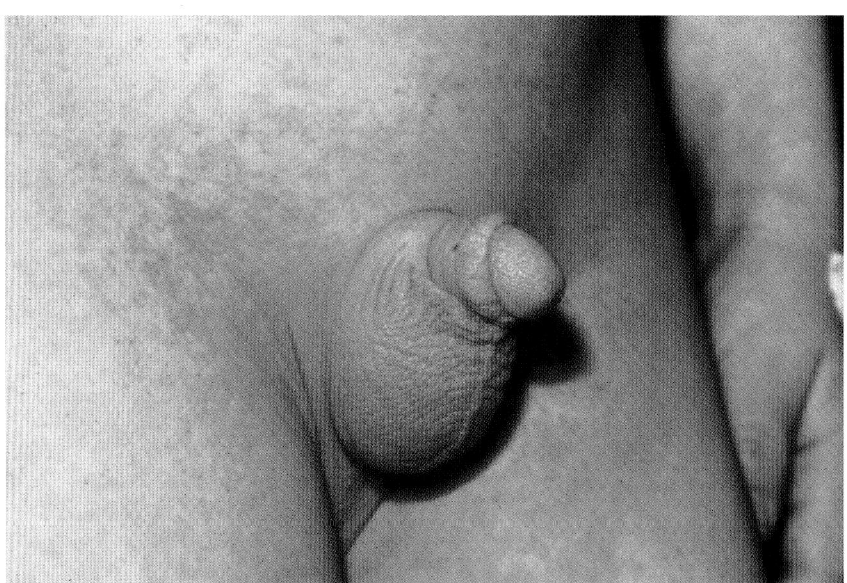

Figure 114.5. Kawasaki disease. Accentuation of erythema in the perineum and genital region is a frequent finding; desquamation also frequently appears in these areas.

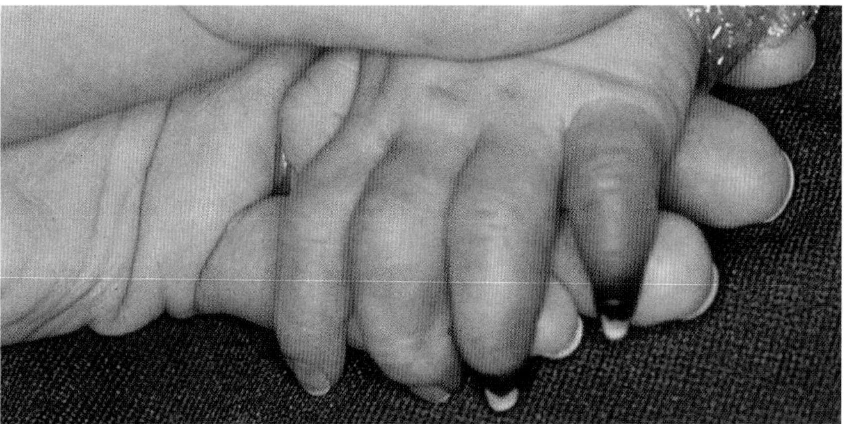

Figure 114.6. Kawasaki disease. Peripheral gangrene involving the fourth and fifth digits occurred in this toddler with the disorder.

Look-alikes

Disorder	Differentiating Features
Serum sickness–like eruption	• History of preceding drug ingestion • Mucous membrane and eye findings usually absent • "Purple urticaria" most characteristic skin finding, in conjunction with periarticular swelling
Viral exanthem (ie, adenovirus, measles)	• Exudative conjunctivitis, Koplik spots, severe cough present (measles). • Rash begins behind ears, does not accentuate in perineum (measles). • Conjunctivitis does not spare perilimbic area and is purulent (adenovirus). • Inflammatory markers (eg, C-reactive protein) minimally elevated (measles and adenovirus).
Scarlet fever	• Exudative pharyngitis present. • Conjunctivae normal. • When facial rash present, circumoral pallor is often present. • Positive test result for *Streptococcus pyogenes.*
Toxic shock syndrome	• Hypotension present. • Renal involvement (elevated serum creatinine), elevation of creatine phosphokinase. • Rash appears as diffuse erythema. • Primary focus of *Staphylococcus aureus* infection present.
Systemic-onset juvenile idiopathic arthritis	• Hepatosplenomegaly often present. • Rash is evanescent, salmon-colored; often correlates with presence of fever. • Quotidian (daily)/double quotidian (twice daily) fever curve with relative wellness between spikes.
Stevens-Johnson syndrome	• Skin blisters, denudation • Mucosal blistering and erosions (mouth, eyes, genitals) • In children, often associated with *Mycoplasma pneumoniae* infection

How to Make the Diagnosis

- The diagnosis is suggested by the presence of prolonged fever and other diagnostic criteria.
- Elevation of inflammatory markers (erythrocyte sedimentation rate, C-reactive protein) is nearly universal in Kawasaki disease; conversely, normal levels of inflammatory markers argue strongly against this diagnosis.
- Other laboratory findings that support diagnosis include sterile pyuria, elevation of serum transaminases, and cerebrospinal fluid pleocytosis.
- Thrombocytopenia, anemia, and hypoalbuminemia may be present during the acute phase; thrombocytosis develops during the second to third week of disease.
- White blood cell count may be normal to elevated, with a neutrophil predominance.
- Cardiac imaging with 2-dimensional (2-D) echocardiography is recommended; investigative modalities include multislice spiral computed tomography and coronary magnetic resonance angiography.
- Patients with fever for 5 days or longer and fewer than 4 principal features can be diagnosed as having Kawasaki disease when coronary artery disease is detected by 2-D echocardiography or coronary angiography.

Treatment

- Treatment most effective at decreasing risk of development of coronary aneurysms when given within the first 10 days of the illness.
- Intravenous Ig (IVIG), 2 g/kg as a single infusion over 10 to 12 hours.
- High-dose aspirin (80–100 mg/kg per day divided into 4 doses) during acute phase.
- After 14 days or minimum of 3 days being afebrile, dose of aspirin reduced (3–5 mg/kg once daily); if no echocardiographic abnormalities present, aspirin is discontinued when laboratory studies normalize (usually within 2 months).
- Some recommend a second infusion of IVIG for nonresponders (or those who only improve transiently). Methylprednisolone pulse therapy may be beneficial in those who do not respond to second dose of IVIG.
- Other potential (albeit controversial) therapeutic options include abciximab, infliximab, etanercept, rituximab, clopidogrel, and pentoxifylline.

Prognosis

- If untreated, 20% to 25% of patients develop coronary aneurysms; giant lesions entail the greatest risk for long-term morbidity.
- Prognosis in those with coronary aneurysms is variable, and patients require lifelong follow-up.
- Patients diagnosed when younger than 6 months or older than 9 years appear to have poorer outcomes.
- Patients with a history of Kawasaki disease may have a more adverse cardiovascular risk profile, predisposing them to premature atherosclerosis.

When to Worry or Refer

- Referral to an experienced specialist in Kawasaki disease should be considered for any patient presenting with prolonged fever and clinical features that fall into the diagnostic spectrum of Kawasaki disease and for whom an alternative diagnosis cannot be confirmed.

Resources for Families

- American Academy of Pediatrics: HealthyChildren.org. **www.HealthyChildren.org/kawasaki**
- American Heart Association: Provides information about Kawasaki disease. **www.heart.org/HEARTORG/Conditions/More/CardiovascularConditionsofChildhood/Kawasaki-Disease_UCM_308777_Article.jsp**
- Kawasaki Disease Foundation: Provides information, including a pamphlet and newsletter, for patients and families. **www.kdfoundation.org**

Langerhans Cell Histiocytosis

Introduction/Etiology/Epidemiology

- One of the "histiocytoses," a group of disorders that share in common the abnormal proliferation of histiocytes (a bone marrow progenitor cell). Langerhans cells are one type of histiocyte; others include dermal dendrocyte and macrophages.
- Langerhans cell histiocytosis (LCH) is the contemporary umbrella term for the disorder known in the past variably as histiocytosis X, eosinophilic granuloma, Letterer-Siwe disease, and Hand-Schüller-Christian syndrome; severities of presentation include unifocal, multifocal, and disseminated disease.
- Langerhans cell histiocytosis may occur at any age but has a peak incidence in children between 1 and 4 years of age.
- The exact pathogenesis remains unclear; proposed etiologies include infection, somatic mutation, or immune dysregulation; somatic mutations in the *BRAF* gene have been identified in some patients with LCH.
- The neoplastic versus reactive nature of LCH continues to be debated.

Signs and Symptoms

- Multiple organ systems may be involved (the most important from the standpoint of prognosis are bone marrow, liver, spleen, and lung); skin and bone are the most common.
- Bone involvement presents as pain, with or without swelling, that affects (in order of decreasing frequency) the skull, long bones of the extremities, and flat bones (pelvis, vertebrae, ribs); radiographs reveal unifocal or multifocal lytic lesions.

- Skin involvement presents with scaly red papules and plaques, with a predilection for the scalp, posterior ear folds (Figure 115.1), axillae, groin (especially inguinal folds; Figure 115.2) and neck folds; LCH may, at times, mimic seborrheic dermatitis, although other features listed in this chapter often help distinguish the conditions.

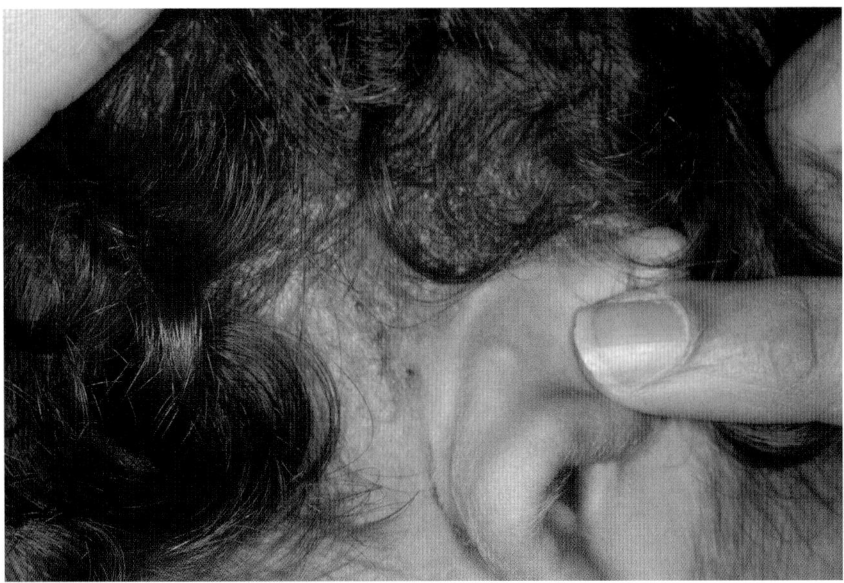

Figure 115.1. Erythema and scaling with some associated hemorrhage in the posterior auricular fold of a child with multisystem Langerhans cell histiocytosis.

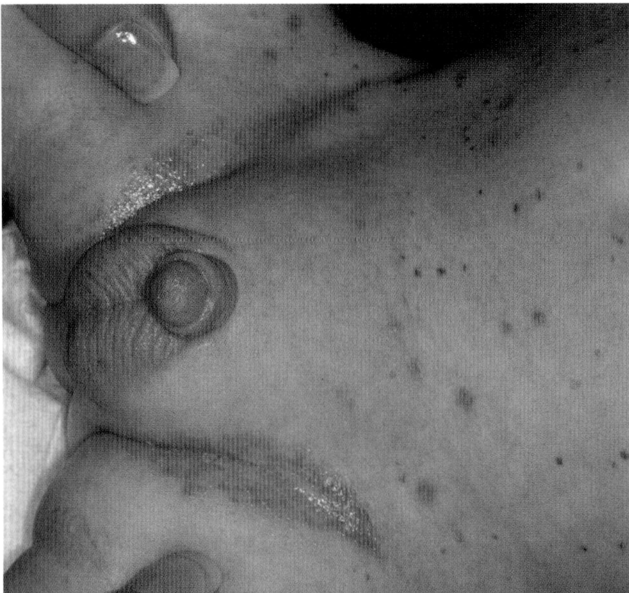

Figure 115.2. Erythema of the inguinal creases with scattered lichenoid, hemorrhagic papules.

- Papules are often red to brown in color and may be accompanied by punctate erosions, crusting (Figure 115.3), and hemorrhage/petechiae; they may occasionally be lichenoid (flat-topped).
- Crusted papules on the palms (Figure 115.4) and soles are common, as is lymphadenopathy.

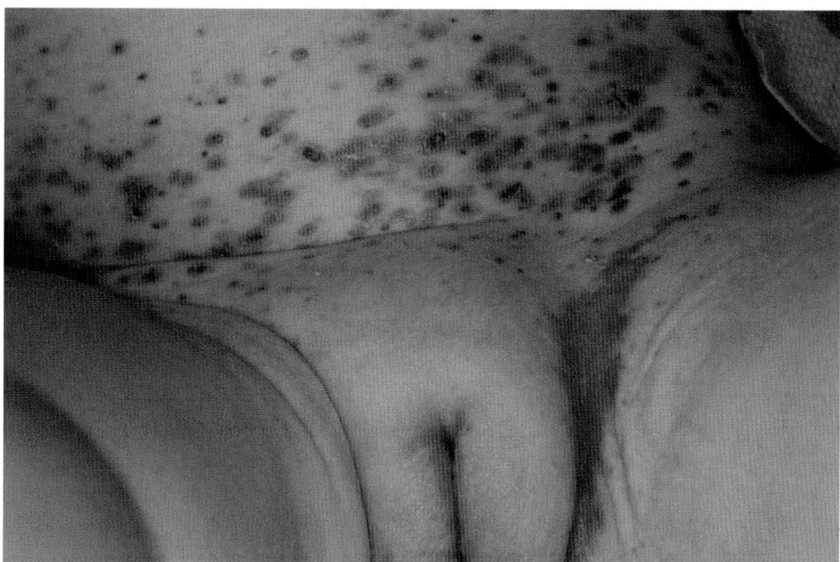

Figure 115.3. Eroded, crusted papules on the lower abdomen and suprapubic area; note the associated involvement of the inguinal crease.

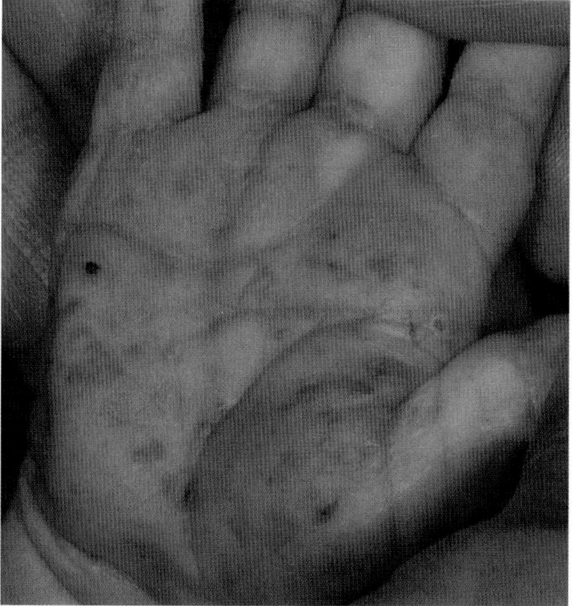

Figure 115.4. Scaly and hemorrhagic papules on the palm of this child with Langerhans cell histiocytosis, who was initially treated for presumed scabies infestation.

- In neonates with LCH, lesions may appear more vesicular or vesiculopustular and may mimic neonatal herpes or varicella; these vesicular lesions often become hemorrhagic or crusted.
- Mucosal involvement may include erosive gingivitis, hemorrhage, and, in infants, premature eruption of deciduous teeth ("natal teeth").
- Involvement of the external auditory canal may result in chronic otitis externa.
- The classic triad (formerly Hand-Schüller-Christian disease, now termed *multifocal LCH*) consists of skull lesions, diabetes insipidus (caused by posterior pituitary involvement), and exophthalmos.

Look-alikes

Disorder	Differentiating Features
Seborrheic dermatitis	• Most often limited to scalp (cradle cap), face, umbilicus, or diaper region • Lacks papules, erosions, crusting, and hemorrhage
Scabies	• Burrows usually present. • Severe pruritus common. • Close contacts often report pruritus/skin lesions. • Mineral oil examination of skin lesion scrapings reveals mites, feces, and eggs.
Atopic dermatitis	• Diaper area spared. • Skin lesions more often plaques with lichenification, rather than papules. • In infants, involvement more likely to be on extensor surfaces (rather than flexural). • Lacks hemorrhage. • Other atopic disorders (keratosis pilaris, ichthyosis vulgaris, allergic rhinoconjunctivitis, asthma, food allergies) or family history of such is often present.
Intertrigo	• Although there is erythema in skinfolds, papules, crusting, and hemorrhage are usually absent. • When secondarily infected with yeast (ie, *Candida*), presents as beefy red color with peripheral satellite papules and pustules. • When secondarily infected with bacteria (eg, *Streptococcus pyogenes, Staphylococcus aureus*), erosive change may be present but is usually diffuse, rather than the punctate erosions seen in LCH.
Diaper dermatitis	• In irritant contact dermatitis, red patches involve lower abdomen, buttocks, and thighs with sparing of the inguinal folds. • Papules, crusting, erosions, and hemorrhage usually absent. • In diaper candidiasis, erythema may involve inguinal creases but crusting, erosions, and hemorrhage are usually absent. • Satellite (peripheral to the primary erythema) papules and pustules may be noted. • In Jacquet erosive diaper dermatitis, well-defined shallow ulcers or ulcerated nodules are present but most often limited to the perianal region.

How to Make the Diagnosis

- Skin biopsy reveals typical histologic changes of a Langerhans cell infiltrate into the epidermis and dermis.
- Diagnostic confirmation is achieved by positive immunostaining with S100, CD1a, or Langerin.
- Electron microscopy (rarely used in the current era) reveals a characteristic organelle, Birbeck granules, within Langerhans cells.
- Other recommended evaluations include complete blood cell count, hepatic function testing, coagulation studies, urine osmolality, radiographic skeletal survey, and chest radiography; more specific studies are performed as clinically indicated.

Treatment

- Therapy depends on the extent of disease.
- With skin-limited LCH, observation alone is often appropriate; when severe, however, therapies for more extensive involvement are often used.
- Unifocal bone lesions may be treated with observation, curettage, excision, or intralesional steroid injection.
- Multifocal and multisystem disease (as well as unifocal lesions in some special sites) requires systemic therapy; first-line treatment includes vinblastine and prednisone.
- Second-line therapies include clofarabine, cytarabine, and cladribine (2-chlordeoxyadenosine).
- Bone marrow transplantation is occasionally indicated; studies of *BRAF* inhibitors for refractory LCH with known *BRAFv600E* mutations are ongoing.

Prognosis

- Prognosis for LCH depends on extent of involvement, degree of organ dysfunction, and initial response to therapy.
- Delayed sequelae may include skeletal defects, dental issues, growth failure and other endocrinopathies (most often diabetes insipidus), hearing loss, and neurodegenerative central nervous system dysfunction.

When to Worry or Refer

- If the diagnosis of cutaneous LCH is being considered, the patient should be referred to a pediatric dermatologist for evaluation and skin biopsy or other specialist (eg, orthopedic surgeon, oncologist) as applicable.
- Treatment and long-term follow-up of patients with LCH are performed by a pediatric oncologist.

Resources for Families

- Histiocytosis Association: LCH in children.
  www.histio.org/lchinchildren
- US National Library of Medicine Genetics Home Reference: Langerhans cell histiocytosis.
  http://ghr.nlm.nih.gov/condition/langerhans-cell-histiocytosis
- National Organization for Rare Disorders: Langerhans cell histiocytosis.
  https://www.rarediseases.org/rare-disease-information/rare-diseases/byID/408/viewAbstract

Lichen Sclerosus et Atrophicus (LSA)

Introduction/Etiology/Epidemiology

- Uncommon chronic inflammatory disease of unknown cause that most frequently involves the anogenital region.
- More common in females (approximately 8:1), especially prepubertal and postmenopausal females (5%–15% of cases occur in children).
- Approximately 70% of prepubertal cases begin before age 7 years.
- Overall prevalence estimated at 1 in 900 girls.

Signs and Symptoms

- Presents as small, pink to white, minimally raised papules that coalesce into plaques with eventual atrophy and small follicular plugs of the surface.
- Anogenital involvement presents as shiny, ivory-colored, hypopigmented atrophic plaques of the vulvar or perianal region in females with a figure 8 or hourglass distribution (ie, affected area surrounds the vulva, perineum, and anus) (Figures 116.1 and 116.2).
  - Associated pruritus (50%) or discomfort of genital region and painful urination or defecation often present. Painful defecation may lead to constipation.
  - Erythema with bullae (occasionally hemorrhagic) may be present before hypopigmentation and atrophy are seen; wrinkling is another clinical feature that may be present.
  - Other symptoms may include pain with urination, bleeding, and vaginal discharge.
- In males, the prepuce becomes sclerotic and difficult to retract (phimosis); the glans may appear shiny and blue-white in color.
  - Involvement in males has been termed *balanitis xerotica obliterans.*
  - Unlike in females, lichen sclerosus et atrophicus (LSA) in males almost always spares the perianal region, and there is rarely involvement of penile shaft or scrotum.
  - Males may experience purpura/hemorrhagic bullae after the trauma of intercourse or masturbation.

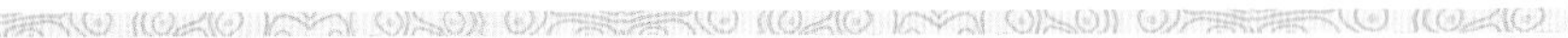

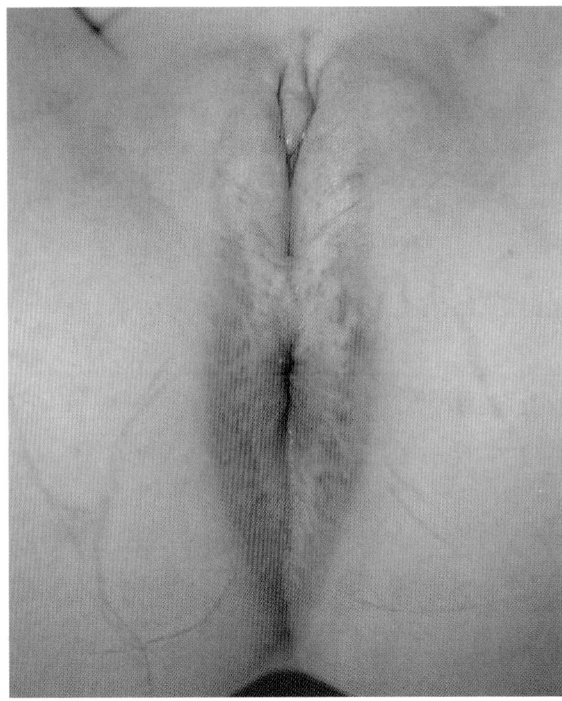

Figure 116.1. Circumferential hypopigmented atrophic patches in a figure 8 configuration characteristic of lichen sclerosus.

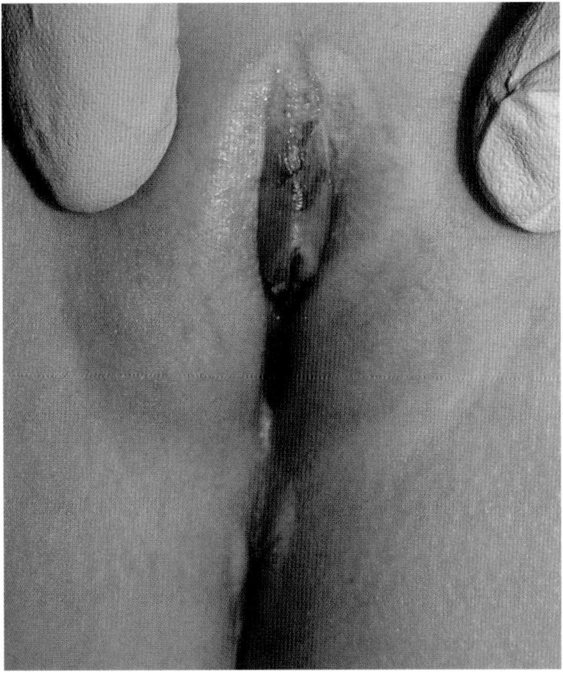

Figure 116.2. Characteristic shiny, hypopigmented, atrophic plaques of the vulvar region with associated ecchymosis.

- Genital LSA may have associated fissures, erosions, hemorrhagic bullae, or purpura of the affected skin; lesions may be predominant in many girls, particularly on the labia minora and clitoris.
- Long-standing LSA can lead to scarring and architectural changes within the anogenital region (in females) and phimosis (in males).
- Extragenital LSA usually is asymptomatic and most commonly occurs in the inframammary region, shoulders, back, neck, and flexural extremities.

Look-alikes

Disorder	Differentiating Features
Erosive lichen planus	• Typical extragenital lesions present (purple, polygonal, flat-topped papules) • White, reticulated patches often present on buccal mucosae • May involve vagina • Less commonly seen in children than LSA
Cicatricial pemphigoid	• Rare in children; an autoimmune blistering disorder • Usually blisters/erosions of mucosal surfaces of eyes, mouth • Distinct histologic findings (subepidermal bullae)
Childhood sexual abuse	• Ivory/shiny atrophic plaques in figure 8 distribution are usually not observed. • May see other physical evidence of physical/sexual abuse. • May have similar findings of purpura, telangiectasias. • Possible to have coexistent LSA and abuse.
Psoriasis	• Well-demarcated erythematous plaques with predilection for intergluteal and hair-bearing regions (may have postinflammatory hypopigmentation after treatment) • Presence of characteristic nongenital lesions (erythematous scaling papules and plaques) or nail changes • Frequently associated with positive family history
Vitiligo	• Occasionally confused with the hypopigmentation of lichen sclerosus. • Lacks the atrophy, wrinkling, bullae, hemorrhage. • Vitiligo is usually depigmented (versus the hypopigmentation of LSA). • Depigmented patches in other sites (especially periorbital and over bony prominences) often present.
Irritant dermatitis or vulvovaginitis	• Severe pruritus often present • Lack of hypopigmentation, atrophy, bullae, hemorrhage • Usually no pain with defecation

How to Make the Diagnosis

- The diagnosis is usually straightforward based on clinical examination.
- If clinical diagnosis is uncertain, a skin biopsy may be used for confirmation.
- Characteristic histologic findings include thinned epidermis, interface dermatitis, and dermal sclerosis.

Treatment

- There is no known cure for LSA.
- First-line treatment usually includes medium- to high-potency topical corticosteroid; many clinicians treat initially or during disease flares with ultra-potent topical steroid (group 1; see Chapter 1) and then gradually taper frequency of medication use or potency of topical steroid as condition improves.
- Generous use of barrier protection, such as zinc oxide–containing products or petrolatum-based emollients, may improve symptoms of pruritus as well as pain with urination or defecation.
- Avoid fragrance-containing soaps, bubble baths, or skin care products.
- Topical calcineurin inhibitors (tacrolimus, pimecrolimus) have been proven effective in the initial treatment of LSA and often are used to maintain remission following initial therapy with a topical corticosteroid.
- Topical testosterone or estrogen products were used frequently in the past; however, untoward side effects make them less desirable in children.

Treating Associated Conditions

- Secondary bacterial or candidal infections must be recognized and treated, as indicated. Maintain a high index of suspicion during disease flares and obtain skin cultures for confirmation.
- Surgical intervention may rarely be necessary to correct narrowing of introitus or reverse burying of clitoris. Male patients may require circumcision if they develop significant phimosis.

Prognosis

- Data are conflicting on the spontaneous involution rate of pediatric LSA at puberty.
- Increased risk of squamous cell carcinoma, as documented in adult cases, not established in pediatric disease.

When to Worry or Refer

- Consider referral to a pediatric dermatologist for confirmation of diagnosis or management of the condition.
- Consider referral to child abuse specialist for full evaluation if any clinical suspicion of abuse is present.

Resources for Families

- Association for Lichen Sclerosus & Vulval Health: Group located in the United Kingdom that provides information and support for patients. **www.lichensclerosus.org**
- WebMD: Information for families is contained in the Health A-Z topics. **www.webmd.com/skin-problems-and-treatments/lichen-sclerosus**

Polymorphous Light Eruption

Introduction/Etiology/Epidemiology

- Polymorphous light eruption (PMLE) is the most common type of photodermatitis in children; it is estimated to occur in 5% to 15% of the population.
- Occurs more often in fair-skinned individuals but may occur in all skin types; it occurs more commonly in females than males (4:1).
- Usually presents in the second or third decade of life; however, 20% of patients present in childhood.
- Occasionally referred to as "sun poisoning" or "sun allergy," the exact etiology of PMLE remains unclear; it is believed to be an immune-mediated delayed hypersensitivity reaction to ultraviolet radiation (290–480 nm wavelength).
- Genetic factors may play a role, and an autosomal-dominant form has been described.

Signs and Symptoms

- The skin lesions are polymorphous or variable in appearance, as the name suggests; however, the appearance tends to be quite monomorphous in individual patients.
- Characteristic findings include small papules or vesicles, urticarial plaques (Figure 117.1), and eczematous eruptions; in some patients, the appearance may mimic erythema multiforme.
- The most commonly involved areas include the face (most prominent), lateral neck, and sun-exposed areas of the hands and arms.
- The lesions of PMLE tend to be quite pruritic; they typically appear 24 to 48 hours after sun exposure and last for 1 to 2 weeks.
- Polymorphous light eruption is most common in the spring and early summer and often improves over the summer months (the phenomenon of "hardening" from continued ultraviolet exposure); it tends to recur yearly in the spring and early summer in affected individuals.

- *Juvenile spring eruption* may be a subtype of PMLE and is characterized by self-limited recurrent outbreaks of papules and papulovesicles, usually localized to the sun-exposed areas of the helices (Figure 117.2); it is seen primarily in young boys, especially those with short hair and larger or protruding ears.
- Juvenile spring eruption also recurs in the spring and early summer, although there are reports of the disorder in the cold winter months as well.

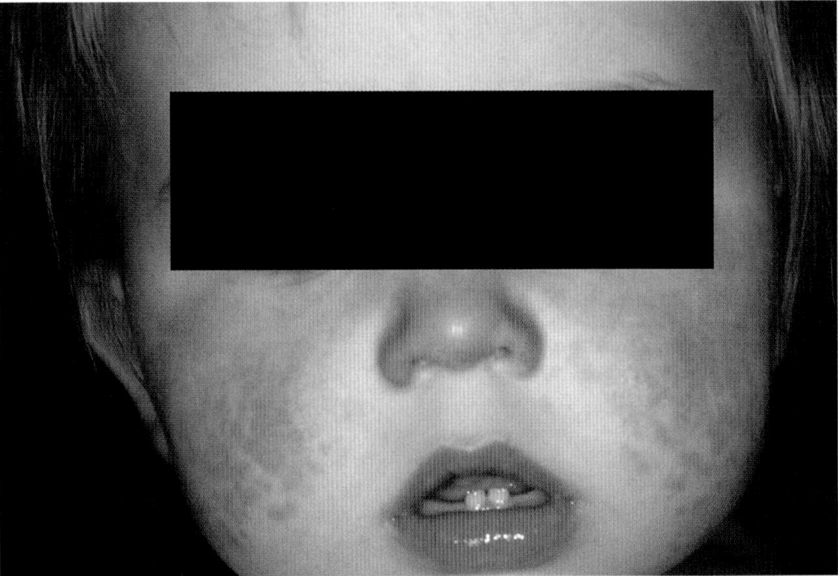

Figure 117.1. Polymorphous light eruption. Urticarial papules and plaques in a toddler following intense sun exposure.

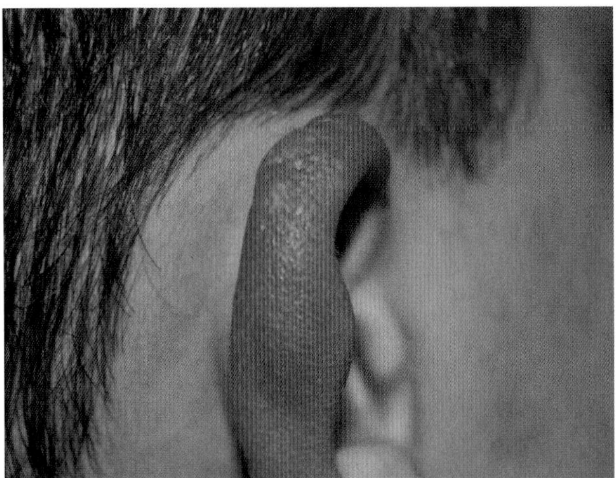

Figure 117.2. Juvenile spring eruption. Erythema of the superior helices with multiple vesicles in a 4-year-old boy following his first significant sun exposure of the spring.

Look-alikes

Disorder	Differentiating Features
Systemic lupus erythematosus (SLE)	• Malar or butterfly eruption (involves cheeks and, classically, the nasal bridge). • May have other characteristic skin findings, including discoid lesions, oral ulcerations, livedo reticularis, bright red to purple papules and plaques on the dorsal hands (often sparing the areas over joints), or panniculitis (inflammation of the fat). • Arthritis, fever, malaise may be present. • Other extracutaneous targets include the hematologic system, lungs, heart, kidneys, and central nervous system. • Positive serologic studies, elevated inflammatory markers, and decreased complement levels may help distinguish SLE from PMLE.
Solar urticaria	• Redness and itching of the skin occurs during or within 30 minutes of sun exposure. • Initial reaction is followed by urticarial lesions in areas of sun exposure. • Lesions typically resolve within hours. • Rare in children; usually presents in third or fourth decade of life.
Actinic prurigo	• Most often affects Indian and mestizo populations of Mexico and Central and South America. • Red, itchy papules and plaques of the face and arms; lower extremities and sun-protected sites (eg, buttocks) may also be involved. • Oral and ocular mucosae are commonly involved; affected individuals often have associated conjunctivitis, photophobia, or cheilitis. • Excoriations and scarring may be present. • More likely than PMLE to persist into winter months.
Hydroa vacciniforme	• Very rare condition; usually beginning in childhood • Eruption characterized by edematous papules or vesicles/bullae that occur hours to days after sun exposure and last for several days • Heals with characteristic varioliform scarring
Juvenile dermatomyositis	• Characteristic skin findings include – Pink to violet discoloration of the eyelids (heliotrope) – Pink to red macules/papules overlying knuckles, especially proximal interphalangeal and metacarpophalangeal joints (Gottron sign/papules) – Dilated capillaries of the proximal nail folds (may need magnification to see) – Calcium deposits over joints (knees, elbows) • Less common skin findings may include lipoatrophy, poikiloderma (hyperpigmentation, hypopigmentation, telangiectasias and atrophy), ulcerations. • Patients often present with fatigue and loss of energy. • Usually associated with proximal muscle weakness (muscle enzymes often elevated); may have associated dysphagia, dysphonia, choking, nasal speech.

How to Make the Diagnosis

- Polymorphous light eruption is usually diagnosed based on clinical features and timing of skin eruption.
- Diagnosis can be confirmed by phototesting, if necessary.
- As clinical features of PMLE may be indistinguishable from lupus erythematosus, serologic testing should be considered.
- Skin biopsy is usually not helpful, as the histologic features are nonspecific and depend on clinical morphology of the lesion biopsied.

Treatment

- Treatment of PMLE is largely aimed at prevention.
- Photoprotective measures should include broad-spectrum sunscreen (with good UV-A protection) and photoprotective clothing, as well as avoidance of significant midday sun exposure.
- Severe cases may benefit from hydroxychloroquine therapy.
- Use of ultraviolet therapy (usually narrowband UV-B or PUVA) 2 to 3 times weekly for several weeks may help to "harden" or desensitize the skin.
- Use of beta carotene may be helpful in some patients.
- Topical or, rarely, systemic steroids may help treat the acute eruption and relieve associated symptoms.

Prognosis

- The condition tends to recur each spring and early summer; in some patients, PMLE may improve or even resolve over time.
- While the condition may significantly affect quality of life, PMLE is not associated with any significant long-term morbidity or mortality.

When to Worry or Refer

- Consider referral to a pediatric dermatologist or rheumatologist if there are concerns about potential lupus erythematosus.
- Consider referral to a pediatric dermatologist for confirmation of diagnosis or management.

Resources for Families

- American Academy of Dermatology: Information on photoprotective measures.
  www.aad.org
- Skin Cancer Foundation: Information on photoprotective measures.
  www.skincancer.org

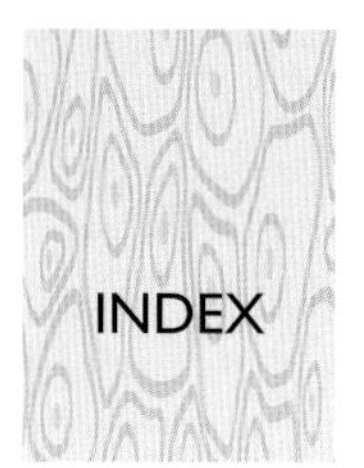

INDEX

Note: Numbers in *italics* indicate figures.

I

J

K

M

N

Q

R

S

T

U